STONE DISEASE

Diagnosis and Management

STONE DISEASE

Diagnosis and Management

Edited by

Stephen N. Rous, M.D.

Professor and Chairman
Department of Urology
Medical University of South Carolina
Charleston, South Carolina

G&S

Grune & Stratton, Inc.
Harcourt Brace Jovanovich, Publishers
Orlando New York San Diego London
San Francisco Tokyo Sydney Toronto

Library of Congress Cataloging-in-Publication Data

Stone disease.

Includes bibliographies and index.
1. Calculi, Urinary. I. Rous, Stephen N. (Stephen Norman), 1931– . [DNLM: 1. Urinary Calculi—diagnosis. 2. Urinary Calculi—therapy. WJ 100 S877]
RC916.S75 1987 616.6′22 87-7554
ISBN 0-8089-1873-7

Grune & Stratton, Inc.
Orlando, Florida 32887

Distributed in the United Kingdom by
Grune & Stratton, Ltd.
24/28 Oval Road
London NW 1 70X

Library of Congress Catalog Number 87-7554
International Standard Book Number 0-8089-1873-7
Printed in the United States of America
87 88 89 90 10 9 8 7 6 5 4 3 2 1

This book is dedicated with much love to my wife, Margot,
always and forever the World's Greatest Woman.

Contents

PART II MEDICAL TREATMENT AND MANAGEMENT OF THE UROLITHIASIS PATIENT

PART III SURGICAL TREATMENT AND MANAGEMENT OF THE UROLITHIASIS PATIENT

Preface

Few conditions in clinical medicine appear as suddenly or as acutely as urolithiasis, and even fewer conditions are more debilitating. It is a disease that is probably as old as man himself, as one needs only to read the Hippocratic Oath to realize.

For hundreds of years little progress was made in the diagnosis or the management of this problem, but within the recent past startling and exciting new progress has been made in both of these directions. It is noteworthy that these dramatic advances have been both medical and surgical. Although the latter tend to make the lay press because they represent exciting new technological advances, it is really the great strides that have been made in the medical management of urolithiasis, both diagnostic and therapeutic, that will benefit far more individuals in the long run.

This book has been written to assist those who care for urolithiasis patients by detailing what is currently known about the clinical aspects of stone disease. Emphasis has been placed on helping the clinician to accurately assess the etiology of the stone formation in a given patient and to plan a medically directed therapeutic approach to that patient. This book also attempts to detail the various surgical options available to the urologist, both emphasizing the current state-of-the-art therapeutic methods and reemphasizing the application of older treatment options where appropriate. The book is therefore intended for those who practice urologic surgery and also for those internists and family physicians who see patients with stone disease. It should be pointed out that this book is not intended for the purist who needs to know the physical chemistry of stone formation or for the basic scientist who relishes knowledge about biochemical or pharmacological interactions as they relate to stones of the urinary tract. It will also not delve in monumental detail into the many theories of stone formation. As noted, this is a book for clinicians and if it is of interest to others, the editor is delighted.

The editor would finally like to express his gratitude and appreciation to Mrs. Susan Pullen, whose boundless energy and unflagging cheerfulness greatly facilitated the work on this book.

Contributors

Alan H. Angell, M.D.
Resident in Urology, School of Medicine, Case Western Reserve University, Cleveland, Ohio

Robert E. Breidenthal, Ph.D.
Assistant Professor, Department of Aeronautics & Astronautics, University of Washington, Seattle, Washington

Robert D. Brooks, Ph.D.
Research Assistant Professor, Department of Aerospace & Energetics Research Program, University of Washington, Seattle, Washington

Robert Campbell, M.D.
Instructor of Urology, Baylor College of Medicine, Houston, Texas

Warren H. Chapman, M.D.
Professor, Department of Urology, School of Medicine, University of Washington, Seattle, Washington

David A. Diamond, M.D.
Assistant Professor of Urology and Pediatrics, Department of Surgery, Division of Urology, University of Massachusetts Medical Center, Worcester, Massachusetts

Stephen P. Dretler, M.D.
Director, Lithotriptor Unit, Department of Urology, Massachusetts General Hospital; Associate Professor of Urology, Harvard Medical School, Boston, Massachusetts

Stephen B. Erickson, M.D.
Consultant, Division of Nephrology and Internal Medicine, Mayo Clinic and Mayo Foundation; Assistant Professor of Medicine, Mayo Medical School, Rochester, Minnesota

Dino N. Frangos, M.D.
Resident in Urology, Department of Urology, Medical University of South Carolina, Charleston, South Carolina

Donald P. Griffith, M.D.
Professor of Urology, Baylor College of Medicine, Houston, Texas

Michael E. Mayo, M.B.B.S., F.R.C.S.
Associate Professor, Department of Urology, School of Medicine, University of Washington, Seattle, Washington

Mani Menon, M.D.
Professor and Chairman, Division of Urology, University of Massachusetts Medical Center, Worcester, Massachusetts

H. Norman Noe, M.D.
Professor of Urology, Department of Urology, The Health Sciences Center, University of Tennessee; Chief, Pediatric Urology, Division of Pediatric Urology, LeBonheur Children's Hospital, Memphis, Tennessee

Barton F. Norton, B.S., M.S., E.E., M.S. Indus. Adminis.
General Manager of Lithotripter, International Biomedics, Inc., Bothell, Washington

Glenn M. Preminger, M.D.
Assistant Professor of Urology, Department of Surgery; Assistant Professor of Internal Medicine, Section on Mineral Metabolism, The University of Texas Health Science Center at Dallas, Southwestern Medical School; Parkland Memorial Hospital; Dallas Veterans Administration Medical Center; Director, North Texas Lithotripsy Center, Dallas, Texas

Martin I. Resnick, M.D.
Professor and Chairman, Division of Urology, School of Medicine, Case Western Reserve University, Cleveland, Ohio

Allen L. Rodgers, M.D.
Senior Lecturer, Department of Physical Chemistry, School of Chemistry, University of Cape Town, Cape Town, Republic of South Africa

G. Alan Rose, M.A., D.M., F.R.C.P., F.R.C.Path., F.R.S.C.
Consultant Chemical Pathologist, St. Peter's Hospital, St. Paul's Hospital, London, England; Royal National Orthopaedic Hospital, Stanmore, Middlesex, England; Honorary Lecturer, Institute of Urology, London, England

Stephen N. Rous, M.D.
Professor and Chairman, Department of Urology, Medical University of South Carolina, Charleston, South Carolina

David A. Russell, Ph.D.
Professor and Chairman, Department of Aeronautics & Astronautics, University of Washington, Seattle, Washington

Colin T. Samuell, M.I.Biol., M.C.B.
Principal Biochemist, Biochemistry Department, St. Peter's Hospital; Honorary Senior Lecturer, Institute of Urology, London, England

Joseph W. Segura, M.D.
Carl Rosen Professor of Urology, Department of Urology, Mayo Medical School, Mayo Clinic, Rochester, Minnesota

M.J. Vernon Smith, M.B., B. Chir. (Cantab), Ph.D., F.A.C.S.
Professor of Urology, Medical College of Virginia, Richmond, Virginia

Myron Spector, Ph.D.
Professor and Director of Research, Department of Orthopedics, Emory University School of Medicine, Atlanta, Georgia

F. Bruder Stapleton, M.D.
Professor of Pediatrics, The Health Sciences Center, University of Tennessee; Head, Division of Pediatric Nephrology, LeBonheur Children's Medical Center, Memphis, Tennessee

Stevan B. Streem, M.D.
Head, Section of Stone Disease and Endourology, Department of Urology, Cleveland Clinic Foundation, Cleveland, Ohio

Christian J. Van Den Berg, M.D.
Associate Professor of Medicine, Mayo Medical School, Rochester, Minnesota; Consultant Physician, Division of Nephrology and Internal Medicine, Mayo Clinic Jacksonville, Jacksonville, Florida

David M. Wilson, M.D.
Consultant in the Division of Nephrology and Internal Medicine; Consultant, Department of Laboratory Medicine, Mayo Clinic, Mayo Foundation; Associate Professor of Medicine, Mayo Medical School, Rochester, Minnesota

Edmund R. Yendt, M.D., F.R.C.P.C.
Professor and Chairman, Division of Endocrinology, Department of Medicine, Queen's University; Attending Physician, Kingston General Hospital, Kingston, Ontario, Canada

STONE DISEASE

Diagnosis and Management

PART I

Incidence, Evaluation, and Fundamental Information

Dino N. Frangos
Stephen N. Rous

1

Incidence and Economic Factors in Urolithiasis

Two exciting bioengineering advances in this decade have wrought a virtual revolution in the management of patients with urolithiasis. First, the percutaneous management of renal and even upper ureteral stones greatly decreased the operative and postoperative morbidity for these patients as compared with the "open" surgical approach, and most recently, the development and implementation of extracorporeal shock-wave lithotripsy (ESWL) has further alleviated the plight of those suffering from kidney and upper ureteral stones. It is all too easy, however, to consider the stone problem as "solved," particularly in view of the anticipation that in the very near future less expensive and better forms of ESWL will greatly reduce the cost of the procedure, eliminate the need for general or regional anesthesia, and very probably permit most lithotripsies to be done on an outpatient basis.

Unfortunately, these exciting new therapeutic advances are really applicable to only about 20 percent of patients with urolithiasis since spontaneous stone passage can be anticipated in the other 80 percent. Thus, even though these new forms of therapy have already decreased the time needed for a postoperative convalescence and in many cases decreased the cost of surgical care, the economic impact of urolithiasis remains unchanged for the great majority of patients who will not be candidates for any of these forms of therapy but will be managed conservatively, as in the past, with every expectation of spontaneous passage of the calculi. Even with the reduced morbidity for those patients who do require the percutaneous or the ESWL form of treatment, the overall impact of the disease remains great in terms of both direct patient care and income lost to the patient and/or to the patient's employer because of continued compensation to the patient even though that patient is not working.

To comprehend the economic magnitude of urolithiasis in the United States, it is necessary to study the incidence or frequency of the condition and discuss this in terms of patient morbidity and cost. It must be well understood in advance that the data to be presented can hardly be construed as "hard" because of the difficulty in determining the precise number of people afflicted with urolithiasis. Certain data are available on a

STONE DISEASE: DIAGNOSIS AND MANAGEMENT
ISBN 0-8089-1873-7

nationwide basis, however, and certain other data have been obtained for the state of South Carolina and by means of interpolation and extrapolation various dollar figures, albeit estimates, can be given so that the economic impact of urolithiasis can be estimated.

INCIDENCE

Studies examining the overall incidence of stone disease in this country have been based largely on hospital records and tend to show striking differences between geographic areas of the country, between blacks and Caucasians, and between males and females. In 1952 Boyce placed the incidence of calculi in the United States at 94.7 persons per 100,000 population.[1] Sierakowski, in 1974, estimated the incidence of urolithiasis at 164.1 per 100,000 population and further calculated that approximately 12 percent of the population will have stone disease at some point in their lives.[2] The most recent study, done in 1984 by the National Center for Health Statistics, noted the rate of hospital discharges for urolithiasis at 140 inpatients per 100,000 population.[3] These studies, however, may not reflect the true incidence of stone disease because they were based only on patients requiring hospitalization and did not attempt to determine the incidence of outpatient urolithiasis. There have, however, also been some studies of inpatient and outpatient urolithiasis within a very specific and defined population. Johnson, in a Mayo Clinic study of all inpatients and outpatients seen from the Rochester, Minnesota area with urolithiasis, calculated an annual adjusted incidence rate over a 25-year period at 68.7 per 100,000 population.[4] Another study within a prepaid medical care program in northern California determined the incidence of a new or a recurrent stone at 122 persons per 100,000 population.[5]

A geographic variation of stone incidence within the United States has been noted by several authors and the southeastern region appears to have a higher rate of lithiasis than other parts of the nation. In an inpatient study done in 1952, Boyce noted the highest incidence of 192.5 and 184.2 persons per 100,000 population for South Carolina and Georgia, respectively.[1] More recently, in another inpatient study done in 1983, the incidence of stone disease in South Carolina was 221 persons per 100,000 population (Table 1-1).[6] Government figures for 1984 confirm the South as the area with the highest incidence of stone disease (Table 1-2).[7] There has been much speculation as to the reason for the high incidence of lithiasis, particularly in South Carolina, North Carolina, and Georgia. This speculation has centered around such diverse etiologies as the soil, the

Table 1-1
Inpatient Discharges for Urolithiasis by Age from Nonfederal Hospitals in South Carolina in 1983

Age (Years)	Discharges	Total Hospital Days	Discharges/ 100,000 Population	Average Length of Stay in Days/Patient
0–14	46	197	6	4.3
15–44	3548	14,882	221	4.2
45–64	2529	14,152	411	5.6
65–	1211	10,081	371	8.3
Total	7334	39,312	221	5.4

Table 1-2
Inpatient Discharges for Urolithiasis Nationwide from Nonfederal Hospitals by Region in 1984

Region	Total Discharges	Region Population	Rate/100,000 Population
Northeast	55,000	49,617,000	111
Northcentral	82,000	58,965,000	139
South	133,000	79,678,000	167
West	58,000	46,192,000	126
Nationwide	328,000	234,452,000	140

weather (hot), and a diet rich in oxalate.[8,9] An extremely interesting and perhaps fruitful lead to the solution of this regional mystery may be found in a recent publication of the U.S. Department of Agriculture showing the considerable content of calcium oxalate in cotton dust.[10] Most urinary tract stones are calcium oxalate, and it is interesting to note that an estimated 750,000 people in the Carolinas and Georgia are employed in the manufacture of textiles, most of which are composed, at least in part, of cotton. Attempts by one of the authors (SNR) to study sample groups of textile workers in South Carolina with reference to urinary levels of calcium and oxalate have been unsuccessful but may well be worth pursuing.

The relative frequency of calculi between Caucasians and blacks has also been noted to be significant. Several large series confirm a lower incidence of urolithiasis in the black population as compared to Caucasians. Because a few of these studies were done in the southern portion of the United States, one author suggests that such results may be biased because of the unclear availability and rate of hospital admissions for the black population.[11] Boyce, however, noted that hospitals devoted entirely to the black population reported the incidence of calculi to be one-fifth to one-twelfth that of other hospitals in the same town.[1] Further, a study in the armed services noted the incidence of urolithiasis to be 10 times greater in Caucasians than in blacks.[12] Discharge data in 1983 from nonfederal hospitals in South Carolina reported white males have a 5 times greater incidence of urolithiasis than nonwhite males (Fig. 1-1).[6] One recent study representing data on races within the same population base noted the rate of stone disease among Caucasians to be only about twice that of blacks and Orientals.[5]

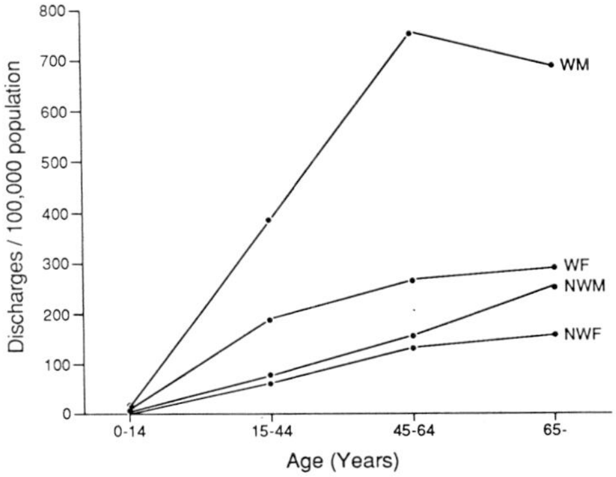

Fig. 1-1. Urolithiasis rates by age, race, and sex in South Carolina nonfederal hospitals in 1983 (WM = white males, WF = white females, NWM = nonwhite males, NWF = nonwhite females).

The frequency of calculi by sex within a defined population as well as nationwide show a male:female ratio between 2:1 and 3:1.[3,4] Hospital records nationally estimate the rate of calculi for males to be 196 per 100,000 population and the rate for females to be 87 per 100,000.[3]

Age-adjusted incidence rates of urolithiasis in South Carolina show the disease to be uncommon under the age of 15, while the highest incidence appears to be in the 45–64-year-old age group (Table 1-1).[6] Similar findings were noted nationwide by the National Center for Health Statistics, which reported the highest rate of urolithiasis in 1984 to be 282 per 100,000 population for the ages 45–64 years (Table 1-3).[3]

Studies of various occupational groups suggest a relationship between the type of work and the frequency of urinary calculi. The highest incidence of stones seems to be found in industrial areas, especially among those workers with a relatively sedentary occupation.[13] Sutor studied the frequency of urolithiasis in occupational groups ranging from professional "nonmanual" work to entirely "manual" work.[14] This study noted the incidence of urolithiasis to be ten times greater among professional workers as compared to the unskilled worker. However, studies of stone disease based on occupation may be misleading and reflect also the influences of socioeconomic status, dietary habits, and working conditions.

ECONOMIC COSTS

The economic costs of illness can be measured in terms of direct and indirect costs. The former represents the cost spent for the detection and treatment of the illness itself, while the indirect costs represent current and future loss of wages and/or salary to the individual or sickness compensation wages or salary lost to the individual's employer. In estimating these economic costs (direct and indirect), only those patients requiring hospitalization will be considered because no hard data exist for patients treated at home. It must be realized, however, that the number of patients hospitalized for urolithiasis is, at most, something less than half the total number of patients with urolithiasis.[15]

Direct Costs

A government study of the number of inpatients discharged from nonfederal hospitals (where the average length of stay is less than 30 days) in 1984 revealed that the total

Table 1-3
Inpatient Discharges for Urolithiasis by Age from Nonfederal Hospitals Nationwide in 1984

Age (Years)	Discharges (000)	Total Hospital Days (100,000)	Discharges/ 100,000 Population	Average Length of Stay (Days/Patient)
0–14	NA	NA	NA	NA
15–44	149	491	135	3.3
45–64	126	529	282	4.2
65–	52	348	185	6.7
Total	328	1378	140	4.2

number of patients discharged including all conditions was 37,162,000. Of these, 3,116,000 patients were listed by first diagnosis on discharge as diseases related to the genitourinary system. Discharge diagnoses of calculi of the kidney and ureter totaled 328,000, representing approximately 0.9 percent of all discharges and 10 percent of discharges from diseases of the genitourinary system.[3]

The diagnostic workup for patients thought to possibly have urolithiasis is, of course, included as direct costs. The evaluation of such patients would include a urine analysis and culture, serum electrolytes, and an excretory urogram (which includes a plain or scout film). The average total costs for these studies is about $200. Noting that 328,000 people were discharged in 1984 from the hospital for stone disease, detection costs for inpatients exceeded $65,000,000.

The average length of hospital stay for inpatients with stone disease for males and females was 4.2 days. Not surprisingly, the average length of stay was longer as the age of each group increased (Table 1-3). Assuming the average cost of a hospital bed is $400 exclusive of physician charges, and that 328,000 patients stayed an average of 4.2 days per admission, the nationwide cost per year of urolithiasis from hospital stay alone exceeds $550,000,000.

Expenditures for physician services are included in direct costs. Of those patients requiring hospitalization, about 22 percent will require surgical intervention.[16] Preminger et al. calculated the average total professional fee (urologist, radiologist, anesthesiologist, and pathologist) for renal stones 2.5 cm or smaller by percutaneous nephrostolithotomy or open renal surgery was just over $2200 (1983–1984).[17] Surgical costs nationwide would thus approach $159,000,000. Physician fees by the urologist for those remaining 78 percent of patients not requiring surgery is estimated at $200, for an expenditure of about $51,000,000.

The yearly total direct cost of stone disease for those patients requiring hospitalization, including detection, hospital stay, and treatment using today's costs (1987), probably exceeds $1 billion (Table 1-4).

Indirect Costs

The indirect costs of stone disease calculated are based on the ages 15–64 years since these years account for 95 percent of total productivity.[18] In 1984, 191,000 men in this large age group were hospitalized for an average of 4.0 days,[3] totaling 2093 work-years lost. In the general population, 87 percent of this male age group actually works, giving a more accurate value for 1821 work-years lost.[18] Using an average income for this group of

Table 1-4
Estimated Direct Costs of Urolithiasis Nationwide for Patients Hospitalized in 1984

Detection	$65,000,000
Hospital stay	$550,000,000
Physician services	
Patients requiring surgery	$159,000,000
Patients not requiring surgery	$51,000,000
Total	$825,000,000

Table 1-5
Estimated Indirect Costs for Urolithiasis Nationwide for Patients Aged 15–64 Years Hospitalized in 1984

Indirect costs from hospital stay	
Males	$35,800,000
Females within the work force	$11,600,000
Females as housewives	$4,060,000
Posthospital discharge costs	
Males	$15,800,000
Females within the work force	$4,330,000
Females as housewives	$1,520,000
Total	$73,110,000

$19,683 (1980 figure),[18] we find that the yearly lost income from hospital stay for males exceeds $35,800,000.

Calculation of the indirect costs for females due to hospitalization necessitated by urolithiasis is somewhat more difficult. For those females within the traditional labor force, it is also necessary to include their value as homemakers, and for those women not "gainfully" employed, it is necessary to calculate their "wages" as homemakers. In 1984, 85,000 females stayed in the hospital for an average of 4.7 days, or 1094 work years, and of this number of patients, 64 percent worked within the traditional labor force, producing approximately 700 work-years lost.[18] The average annual traditional work force earning for women is $9300, while their value as homemakers is about $7200, for a total income of about $16,500.[18] The indirect cost, then, for this group of "traditional" work force women approaches $11,600,000. For the remaining 36 percent of female urolithiasis patients *not* within the traditional work force the earned value of work in the home is about $10,300. Their costs are about $4,060,000, giving a yearly total morbidity value for females from hospitalization of over $15,600,00.

Another source of indirect costs resulting from hospitalization for urolithiasis is the posthospital discharge time until the patient returns to work. Preminger noted that the average number of days following hospital discharge before patients returned to work after removal of kidney stones 2.5 cm or smaller by percutaneous nephrostolithotomy or by open surgery was 2 and 14 days, respectively, or an average of 8 days.[17] Assuming that 22 percent of patients hospitalized for stone disease will have some type of surgical procedure and calculating the losses in a fashion similar to those above, the cost in lost wages is about $15,800,000 in males and in females about $5,850,000 for a total additional indirect cost, exceeding $21,600,000.

Thus, adding the morbidity cost of hospital stay and recovery time following surgery, the yearly total indirect costs from stone disease is roughly $73,100,000 (Table 1-5).

Not even mentioned in *any* of the above calculations are the direct and indirect costs of urolithiasis treated on an outpatient basis. This is because of the extreme difficulty and lack of reliability in obtaining figures about numbers of patients affected; however, most urologists will confirm that there are *at least* as many patients with urolithiasis who are *not* hospitalized as there are who *are* hospitalized.

CONCLUSION

During the last 20 years there has been a dramatic rise in the cost of health care. From 1963 to 1980 a growth rate of almost 350 percent in economic costs has occurred, but in this same time period direct medical costs rose by an extraordinary 837 percent. Indirect medical costs have risen about 189 percent over this same period.[18]

Based on 1984 figures, it appears that in terms of current (1987) dollars, the amount of money spent on the detection and treatment of urolithiasis (and its convalescence) exceeds $1 billion. Stated in other terms, over $3000 of resources potentially allocated toward other means were expended on each patient hospitalized for stone disease. Perhaps a more cogent point is that these figures are most likely an underestimate of the total costs since they are only for inpatients and about 50 percent of patients with urinary stones are never hospitalized. The expenditures, however, for outpatient physician charges, diagnostic tests, medication, and home convalescence are very significant.

Careful perusal of the incidence rates of stone disease give us several clues about future economic costs. Age-adjusted incidence rates of urolithiasis are highest in the age group 45–64 years. With the exception of those over 65 years, this group has the longest length of hospital stay and requires the longest recovery period. As the average age of our population and those within the working force increases, we can only expect the costs of stone disease to increase. The effects of the present population shifts to the relative stone prevalence of the Sun Belt areas as well as the increasing industrialization of America remain to be seen.

The increasing number of women entering the labor force may have a profound effect on the costs of stone disease. During the 1950s only one-third of working-age women were employed as compared to more than one-half of women today. Further, as these women become increasingly skilled, the potential losses of their earnings will become more significant.

Newer methods of treatment, including endourology and ESWL, may help to lower the costs of illness but will certainly not prevent them. The Health Planning Council for greater Boston estimated that the use of ESWL could save approximately $2000 per case, which includes a reduction in hospital stay.[16] The United States Department of Health and Human Services projects a yearly savings of $160,000,000 nationwide for stone disease.[16] Although this savings is significant, it must be remembered that this procedure probably will be useful only in those 22 percent of patients requiring surgical intervention and does not address the problem of stone recurrence. Williams reviewed several studies in which recurrence rates ranged from 28 to 63 percent following nephrolithotomy. His study, averaging 18.5 years' follow-up, revealed a recurrence rate of 80 and 60 percent for males and females, respectively.[19]

The real key to the huge economic—direct and indirect—costs of urolithiasis remain with the diagnostic workup and medical management of this disease. If knowledgeable physicians take the time and expend the effort to find out why a patient has urolithiasis and then prescribe the correct medication, urolithiasis recurrence can be prevented or dramatically decreased in 90 percent of patients.

In summary, there have not been any previously detailed estimates on the economic costs of urolithiasis nationwide. These statistics have been presented to illustrate the enormous amount of lost resources from stone disease and to thereby stress the need for diligent application of modern medical methods of diagnosis and therapy in urolithiasis patients.

REFERENCES

1. Boyce WH, Garvey FK, Strawcutter HE: Incidence of urinary calculi among patients in general hospitals, 1948 to 1952. JAMA 161:1437, 1956
2. Sierakowski R, Finlayson B, Landes RR, et al: The frequency of urolithiasis in hospital discharge diagnoses in the United States. Invest Urol 15:438, 1978
3. National Center for Health Statistics, CF Dennison: 1984 Summary: National Hospital Discharge Survey. Advance data from Vital and Health Statistics. No. 112. DHHS Publication No. (PHS) 85-1250. Public Health Service, Hyattsville, MD, September 27, 1985
4. Johnson CM, Wilson DM, O'Fallon WM, et al: Renal stone epidemiology: A 25-year study in Rochester, Minnesota. Kidney International 16:624, 1979
5. Hiatt RA, Dabs LG, Friedman GD, et al: Frequency of urolithiasis in a pre-paid medical care program. Am J Epidemiol 115:255, 1982
6. Division of Research and Statistical Services for South Carolina. Columbia, South Carolina
7. National Center for Health Statistics 1984. Unpublished data
8. Prince CL, Scardino PL, Wolan CT: The effect of temperature, humidity and dehydration on the formation of renal calculi. J. Urol 75:209, 1956
9. Elliot JP Jr, Gordon JO, Evans JW, et al: A stone season. A 10-year retrospective study of 768 surgical stone cases with respect to seasonal variation. J Urol 114:574, 1975
10. Goynes WR, Ingber BF, Berni RJ: Occurrence of calcium oxalate crystals in cotton plants and cotton-related dusts. Textile Res J 54:9, 1984
11. Scott R: Epidemiology of stone disease. Br J Urol 57:491, 1985
12. Pierce LW, Bloom B: Observations on urolithiasis among American troops in a desert area. J Urol 54:466, 1945
13. Wickham JEA: Urinary Calculous Disease. Edinburgh, Churchill Livingstone, 1979, p 21
14. Sutor DJ, Wooley SE, Illingworth JJ: Some aspects of the adult urinary stone problem in Great Britain and Northern Ireland. Br J Urol 46:275, 1974
15. Prince CL, Scardino PL: A statistical analysis of ureteral calculi. J Urol 83:561, 1960
16. National Kidney Foundation Position Paper on Extracorporeal Shockwave Lithotripsy. Approved by the National Kidney Foundation Health and Scientific Affairs Committe, March 1, 1985
17. Preminger GM, Clayman RV, Hardeman SW, et al: Percutaneous nephrostolithotomy vs. open surgery for renal calculi: A comparative study. JAMA 254:1054. 1985
18. Rice DP, Hodgson TA, Kopstein AN: The economic costs of illness: A replication and update. Health Care Finan Rev 7:61, 1985
19. Williams RE: Long term survey of 538 patients with upper urinary stone. Br J Urol 35:416, 1963

Stephen N. Rous

2

Evaluation of the Urolithiasis Patient

THE FIRST-TIME STONE FORMER

The purpose of doing a complete and meticulous metabolic evaluation of a stone-forming patient is to determine the etiology of the stone-forming process so as to prescribe a prophylactic regime, often consisting of medication, that will prevent or greatly minimize future stone formation. Since the author feels that the first-time stone former may well turn out to be a one-time stone former, it is obvious that such an individual represents a different clinical problem than the recurrent stone former, and these two clinical situations call for different diagnostic approaches. The author does not feel that a full and complete metabolic evaluation is warranted in the first-time stone former, and there are two reasons for this: (1) a very significant percentage of first-time stone formers and possibly even a majority will not form another stone in the forseeable future,[1,2] and (2) it is a very rare patient indeed who will comply with a medication program of 2, 3, 4 times daily medication for an indefinite period of time after only one bout of lithiasis.

Although it is true that many first-time stone formers have demonstrable metabolic abnormalities,[3] the author concurs with those[4] who feel that such metabolic abnormalities are not necessarily any more clinically significant than similar metabolic abnormalities found in the non-stone-forming population, and thus detecting such abnormalities does not necessarily mean that treatment is indicated. For this reason, performing a complete stone workup is very likely not indicated, either.

For the first-time stone former, therefore, the author obtains only a few tests: a urine analysis; a urine for culture and sensitivity; an excretory urogram (intravenous pyelogram [IVP]); a serum calcium (×3); and also a serum creatinine, electrolytes, uric acid,

STONE DISEASE: DIAGNOSIS AND MANAGEMENT
ISBN 0-8089-1873-7

and phosphorus. If the patient is seen during the time that the stone is being passed, the excretory urogram is necessary to confirm the diagnosis of stone and also to assist the clinician in managing the patient since the excretory urogram should demonstrate the size and position of the stone and the degree of obstruction above it. Moreover, if the excretory urogram is totally normal, it might direct the clinician to other possible sources of the continuing pain, particularly in the absence of any red blood cells in the urine. Should there be a contraindication to the excretory urogram, a KUB (film of kidneys, ureters, and bladder), a renal scan, and a renal ultrasound should serve almost the same purpose. The routine urine is obtained, particularly to look for red blood cells and crystals, and the culture is obtained because the presence of bacterial infection, particularly above an obstructing stone, removes much of the flexibility from patient management. The creatinine is obtained for baseline purposes and the uric acid to rule out hyperuricemia, which may or may not be related to the stone problem. The electrolytes are obtained as a screening test for the complete form of type I renal tubular acidosis (RTA), which, if present, will often show a hyperchloremic acidosis. Most important of all in this very preliminary screening process are the serum calciums (×3), which are performed to detect a hyperparathyroid condition, which, in the author's opinion, is best diagnosed by a serum calcium elevation over 10.1 mg percent, particularly in the presence of an elevated parathyroid hormone assay. Hyperparathyroidism, when found, should be treated surgically, even if the stone episode is a first-time one, because this disease is a progressive, systemic one best treated surgically regardless of whether urolithiasis is a complicating factor.[5] The serum phosphorus is obtained because a low level is helpful (but not essential) in the diagnosis of hyperparathyroidism.

The author additionally examines the patient's urine sediment in both the evaporated and unevaporated form (see Chapter 17) to look for crystals, particularly clumping and aggregation of crystals, as well as large crystals since these findings, when present, suggest the likelihood of recurrent problems with calculi.[6,7] Also, examination of the urine sediment often permits detection of the hexagonal crystals of cystine, which, if present, strongly suggest the etiology of the lithiasis.

Whether the patient is hospitalized or followed as an outpatient, the author likes to have the patient note and record the urinary pH following each voiding for a 24-hour period. This study is often helpful in tentatively establishing the composition of the stone since cystine and uric acid stones tend to be found when the urinary pH is quite consistently around 5.5 or lower, calcium phosphate stones tend to be present when the pH is persistently on the alkaline side of 6.5, "infected" stones are usually present in a persistent alkaline medium, and only the ubiquitous calcium oxalate stones—which are the most prevalent of all stones—will be found in a pH that mirrors the normal diurnal variation. Recovery of the stone for definitive crystallographic analysis is critically important for its role in stone prevention (see Chapter 4), and the author generally obtains this analysis by sending the stone to the Louis Herring Company in Orlando (Florida) or Calculab in Richmond (Virginia).

In general, additional studies are not carried out for the first-time stone former except under unusual circumstances such as the presence of a solitary kidney, a very strong family history of lithiasis, or other situations in which stone recurrence is felt to be likely (such as persistent clumping or aggregation of crystals in the urine sediment). In such special situations the first-time stone former will have the additional studies noted below in order to establish an etiology for the lithiasis so that appropriate therapy may be started.

THE PATIENT WITH RECURRENT UROLITHIASIS

Obstruction in the urinary tract, in the absence of infection, is not nearly as common a cause of urolithiasis as was formerly thought.[8] Infection as a cause of stone disease is covered in Chapter 15. This section discusses metabolic causes for recurrent urolithiasis.

The group of patients in whom the author feels a full metabolic workup is indicated in order to assign an etiology for the stones and thereby derive a therapeutic regime consists of those individual patients who have had more than one episode of clinical lithiasis and also those patients who have evidence of metabolically active disease.[9] This latter is defined as—in a 1-year period—documented growth of a preexisting stone in the kidney, formation of additional renal stones, or documented passage of gravel. Note that metabolically active disease and clinical lithiasis may be, but are not necessarily, the same. The protocol outlined below, then, is used for the evaluation of patients with clinically recurrent urolithiasis and/or those with metabolically active disease.

The evaluation includes the same blood studies as for the initial stone former and these include a serum calcium ×3, and a serum creatinine, electrolytes, uric acid, and phosphorus and the information to be gained from these studies relates to the same conditions as noted for the first-time stone formers. A discussion of these conditions is found in Chapters 9–12. In the majority of stone formers, however, all the blood studies will be normal, and so a very major part of the evaluation for the recurrent stone former lies in two or three meticulously carried out 24-hour urine collections for calcium, uric acid, oxalate, citrate, sodium, and probably a creatinine clearance as well that is done for baseline purposes should the patient undergo deterioration of renal function in the future. It has been debated as to whether these 24-hour urine values obtained would be accurate if an obstructing stone were present in the ureter. Recent studies suggested that the most accurate results will probably be obtained by waiting for several weeks after the patient has left the hospital and after the stone has been passed or removed.[10] Certainly, at the least, the patient must have been on a regular diet for a week or two, and therefore these 24-hour urine studies cannot possibly be done while the patient is hospitalized and ideally should not be done while any lingering pain is present. For these additional reasons the author agrees that it is best to delay the urine collections until the stone is no longer present.

The author will usually give to each patient four containers, each of 3-liter size, and two of these are acidified for collection of calcium and oxalate, and the other two have a preservative such as toluene for collection of the uric acid, citrate, and sodium. (The creatinine clearance is done on the containers with toluene.) It is extremely important that the calcium and oxalate be collected in a pH of 2–3, and this can be done by adding 20 ml of 6 *N* hydrochloric acid to each of the two containers that are to be studied for calcium and oxalate. If these urines are not collected in this highly acid pH, the ascorbate present in the urine and normally converted to oxalate in an alkaline pH will do precisely that in varying amounts, leading to spuriously high oxalate levels. Moreover, calcium oxalate and calcium phosphate will precipitate in unacidified urine, and it is not possible to drive these precipitated substances completely back into solution by acidifying the containers *after* they arrive in the laboratory. This will lead to false low values of calcium and oxalate. The importance of this acidification of the containers in which the calcium and the oxalate are to be measured is not generally appreciated and cannot be emphasized strongly enough. For the citrate, uric acid, and sodium collections, all that is needed is a preservative and approximately 10 ml of toluene or thymol are satisfactory.

It is most probable that the oxalic acid level in a 24-hour urine is even more important than that of the calcium level as a major factor in urolithiasis, and this has not generally been appreciated.[11] Historically, this importance has gone unrecognized because of the great difficulty in accurately performing urinary oxalate levels, a situation changed only quite recently.[12,13] In 1985 the Sigma Diagnostics Company of St. Louis introduced an accurate and reproducible oxalate kit that is inexpensive and very rapid and easy to perform. Determination of the urinary citrate level, although not commonly done in laboratories, is not difficult and also is quite accurate and very reproducible.[14]

In evaluating the patient with recurrent lithiasis and/or metabolically active stone disease it is helpful to realize that there are several possible etiologies, and these have approximately the following distribution: (1) "idiopathic" nephrolithiasis—±40 percent of patients; (2) Hypercalciuric nephrolithiasis—±30 percent of patients; (3) tubular and/or enzymatic disorders—±2 percent of patients; (4) primary hyperparathyroidism—±5 percent of patients; and (5) other disorders leading to lithiasis, such as the various hypercalcemic states (but not including hyperparathyroidism), uric acid lithiasis, and the gastrointestinal (GI) disorders that produce urolithiasis—±20 percent of patients. The therapy of each of these conditions is discussed in subsequent chapters.

Idiopathic Nephrolithiasis

In the author's experience this is the most common single finding in the etiologic workup of patients with recurrent urolithiasis, although others find it less common than hypercalciuric nephrolithiasis.[9] It is really a diagnosis of exclusion because all the patients' blood values are normal, as are all the 24-hour urine studies. The author feels that the most likely reason for this normocalcemic, normocalciuric (idiopathic) form of nephrolithiasis is a defect of one or more of the various urinary inhibitors of crystallization, some of the better known of which are magnesium, citrate, pyrophospate, RNA-like substances, heparin-like substances and glycosaminoglycans (GAGs). If the defect is in the readily measurable urinary citrate level, it will be noted to be below the usual norm of 400–600 mg per 24-hour period. The determination of a low magnesium level in the urine is also easily determined. However, more often than not in this "idiopathic" group of stone formers both of these levels will be found to be within normal limits and the determination of the levels of the other known inhibitors is just not done in most hospital and commercial laboratories because it is tedious, technically difficult, and thus very costly.

Although obviously not "idiopathic" by definition, there are three other known causes of urolithiasis that the author frequently includes in the "idiopathic" category for convenience sake, and these are all diagnosed by examination of the urine and they all show normocalcemia and normocalciuria. One is a hyperuricosuria, otherwise asymptomatic, in which the presence of increased amounts of uric acid in the urine leads to an increased precipitation of calcium oxalate crystals; the second is a hyperoxaluria (secondary) due to dietary oxalate overload or even to a mild metabolic hyperoxaluria (see Chapter 16) in which the oxalate level is minimally elevated for unknown reasons. The third is an increased urinary alkalinity that is fairly persistent in the region of pH 6.5–7.0 and that leads to precipitation of calcium phosphate crystals with resulting calcium phosphate lithiasis. This situation, in which the usual diurnal pH variations do not occur, may be due to the ingestion of large amounts of citrus fruit juice (which is metabolized to bicarbonate) and/or to a nonmeat vegetarian diet.

Hypercalciuric Nephrolithiasis

In this disease category the serum calcium remains normal while the 24-hour urinary calcium is elevated to greater than 300 mg per 24-hour period in men and greater than 275 mg per 24-hour period in women. All other blood and urine parameters are normal. Inasmuch as the urinary calcium is largely dependent on the dietary calcium intake, it is important that the 24-hour urinary calcium be measured while the patient is on a regular diet and it is distinctly advantageous to measure it on two or even three separate occasions because there are certain individuals that are "binge" calcium eaters, and this could be missed by relying on a solitary 24-hour urine calcium determination.

After it has been determined that hypercalciuria exists, the next step is to determine the reason for it. In the author's experience, a renal tubular "leak" is the most common finding and the absorptive (from the gut) hypercalciuria is the next most common cause. It should be noted, however, that in some series "absorptive" hypercalciuria is more common than renal tubular "leakage" of calcium.[15] Also to be considered, although infrequently of clinical significance, is the resorptive hypercalciuria such as seen with prolonged immobilization and resulting calcium resorption from the skeletal system.

It is advantageous to try to separate the renal tubular leak patients from the absorptive patients because the therapy for these two conditions is not necessarily the same and because adequate therapy for the absorptive hypercalciuria can sometimes be confined to dietary limitation of calcium. There are many suggested methods, some complex and some simple, for separating the leakers from the hyperabsorbers, and the author has found the simplest reliable method to be the one that is the easiest for the patient and the physician as well. It requires an overnight fast of something over 14 hours, with the patient on a regular diet prior to the fast, followed by a 2-hour urine collection immediately following the fasting period. If there is less than 20 mg of calcium in this 2-hour urine then the patient most likely has the absorptive type of hypercalciuria. On the other hand, if there is more than 30 mg of calcium present in the two-hour urine, the patient is a renal tubular leaker. If the 2-hour urine specimen contains more than 20 mg but les than 30 mg of calcium, the overnight fasting period should be repeated and lengthened. A persistent hypercalciuria (over 20 mg) suggests that the etiology of the hypercalciuria is *not* absorptive but is most likely due to a renal tubular leak. In the author's experience the renal tubular leakers outnumber the hyperabsorbers by about a 3:1 margin.

Renal Tubular and Enzyme Disorders

Cystinuria

This will be a clinical problem if there is more than 400 mg of cystine per 24 hour of urine, and if this situation exists, microscopy will reveal hexagonal crystals, which are almost never seen in the absence of clinical cystinuria. The sodium nitroprusside test is also positive with clinically significant cystinuria, and this test is done by adding equal volumes of the patient's urine and 5 percent sodium cyanide and allowing this mixture to stand for 5 minutes. This reduces the cystine to cysteine, and the addition of a few drops of freshly prepared sodium nitroprusside will lead to an immediate purple color that soon fades. This positive reaction, indicative of clinically significant cystinuria, will revert to negative when the patient is under adequate therapy for cystinuria.

Renal Tubular Acidosis (RTA), Type I

This (type I) is the only really significant form of renal tubular acidosis as a cause of urolithiasis, and when it is in its complete form, a screening battery of blood tests will reveal a hyperchloremic acidosis that should suggest (but not prove) the presence of this condition. Unfortunately, the incomplete form of RTA is frequently present, and this may be screened for in one of two ways after first checking the fasting urine, which should normally be of pH 5.5 or less. If it is not, an ammonium chloride load (100 mg/kg per 24-hour period) should produce a urine ph of 5.5 or less; if it does not, RTA may be said to exist. More simply, and possibly preferable to the ammonium chloride loading test, is the 24-hour urine citrate level, which will be less than 50 mg when a type I RTA exists. The normal 24-hour urine citrate level is 400–600 mg, and the low urinary citrate level seen with RTA exists because citrate production falls dramatically in the presence of renal intracellular acidosis. A low urinary citrate level by itself, however, can be found in the presence of conditions other than RTA.

Primary Hyperoxaluria

This is an inborn error of metabolism, is dependent for diagnosis on an accurate 24-hour urine oxalate measurement, and when hyperoxaluria (over 40 mg per 24-hour period) is found, must be differentiated from the secondary hyperoxaluria caused by dietary excesses. This differentiation is usually not difficult since the primary form of hyperoxaluria will usually be manifest in the first or second decade of life while secondary hyperoxaluria will occur at a later time. A dietary history of ingesting foods or liquids high in oxalate concentration would be helpful, but the definitive diagnosis of primary versus secondary hyperoxaluria may require measuring the urinary glycollate level,[16] which is normally less than 0.33 mmol/liter in adults and children. Glycollate is an intermediate metabolic product in the normal metabolism of oxalic acid, and if it is elevated, it suggests a primary problem, whereas a normal urinary glycollate level in the face of elevated 24-hour urinary oxalate levels suggests a secondary hyperoxaluria.

The upper limit of normal is 40 mg of oxalate per 24 hours of urine, and primary hyperoxalurias usually yield values between 80 and 400 mg or even higher per 24-hour period. Secondary oxaluria, from dietary overload, can give values that do not usually exceed 60 mg per 24-hour period.

Mild Metabolic Hyperoxaluria

This is a recently described entity[17] in which there is an elevated urinary oxalate level that is not as high as with primary hyperoxaluria and there is also an elevated urinary glycollate level since this is a metabolic problem and not a result of excess dietary oxalates. Urinary 24-hour oxalate levels will generally not exceed 60 mg with this newly described entity of mild metabolic hyperoxaluria.

Hypercalcemic Nephrolithiasis

By far the most common entity in this broad category of disease causing recurrent nephrolithiasis is hyperparathyroidism, and the diagnosis is most commonly made by repeated measurements of the serum calcium levels, which, if higher than 10.1 mg percent, strongly suggest the presence of hyperparathyroidism. This may be confirmed with parathormone assays, and it is helpful, but not necessary, for the serum phosphorus level to be depressed. Other far less common causes of hypercalcemic states that should be considered are prolonged imobilization, milk-alkali syndrome, sarcoidosis, hypervitaminosis D, neoplasms (particularly those of the bladder and urethra that are already metastatic), steroid use, and hyperthryroidism.

Uric Acid Lithiasis

The diagnosis of this condition rests entirely on the recovery and crystallographic analysis of the patient's stone (see Chapter 4) inasmuch as most patients with uric acid lithiasis have normal blood and urine uric acid levels. A clue to the presence of a uric acid stone can be gained from the fact that most (but not all) patients with this condition will run fairly constant urinary pH levels of 5.5 or lower. Also, the presence of an elevated blood or urine (or both) uric acid level or the clinical presence of gout can be helpful clues (but by no means definite proof) that the offending stone is one of uric acid.

Gastrointestinal Disorders

The most common form of stone in this disease category is calcium oxalate that is produced as a result of the secondary hyperoxaluria present in patients who have had surgical bypass operations for morbid obesity as well as other entities involving small bowel disease and/or resection. In these conditions it is felt that there is an excess of fatty acids present in the gut that binds the calcium thereby leaving a surplus of oxalate free to become absorbed and to bring about a secondary hyperoxaluria with resulting calcium oxalate lithiasis.[9] In this type of secondary hyperoxaluria the 24-hour urine oxalate level is quite high, usually well over 80–100 mg per 24-hour period. It is interesting to note that apparently an intact and normal large bowel must be present for this type of secondary hyperoxaluria to result.

Ileostomies and other small bowel disease states leading to protracted diarrhea will result in an excess loss of water and bicarbonate with a resulting low urine volume and very acid pH. This, in turn, may result in a uric acid lithiasis. Whether a given patient's intestinal problem is producing a uric acid or an oxalate lithiasis cannot always be determined by the clinical findings of the history; therefore, a crystallographic analysis of a recovered stone is mandatory prior to the institution of any therapy.

In this chapter, the various metabolic and idiopathic factors in recurrent urolithiasis have been discussed and an approach to the accurate determination of the stone etiology presented. Almost all of the causes of recurrent lithiasis have been covered, and those other factors not covered such as obstruction and/or infection, bladder calculi, and stones in the pediatric age group will be covered in succeeding chapters. This chapter also did not discuss medical management of recurrent lithiasis since this will be discussed in detail in subsequent chapters.

REFERENCES

1. Johnson CM, Wilson D, O'Fallon WM, et al: Renal stone epidemiology: A 25-year study in Rochester, Minnesota. Kidney Internat 16:624, 1979
2. Williams RE: Long-term survey of 538 patients with upper urinary tract stone. Br J Urol 35:416–437, 1963
3. Pak CYC: Should patients with single renal stone occurrence undergo diagnostic evaluation? J Urol 127:855–858, May 1982

4. Hosking DH, Ericson SB, Van den Berg CJ, et al: The stone clinic effect in patients with idiopathic calcium urolithiasis. J Urol 130:1115–1118, 1983
5. Van Heerden J, Kent RB III, Sizemore GW, et al: Primary hyperparathyroidism in patients with multiple endocrine neoplasia syndrome: Surgical Experience. Arch Surg 118:533–536, May 1983
6. Robertson WG, Peacock M: Calcium oxalate crystalluria and inhibitors of crystallization in recurrent renal stone formers. Clin Sci 43:499–506, 1972
7. Robertson WG, Peacock M, Nordin BEC: Calcium crystalluria in recurrent renal stone formers. Lancet 2:21–24, 1969
8. Boyce WH: Diagnosis of renal calculi, in Glenn JF (ed): Diagnostic Urology. New York, Harper & Row, 1964, pp 290–311
9. Smith LH: Urolithiasis, in Early LE, Gottschalk CW (eds): Strauss & Welt's Diseases of the Kidney, 3d ed. Vol II, Boston, Little Brown, 1979, pp 893–931
10. Norman RW, Bath SS, Robertson WG, et al: When should patients with symptomatic urinary stone disease be evaluated metabolically? J Urol 132:1137–1139, 1984
11. Robertson WG, Peacock M: The cause of idiopathic calcium stone disease: Hypercalciuria or hyperoxaluria. Nephron 26:105–110, 1980
12. Kasidas GP, Rose GA: Continuous flow assay for urinary oxalate using immobilized oxalate oxidase. Ann Clin Biochem 22:412–419, 1985
13. Kasidas GP, Rose GA: Measurement of plasma oxalate in healthy subjects and in patients with chronic renal failure using immobilized oxalate oxidase. Clin Chim Acta 154:49–52, 1986
14. Hosking DH, Wilson JWL, Liedtke RR, et al: Urinary citrate excretion in normal persons and patients with idiopathic calcium urolithiasis. J Lab Clin Med 106:682–689, 1985
15. Nordin BEC: Hypecalciuria. Clin Sci Molec Med 52:1–8, 1977
16. Kasidis GP, Rose GA: A new enzymatic method for the determination of glycollate in urine and plasma. Clin Chim Acta 96:25–36, 1979
17. Kasidis GP, Rose GA: Metabolic hyperoxaluria and its response to pyridoxine, in Ryall R, Brockis JG, Marshall V, et al (eds): Urinary Stone. Churchill Livingstone, 1984, pp 138–147

Alan H. Angell
Martin I. Resnick

3

Urinary Inhibitors and Promoters of Stone Formation

There has long been an interest in promoters and inhibitors in urine. It has long been known that urine is a supersaturated solution. Joly wrote that normal urine was able to contain 3–4 times the concentration of calcium oxalate obtainable in water,[51] and uric acid was also known to be more soluble in urine than in plain water. Lichtwitz noted the presence of colloids in urine that were not dialyzable.[57] When urine was dialyzed against water, the crystalloid component would form calcium oxalate, calcium phosphate, and uric acid deposits when the water was evaporated. It has long been known that colloids have a protective action tending to prevent the precipitation of salts or other colloids. The colloid was thought to surround the inorganic salts with a thin layer and thereby increase their solubility.[51]

It was long thought some colloids present in urine exerted a protective effect. Butt reasoned that increasing these protective colloids would be beneficial in stone formers.[20] He treated patients with injections of hyaluronidase and noted a significant increase in the excretion of colloid in 82 percent of the subjects. Hyaluronidase was used because of its spreading properties.

Calculi form by a combination of three processes: nucleation, growth, and aggregation. Promoters and inhibitors can affect any or all of these three processes. It is possible that substances can promote at one stage while inhibit at another. Strictly speaking, promoters and inhibitors of urolithiasis work not by changing the concentration of the constituent ions, but "on an action at the developing surface of the embryo or crystal itself."[31]

Research in the last 35 years has contributed much to the understanding of how one class of molecules can vary the interactions of other molecules. Most of the work has involved calcium oxalate and calcium phosphate stones. There are several ways that inhibitors and promoters can be classified: molecular size, molecular class, the mode of action, the stage of calculus formation at which they are active, the quantity present in urine, by the stone composition they affect, naturally occurring versus synthetic, and

STONE DISEASE: DIAGNOSIS AND MANAGEMENT
ISBN 0-8089-1873-7

other factors. Several in vitro methods also exist for testing the effectiveness of promoters and inhibitors. They each have drawbacks and advantages, and no perfect model exists as yet that duplicates the complex interactions involved in calculus formation in the urinary tract.

TESTING METHODS

An early model involved incubating rachitic rat cartilage in urine. Urine from healthy individuals did not calcify the cartilage, whereas urine from stone formers did.[46,113] Different substances could then be added to the urine of stone formers to determine whether the formation of calcified cartilage was prevented. Inhibitors had the property of turning "evil" urine into "good" urine.[48]

Robertson et al. developed a methodology that enabled the growth and aggregation of calcium oxalate to be quantitatively measured.[87] A metastable solution had calcium oxalate monohydrate seed crystals added, and the solution was then incubated for several hours. At regular intervals a small sample was removed, and a Coulter counter measured the crystal size between 6 and 40 μm. The number of particles measuring over 20 μm was measured and an increase was indicative of enhanced growth and aggregation. Later this was further refined to separate growth and aggregation. An increase in crystal diameter represented growth while a decrease in crystal number indicated aggregation was taking place. Their model has recently undergone criticism in that it does not take into account crystals that grow or aggregate into the range of detection of the Coulter counter. A computer model has been developed that excludes these crystals.[99]

Meyer and Smith developed a seeded crystal system whereby calcium oxalate crystals were added to a supersaturated solution containing calcium and oxalate ions.[64] At predetermined intervals some of the solution was filtered to remove the crystals. The concentration of Ca^{2+} in the filtrate was then measured by atomic absorption and crystal growth was determined by using a 1:1 stoichiometric relationship between calcium oxalate and calcium and oxalate ions. Modifications that exist include using radioactive calcium ions. The decrease in oxalate concentration can also be followed and ^{14}C-oxalate may be a more sensitive molecule to measure.[58] Crystal aggregation can be measured by use of a Coulter counter that measures the size of the crystals at specific time intervals. This technique is precise and reproducible; however, it is too sensitive to be used with whole urine; where dilutions of 1–5 percent v/v must be made.[31] The problem of testing with diluted urine samples will be discussed later.

Workers in Israel have developed a *discriminating index* that standardizes the calcium concentration in urine and then adds a known amount of oxalate such that a supersaturated solution is created and precipitation begins immediately. The calcium ion concentration is measured at 30 seconds and again at 10 minutes. The index is then calculated. The lower the number, the greater the potential of the urine or test solution to inhibit aggregation.[102]

Recently it has become apparent that it is important to work with undiluted urine.[31] In 1979 Hallson and Rose described the use of a rotary evaporator in which whole urine was evaporated to a standard osmolarity.[42] The pH was adjusted to 5.3 to study calcium oxalate or 6.8 to study calcium phosphate crystal formation. The crystals formed were then quantitated. The technique has been used primarily to study promoters because their effectiveness may depend on ionic strength.[92]

Pak has used the formation product ratio (FPR) to obtain information on the modifying effect of inhibitors and promoters on spontaneous precipitation. It is the ratio of the activity product "necessary to form a precipitate from a given urine specimen to that of another aliquot of the same urine specimen after equilibration with brushite," or any crystal.[78] It gives a measure of the state of supersaturation and "provides a quantitative measure of the risk of spontaneous precipitation."[31]

Newer methods have been developed to better approximate the in vivo environment. The continuous mixed-suspension–mixed-product-removal crystallizer[68] allows one to work with whole urine. It provides information on the nucleation and growth rates as well as total crystal mass produced. The results are reproducible.

INHIBITORS

Molecular Inhibitors

Early work on inhibitors examined the supersolubility of calcium phosphate in natural urine when compared to water or artificial urine. The presence of magnesium and citrate were known to contribute to the inhibitory effect, but the mode of action was unknown. Furthermore, not all the inhibitory effect could be attributed to the two ions. An unidentified, dialyzable substance was reported as being responsible for maintaining calcium phosphate in solution.[118]

Pyrophosphate

In 1962 Fleisch and Bisaz noted that the addition of 2 percent dilute urine approximately doubled the formation product of calcium phosphate.[32] The addition of citrate to the solution had no effect on the formation product. If urine was passed through an anion exchanger before being added to the test solution, the urine lost all its inhibiting power. Addition to a cation exchanger, however, only partially diminished this ability. They isolated the responsible molecule and identified it as pyrophosphate and predicted that the oral feeding of polyphosphates (changed by the intestine and absorbed as orthophosphate) could be used to prevent hydroxyapatite stone formation. Later studies indeed showed that the feeding of inorganic orthophosphates to patients raised the pyrophosphate concentration in urine whereas suppression reduced the concentration.[34] The in vitro range of maximal inhibition was at the concentration found in urine.[33] Pyrophosphate was found to have no effect on the crystallization of uric acid and magnesium ammonium phosphate.[35]

Diphosphonates

The search for an oral agent that would be resistant to the action of phosphatases led to the synthesis of disphosphonates. The most commonly used diphosphonate is disodium ethane-1-hydroxy-1, 1-diphosphonate (EHDP, Didronel®, Norwich Eaton). The EHDP compound is used primarily in the treatment of Paget's disease and heterogeneous ossification. The structural similarity of EHDP to inorganic pyrophosphate (PPi) led to in vitro testing, and it was found to be similar as PPi in effect. It inhibited the precipitation of calcium phosphate from metastable solutions, slowed the phase transformation of calcium phosphate into hydroxyapatite, and inhibited the formation of brushite. The effects on calcium oxalate were similar, increasing the formation product ratio of calcium oxalate and preventing in vitro aggregation.[36] The EHDP compound was resistant to kidney pyrophosphatase. It prevented calcium phosphate, calcium oxalate monohydrate (COM), and calcium oxalate dihydrate (COD) zinc pellet induced bladder stones in rats.[37] In clinical trials, oral EHDP resulted in a decreased incidence of stone passage in calcium oxalate or calcium oxalate–calcium phosphate stone formers; however, the potential side effects (muscle weakness, skeletal pain, increased serum alkaline phosphatase, decreased bone density, inducement of osteomalacia) may limit its usefulness.[7]

Citrate

The role of citrate in preventing stone formation may be ascribed to its ability to work as an inhibitor as well as form soluble complexes with Ca^{2+}. Citrate was shown to change evil urine into good urine.[113] Recent work involves the complexation of citrate to metal ions. Using a high ratio of citrate to ferric ion at neutral pH, a low-molecular-weight (LMW) Fe(III)–citric acid complex forms. This complex inhibited the growth of calcium phosphate in a seeded crystal system. This was also observed for Al(III) and Cr(III)–citrate complexes. The Al(III) and Cr(III) were inhibitors by themselves but worked much better as inhibitors when complexed to citrate. Iron(III) had no effect by itself on calcium phosphate.[66] A high-molecular weight (HMW) complex could be formed with a low ratio of citrate to ferric ion. This formed an inhibitor effective on the growth of calcium oxalate. No effect was seen when Cr(III) or Al(III) was combined with citrate.[67] Seventy to eighty percent of Al(III), Fe(III), and Cr(III) in urine is complexed to citrate.[112]

Phosphocitrate

In 1976 Howard isolated a potent in vitro inhibitor of urinary stone calcification. At pH 1, citrate and pyrophosphate interacted to form an agent that had stronger anticalcifying properties than did pyrophosphate and citrate combined. The compound, phosphocitrate, had been found in liver, kidney mitochondria, and human urine. It is small in molecular size, highly acidic, and has an organic moiety. It inhibited the growth of hydroxyapatite in a seeded crystal system. Hydroxyapatite adsorbs the phosphocitrate rapidly.[110] This is probably due to the selective absorption of phosphocitrate at active crystal growth sites. Small doses of PC have been very effective at reducing stone formation produced in mice with large doses of parathyroid hormone.[111] Phosphocitrate also inhibited the formation of calcium oxalate crystal growth on glass fibers. However, the importance of phosphocitrate as an inhibitor must be questioned as it is rapidly hydrolyzed by enzymes in the kidney. Its role may be to prevent intracellular or intramitochondrial deposition of calcium salts.[122]

SAT

The liability of PC led to the synthesis of *N*-sulfo-2-amino-tricarballylate (SAT). This molecule has a similar structure to PC yet is resistant to the enzymatic hydrolysis. It has the ability to inhibit the change of amorphous calcium phosphate into hydroxyapatite; it was less effective than PC but more effective than PPi [PPi $<$ SAT $<$ PC]. A calcium oxalate seeded crystal in vitro study revealed SAT to be less effective than PPi and PC. Nevertheless, the effect of all three inhibitors in both systems was "potent and significant."[17] In vivo studies in rats revealed that 70 percent of orally administered SAT was absorbed, had no toxic short-term effects, was resistant to enzymatic degradation, and was rapidly cleared by the kidney (80 percent excreted unchanged after 24 hours). It was more effective in preventing calcium oxalate formation than PC, whereas PC was more effective at preventing hydroxyapatite crystal deposition.[18] Even though SAT may be weaker than PC, it probably has more overall effect as it is not susceptible to enzymatic degradation.

Magnesium

Magnesium has been shown to decrease the incidence of calcium oxalate calculus formation. This is due, in part, to its ability to form soluble complexes with oxalate and thereby increase the solubility of calcium oxalate. The interaction is Ph dependent and alkalinization increases the effect. Magnesium does exhibit inhibitory ability.[8] It has been shown to retard the growth rate of COM in a continuous mixed-suspension–mixed-product-removal crystallizer.[56]

Dyes

A number of dyes, such as safranin O, have been known to interact with crystals and inhibit mineralization of bone at active sites of growth, as well as inhibit calcification of rachitic rat cartilage. Most of the work has been done with methylene blue. Bladder calculi in rats were inhibited and dissolved by methylene blue.[116] Methylene blue was picked as it is excreted unchanged in the urine. Using a model of zinc bladder disks in rats fed ethylene glycol (to assure the formation of calcium oxalate stones), it was felt that without the addition of vitamin C to the diet methylene blue was ineffective. Patients on oral methylene blue were noted to have no new stone formation, dissolution of preexisting calculi, and clearance of recurrent action.[14] Another dye, copper chlorophyllin (used as a coloring agent for food and drugs), has been shown to be a powerful in vitro inhibitor of COM growth. It is 20 times more powerful as a COM inhibitor than as a COD inhibitor.[109]

Tamarind Fruit

In southern India there is an unusually decreased incidence in stone formation. This was attributed to people eating the tamarind fruit, which contains tartaric acid. Tartaric acid has inhibitory activity on dilute urine. In concentrated, whole urine, tartaric acid and its stereoisomers were effective in inhibiting calcium oxalate crystallization.[43] Others corroborate the growth inhibition data in dilute or artificial urine. In natural urine, they found an insignificant decrease in reduction of precipitation and concluded that the tamarind fruit did not have a protective effect.[21]

Macromolecular Inhibitors

Glycosaminoglycans

The identification of macromolecular inhibitors began with the finding that 1 percent urine from healthy people was significantly better at inhibiting crystal growth and aggregation in vitro than was urine from recurrent calcium oxalate stone formers. This activity persisted despite the addition of pyrophosphatase to the urine (which inactivated PPi). An anionic inhibitor with molecular weight of 10,000–50,000 was identified; it was a sulfated polysaccharide and highly charged.[85] Positive ions such as magnesium and methylene blue had no effect as inhibitors in the system.

Glycosaminoglycans (GAGs) are found in urine and are polysulfated, polyanionic substances. It is unclear where GAGS are produced. It is thought that they are filtered from blood with some contribution from the kidney. Some researchers feel that little is contributed by the bladder.[10] If they were simply filtered by the kidney from serum, however, urine would contain heparin. Human kidneys contain primarily heparan sulfates, hyaluronic acid, and dermatan sulfate. Chondroitins A and C, an oversulfated chondroitin sulfate, and a nonsulfated chondroitin represent about one-sixth of the kidney GAG content.[69] Glycosaminoglycans may be secreted by the peritubular cells.

Normal urine contains approximately 60 percent chondroitin sulfate (both chondroitin-4-sulfate, or chondroitin A; and chondroitin-6-sulfate, or chondroitin C), 2 percent unsulfated chondroitin, 15 percent heparan sulfate, 18 percent keratan sulfate, 4 percent hyaluronic acid, and 1 percent dermatan sulfate. Heparin is not found in urine.[40,119] Heparin and chondroitin A were found to be very strong inhibitors of growth and aggregation, working in a range down to 0.001 μM. In contrast, highly charged anions only inhibited in a range down to 0.1–1 μM.[87] They were 1000 times more potent than EHDP and PPi at inhibiting calcium oxalate crystallization.[85] Sallis and Lumley isolated GAGs from the urine of healthy volunteers.[101] Using a test system of glass rods in a metastable solution of sodium oxalate and calcium chloride, they tested for the inhibition of precipitation after an incubation period of 24 hours. Three peaks of activity were found that corresponded to hyaluronic acid, heparan sulfate, dermatan sulfate, and chondroitins A and C.

Recently, two-dimensional electrophoresis of GAGs extracted from stone matrix has shown that heparan sulfate and hyaluronic acid are present in fractions disproportionate to their excretion in urine.[76] These workers argue that these GAGs must play an important role in stone formation and that must be one of promoters; however, this argument is less than convincing.

Sodium Pentosan Polysulfate

The usefulness of an oral anticoagulant similar to heparin led to the synthesis of the sulfated, polyanionic GAG-like molecule of sodium pentosan polysulfate (SP 54, Elmiron,® Pharmacia). When taken orally, SP 54 is excreted unchanged in urine. In bladder mucosa stripped of its glycocalyx coat, SP 54 restores its ability to prevent adherence of bacteria.[80] It decreases the growth rate, agglomeration, and total amount of calcium oxalate precipitated in in vitro systems. Oral SP 54 contributes to increased urinary polyanionic inhibitory activity against calcium oxalate crystallization.[77]

Ribonucleic Acid

Alcian blue has been used to precipitate macromolecules in urine [known as alcian blue precipitatable proteins, (ABPP)]. Glycosaminoglycans are known to be part of the alcian blue precipitate.[9] Ribonucleic acid (RNA) also is precipitated by alcian blue. Ribonucleic acid and four related homopolyribonucleotides have been shown to inhibit calcium oxalate crystal growth and aggregation. They are all polyanionic molecules. Deoxyribonucleic acid, or DNA, is much less inhibitory than RNA in the same system. In testing of the effect of ribonuclease on urine, however, only 3 of 17 samples had decreases in inhibitory strength.[50] Others have shown that human urine is susceptible to the effects of bovine pancreatic ribonuclease and that RNA and RNA-like material in urine contributes to inhibition. The enzymatic inactivation results in a 25 $\pm$ 12 percent loss of inhibition.[103]

Peptides, Polypeptides, Glycopeptides, and Glycoproteins

Glutamic acid has been shown to be an inhibitor.[3] Selective ultrafiltration indicates that amino acids or small peptides exist in the 500–1000-dalton range that also have function.[1] The anionic homopolypeptides of aspartic acid and glutamic acid have also been shown to inhibit calcium oxalate growth in dilute human urine. Urine is sensitive to pronase digestion, and peptides appear to be responsible for some of the inhibitory action in urine.[50]

Acid polypeptides in human urine have been shown to be good in vitro inhibitors of calcium oxalate growth. Two were isolated and found to be glycoproteins; they also contained γ-carboxyglutamic acid.[73] Human kidney tissue culture medium has been shown to contain a glycoprotein that is a very potent inhibitor of COM growth. The molecular weight was 1.33×10^{4}, and it contained 73 amino acid residues. Unlike the glycoproteins isolated from urine, this one had little, if any, mannose content and also contained no γ-carboxyglutamic acid. This glycoprotein could also form dimers, trimers, and tetramers via a Ca^{2+}-dependent process that may explain the presence of several glycoproteins that were found in earlier studies.[74]

The glycoprotein inhibitor was purified from human urine and found to be highly acidic. It has a molecular weight of 1.4×10^4 and contains γ-carboxyglutamic acid. It can exist in monomeric as well as oligomeric forms. Carbohydrates are responsible for 10.3 percent of the weight, and no glucuronic acid is present.[71]

Glycoproteins were purified from rat kidney and urine and both were found to have a molecular weight of 1.4×10^4 and contained γ-carboxyglutamic acid. There was no glucuronic acid content to the glycoproteins isolated (thus ruling out the possibility that these were GAGs). They were found to be extremely potent COM growth inhibitors. The amino acid residues were similar, but the carbohydrate content different; this may have been due to an enzymatic degradation during homogenization of kidney tissue.[70]

Different glycopeptides containing glucuronic acid also appear to exhibit inhibitory properties against calcium oxalate precipitation, although they have been less well characterized. They are relatively small in size and may be degradation products from larger glycoproteins or GAGs.[54]

Other Inhibitors

At physiologic concentrations, urea has a small but significant inhibitory action.[87] Urine also has enzymes present. Urinary glutamic oxalacetic transaminase (UGOT) contributes to the production of glutamic acid, which has antiinhibitory activity against the precipitation of calcium oxalate.[3]

In 1967 two LMW substances were isolated. They were acid, heat, and cold-stable and prevented the calcification of rachitic rat cartilage. The molecules were thought to be anions because of their affinity for anion-exchange columns. They were further found to be polypeptides with common residues of aspartic acid, serine, glutamic acid, and glycine. Their molecular weights were approximately 580 and 950 daltons (D). The mechanism of action was thought to be similar to PPi, but on a molar basis it was 1000 times stronger (50 times stronger on a weight basis) than PPi. These peptides were termed *substance 1*.[47,107]

It is felt that this LMW inhibitor plays an important role in calcium phosphate inhibition.[63] Selective ultrafiltration also argues for the existence of a LMW inhibitor in calcium oxalate formation.[1] Zinc and manganese are also recognized inhibitors.[38]

PROMOTERS

Foreign substances in the urinary tract have long been known to promote the formation of calculi. While bacterial infection of the offending agent is usually involved, calculi do form in sterile urine by heterogeneous nucleation on such materials as suture, metal, and indwelling stents and catheters.[15,45,108] Heterogeneous nucleation can be caused by crystals of another composition. Sodium urate can form a nidus for calcium oxalate crystallization. Other promoters can be divided by size into molecular and macromolecular categories.

Uromucoid; Tamm-Horsfall Mucoprotein

Research in this area has concentrated on whole urine. With the use of a rotary evaporator at 37°C, fresh undiluted urine was evaporated to a standard osmolality of 1250 mosm; pH must first be adjusted to 5.3 to precipitate calcium oxalate or 6.8 to precipitate calcium phosphate crystals. If the urine is first ultrafiltered to remove molecules over 12,000 daltons (mostly uromucoid), the total crystal mass produced is significantly less than that precipitated from unfiltered urine. This was found for both calcium oxalate and calcium phosphate, with the macromolecules acting as promoters in the formation of these crystals.[42]

The fraction responsible for 90 percent of the promoter function was found to weigh (in its monomeric form) 4.17×10^7 daltons and is thought to be the Tamm-Horsfall mucoprotein (THM). Calcium phosphate crystallization from whole urine was reduced approximately 77 percent when the THM was removed by ultrafiltration. Addition of the THM back to ultrafiltered urine restored most of the promoting ability, although the crystal yield was not as large as that from unfiltered urine. The THM also caused crystal clumping, which disappeared after ultrafiltration.[91]

Tamm-Horsfall mucoprotein works better as an polymer. Sodium dodecyl sulfate (SDS) was added to a final concentration of 0.3 percent in the evaporator. The SDS caused dissociation of THM into monomers. Calcium oxalate and calcium phosphate crystal production were reduced by 64 percent and 53 percent, respectively.[89] The workers state that their findings are in agreement with Boyce's finding that fraction 1 mucoprotein from urine of recurrent stone formers binds calcium and forms an insoluble complex. Phosphate then binds to the calcium ions and forms calcium phosphate.[91] Rose and Sulaiman also note that a second promoter with a molecular weight between 100,000 and 300,000 D exists and contributes the other 10 percent in promoting crystal formation.[90]

Tamm-Horsfall mucoprotein does not appear to work by causing spontaneous nucleation. An eightfold increase in the level of saturation would be required to cause spontaneous precipitation of calcium oxalate.[53]

These is some evidence for an inhibitory function in THM. In metastable solutions incubated with seeded crystals, THM was equal in strength to chondroitin sulfates in calcium oxalate growth inhibition.[28] Kitamura and Pak reported that THM isolated from the urine of stone formers and non–stone formers inhibited crystal growth of calcium oxalate; as the concentration of THM increased, the rate of growth decreased.[53]

Matrix

Boyce discovered at least two urinary mucoproteins that were capable of binding calcium and were increased in the urines of patients with calculous disease.[12] The matrix from calcigerous calculi was found to contain a mucoprotein and a mucopolysaccharide.

It was believed that matrix was necessary for calculus formation and that the initial phase involved the condensation of the organic molecules, the deposition of crystals, and more deposition of matrix.[11] The most prominent molecule, as detected by immunological methods, from matrix is matrix substance A (MSA). Only recurrent stone formers have MSA in their urine.[13]

More recent work indicates that MSA may be partly inhibitory. Soluble fractions from calculi and macromolecular fractions from urine cause net inhibition of calcium oxalate growth. The greatest inhibition occurred in the fractions that contained GAGs; this fraction may promote aggregation.[39] The soluble fraction of MSA is a good inhibitor of growth and aggregation, but it must be remembered that the effects of the insoluble fraction depend upon the experimental system used to test it.[105]

HOW INHIBITORS WORK

Inhibitors poison the crystal surface.[9] They become adsorbed to the crystal surface at sites of defects or dislocations where growth occurs and prevent the further growth of the crystal.[107] Incomplete occupation of these sites could result in slower growth, affecting crystal morphology.[75] Ethane-1-hydroxy-1, 1-diphosphonate leads to the formation of defective crystals.[44] All of the crystalline surface does not need to be bound by inhibitors in order to prevent growth. Adsorbtion of inhibitors at growth sites may be sufficient to prevent growth; this may represent less than 1 percent of the total binding sites.[30] This adsorption prevents the further incorporation of ions in the lattice.[65] The binding of glycoprotein and other inhibitors to the crystal surface appears to be irreversible. Inorganic pyrophosphate binds strongly to hydroxyapatite.[36]

Many inhibitors, including glycoprotein, pyrophosphate, GAGs, and whole urine, work by binding to the surface according to the principles of the Langmuir theory of adsorption equilibrium.[19,65,74] Glycoprotein binds to ionic sites on the crystal surface and prevents further growth by hydrophobic properties.[71] The inhibitory effects of magnesium on COM also appear to be related to adsorption onto the crystal surface; its mode of action may be slightly different, competing for a lattice position and thereby preventing growth.[107] The fractional rate of reduction by Mg^{2+} is proportional to the fraction of the surface covered by the ion. The adsorption can be plotted on a Langmuir adsorption isotherm as well.[22]

The effectiveness of inhibitors is also charge-related. Aggregation is influenced by molecules that alter the zeta (or electrokinetic) potential of the crystal surface. The more negative the zeta potential, the better the inhibition. Polyanions are effective inhibitors.[30,97] Studies on anionic homopolypeptide inhibitors indicate a positive correlation between the length of the chain and inhibitory strength.[50] At low concentrations, only polyanionic substances exhibited inhibitory activity against calcium oxalate crystal growth.[52] Zeta potential is dependent on the relative concentrations of inhibitors, ionic strength of urine, and THM.[106]

Chondroitin sulfate is a poorer inhibitor than heparin, probably because of its decreased charge and affinity for calcium oxalate molecules.[28] The SP 54 compound increases the negative zeta potential produced on the crystal surface.[77] Metals with a high charge:diameter ratio are inhibitors.[112] Aggregation inhibition may be a function of molecules that alter the zeta potential and growth inhibition dependent on adsorption of molecules onto the growth sites.[97]

Phase Transformation

Some inhibitors may not work entirely by preventing crystallization. Calcium oxalate dihydrate is thermodynamically less stable than COM; it is difficult to form in vitro except in whole urine. It could, however, be a transition state to COM.[60] Calcium oxalate dihydrate will eventually undergo transformation to COM unless it is stabilized by a foreign ion or molecule.[82] Mixed COM–COD stones also dissolve faster as the fraction of COD contained in the stone rises.[55] Inhibitors may form COD preferentially over COM. Increasing urine pH increases the percentage of COD formed. Heparin, citrate, RNA, and PPi all increase the fraction of COD precipitated. Increasing concentrations of each compound increase the percentage of COD formed. A maximal concentration is reached by each inhibitor, after which the fraction of COD formed does not increase. This effect has not been noted with chondroitin sulfate or magnesium.[60] Similarly, PPi, EHDP, and SAT slow or inhibit the transformation of amorphous calcium phosphate into a more stable hydroxyapatite.[36]

Other factors play a role. The degree of sulfation of GAGs appears to affect their inhibitory ability.[100] Methylene blue changes crystal lattice surface dimensions. After it adsorbs to the surface, a portion of the crystal breaks off, allowing more adsorption of methylene blue; the process then starts again. It may also work by preventing crystal nucleation.[116] Citrate works in an unknown way to inhibit growth.[107]

ASPECTS OF CRYSTAL FORMATION

Hydroxyapatite growth is completely inhibited by PPi, while citrate and magnesium slow the growth rate without completely inhibiting it.[63] Citrate, PPi, diphosphonates, and GAGs (specifically heparin, hyaluronic acid, and dermatan sulfate) inhibit calcium phosphate aggregation. Calcium phosphate formation is inhibited by PPi, fluoride, zinc, magnesium, citrate, and stannous ions.[30] Heparin stimulated disaggregation at low concentrations. At concentrations of 0.1–1.0 μg/ml hyaluronic acid stimulated aggregation. At concentrations above 10 μg/ml it induced disaggregation.[29]

Diphosphonates, GAGs (especially chondroitin sulfates and heparin), and PPi inhibit aggregation of calcium oxalate crystals. Also effective in preventing crystal formation are PPi, citrate, dyes, metal ions, and various macromolecules.[36,104] Pentosan polysulfate decreases the rate of calcium oxalate crystallization, probably by growth inhibition.[61,115] It also decreases the degree of agglomeration and total amount of crystal precipitated at low concentrations.[77] At physiologic concentrations magnesium promotes growth but inhibits aggregation. At elevated concentrations it inhibits growth completely. Urine diluted to 10 percent causes disaggregation of calcium oxalate crystals in vitro. Dilution to 1 percent cancels this effect.[97] At low concentrations of RNA (a polyanion), aggregation occurs as a result of polymeric bridging. At concentrations of RNA above 5 mg/dl a denser layer forms and aggregation is prevented by steric repulsion.[16]

It was first thought that inhibitors would not be able to prevent nucleation because the rate of nucleation was so rapid that the inhibitors had little, if any, effect on the formation of new crystals.[87] More recent work seems to show that inhibitors may actually *cause* heterogeneous nucleation while inhibiting aggregation and growth. Smaller crystals would be more easily washed out of the collecting system.

With the use of a model of COD in an artificial urine, polymeric molecules were added to determine their effect on crystal precipitation, growth, and aggregation. Polyglutamic acid and heparin (both polyanions), as well as 5 percent natural urine yielded crystals of smaller size, decreased the linear growth rate, and also resulted in a lower total yield of crystals. Polylysine did not have this effect. The effect correlates with the number of carboxylic groups on the inhibiting molecule. The γ-carboxyglutamic acid residues may serve as the substrate for heterogeneous nucleation. The acidic polymers thus work at extremely low concentrations (10^{-8}–$10^{-7}M$) to enhance nucleation of smaller crystals while inhibiting the total amount of crystal precipitated. Reduction was by a factor of 3.6. The defect in stone formers may be due to an excess of inhibitory macromolecules, causing aggregation that results in calculi formation.[23] Ribonucleic acid, GAGs (including chondroitin A), and PPi all increased nucleation while inhibiting aggregation. Their relative abilities in causing this were: RNA > GAGs > PPi; this is consistent with their inhibitory potential on growth and aggregation.[82,88]

WHICH INHIBITORS ARE IMPORTANT

In whole urine, the inhibitory activity against calcium phosphate appears to be citrate, 50 percent; magnesium, 20 percent and PPi, 10 percent. The concentration of PPi is variable in urine due to the presence of pyrophosphatases.[30,100] It may be most important near sites of its production where elevated concentrations are possible. Its effect is primarily on calcium phosphate and not calcium oxalate. Glycosaminoglycans also inhibit hydroxyapatite crystal aggregation; in descending order of inhibitory potential they are: heparin > hyaluronic acid > dermatan > chondroitin A > chondroitin C.[29]

The contribution by PPi could be more significant than is generally believed. With the use of a constant composition technique, PPi has the least change in activity against hydroxyapatite. The effect of citrate increases with a decrease in pH, while magnesium activity has just the opposite reaction.[123]

There is insufficient chromic ion in urine to alter hydroxyapatite stone formation. Ferric and Al(III) ions are present in sufficient quantities to complex with citrate, although their role in inhibition is uncertain.[112]

In calcium oxalate crystallization, GAGs, RNA, and acidic glycoproteins are the main inhibitors of crystallization. Nancollas and coworkers note that over 76 percent of the inhibitory activity is between 10,000 and 50,000 daltons.[55] When urine was applied to a Sephadex G-200 column, the maximal inhibitory activity (for molecules >10,000 daltons) against growth, as measured in a seeded crystal system, correlated with the peaks of chondroitin sulfate and ABPP. There was also activity associated with a LMW unknown but considered possibly to be glycoproteins.[27] Ribonucleic acid, citrate, and acidic glycoprotein inhibit growth.[106] Glycosaminoglycans are primarily an inhibitor of aggregation. Ryall and Marshall believe that since urine is a better inhibitor of aggregation than of growth, the primary inhibitors in urine are GAGs.[96]

The relative strength needed for 50 percent reduction on calcium oxalate crystal growth is: RNA > heparin > chondroitin S and (SP 54) > PPi > THM. Calcium oxalate aggregation inhibitors are: RNA > GAGs > THM > PPi.[61,82] When activity was measured at concentrations likely to be found in 1 percent urine, heparin was 25 times more potent than chondroitin sulfate at inhibiting aggregation and 2000 times more potent at inhibiting growth.[93] Other data suggest a decreased importance of heparin. Heparin was the most effective GAG in inhibiting growth; chondroitin A had 16 percent the activity of heparin; chondroitin C, 19 percent, SP 54, 40 percent PPi, 70 percent and THM, 17 percent.[28]

Coe and coworkers believe that their acidic glycoprotein is responsible for 90 percent of the growth inhibition of calcium oxalate in urine.[71,74] It is as powerful as RNA in achieving 50 percent in calcium oxalate growth, yet it is present in 100 times this concentration.[71,74]

In a metastable seeded crystal system, magnesium, citrate, and PPi did little to inhibit the growth and aggregation of calcium oxalate, although they were effective for calcium phosphate.[65] Both PPi and citrate exert a small effect on calcium oxalate in concentrations found. The effects of PPi (and EHDP) are pH-dependent and improve with an alkaline pH.[30] Chondroitin sulfate is about 100 times as powerful, and heparin is approximately 1000 times as powerful as PPi and EHDP in inhibition of calcium oxalate growth.[121]

Chondroitin sulfates are responsible for the major inhibitory effect on calcium oxalate seen in 1 percent urine; it inhibits aggregation better than growth.[93] Whole urine was found to be very strong, with a 1:62 dilution resulting in a 50 percent reduction in the calcium oxalate growth rate.[65] Work in the continuous crystallizer system approximating the conditions in whole urine has shown that at normal concentrations, citrate and chondroitin A are weak inhibitors of calcium oxalate growth and agglomeration.[88]

The role of magnesium in inhibition of calcium oxalate crystallization is unknown. Depending on its concentration, it can either promote or inhibit growth. At physiologic concentrations it promotes growth but inhibits aggregation.[97] In a continuous crystallizer magnesium had weak inhibition of growth and no effect on agglomeration.[88]

DO STONE FORMERS HAVE LESS INHIBITORY ABILITY IN THEIR URINE?

In the quest for solutions to why idiopathic stone formers form stones, one of the major areas where researchers turned has been inhibitors. Is there any differentiating characteristic in the inhibitors (and promoters) in the urine of healthy individuals who have compared to stone formers? The answer is not a simple yes or no. It depends on the test system used, dilute versus whole urine, artificial versus natural urine, crystal composition and morphology, and other factors.

The early work of Boyce and his fellow workers explained stone formation by the presence of MSA in calculi and in the urine of recurrent stone formers.[13] Matrix substance A is a complex and heterogeneous mixture of macromolecules that probably promote and inhibit stone formation.

In seeded crystal metastable solutions, 1 percent urine from stone formers was significantly poorer at inhibiting the aggregation and growth of calcium oxalate when compared to urine from controls. The explanation was that stone formers had less inhibitory material in their urine.[84,85] Citrate excretion has been found to be lower in recurrent calcium stone formers when compared to controls.[104] Male stone formers were noted to have a reduction in the excretion of PPi with a concomitant decrease in their ability to inhibit calcium phosphate precipitation. This may have been age related, occurring after the fourth decade; however, there was no difference between stone formers and healthy individuals in the inhibition of calcium oxalate aggregation.[5] Using a more sensitive technique, Ligabue et al. Found the inhibitory activity of urine from 12 recurrent calcium oxalate stone formers to be significantly lower than age-matched controls.[58]

Kitamura et al. characterized the molecular material in the urine of stone formers and non–stone formers.[54] There were three main classes. The large material consisted of uromucoid; this was found in both groups, although stone formers had more uromucoid. Glycosaminoglycans of large and medium size were found in both groups as well. The small material, believed to be glycoproteins, were present in more quantity in the healthy group. While the large material from the stone formers group had no inhibitory activity, all the other molecules inhibited the precipitation of calcium oxalate. Inhibition was found to increase in inverse proportion to the size of the molecule. The total inhibitory activity for stone formers was 36 percent less than that for the non–stone formers.

Others confirm these findings; using the discriminating index and studying different fractions, Azoury et al. found that stone formers have inhibitors that are absent or inactivated above 10,000 daltons.[2] Removal of this fraction from normal urine significantly decreases its inhibitory potential.[2] There may be a qualitative difference in the GAGs, with GAGs from recurrent stone formers causing more in vitro aggregation than GAGs from single stone formers.[49]

One study using a continuous crystallizer revealed that stone formers had no decrease in their daily excretion of PPi, magnesium, or citrate. Alcian blue precipitatable proteins, GAGs, THM, and RNA were all found to be significantly decreased. Protection from calcium oxalate appeared to be from these macromolecular inhibitors, and they were all decreased.[82]

Ryall and Marshall found that there was no difference between the urine of stone formers and non–stone formers in the ability to inhibit calcium oxalate growth and aggregation in seeded crystal systems.[96] There was no difference in the total daily excretion of GAGs during a 24-hour collection. Among individuals (stone and non–stone formers), however, there was a significant relationship between concentrations of GAGs, uric acid, creatinine, and osmolality in inhibitory capability.[98] This suggests a dilutional factor may be playing a role. In comparing the GAG excretion among patients of different stone composition, only patients with struvite stones had decreased GAG excretion when compared to controls.[6]

Using whole urine and testing its ability to withstand increasing concentrations of oxalate before undergoing spontaneous nucleation, the urine from stone formers had lower metastable limits. The concentration of GAGs were found to be significantly lower, however, as were the concentrations of oxalate, calcium, and urate. The stone formers all had higher urine volumes than did the controls. The total output of inhibitors was not different, but the concentrations were lower as a result of the increased volume. This lowered the metastable limit, thus rendering the urine more likely to undergo spontaneous nucleation.[95]

Urate

Sodium urate can act as a heterogeneous nucleator for calcium oxalate. Its effect is dependent on the saturation of calcium oxalate. In highly supersaturated and highly metastable solutions it had no effect. Only in low metastable solutions did high concentrations of urate crystals promote crystallization.[114] The problem is that the formation product of urate is never exceeded in urine, and that sodium and urate must be excreted in concentrations unobtainable in urine.[62,83] The inhibition of crystallization by acid mucopolysaccharides is dependent on the concentration of urate; the higher the concentration of urate, the less effective the inhibition. Therefore, while urate has the possibility to work as a nucleator, it is more likely that it binds the inhibitor modulating its ability to work.[81,114]

Urate has been shown to bind radioactive heparin.[79] The effect is potentiated by calcium and magnesium ions.[26] Preincubation of heparin with crystalline sodium urate decreases the ability of heparin to increase the formation product ratio of calcium oxalate. The effects of heparin could be entirely inhibited.[79] In a seeded metastable crystal system, colloidal urate decreased the inhibition of aggregation and growth by heparin.[94]

The interaction between chondroitin sulfates and urate is not as clear. Some feel that chondroitin sulfate is bound to urate, but with less affinity.[26] Others note no binding between urate and chondroitin A.[62] Pak and coworkers report that urate does not decrease the inhibition caused by chondroitin sulfate.[79] More recent work has shown that urate decreases the inhibition of aggregation caused by chondroitin sulfate, but not the inhibition of growth. Urine was noted to have a similar outcome in the metastable system; urate attenuated the inhibition of aggregation, but the results with growth rates were inconclusive.[94]

Uric Acid

Colloidal uric acid appeared to have little effect in modifying nucleation of crystals.[4,114] Uric acid does not bind heparin or chondroitin sulfates.[26] No difference has been noted between stone formers and non–stone formers in terms of the concentration of uric acid or the 24-hour excretion of GAGs and uric acid.[96,98] Using the discriminating index, Godwasser et al. found that uric acid does not appear to be a factor in idiopathic calcium oxalate calculi formation.[41]

Crystal Size

Robertson, et al. noted that at low pH, warm fresh urine maintained at 37°C resulted in the crystallization of calcium oxalate.[86] At a pH of over 6.2, amorphous calcium phosphate and occasional calcium oxalate formed. This occurred in urine from both recurrent stone formers and healthy individuals. At the low pH, the crystals from the stone formers were larger in individual volume and a greater volume of crystals per volume of urine was formed. Robertson and coworkers felt aggregation was responsible for part of this observation as no aggregation occurred in urine from non–stone formers. This effect was not seen at the higher pH. They were unsure as to whether the effect was due to $[Ca^{2+}]$ $[\text{oxalate}^{2-}]$, or inhibitors.

Crystalluria is not common in the urine of healthy individuals and nonrecurrent stone formers. Urine from these individuals contains crystals of approximately 6-μm diameter. Recurrent stone formers pass crystals more often, and their crystals are larger in size and tend to aggregate. There is a bimodal distribution in crystal size; the first peak is at the same size as crystals in healthy urine, while the second peak is over 12.2 μm. Calcium oxalate crystals in metastable solutions are known to increase in size with time; larger aggregates form as well.[87]

COM and COD

Calcium oxalate monohydrate crystalluria is significantly more likely to occur in stone formers than in non–stone formers.[95] Urine from stone formers also retards the growth of COM to a lesser extent than does healthy urine.[52]

Molecular Abnormality

There is evidence for a molecular abnormality in inhibitors. Nakagawa et al. found that glycoprotein from stone formers contained no γ-carboxyglutamic acid.[72] Also two of the four subgroups of glycoprotein were less active (4 and 20 times) than glycoprotein from normal individuals in inhibition of calcium oxalate growth by use of a metastable seeded crystal system. Also, the surface properties of the defective molecules were different with a film collapse pressure of glycoprotein from stone formers one-half from healthy urine.

LMW Modulators

Another example of modulation may be seen with LMW substances. Calcium oxalate and carbon were used to adsorb a synthetic inhibitor (ethylene–diamine–tetramethylene–phosphonic acid) and naturally occurring polyanionic inhibitors. This adsorption reduced the strength of the inhibitors; however, this occurred only when LMW molecules were first removed by dialysis. This suggests that the LMW molecules have a protective effect for the macromolecular inhibitors, preventing them from being adsorbed onto surfaces and being rendered inactive.[120]

LOCATIONAL CONSIDERATIONS

It has recently been shown that voided urine may not be representative of the GAG content of urine at the level of the kidney. Transitional epithelial cells of the bladder secrete GAG. It has been shown to protect against the adherence of bacteria, calcium, and protein.[80] Saline washout of the bladders of patients undergoing cystoscopy has been found to have a much greater inhibitory effect on calcium oxalate growth and aggregation (in a seeded crystal system) than urine diluted to the same creatinine concentration.[24] No GAG was detected in the bladder washout, however; the saline was in contact with the bladder mucosa for only 30 seconds, and hence GAG, if present, may have been in too low a concentration to be detected.,[25]

Canine urine was evaluated before and 10 days after bilateral ureterostomies were performed. Inhibitory activity of calcium oxalate growth was significantly increased as urine progressed from the kidney to the bladder. There was also a significant increase in the amount of ABPP in bladder urine. The material could be RNA, GAGs, and/or glycoprotein; therefore, the LMW inhibitors may be more important in protecting the kidney tubule (where they are excreted) than first believed.[59]

CONCLUSIONS

Investigations on promoters and inhibitors have increased our understanding in the pathogenesis and pathophysiology of calculus formation. It has led to the institution of effective medical therapies, as well as the synthesis of new agents possibly helpful in the prevention of stone recurrence. Most of the work has centered on calcium phosphate and calcium oxalate. Much of the work has been carried out in systems that do not mimic in vivo conditions very well. Further research needs to be continued to better understand lithogenic mechanisms and also to involve work on stones of other composition(s).

REFERENCES

1. Azoury R, Goldwasser B, Perlberg S, et al: The relative inhibitory potential of urinary macromolecular fractions on calcium oxalate precipitation, in Schwille PO, Smith LH, Robertson WG, et al (eds): Urolithiasis and Related Clinical Research. New York, Plenum Press, 1985, pp 839–842
2. Azoury R, Goldwasser B, Wax Y, et al: Evaluation of the relative inhibitory potential of fractionated urinary macromolecules. Urol Res 13:199–205, 1985
3. Azoury R, Sarig S, Garti N, et al: Retardation of calcium oxalate precipitation by glutamic-oxalacetic-transaminase activity. Urol Res 10:169–172, 1982
4. Baggio B, Bambaro G, Cicerello E, et al: Further studies on the possible lithogenic role of uric acid in calcium oxalate stone disease, in Schwille PO, Smith LH, Robertson WG, et al (eds): Urolithiasis and Related Clinical Research. New York Plenum Press, 1985, pp 863–866
5. Baumann JM, Bisaz S, Felix F, et al: The role of inhibitors and other factors in the pathogenesis of recurrent calcium-containing renal stones. Clin Sci Molec Med, 53:141–148, 1977
6. Bichler K-H, Sallis J, Bröring S: Observations on urinary glycosaminoglycan concentration in relation to the type of calculus and its tissue location, and to tissue tumors, in Brockis JG, Finlaysons B (eds): Urinary Calculus. Littleton, MA: PSG Publishing, 1981, pp 335–340
7. Bone HG III, Zerwekh JE, Britton F, et al: Treatment of calcium urolithiasis with diphosphonate: Efficacy and hazards. J Urol, 121(5):568–571, 1979
8. Borden TA, Lyon ES: The effect of magnesium and pH on experimental calcium oxalate stone disease. Invest Urol, 6(4):412–422, 1969
9. Bowyer RC, Brockis JG, McCulloch RK: Glycosaminoglycans as inhibitors of calcium oxalate crystal growth and aggregation. Clinica Chimica Acta, 95:23–28, 1975
10. Bowyer RC, Brockis JG, McCulloch RK: The role of glycosaminoglycans in the inhibition of calcium oxalate crystal growth and aggregation in urine, in Brockis JG, Finlaysons (eds): Urinary Calculus. Littleton, MA: PSG Publishing, 1981, pp 329–334
11. Boyce WH, Garvey FK: The amount and nature of organic matrix in urinary calculi: A review. J Urol, 76(3):213–227, 1956
12. Boyce WH, Garvey FK, Norfleet CM: Ion-binding properties of electrophoretically homogeneous mucoproteins of urine in normal subjects and in patients with renal calculus disease. J Urol, 72(6):1019–1034, 1954
13. Boyce WH, King JS Jr, Fielden ML: Total nondialyzable solids (TNDS) in human urine. XIII. Immunological detection of a complnent peculiar to renal calculous matrix and to urine of calculous patients. J Clin Invest, 41(5):1180–1189, 1961
14. Boyce WC, McKinney WM, Long TT, et al: Oral administration of methylene blue to patients with renal calculi. J Urol 97(5):783–789, 1967
15. Brenner M, Johnson DE: Ileal conduit calculi from stapler anastomosis: A long-term complication? Urology, 26(6):537–540, 1985
16. Brown CM, Senior P, Charest H, et al: Adsorption of RNA onto aged calcium oxalate monohydrate (COM), in Schwille PO, Smith LH, Robertson WG, et al (eds): Urolithiasis and Related Clinical Research. New York, Plenum Press, 9185, pp 843–846
17. Brown MR, Sallis JD: The synthesis and characterization of *N*-sulfo-2-amino tricarballylate: An analogue of phosphocitrate and inhibitor of calcification. Anal Biochem 132:115–123, 1983
18. Brown MR, Sallis JD: *N*-sulfo-2-amino tricarballylate. A new analogue of phosphocitrate: Metabolism and inhibitory effects on renal calcification, in Schwille PO, Smith LH, Robertson WG, et al (eds): Urolithiasis and Related Clinical Research New York, Plenum Press, 1985, pp 891–894
19. Brunauer S, Copeland LE, Kantro DL: The Langmuir and BET theories, in Flood EA (ed): The Solid–Gas Interface, Vol 1. New York, Marcel Dekker, 1967, Chapter 3, pp 77–103

20. Butt AJ: Role of protective urinary colloids in prevention of renal lithiasis. J Urol, 69(4):450–459, 1952
21. Croft K, Adair JH, Bowyer R, et al: An evaluation of tamarind and tartaric acid as inhibitors of calcium oxalate crystallisation in urine, in Ryall R, Brockis JG, Marshall V, et al (eds): Urinary Stone. Melbourne, Churchill Livingstone, 1984, pp 189–197
22. Desmus JF, Tawashi R: Dissolution and growth of calcium oxalate monohydrate. I. Effect of magnesium and pH. Biochimica et Biophysica Acta 313:256–267, 1973
23. Drach GW, Sarig S, Randolph AD, et al: The paradox of inhibition and enhancement of the formation of urinary stones. Urol Res 10:165–168, 1982
24. Edyvane KA, Ryall RL, Marshall VR: Does the bladder mucosa contribute to urinary inhibitory activity? in Schwille PO, Smith LH, Robertson WG, et al (eds): Urolithiasis and Related Clinical Research. New York, Plenum Press, 1985, pp 867–870
25. Edyvane KA, Ryall RL, Marshall VR: The effects of saline bladder washings on calcium oxalate crystal growth and aggregation. J Urol, 134(1):158–161, 1985
26. Fellström B, Danielson BG, Karlsson FA, et al: Crystal inhibition: Binding of heparin and chondroitin sulfate of calcium oxalate, sodium urate, and uric acid crystals in Schwille PO, Smith LH, Robertson WG, et al (eds): Urolithiasis and Related Clinical Research. New York, Plenum Press, 1985, pp 831–834
27. Fellström B, Danielson BG, Ljunghall S, et al: Gel filtration of concentrated urine: The relation between calcium oxalate crystal growth inhibition and glycosaminoglycan chromatograms, in Schwille PO, Smith LH, Robertson WG, et al (eds): Urolithiasis and Related Clinical Research. New York, Plenum Press, 1985, pp 823–826
28. Fellström B, Danielson BG, Ljunghall S, et al: The inhibition of calcium oxalate crystal growth by chondroitin sulphates, heparin, pentosan polysulphate and Tamm-Horsfall glycoprotein, in Schwille PO, Smith LH, Robertson WG, et al (eds): Urolithiasis and Related Clinical Research. New York, Plenum Press, 1985, pp 887–890
29. Felix R, Bisaz S, Hansen NM, et al: Aggregation and disaggregation of hydroxyapatite crystals, in Fleisch H, Robertson WG, Smith LH, et al (eds): Urolithiasis Research. New York, Plenum Press, 1976, pp 265–268
30. Fleisch H: Inhibitors and promoters of stone formation. Kidney Internatl, 13:361–371, 1978
31. Fleisch H: Round table discussion on the comparison of models for the study of inhibitory activity in urine, in Schwille PO, Smith LH, Robertson WG, et al (eds): Urolithiasis and Related Clinical Research. New York, Plenum Press, 1985, pp 903–908
32. Fleisch H, Bisaz S: Isolation from urine of pyrophosphate, a calcification inhibitor. Am J Physiol, 203:671–675, 1962
33. Fleisch H, Bisaz S: The inhibitory effect of pyrophosphate on calcium oxalate precipitation and its relation to urolithiasis. Experientia, 20(5):276–277, 1964
34. Fleisch H, Bisaz S, Care AD: Effect of orthophosphate on urinary pyrophosphate excretion and the prevention of urolithiasis. Lancet 1:1065–1067, 1964
35. Fleisch H Bisaz S, Russell RGG: Influence of pyrophosphate on the crystallisation of uric acid and magnesium ammonium phosphate and its implications in phosphate therapy for urolithiasis. Urologica Internationalis, 22:483–491, 1967
36. Fleisch H, Russell RGG: Inhibitors in urinary stone disease: Role of diphosphonates, in Cifuentes Delatte L, Rapado A, Hodgkinson A (eds): Urinary Calculi, Recent Advances ;in Aetiology, Stone Structure, and Treatment. Basel, S Karger, 1973, pp 296–301
37. Fraser D, Russell RGG, Pohler O, et al: The influence of disodium ethane-1-hydroxy-1, 1-diphosphonate (EHDP) on the development of experimentally induced urinary stones in rats. Clin Sci, 42:197–207, 1972
38. Gill WB, Karesh JW, Garsin L, et al: Inhibitory effects of urinary macromolecules on the crystallization of calcium oxalate. Invest Urol, 15(2):95–99, 1977
39. Gjaldbaek JC, Robertson WG: Does urine from stone-formers contain macromolecules

which promote the crystal growth rate of calcium oxalate crystals in vitro? Clinica Chimica Acta, 108:75–80, 1980
40. Goldberg JM, Cotlier E: Specific isolation and analysis of mucopolysaccharides (glycosaminoglycans) from human urine. Clinica Chimica Acta, 41:19–27, 1972
41. Goldwasser B, Sarig S, Azoury R, et al: Hyperuricosuria and calcium oxalate stone formation, in Schwille PO, Smith LH, Robertson WG, et al (eds): Urolithiasis and Related Clinical Research. New York, Plenum Press, 1985, pp 859–862
42. Hallson PC, Rose GA: Uromucoids and urinary stone formation. Lancet, 1:1000–1002, 1979
43. Hallson PC, Rose GA: The additive effects of magnesium and tartrate upon inhibition of calcium oxalate crystal formation in whole urine, in Schwille PO, Smith LH, Robertson WG, et al (eds): Urolithiasis and Related Clinical Research. New York, Plenum Press, 1985, pp 847–850
44. Hallson PC, Rose GA, Samuell CT: Inhibitors of calcium oxalate and calcium phosphate crystal formation in urine—a critique and reappraisal, in Smith LH, Robertson WG, Finlayson B (eds): Urolithiasis, Clinical and Basic Research. New York, Plenum Press, 1981, pp 589–599
45. Hedelin H, Eddelin A, Larsson L, et al: The composition of catheter encrustations, including the effects of allopurinol treatment. Br J Urol, 56(3):250–254, 1984
46. Howard JE: Studies on urinary stone formation: A saga of clinical investigation. Johns Hopkins Medical Bull, 139:239–252, 1976
47. Howard JE, Thomas WC Jr, Barker, LM, Smith LH, et al: The recognition and isolation from urine and serum of a peptide inhibitor to calcification. Johns Hopkins Med Bull, 120:119–136, 1967
48. Howard JE, Thomas WC Jr, Mukai T, et al: The calcification of cartilate by urine, and a suggestion for therapy in patients with certain kinds of calculi. Trans Assoc Am Physicians, 75:301–306, 1962
49. Itatani H, Koide T, Sonoda T: Calcium oxalate crystal aggregation study in an experimental model and human, in Ryall R, Brockis JG, Marshall V, et al (eds): Urinary Stone. Melbourne, Churchill Livingstone, 1984, pp 207–211
50. Ito H, Coe FL: Acidic peptide and polyribonucleotide crystal growth inhibitors in human urine. Am J Physiol, 233:F455–463, 1977
51. Joly JS: Stone and Calculous Disease of the Urinary Organs. St. Louis, CV Mosby, 1931
52. Joost J, Lusser M, Kleboth K: Calcium oxalate crystal growth: Investigations on inhibitory activity of model compounds and urine samples, in Schwille PO, Smith LH, Robertson WG, et al (eds): Urolithiasis and Related Clinical Research. New York, Plenum Press, 1985, pp 851–854
53. Kitamura T, Pak CYC: Tamm and Horsfall glycoprotein does not promote spontaneous precipitation and crystal growth of calcium oxalate in vitro. J Urol, 127(5):1024–1026, 1982
54. Kitamura T, Zerwekh JE, Pak CYC: Partial biochemical and physicochemical characterization of organic macromolecules in urine from patients with renal stones and control subjects. Kidney Internatl, 21:379–386, 1982
55. Lanzalco A, Coyle M, Gaur S, et al: Natural inhibitors of formation and dissolution of stone minerals, in Schwille PO, Smith LH, Robertson WG, et al (eds): Urolithiasis and Related Clinical Research. New York, Plenum Press, 1985, pp 815–818
56. Li MK, Blacklock NJ, Garside J: Effects of magnesium on calcium oxalate crystallization. J Urol, 133(1):123–125, 1985
57. Lichtwitz L: Über die bildung von niederschlägen un konkrementen im harn und in den harnwegen, in Spezielle Pathogie und Therapie Innerer Krankheiten, Kraus and Brugsh, Vol I, 1919, quoted in Joly JS: Stone and Calculous Disease of the Urinary Organs. St Louis, CV Mosby, 1931
58. Ligabue A, Fini M, Robertson WG: Influence of urine on "in vitro" crystallization rate of

calcium oxalate: Determination of inhibitory activity by a [^{14}C] oxalate technique. Clinica Chimica Acta, 98:39–46, 1979

59. Martin X, Opgenorth TJ, Werness PG, et al: Bladder secretion of inhibitors of calcium oxalate crystal growth. Kidney Internatl, 28:636–639, 1985
60. Martin X, Smith LH, Werness PG: Effect of additives and whole urine on calcium oxalate dihydrate formation, in Schwille PO, Smith LH, Robertson WG, et al (eds): Urolithiasis and Related Clinical Research. New York, Plenum Press, 1985, pp 827–830
61. Martin X, Werness PG, Bergert JH, et al: Pentosan polysulfate as an inhibitor of calcium oxalate crystal growth. J Urol, 132(4):786–788, 1984
62. McCulloch RK, Bowyer RC, Brockis JG: Possible roles of urate in calcium urolithiasis, in Brockis JG, Finlaysons B (eds): Urinary Calculus. Littleton, MA, PSG Publishing, 1981, pp 347–352
63. Meyer JL: The relative importance of calcium phosphate urinary inhibitors, in Schwille PO, Smith LH, Robertson WG, et al (eds): Urolithiasis and Related Clinical Research. New York, Plenum Press, 1985, pp 811–814
64. Meyer JL, Smith LH: Growth of calcium oxalate crystals. I. A model for urinary stone growth. Invest Urol, 13(1):33–35, 1975
65. Meyer JL, Smith LH: Growth of calcium oxalate crystals. II. Inhibition by natural urinary growth inhibitors. Invest Urol, 13(1):36–39, 1975
66. Meyer JL, Thomas WC Jr: Trace metal–citric acid complexes as inhibitors of calcifications and crystal growth. I. Effects of Fe(III), Cr(III), and Al(III) complexes on calcium phosphate crystal growth. J Urol, 128(6):1372–1375, 1982
67. Meyer JL, Thomas WC Jr: Trace metal–citric acid complexes as inhibitors of calcifications and crystal growth. II. Effects of Fe(III), Cr(III), and Al(III) complexes on calcium oxalate crystal growth. J Urol, 128(6):1376–1378, 1982
68. Miller JD, Randolph AD, Drach GW: Observations upon calcium oxalate crystallization kinetics in simulated urine. J Urol, 177(3):342–345, 1977
69. Murata K: Acidic glycosaminoglycans in human kidney tissue. Clinica Chimica Acta, 63:157–169, 1975
70. Nakagawa Y, Abram Y, Coe FL: Isolation of calcium oxalate crystal growth inhibitor from rat kidney and urine. Am J Physiol, 247(5, Pt 2):F765–772, 1984
71. Nakagawa Y, Abram V, Kézdy FJ, et al: Purification and characterization of the principle inhibitor of calcium oxalate monohydrate crystal growth in human urine. J Biol Chem, 258(20):12594–12600, 1983
72. Nakagawa Y, Abram V, Parks JH, et al: Urine glycoprotein crystal growth inhibitors. Evidence for a molecular abnormality in calcium oxalate nephrolithiasis. J Clin Invest, 76(4):1455–1462, 1985
73. Nakagawa Y, Kaiser ET, Coe FL: Isolation and characterization of calcium oxalate crystal growth inhibitors from human urine. Biochem Biophys Res Commun, 84(4):1038–1044, 1978
74. Nakagawa Y, Margolis HC, Yokoyama S, et al: Purification and characterization of a calcium oxalate monohydrate crystal growth inhibitor from human kidney tissue culture medium. J Biol Chem, 256(8):3936–3944, 1981
75. Nancollas GH: The kinetics of crystal growth and renal stone-formation, in Fleisch H, Robertson WG, Smith LH, et al (eds): Urolithiasis Research. New York, Plenum Press, 1976, pp 5–23
76. Nishio S, Abe, Y, Wakatsuki A, et al: Matrix glycosaminoglycans in urinary stones. J Urol, 134(3):503–504, 1985
77. Norman RW, Scurr DS, Robertson WG, et al: Inhibition of calcium oxalate crystallisation by pentosan polysulphate in control subjects and stone formers. Br J Urol, 56:594–598, 1984
78. Pak CYC, Eanes ED, Ruskin B: Spontaneous precipitation of brushite in urine: Evidence that

brushite is the nidus of renal stones originating as calcium phosphate. Proc Natl Acad Sci, 68(7):1456–1460, 1971

79. Pak CYC, Holt K, Zerwekh JE: Attenuation by monosodium urate of the inhibitory effect of glycosaminoglycans on calcium oxalate nucleation. Invest Urol, 17(2):138–140, 1979
80. Parsons CL, Stauffer C, Schmidt JD: Bladder-surface glycosaminoglycans: An efficient mechanism of environmental adaption. Science, 208(9):605–607, 1980
81. Robertson WG, Knowles F, Peacock M: Urinary acid mucopolysaccharide inhibitors of calcium oxalate crystallisation, in Fleisch H, Robertson WG, Smith LH, et al (eds): Urolithiasis Research. New York, Plenum Press, 1976, pp 331–334
82. Robertson WG, Latif AB, Scurr, DS, et al: Inhibitors of calcium oxalate crystallization in urine from stone-formers and normals, in Ryall R, Brockis JG, Marshall V, et al (eds): Urinary Stone. Melbourne, Churchill Livingstone, 1984, pp 167–172
83. Robertson WG, Marshall RW, Peacock M, et al: The saturation of urine in recurrent idiopathic calcium stone formers, in Fleisch H, Robertson WG, Smith LH, et al (eds): Urolithiasis Research. New York, Plenum Press, 1976, pp 335–338
84. Robertson WG, Peacock M: Calcium oxalate crystalluria and inhibitors of crystallization in recurrent renal stone-formers. Clin Sci, 43:499–506, 1972
85. Robertson WG, Peacock M, Knowles CF: Calcium oxalate crystalluria and inhibitors of crystallisation in recurrent renal stone formers, in Cifuentes Delatte L, Rapado A, Hodgkinson A (eds): Urinary Calculi, Recent Advances in Aetiology, Stone Structure, and Treatment. Basel, S Karger, 1973, pp 302–306
86. Robertson WG, Peacock M, Nordin BEC: Calcium crystalluria in recurrent renal stone-formers. Lancet, 2:21–24, 1969
87. Robertson WG, Peacock M, Nordin BEC: Inhibitors of the growth and aggregation of calcium oxalate crystals. Clinica Chimica Acta, 43:31–37, 1973
88. Robertson WG, Scurr DS: Modifiers of calcium oxalate crystallization found in urine. I. Studies with a continuous crystallizer using an artificial urine. J Urol, 135(6):1322–1326, 1986
89. Rose GA, Sulaiman S: Effect of macromolecules and of sodium dodecyl sulphate upon precipitation of calcium oxalate and phosphate from whole urine. Urologica Internationalis, 39:68–72, 1984
90. Rose GA, Sulaiman S: Effect of different fractions of macromolecules upon triggering of calcium oxalate and calcium phosphate crystal formation in whole urine. Urologica Internationalis, 39:147–149, 1984
91. Rose GA, Sulaiman S: Tamm-Horsfall mucoprotein promotes calcium phosphate crystal formation in whole urine: Quantitative studies. Urol Res, 12:217–221, 1984
92. Rose GA, Sulaiman S: Macromolecules in whole urine that promote calcium oxalate and phosphate crystal formation, in Schwille PO, Smith LH, Robertson WG, et al (eds): Urolithiasis and Related Clinical Research. New York, Plenum Press, 1985, pp 883–886
93. Ryall RL, Harnett RM, Marshall VR: The effect of urine, pyrophosphate, citrate, magnesium, and glycosaminoglycans on the growth and aggregation of calcium oxalate crystals *in vitro*. Cinica Chimica Acta, 112:349–356, 1981
94. Ryall RL, Harnett RM, Marshall VR: The effect of monosodium urate on the capacity of urine, chondroitin sulphate, and heparin to inhibit calcium oxalate crystal growth and aggregation. J Urol, 135(1):174–177, 1986
95. Ryall RL, Hibberd CM, Mazzachi BC, et al: Inhibitory activity of whole urine: A comparison of urines from stone formers and healthy subjects. Clinica Chimica Acta, 154:59–68, 1986
96. Ryall RL, Marshall VR: The effect of normal and stone-forming urine on the growth and aggregation of calcium oxalate crystals in relation to urinary glycosaminoglycan and urate concentrations, in Smith LH, Robertson WG, Finlayson B (eds): urolithiasis, Clinical and Basic Research. New York, Plenum Press, 1981, pp 611–618
97. Ryall RL, Marshall VR: The effect of urine and other inhibitors on the growth and aggrega-

tion of calcium oxalate crystals in vitro, in Smith LH, Robertson WG, Finlayson B (eds): Urolithiasis, Clinical and Basic Research. New York, Plenum Press, 1981, pp 631–635

98. Ryall RL, Marshall VR: The relationship between urinary inhibitory activity and endogenous concentrations of glycosaminoglycans and uric acid: Comparison of urines from stone-formers and normal subjects. Clinica Chimica Acta, 141:197–204, 1984
99. Ryall RL, Ryall RG, Marshall VR: The interpretation of the effects of urinary inhibitors on the growth and aggregation of calcium oxalate crystals, in Ryall R, Brockis JG, Marshall V, et al (eds): Urinary Stone. Melbourne, Churchill Livingstone, 1984, pp 178–184
100. Sallis JD: Inhibitors of the precipitation of stone-forming urinary constituents: Are the established inhibitors effective in preventing stone formation and growth or is a moss-covered stone inevitable? in Schwille PO, Smith LH, Robertson WG, et al (eds): Urolithiasis and Related Clinical Research. New York, Plenum Press, 1985, pp 803–809
101. Sallis JD, Lumley MF: On the possible role of glycosaminoglycans as natural inhibitors of calcium oxalate stone. Invest Urol, 16 (4):296–299, 1979
102. Sarig S, Garti N, Azoury R, et al: A method for discrimination between calcium oxalate kidney stone formers and normals. J Urol, 128(3):645–649, 1982
103. Schrier EE, Rubin JL, Lee KE, et al: Characterization of the calcium oxalate crystal growth inhibitors in human urine, in Smith LH, Robertson WG, Finlayson B (eds): Urolithiasis, Clinical and Basic Research. New York, Plenum Press, 1981, pp 579–588
104. Schwille PO, Scholz D, Paulus M, et al: Citrate in daily and fasting urine. Results of controls, patients with recurrent idiopathic calcium urolithiasis and primary hyperparathyroidism. Invest Urol, 16(6):457–462, 1979
105. Scurr DS, Bridge CM, Robertson WG: Studies on inhibitors and promoters of the crystallization of calcium oxalate in urine and in matrix from calcium oxalate stones, in Smith LH, Robertson WG, Finlayson B (eds): Urolithiasis, Clinical and Basic Research. New York, Plenum Press, 1981, pp 601–605
106. Scurr DS, Robertson WG: Studies on the mode of action of polyanionic inhibitors of calcium oxalate crystallization in urine, in Schwill PO, Smith LH, Robertson WG, et al (eds): Urolithiasis and Related Clinical Research. New York, Plenum Press, 1985, pp 835–838
107. Smith LH, Meyer JL, McCall JT: Chemical nature of crystal inhibitors isolated from human urine, in Cifuentes Delatte L, Rapado A, Hodgkinson A (eds): Urinary Calculi, Recent Advances in Aetiology, Stone Structure, and Treatment. Basel, S Karger, 1973, pp 318–327
108. Spirnak JP, Resnick MI: Stone formation as a complication of indwelling ureteral stents: A report of 5 cases. J Urol, 134(2):349–351, 1985
109. Tawashi R, Cousineau M, Denis G: Crystallisation of calcium oxalate dihydrate in normal urine in presence of sodium copper chlorophylline. Urol Res, 10:173–176, 1982
110. Tew WP, Mahle C, Benavides J, et al: Synthesis and charcterization of phosphocitric acid, a potent inhibitor of hydroxylapatite crystal growth. Biochemistry, 19:1983–1988, 1980
111. Tew WP, Malis CD, Lehninger AL, et al: Inhibition of PTH-induced nephrocalcinosis by phosphocitrate, in Smith LH, Robertson WG, Finlayson B (eds): Urolithiasis, Clinical and Basic Research. New York, Plenum Press, 1981, pp 559–568
112. Thomas WC Jr: Recently identified inhibitors of crystal growth in urine of calculous patients, in Ryall R, Brockis JG, Marshall V, et al (eds): Urinary Stone. Melbourne, Churchill Livingstone, 1984, pp 173–177
113. Thomas WC Jr, Howard JE: Studies on the mineralizing propensity of urine from patients with and without renal calculi. Trans Assoc Am Physicians, 72:181–187, 1959
114. Tiselius H-G: Effects of sodium urate and uric acid crystals on the crystallization of calcium oxalate. Urol Res, 12:11–15, 1984
115. Tiselius H-G: The effect of sodium sulfopentosan on the crystallization of calcium oxalate, in Schwille PO, Smith LH, Robertson WG, et al (eds): Urolithiasis and Related Clinical Research. New York, Plenum Press, 1985, pp 895–898

116. Van't Riet B, McKinney WM, Brandt EA, et al: Dye effects on inhibition and dissolution of urinary calculi. I. Invest Urol, 1(5):446–456, 1964
117. Van't Riet B, O'Rear CE, Smith MJV: Methylene blue and other agents as inhibitors of calcium oxalithiasis *in vivo*. Invest Urol, 16(3):201–203, 1978
118. Vermeulen CW, Lyon ES, Miller GH: Calcium phosphate solubility in urine as measured by a precipitation test: Experimental urolithiasis XIII. J Urol, 79(3):596–606, 1958
119. Wessler J: The nature of the non-ultrafilterable glycosaminoglycans of normal human urine. Biochem J, 122:373–384, 1971
120. White DH Jr, Christoffersen J, Herman TS, et al: Effects of urine pretreatment on calcium oxalate crystallization inhibition potentials. J Urol, 129(1):175–179, 1983
121. Will EJ, Bijvoet OLM, te-Brake van der Linden H: Inhibition of calcium oxalate crystal growth—a simple method of measurement and preliminary results, in Fleisch H, Robertson WG, Smith LH, et al (eds): urolithiasis Research. New York, Plenum Press, 1976, pp 367–370
122. Williams G, Sallis JD: The sources of phosphocitrate and its role as an inhibitor of calcium phosphate and calcium oxalate crystallization, in Smith LH, Robertson WG, Finlayson B (eds): Urolithiasis, Clinical and Basic Research. New York, Plenum Press, 1981, pp 569–577
123. Wilson JWG, Werness PG, Smith LH: Urinary inhibitors of hydroxyapatite crystal growth: A constant composition approach, in Schwille PO, Smith LH, Robertson WG, et al (eds): Urolithiasis and Related Clinical Research. New York, Plenum Press, 1985, pp 819–822

Allen L. Rodgers
Myron Spector

4

Crystallographic Analysis of Urinary Calculi

Importance of Stone Analysis

Analysis of urinary calculi offers a somewhat unique challenge to the clinical scientist in that the very complex composition and structure of these entities impose practical limitations on the applied procedures. The stones usually are multicomponent systems containing crystalline and noncrystalline material, which, in turn, can be organic and/or inorganic in composition. Many different morphologies, sometimes of the same chemical species, are observed. Identification of all the constituents in a urinary calculus enables investigators to accurately characterize the chemical conditions prevailing at the time of nucleation and growth. A detailed analysis is important since very often the component present in high relative concentrations is deposited in secondary processes while deposition of the less concentrated component occurs in a primary event.

Once a stone has been properly analyzed, etiology can be postulated and treatment of the disease can be prescribed. This is particularly true in the case of urinary stones, where several etiologic factors govern their formation.[1,2] These include inherited metabolic disorders such as cystinuria, gout and renal tubular acidosis (RTA); diseases that cause uricosuria, hyperuricemia, hypercalciuria, or hypercalcemia; and urinary tract infections. Each of these requires its own specific kind of treatment. Analysis of a stone yields information that may enable the clinician to ascertain which of the above conditions are operative and whether the patient is at risk for recurrent stone forming episodes and so prescribe appropriate treatment. Comprehensive analysis in which the minor components are all identified is essential for accurate etiologic hypotheses. Moreover, careful analysis with respect to the sequential deposition of the various components is also of importance to the clinician. For example, Figures 4-1 and 4-2 depict a mixed calcium oxalate–uric acid stone, yet different etiologies are involved. In the former (calcium oxalate core) the condition requiring treatment may have originally led to the deposition of calcium oxalate, such as hypercalciuria or hyperoxaluria. In the latter case,

STONE DISEASE: DIAGNOSIS AND MANAGEMENT
ISBN 0-8089-1873-7

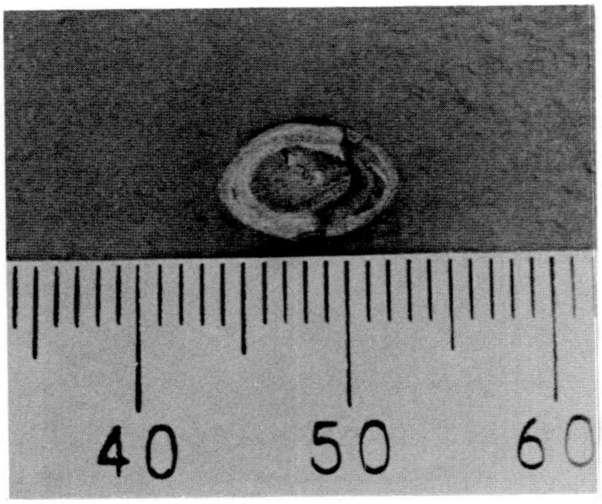

Fig. 4-1. Mixed calcium oxalate–uric acid stone (calcium oxalate core).

however (uric acid core), the condition requiring treatment may be associated primarily with uric acid deposition such as uricosuria.

Several techniques have developed over the years and are available for the qualitative and quantitative analysis of urinary calculi. Whereas chemical analysis has been used for many years, other physicochemical procedures have enjoyed much success in the analysis of stones. In this chapter, crystallographic studies of calculi are described. Because the large majority of the composition of most stones comprise crystalline material, methods enabling their identification have been of utmost importance in stone analysis.

X-ray Powder Diffraction (XRD) Analysis

Crystallographic studies of stones are of two main kinds: x-ray diffraction and optical. Both depend on the fact that crystalline substances have definite crystal structures and thus will give unique x-ray diffraction patterns and optical properties. Constituents within a particular stone can therefore be identified by comparison with a reference set of standard values for known calculus constituents.

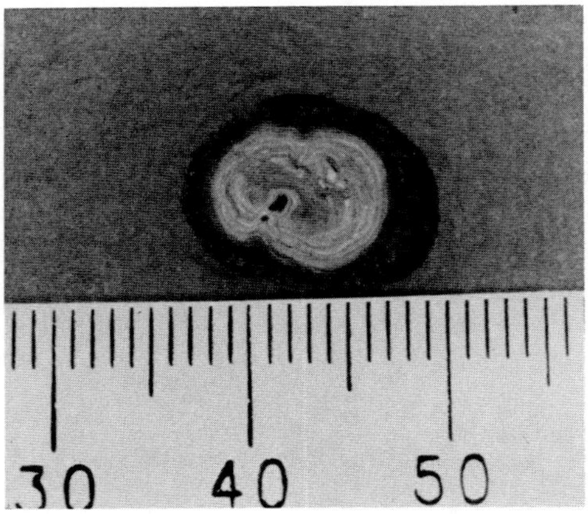

Fig. 4-2. Mixed calcium oxalate–uric acid stone (uric acid core).

In the XRD method, one of two procedures is followed. Either the entire stone is crushed to form a single powder specimen, or samples are obtained from the center, interior, and outer regions of a stone's exposed surface. These selected samples are obtained by using a lancet point metal probe and are ground to a fine powder with mortar and pestle. The advantages of the former technique are (1) the inclusion of all stone constituents in the powder and (2) the rapidity with which the specimen is prepared for analysis. The disadvantage of powdering the entire stone is that crystallite identity cannot be directly correlated with location in the stone. Moreover, since XRD techniques cannot detect crystalline constituents constituting less than 10 percent of the powder, important stone components might be missed by the analysis.

The x-ray diffraction patterns of the powdered specimens can be recorded on film or in a diffractometer employing a proportional counter (able to detect x-ray photons) mounted on a goniometer. The advantage of the photographic technique is that very small samples (0.1–0.3 mg) are sufficient for analysis, whereas 10–15 mg of powder is required for the diffractometer technique. However, the advantage of the diffractometer is that a line tracing of the pattern can be produced in a shorter time than a film recording. Furthermore, identification of the x-ray diffraction peaks and measurement of their "reflection" angles is easier in the strip chart recording from the diffractometer.

In the photographic procedure the powdered specimen is sealed in a short length of capillary tubing and clamped in a Debye-Scherrer XRD camera. Guinier XRD cameras employ a different configuration that permit the simultaneous irradiation of four powdered samples. While this camera has the obvious advantage of multiple analyses, a serious shortcoming is the need for relatively large sample quantities. In either case the sample is slowly rotated in a beam of monochromatic x-rays. The various planes of atoms within the crystalline lattices diffract the x-ray beam at characteristic angles. The diffracted rays are allowed to impinge on an x-ray sensitive film, and these give rise to the so-called diffraction pattern. In the case of the Debye-Scherrer camera, a series of arcs of varying intensity is obtained (Fig. 4-3), while the Guinier camera gives a series of lines for each of the four specimens. When a diffractometer is employed, the powder is dispersed

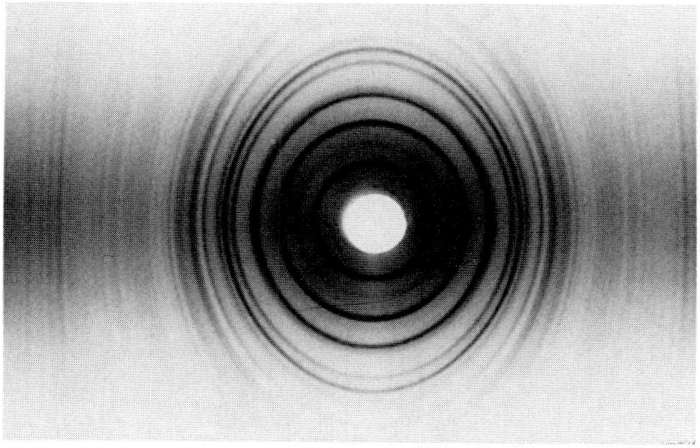

Fig. 4-3. X-ray powder diffraction photograph of a pattern of calcium oxalate monohydrate (whewhellite). The spacing and intensity of each line (reflection) is the fingerprint of a particular substance and identifies it absolutely.

onto a flat metal platen to cover an area approximately 5 × 12 mm. If sufficient material is available, it is impacted in a well (approximately 1 mm deep) with the rectangular dimensions given above. Otherwise, the powder is dispersed onto an adhesive binder applied to the surface of the metal platen. Recording of the diffraction profile is achieved by linking a strip chart recorder to the diffractometer. The reflections then appear as a spectrum of peaks of varying intensity (Fig. 4-4).

Whatever the particular configuration used for the collection of reflection data, the diffraction pattern so obtained (i.e., the relative position and intensity of each "reflection") is unique for the particular crystalline constituent(s) present in the sample and is referred to as the "fingerprint" of that substance.[3] The locations of the peaks on the x-ray film or strip chart recording (from the diffractometer) are related to the symmetry and dimensions of the latticework on which the atoms and molecules are arranged to form the crystal. The relative intensity of the peaks is dependent on the specific atoms or molecules present. Simple measurements permit the calculation of the characteristic distance between various lattice planes (*d*) of atoms or molecules that together with the relative intensities (*I*) enable the investigator to identify (within certain limits) the crystalline constituents present in the sample by comparison with published reference standards.

Application of XRD

This technique was first reported for the analysis of stones by Jensen and Thygesen in 1938[4] and by Prien and Frondel in 1947.[5] Since then it has been extensively used for this purpose, including several studies involving thousands of stones. For example, Herring successfully employed the procedure in the analysis of 10,000 calculi,[6] while Gibson has reported using XRD for the analysis of 15,000 stones.[7] Prien, in turn, analyzed 25,000 calculi with this method.[8] Sutor has reported XRD analyses on collections of stones from all over the world.[9–12]

What is it that makes this technique so popular and successful? Indeed, it is generally

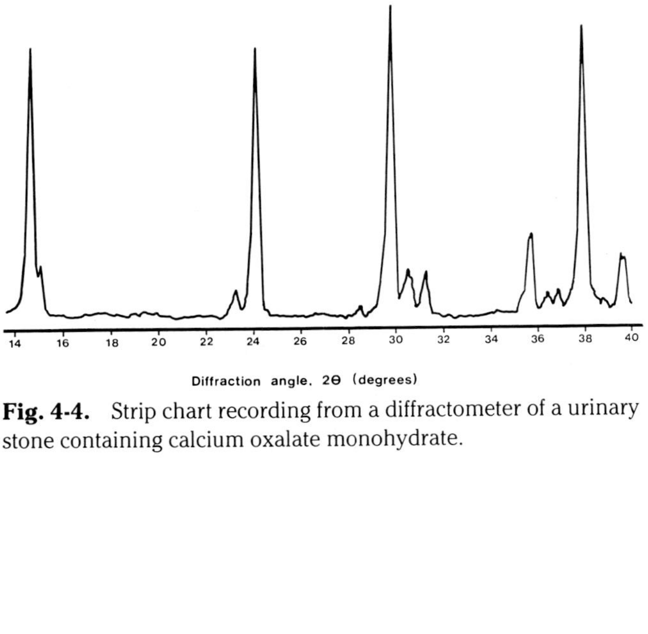

Fig. 4-4. Strip chart recording from a diffractometer of a urinary stone containing calcium oxalate monohydrate.

regarded as the method of first choice in urinary stone analysis for the following three reasons: (1) the technique affords unambiguous identification of crystalline constituents; (2) small sample sizes are sufficient, and specimens are not destroyed during analysis; and (3) representative specimens from throughout the sample may be easily selected for analysis.

Despite these advantages, several serious shortcomings have been identified, the principal one of which is the failure of XRD to reveal the presence of constituents in minor concentrations.[13–15] Sutor has shown that a constituent whose concentration is less than about 10 percent will give only a weak diffraction pattern that may be partly obscured by the major component. The situation is aggravated in those cases where stone constituents have common reflections in the diffraction pattern. Apatite, for example, has several *d* spacings that coincide with *d* spacings in struvite and weddellite. As a result, the presence of apatite in such stones is very often difficult to detect, even when its concentration level is significantly high. Biologic apatites, in general, have a poor diffraction pattern because of the small size of the crystallites that may contain noncrystalline regions. As a result, apatites in calculi are often difficult to identify in diffraction patterns. A further source of error associated with XRD analysis lies in the very nature of selecting representative samples for analysis from the interior of a stone. Constituents, present as distinct but possibly isolated grains, can be physically missed by the sampling process. Limitations are also imposed by the equipment employed. The resolution of reflections is directly dependent on camera radius and inversely proportional to the wavelength of the radiation. Finally, it should be pointed out that all stones contain about 2.5 percent amorphous organic material commonly referred to as *matrix*. Because of its very nature such material does not give x-ray diffraction patterns. Studies of this most important component of urinary calculi must thus be undertaken by use of a technique other than XRD.

Notwithstanding these various shortcomings and limitations, XRD has emerged as the most widely used routine analytical procedure in the study of urinary calculi.

Analysis by Optical Methods

The external habit (morphology) and the internal molecular structure of crystals are distinct, constant, and characteristic for any particular substance. As such, light passing through transparent crystalline material is influenced by the crystal structure according to the laws of optics. The polarizing microscope enables researchers to measure the so-called optical constants of the crystalline material under investigation, such as refractive index, optical sign, axial angle, dispersion, and extinction angle. Following determination of these parameters for a series of "control substances," that is, compounds of known chemical composition, it is possible to identify unknown substances by measurement of their optical constants and comparision with prepared tables.

The experimental procedure is relatively simple. A minute quantity of powdered crystalline material (approximately 1 mg) is placed on a glass slide and immersed in a succession of liquids of known refractive index until a match is found. In an alterative approach sections of the stone are ground thin enough to transmit light. This is generally facilitated by prior embedment in a plastic medium. In this technique the location of the crystallites in the stone is retained. In addition, sufficient optical information for identification of the crystallites can often be obtained.

In the context of urinary stone analysis, Prien and Frondel have described the principles and application of this technique in some detail.[5] Since then the procedure has been widely used with much success in a number of different analytical studies.[3,5,6,16,17]

Summary

Crystallographic methods of analysis, particularly XRD, have proved to be of the utmost value in the identification of the predominant constituents of urinary stones in the clinical workup of the stone-forming patient and in research investigations into urolithiasis. Identification of the crystalline substances constituting calculi has greatly facilitated treatment of urolithiasis.

REFERENCES

1. King JS: Etiologic factors involved in urolithiasis: A review of recent research. J Urol 97:583–591, 1967
2. Lien J: Nephrolithiasis: Investigation and clinical management. Mod Med, 49–57, 1981
3. Sutor DJ, Schiedt S: Identification standards for human urinary calculus components using crystallographic methods. Br J Urol 40:22–28, 1969
4. Jensen AT, Thygesen JE: Über die phosphatkonkremente der Harnwege. Z Urol 32:659–666, 1938
5. Prien EL, Frondel (1947). Studies in urolithiasis: The composition of urinary calculi. J Urol, *57,* 949-994
6. Herring L: Observations on the analysis of ten thousand urinary calculi. J Urol 88:545–562, 1962
7. Gibson R: Descriptive human pathological mineralogy: Am Mineral 59:1177–1182, 1974
8. Prien EL: The analysis of urinary calculi. Urol Clin N Am 1:229–240, 1974
9. Sutor DJ, Wooley SE: Composition of urinary calculi by x-ray diffraction. Collected data from various localities. Part VII. Br J Urol 41:397–400, 1969
10. Sutor DJ, Wooley SE: Composition of urinary calculi by x-ray diffraction. Collected data from various localities. Part VIII. Leeds, England. Br J Urol 42:302–305, 1970
11. Sutor DJ, Wooley SE: Composition of urinary calculi by x-ray diffraction. Collected data from various localities. Parts IX–XI. Glasgow, USA, and Sudan. Br J Urol 43:268–272, 1971
12. Sutor DJ, Wooley SE: Composition of urinary calculi by x-ray diffraction. Collected data from various localities. Parts XII–XIV. Northern Ireland, South Africa, and Kuwait. Br J Urol 44:287–291, 1972
13. Rodgers AL: Analysis of renal calculi by x-ray diffraction and electron microprobe: A comparision of two methods. Invest Urol 19:25–28, 1981
14. Rodgers AL, Nassimbeni LR, Mulder KJ: A multiple technique approach to the analysis of urinary calculi. Urol Res 10, 177–184, 1982
15. Sutor DJ: Difficulties in the identification of components of mixed urinary calculi using the x-ray powder method. Br J Urol 49:29–32, 1968
16. Beeler MF, Verth DA, Morriss RH, et al: Analysis of urinary calculus. Am J Clin Pathol 41:553–560, 1964
17. Hicking W, Hesse A, Gebhardt M, et al: Investigation with polarizing microscopy for the classification of urinary stones from humans and dogs, in Smith LH, Robertson WG, Finlayson B (eds): Urolithiasis: Clinical and Basic Research. New York, Plenum Press, 1981, pp 901–906

Allen L. Rodgers
Myron Spector

5

Crystalluria

Although the existence of crystals in urine has been known for a very long time, it has been appreciated only recently that the study of crystalluria may yield some valuable clues in the never-ending search for solutions to the many riddles of urinary stone formation. Moreover, the analysis of crystalluria might prove to be valuable as a diagnostic aid to assess the propensity toward stone formation in individuals.

Since the days of Hippocrates, scientists and clinicians have suggested that there may be a relationship between crystalluria and stone disease. Hippocrates himself observed that the passage of sand in the urine was often indicative of the presence of stone in the kidneys and bladder.[1] Since those days a variety of crystalline substances have been identified in urine. These include oxalates, urates, and phosphates.[1] Indentification of the crystal types in urine is facilitated by the distinctly different morphologies (Fig. 5-1–5-5) and optical properties of the substances. Care must be taken to prevent introduction of artifacts during handling of urine. One of the problems in previous studies of crystalluria is that experiments were conducted in such a manner that the urine specimens under investigation were often allowed to stand for long periods and to cool to room temperature without any precautions taken to keep the pH constant. In more recent times the experimental procedures have improved. In order to conduct studies at body temperature, the patient is required to void urine directly into a vacuum flask that has been preheated to the desired temperature. The specimen is subsequently centrifuged or filtered in equipment held at 37°C, and the deposited crystals are examined shortly thereafter under an optical microscope equipped with a temperature-controlled stage or under a scanning electron microscope (SEM).

Dyer and Nordin showed that if crystalluria is studied at 37°C, the number of crystal types is very much less than previously reported.[2] They found that the only crystalline substances observed were calcium oxalates, mainly as the dihydrate, and an "irregular" form of basic calcium phosphate.

Robertson and Peacock, in their examination of random fresh urine samples collected and maintained at 37°C from nonrecurrent idiopathic stone formers and normal

STONE DISEASE: DIAGNOSIS AND MANAGEMENT

ISBN 0-8089-1873-7

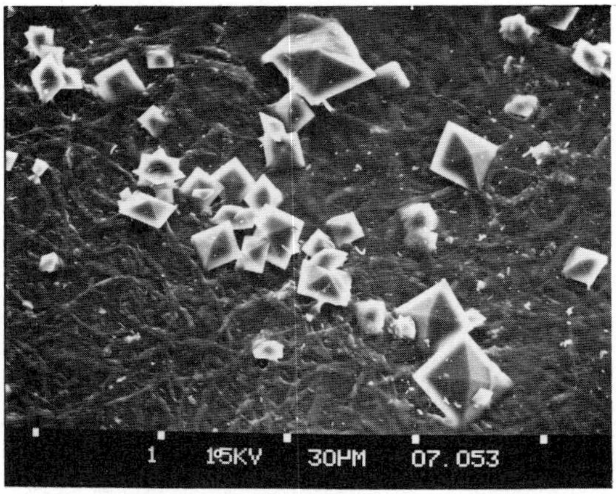

Fig. 5-1. Envelope-shaped crystals of calcium oxalate dihydrate (magnification 750×).

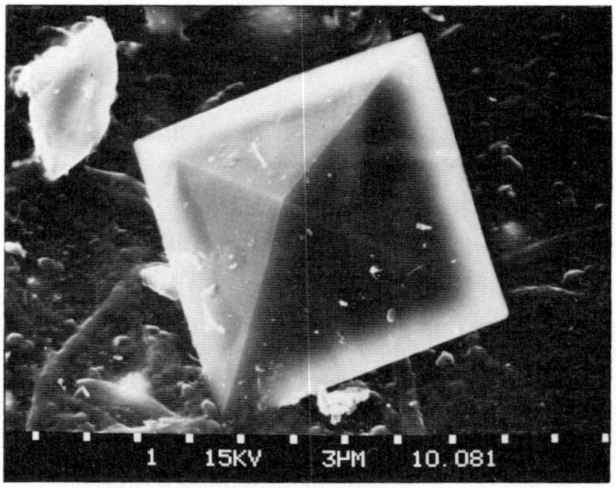

Fig. 5-2. High magnification of a calcium oxalate dihydrate crystal (magnification 3300×).

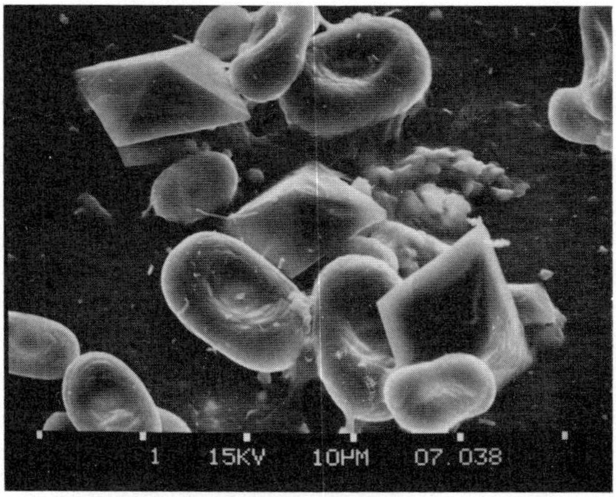

Fig. 5-3. Calcium oxalate dihydrate (envelope shape) and monohydrate (oval, hollowed shape) crystals (magnification 2000×).

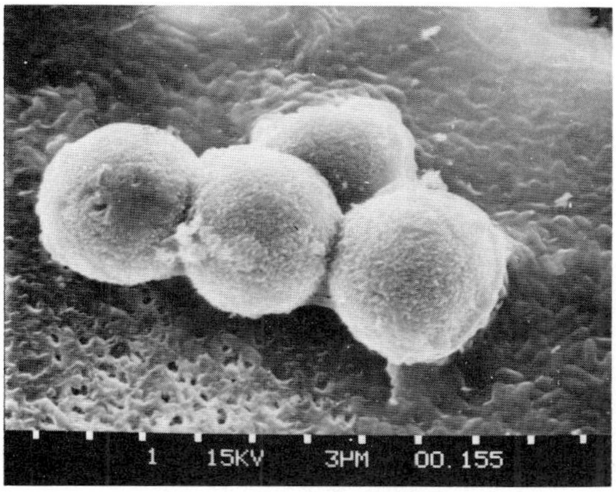

Fig. 5-4. Spherular cluster of tiny, hair-like crystals of apatite (magnification 3600×).

healthy controls, identified only calcium oxalate crystals.[3] However, other studies have shown that normal subjects as well as stone-forming patients frequently void urines supersaturated with one or more of several sparingly soluble salts.[4–6] Werness et al. studied crystalluria in a group of subjects made up of patients with primary hyperparathyroidism (with and without stones), primary hyperoxaluria, and idiopathic calcium urolithiasis.[7] Normal subjects were also included in the study. They reported that crystalluria was observed in all these groups and that the stone-forming patients had a greater number of crystals in their urine than did normal subjects. The hypothesis that there exists some link between crystalluria and stone disease thus persists. Indeed, Rose of the St. Peter's Hospitals, London, states that he and his group have been employing crystalluric studies since 1975,[8] and that these have proved of particular value with regard to both the practical and theoretical aspects of urinary stone formation.

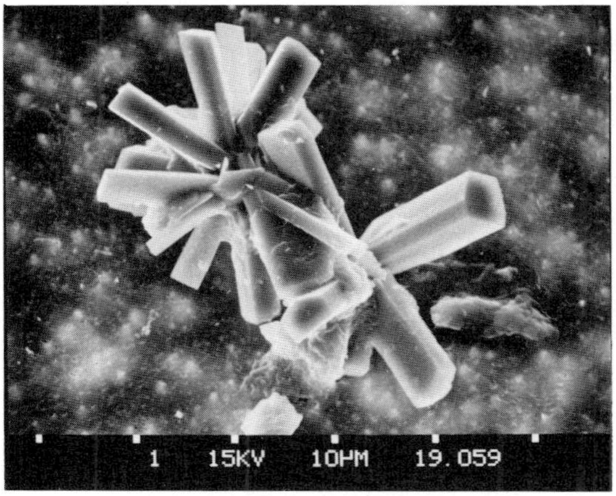

Fig. 5-5. Aggregate of rod-shaped crystals of brushite (magnification 2000×).

CRYSTAL TYPE, SIZE, AND NUMBERS

Robertson was the first to suggest that if the hypothesis is correct that the processes of precipitation, aggregation and crystal growth determine the initiation of urinary tract calculi, then crystals of the salts concerned ought to be detectable in greater numbers or size, or with greater frequency in the urine of stone formers than in the urine of normal subjects.[1] Indeed, Robertson and coworkers subsequently showed that there is a qualitative and quantitative difference in the crystalluria of recurrent, idiopathic stone formers and their controls under the same conditions of dietary and fluid intake.[3,9] They found that crystals excreted by controls are small (3–4 μm in diameter) and belong to a unimodal distribution whereas those excreted by stone formers belong to a distribution that contains, in addition to the 3–4 μm peak, a second peak of much larger particles (20–40 μm in diameter). These particles were identified as calcium oxalate dihydrate and were found to occur in aggregates up to 200 μm in diameter. Crasweller et al., in their studies of size distribution patterns,[10] reported similar profiles to those determined by Robertson and coworkers.[3,9] A typical particle volume–size distribution curve for normal male subjects is shown in Figure 5–6.

Hallson and Rose also found that stone formers show a much higher degree of aggregation of calcium oxalate dihydrate crystals than do controls but reported that the main difference between normal subjects and stone formers was an increased incidence of phosphate crystals in the latter.[11] Other clinical studies noted that calcium oxalate dihydrate predominates in the urine of normals as well as stone formers.[12]

One of the most extensive studies of the different kinds of crystalluria was recently reported by Werness et al.,[7] who analyzed a total of 4835 voidings from 162 subjects. Not unexpectedly, the incidence and type of crystal observed varied with the particular group investigated. Hydroxyapatite, calcium oxalate monohydrate (COM), and uric acid were observed in the normal subjects. The patients with primary hyperparathyroidism were

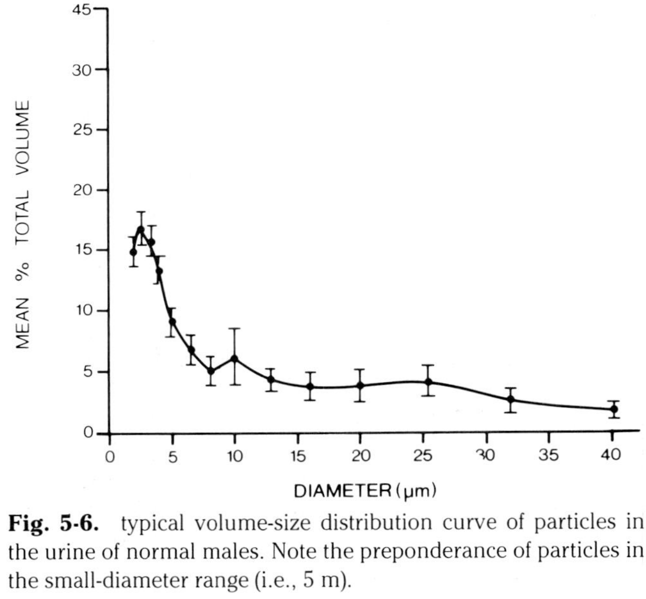

Fig. 5-6. typical volume-size distribution curve of particles in the urine of normal males. Note the preponderance of particles in the small-diameter range (i.e., 5 m).

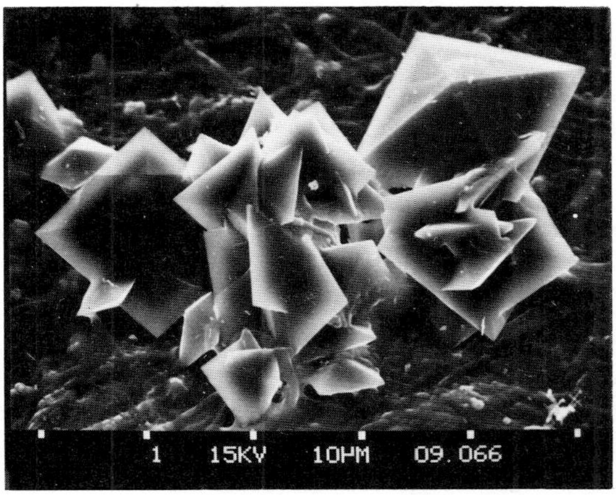

Fig. 5-7. Aggregate of calcium oxalate dihydrate crystals typical of stone formers' urine (magnification 2000×).

divided into two groups—those with stones and those without. Both groups displayed the same kind of crystalluria as the normal subjects, but, in addition, calcium oxalate dihydrate (COD) and brushite were observed in urine specimens from those subjects with stones. Patients with primary hyperoxaluria had COM and COD crystals only, while those individuals with idiopathic calcium urolithiasis had crystals of hydroxyapatite, both hydrates of calcium oxalate, uric acid, and brushite.

It is of some interest that an earlier study by Dent and Sutor showed that when normal urine is slowly saturated with calcium and oxalate ions at pH 5.5–6.2, the crystals that form first are those of the monohydrate.[13] Stone formers' urine, however, was found to crystallize COD first. These results, together with those described above, tend to suggest that the urine of normal subjects is characterized by COM crystals, the sizes of which are generally small (approximately 5 μm), while in stone formers' urine the crystals are large (approximately 30 μm) and of the dihydrate type. An example of the latter is shown in Figure 5-3. Aggregation of calcium oxalate dihydrate crystals appears to be another feature of stone formers' urine. A typical example is shown in Figure 5-7.

The proposition that calcium oxalate dihydrate predominates in the urines of stone formers is somewhat confounding in that (1) COM is a more common urinary stone constituent and (2) the dihydrate phase is thermodynamically unstable with respect to calcium oxalate monohydrate.[14]

ANIMAL STUDIES OF CRYSTALLURIA

There are few reports in the literature of animal investigations of crystalluria. In one such study intratubular calcium oxalate formation and crystalluria was investigated in rats made hyperoxaluric and hypomagnesuric.[15] Whereas the control animals displayed no crystalluria, after only 1 day the experimental group had crystalluria consisting predominantly, and often exclusively, of COM crystals ranging from 2 to 15 μm. Individual monohydrate crystals and crystal aggregates were observed. A few animals from this group also displayed COD crystals that were considerably fewer in number and smaller in size, ranging from 2 to 5 μm. These animals also had intratubular crystalline deposits and a propensity toward urolithiasis.

In another test group of animals that were maintained hyperoxaluric only with a less lithogenic protocol, a degree of crystalluria similar to that seen in the test group in the combined protocol was noted; however, the crystalluria in this hyperoxaluric group initially consisted primarily of COM. Urine aspirated from the bladders of these animals 2 days after the hyperoxaluric treatment was initiated consisted exclusively of dihydrate crystals ranging from 1 to 40 μm. It was only later (after 4 days) that COM crystals (ranging from 2 to 25 μm) also began to appear in the urine. With time there was a tendency toward crystal aggregation.

The results of these animal investigations suggested a correlation between the type of urinary crystals and intratubular crystal formation and urolithiasis. Calcium oxalate monohydrate crystals predominated in the urine of the animals that had intratubular COM deposition and, perhaps, a predisposition to stone formation. Calcium oxalate dihydrate crystalluria was found in animals that did not display signs of intratubular calcium deposition. The difference in the crystalluria in the test groups could be related to differences in the degree of supersaturation with respect to the calcium oxalate in the renal pelvis and/or bladder. One effect of decreasing urinary magnesium may be to increase the available oxalate for precipitation with calcium and, hence, increase the degree of supersaturation.

This animal investigation suggests that, at least in the rat kidney, the identification of COM crystalluria is an important indicator of intranephronic calcium oxalate formation and propensity toward stone formation. A similar correlation has been suggested by preliminary clinical data that show greater amounts of monohydrate in the crystalluria of stone formers than in urines of non-stone-forming individuals.[16,17] This is counter to other clinical and experimental observations suggesting a correlation between calcium oxalate dihydrate precipitation and urolithiasis.

Examination of the crystalluria in animal studies[15] has begun to reveal the mechanisms by which aggregates of COM and COD crystals form in urine. The dumbbell-shaped monohydrate clusters and most dihydrate aggregates result from the growth of one crystal from the surface of another, often producing a fused appearance. The monohydrate dumbbells appeared to result from "twinning" of the flat hexagonal crystalline plates during growth from the surface of other plates. In the case of monohydrate cast-like aggregates and some dihydrate aggregates, the clustering of crystals appeared to be due to a second mechanism related to the presence of an organic, mucoidlike cementing substance. The presence of the cast-like aggregates of cemented monohydrate crystals in the nidi of renal stones in the rats suggested their potential importance in urolithiasis.

EFFECT OF TREATMENT ON CRYSTALLURIA

Hallson and Rose studied a group of adult subjects comprising normal volunteers and stone formers in whom a diagnosis of idiopathic hypercalciuria had been made and who were either untreated or receiving treatment with thiazide diuretics (bendrofluazide) and/or cellulose phosphate. They found that the main difference between normal subjects and stone formers was an increased incidence of phosphate crystals in the latter. Treatment with thiazide considerably reduced the incidence of phosphate crystals but slightly increased the incidence of oxalate crystals. Cellulose phosphate therapy resulted in an almost complete disappearance of phosphate crystals but a striking increase of oxalate crystals. The overall percentage of samples showing aggregation was, however, virtually unchanged by these treatments. The treatment most effective in reducing crystal incidence as a whole was the combination of cellulose phosphate and thiazide.

In another study, patients with primary hyperoxaluria were treated with orthophosphate or thiazide duretics.[7] It was found that these treatments reduced the crystalluria significantly to levels compatible with those occurring in normal subjects. Dramatic scanning electron micrographs showing the quantitative differences in crystalluria before and after treatment are presented by these workers.[7]

EFFECT OF URINARY pH ON CRYSTALLURIA

Robertson et al. showed that two types of crystal were observed depending on the urinary pH.[9] Between pH 5.0 and 6.2 only calcium oxalate was present, while above pH 6.2, amorphous calcium phosphate was the main substance detected, occasionally mixed with calcium oxalate. These findings were subsequently confirmed by the work of Hallson and Rose.[11] Since crystal type is thus pH-dependent, it was important to establish whether changes from one type to another during treatment was due to the treatment, per se, or to a change in pH. This was investigated by Hallson and Rose, who showed that thiazide or cellulose phosphate treatment did not, in fact, alter urine pH.[11] They therefore concluded that the striking changes in crystal type brought about by treatment with these substances were not due to pH changes.

CLINICAL SIGNIFICANCE OF CRYSTALLURIA

According to Rose, one of the most difficult tasks of the clinician treating urolithiasis in a patient is to decide whether the condition is "active" at the time of investigation.[8] Rose has pointed out that urinary calcium is not a good guide as many normal subjects show hypercalciuric levels. On the other hand, hyperoxaluria is a good indicator of high risk, but this condition seldom occurs in stone formers. Rose and others have thus concluded that there does not exist a single factor that is a good predictor of stone disease.[7]

Despite these findings, a number of physicochemical factors have been identified as playing some or other role in the formation of urinary stones. These include state of saturation, presence of inhibitors or promotors of crystal growth and aggregation, organic matrix and/or mucoid material, epitaxy or heterogeneous nucleation, and site of crystal formation and retention. Werness et al. have made the point that since all these factors should also affect crystalline material passed in the urine, the study of crystalluria can provide clues as to which of these factors are actually involved in stone formation.[7]

Finlayson has considered the significance of crystalluria from a different point of view but has arrived at the same conclusion.[18] He has drawn attention to the fact that other workers have suggested that crystalluria particles are truly microstones and has calculated the relationship between particle size and the probability of unhindered passage through a pericalyceal lymphatic, a duct of Bellini, and a ureter. These calculations show that there is a size difference of less than an order of magnitude between large crystalluria particles and small conventional stones, suggesting that crystals and calculi

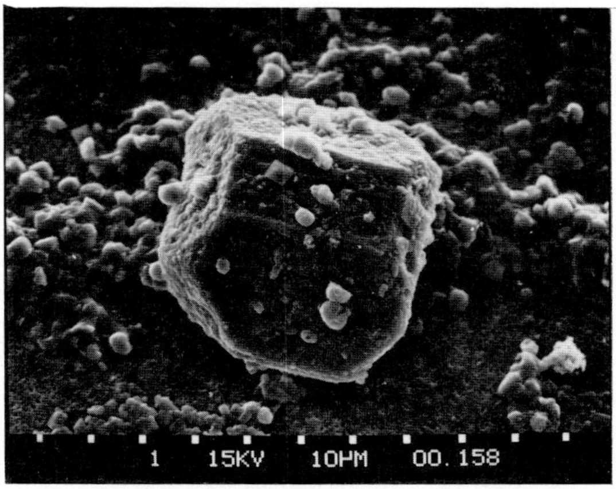

Fig. 5-8. Large struvite crystal with several spherular clusters of apatite (magnification 1060×).

are part of the same continuum. He concludes that, regardless of its precise role in urolithiasis, crystalluria is a useful indication of the stone-forming potential of urine.

Let us briefly examine and summarize the crystalluric factors that may be of value as a guide for assessing the propensity toward stone formation. In the first instance it appears that under the same conditions of urinary concentrations, most studies suggest that normal subjects have COM crystalluria while patients with recurrent idiopathic calcium oxalate stone disease who are between episodes have calcium oxalate dihydrate crystalluria.[3,13] Moreover, independent laboratories have reported that aggregated dihydrate crystals (sometimes up to 200 μm in size) are virtually confined to the urine of recurrent stone formers.[9,11] It has also been shown that the particle size distributions in the urine of normal and stone forming patients are different.[3,9] The distribution in the former is unimodal (approximately 4 μm), while that of the latter is bimodal (4 and 30 μm). These criteria should serve as a guide instead of a fixed diagnostic schema since our understanding of the correlation between the hydrated forms of calcium oxalate and urolithiasis is incomplete.

Struvite crystalluria is a strong indicator of urinary infection. For crystallization of this substance to occur, high levels of ammonia are required at elevated pH levels. These conditions prevail in the presence of urease-producing bacteria that split urea (thereby releasing ammonia) and increase urinary pH. An example of struvite crystals isolated from infected urine is shown in Figure 5-8.

It can therefore be appreciated that quantitative and qualitative tests of crystalluria can be applied in order to assess whether treatment of a particular patient is effective. According to Finlayson, an antistone therapy that arrests crystalluria can be expected to retard urolithiasis,[18] while Rose states that if treatment of a calcium oxalate stone former results in the disappearance of large crystal aggregates from the urine, further stone formation in such a patient is unlikely to occur.[8] It is thus conceivable that simple crystalluria tests could be conducted in hospital laboratories and be included in the routine workup of stone patients. Such tests would undoubtedly reveal informative and useful data to the attending clinician.

REFERENCES

1. Robertson WG: A method for measuring calcium crystalluria. Clin Chim Acta 26:105–110, 1969
2. Dyer A, Nordin BEC: Urine crystals and their relations to stone formations. Nature 215:751, 1967
3. Robertson WG, Peacock M: Calcium oxalate crystalluria and inhibitors of crystallization in recurrent renal stone-formers. Clin Sci 43:499–506, 1972
4. Robertson WG, Peacock M, Nordin BEC: Calcium oxalate crystalluria and urine saturation in recurrent renal stone formers. Clin Sci 40:365, 1971
5. Pak C: Physicochemical basis for formation of renal stone of calcium phosphate origin. Calculation of the degree of saturation of urine with respect to brushite. J Clin Invest 48:1914, 1969
6. Robertson WG, Peacock M, Nordin BEC: Activity products in stone forming and non stone forming urine. Clin Sci 34:579–594, 1968
7. Werness PG, Bergert JH, Smith LH: Crystalluria. J Cyst Growth 53:166–181, 1981
8. Rose GA: Crystalluria as an aid to the study of urinary stones. Lab-Lore (Wellcome Diagnostics) 9:738–740, 1982
9. Robertson WG, Peacock M, Nordin BEC: Calcium crystalluria in recurrent renal stone formers. Lancet 2:21–24, 1969
10. Crassweller PO, Brandes L, Katirtzoglou A, Oreopoulos DG: Studies of crystalluria in recurrent calcium lithiasis. Can J Surg 22:527–529, 1979
11. Hallson PC, Rose GA: Crystalluria in normal subjects and in stone formers with and without thiazide and cellulose phosphate treatment. Br J Urol 48:515–524, 1976
12. Elliot JS, Rabinowitz IN, Silvert M: Calcium oxalate crystalluria. J Urol 116:773–775, 1976
13. Dent CE, Sutor DJ: Presence or absence of inhibitor of calcium oxalate crystal growth in urine of normals and of stone formers. Lancet 775–778, 1971
14. Hodgkinson A: Oxalic Acid in Biology and Medicine. New York, Academic Press, 1977, p 46
15. Rushton HC, Spector M: Effects of magnesium deficiency on intratubular calcium oxalate formation and crystalluria in hyperoxaluric rats. J Urol 127:598–604, 1982
16. Elliot JS, Rabinowitz IN: Calcium oxalate crystalluria: Crystal size in urine. J Urol 123:324–317, 1980
17. Hesse A, Bach D, Strenge A, et al: The effect of dietary oxalate loads on urinary oxalate excretion, in Oxalate in Human Biochemistry and Clinical Pathology. London, The Wellcome Foundation Ltd, 1979, p 100
18. Finlayson B: Renal lithiasis in review. Urol Clin N Am 1:181–212, 1974

Allen L. Rodgers
Myron Spector

6

Morphogenesis and Pathogenesis of Urolithiasis

Stones are an age-old anguish of the human body and occur at several sites, in particular the kidney, urinary bladder, gallbladder, prostate gland, salivary gland, and pancreas.[1–3] Reports from antiquity as well as from modern-day clinicians reveal that, although not necessarily life-threatening, stones were—and still are—a source of considerable pain.[4–6] Many techniques have been developed over the years to investigate this disease, therefore, and today the most sophisticated of these are utilized in concerted efforts directed at gaining insight into the mechanism of stone growth.

Among these different stone afflictions, urinary calculus disease is one of the oldest known medical disorders of humankind. As early as the third century B.C. the Greek physician Ammonios used the technique of lithotrity to break up bladder stones mechanically so that they could be passed in the urine. The bladder stone was the typical urinary concrement of history. Today, a fundamental change in the pattern of calculus disease reveals renal and ureteric stones to be the characteristic clinical manifestation of the ailment. Over the past 30 years, worldwide prevalence of renal calculi in particular has multiplied, paralleled by generally increasing prosperity. It is reported that in 1979 about 5 percent of the entire (West) German population contracted one or more stones during their lifetime.[7] In the United States about 200,000 kidney stone patients are admitted to hospital annually. Since figures of stone frequency are usually based on hospital statistics only, many more people might be potential stone sufferers; hence, some researchers believe that kidney stones are as common as diabetes and high blood pressure. This has led to the ailment of urinary stones being designated a "public disease."[8]

It is thus not surprising that a great deal of scientific effort has been directed at investigating the prevention and dissolution of calculi. The hope that such studies would reveal the cause of urinary lithiasis has not yet been realized, however; the main difficulty is the multiplicity of factors contributing to the formation of stones. As a result, the

STONE DISEASE: DIAGNOSIS AND MANAGEMENT
ISBN 0-8089-1873-7

specific combination of these factors has to be determined separately in each individual case.

Among the causal factors, pathologic changes of the kidney and metabolic disorders such as hypercalciuria, hyperoxaluria, and cystinuria,[9] in addition to geographic, environmental, ethnic, and familial parameters, have been shown to predispose certain people to stone disease.[10]

Geographic correlations of urolithiasis show differences in incidence related to the development and economy of countries and communities. According to Robertson et al., the prevalence of renal calculi is correlated with the net income of a population group, probably as a result of increased ingestion of animal protein with increasing wealth.[11] Sutor observed changes in stone type and composition, as countries become technologically developed.[12] Further evidence in support of the suggested role of diet in urolithiasis is provided by the occurrence of stone waves in times of prosperity.[13]

Environmental variables include climate, occupation, and personal circumstances. An increased incidence of renal stones with a rise in atmospheric temperature has been observed, and a high prevalence of stones in persons with occupations that entail exposure to high environmental temperatures (e.g., chefs, shipboard engineers) is well documented.[10] Another factor is the physical activity associated with certain occupations—the more sedentary a job, the higher the frequency of stones.

Regarding other "personal" parameters, a positive family history also seems to be correlated with multiple occurrences of calculi.[14] The observation that calculi are rare amongst certain racial groups further raises the question of the importance of genetic influences and heredity. Most studies, however, point more to the involvement of nutritional and dietary factors that are now considered to represent the most significant determinant in the epidemiology of stones.

It is thus understood that urinary stone formation is a complex process involving many variables, the pathogenesis of which is not completely clear. Of the multitude of factors, only a few are well known, and in only two cases, hyperparathyroidism and uric acid stone formation, has consensus about the underlying principles been reached.

Three mechanisms are important in stone formation: nucleation, growth, and aggregation.[15,16] *Nucleation* refers to the "birth" of submicroscopic molecular species of "critical size" within the supersaturated solution.[17] This initial event can be of either the homogeneous type, where particles of the same compound nucleate on each other, or the heterogeneous type, involving nucleation of one compound on another. Once nuclei are present, the second mechanism becomes operative (i.e., growth).[18] As a consequence of ongoing or recurrent supersaturation and other factors, aggregation of the formed crystals may occur, by either "sintering" or interparticle bridging of polymeric material.[19] With the subsequent trapping of the resulting polycrystalline mass in the kidney, a stone is formed.

Investigation of the fundamental causes that trigger the above-mentioned mechanisms involves both clinical and scientific approaches. On one hand, the clinician is mostly concerned with in vivo characterization of the primary etiologic and biologic factors of the various metabolic disorders contributing to the disease. From such studies new (empirical) measures for the treatment of the clinical picture of stones can be derived. On the other hand, scientific approaches to urolithiasis essentially embrace three areas: stone analysis, crystallization experiments, and animal models. These approaches are discussed in this chapter.

STONE ANALYSIS

The importance of stone analysis and the role it plays in assisting the clinician to accurately characterize the chemical conditions prevailing at the time of initiation and hence to prescribe effective treatment has already been discussed in Chapter 4. These analyses, however, are essentially of a chemical nature. Analyses of structure and ultrastructure, on the other hand, yields for the investigator much useful data that can provide insights into the various mechanisms that govern stone morphogenesis. The technique of scanning electron microscopy (SEM) has been widely used in this regard[20–31] and has proved to be of great value with respect to at least two aspects of stone growth and etiology: (1) the role of epitaxy and (2) the role of apatite in stone formation. It has been hypothesized that the former might provide a crystallographic explanation of stone growth mechanism[32] while the latter is the most prevalent crystalline constituent of urinary calculi. It is of some interest to consider each of these aspects in turn.

The phenomenon of epitaxy was first demonstrated by Lonsdale, who showed that in urinary and biliary calculi certain constituents will grow on each other if there is a good geometric fit between the respective two-dimensional lattice networks that are in contact.[32] According to Lonsdale, the degree of misfit that can be tolerated for an epitaxial interaction must not exceed "a few percent." This concept is diagramatically illustrated in Figure 6-1, in which four such interactions are shown. In each case two different kinds of "unit cell" (i.e., building block) are shown in contact. In case 1 the geometric match of the two interacting faces is perfect, while in cases 2 and 3, a small degree of misfit occurs. Case 4 shows that simple integral multiples of the unit cells can also lead to an epitaxial situation. Tables 6-1 and 6-2 illustrate the phenomenon for uric acid and calcium oxalate monohydrate and show that their respective lattice dimensions agree very well and favor epitaxial growth. The frequent occurrence of these two components within the same calculus tends to support Londale's hypothesis that epitaxy is a key factor in the morpho-

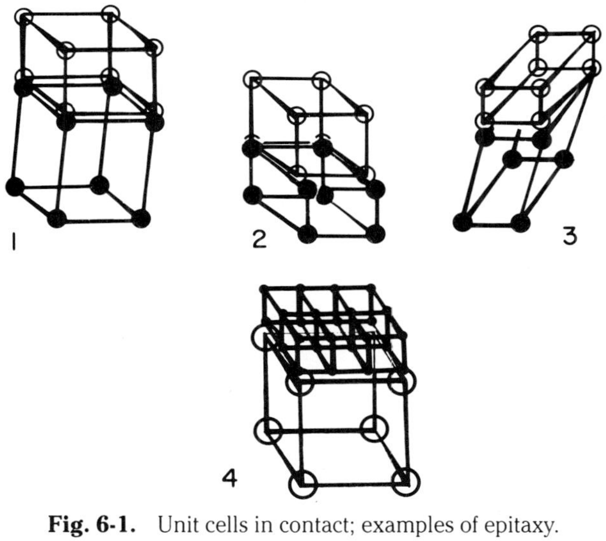

Fig. 6-1. Unit cells in contact; examples of epitaxy.

Table 6-1
Unit Cell Dimensions, Å

	a	*b*	*c*
Uric acid	13.12	7.40	6.21
COM	6.28	14.57	10.11

genesis of stones. Indeed, she has shown that several other components satisfy the geometric criteria for epitaxy as well.

Scanning electron microscopic studies of urinary calculi have provided further evidence in support of this hypothesis. Examples are shown in Figures 6-2–6-5. In Figure 6-2, bipyramidal crystals of calcium oxalate dihydrate (COD) are seen protruding from a calcium oxalate monohydrate (COM) substrate or base as is often observed on the exterior surface of calcium oxalate calculi. The COD crystal in Figure 6-3 appears to be spawning a number of apatite entities. Apatite deposits are shown in intimate contact with large struvite crystals in Figure 6-4, while Figure 6-5 depicts a large aggregate of uric acid needle crystals in contact with COM bodies. It must be pointed out that these micrographs do not *prove* that epitaxial growth has taken place between the contacting substances. Indeed, their presence might simply have resulted from a mechanical process in which one material was deposited on another; however, the micrographs do provide evidence that epitaxy *might* have occurred. Since all the above-mentioned commonly occurring two-component systems possess, according to Lonsdale, matching geometric lattices, the phenomenon of epitaxy cannot be discounted. As far as the role of apatite is concerned, SEM studies of this material have provided insight into the similarity of the morphogenesis of uroliths and other types of pathologic tissue calcification in which it is the primary constituent. Spector and Jamieson showed in their SEM studies of urinary calculi[30] that apatite crystallites occur in spherical aggregates of diameter 2–10 μm such as those shown in figures 6-6 and 6-7 and that the spheres themselves were made up of concentric spherical lamellae that appeared to have been produced by successive stages of growth. Spector et al. have pointed out that the spherical apatite deposits in urinary calculi are remarkably similar to apatite deposits identified in a variety of calcified tissues such as nephrocalcinosis.[28,29] These workers suggest that in some cases, urinary apatite deposits might be derived from renal calcification. Rodgers has shown that the morphology of apatite–spherular clusters (10 μm in diameter) of hairlike crystallites are very similar in urinary, prostatic, biliary, and salivary calculi and has suggested that this might be indicative of similar morphogenetic mechanisms in the different calculi.[33]

Table 6-2
Test of Epitaxial Fit for Uric Acid and COM*

	p, Å	q, Å	$m \times n$	Dimensions of Net	Percent Misfit Δmp	Percent Misfit Δnq
Uric acid	7.40	6.21	2×1	14.80×6.21	1.6	1.1
COM	6.28	14.57	1×1	14.57×6.28		

*The translations in the net on which epitaxy occurs are p and q; m and n are the integral multiples of p and q involved in the epitaxial contact; Δmp and Δnq are the percentage misfits in the linear dimensions of mp and nq as they occur in the respective nets.

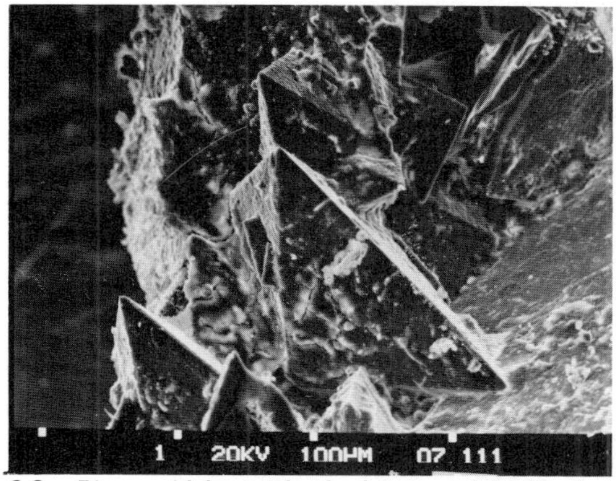

Fig. 6-2. Bipyramidal crystals of calcium oxalate dihydrate protruding from a calcium oxalate monohydrate concrement.

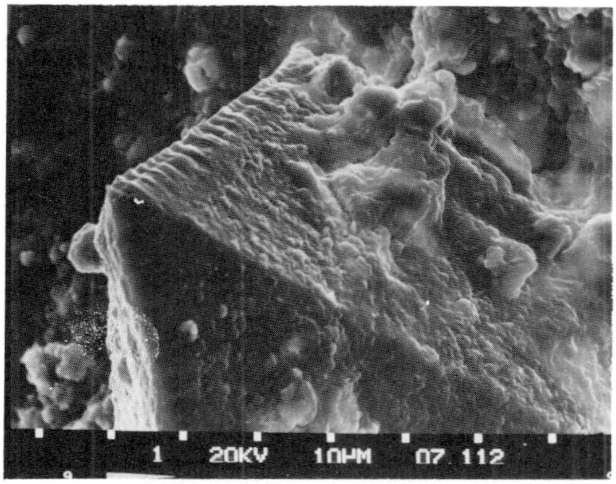

Fig. 6-3. Apatite entities growing on a calcium oxalate dihydrate crystal face.

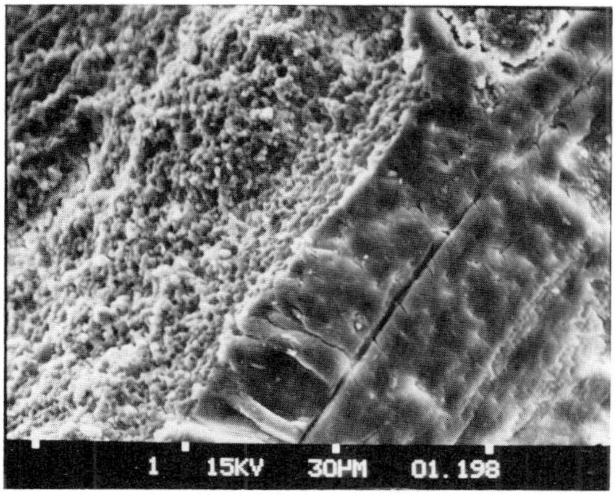

Fig. 6-4. Apatite deposits in contact with large struvite concrement.

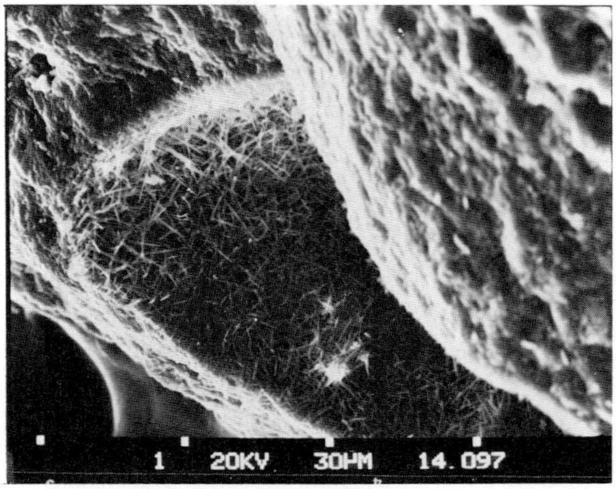

Fig. 6-5. Large aggregate of uric acid needle crystals in contact with calcium oxalate monohydrate concrements.

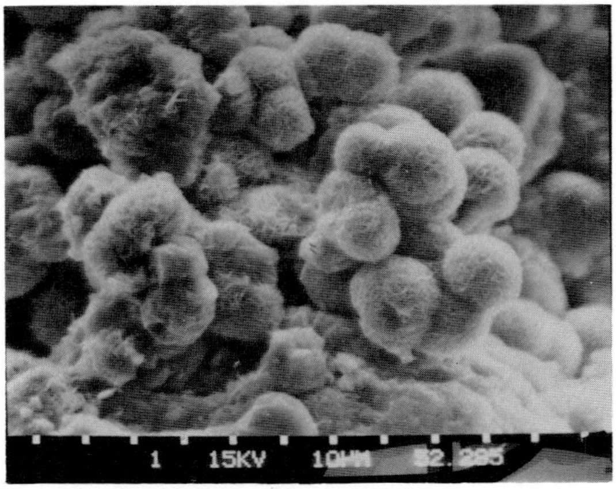

Fig. 6-6. Spherular aggregates of tiny hair-like crystals of apatite.

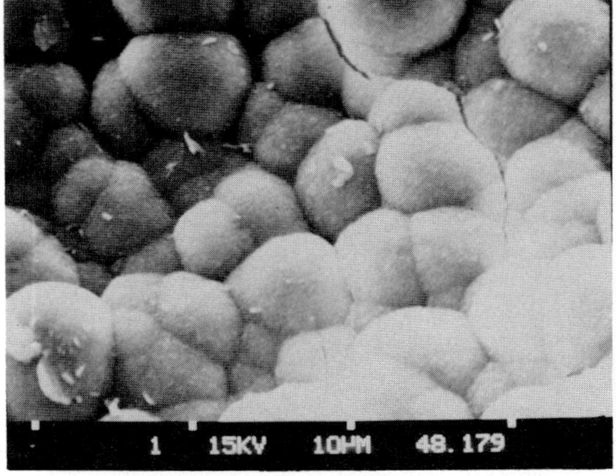

Fig. 6-7. Spherular aggregates of tiny hair-like crystals of apatite.

Another aspect of stone morphogenesis concerns the role of the so-called matrix component of urinary calculi. Analysis has revealed that all stones formed within the urinary tract, irrespective of cause or composition, have, in addition to the crystalline inorganic substances, an amorphous organic phase admixed with the crystal aggregates. This matrix component constitutes about 2–10 percent of the total mass and is believed to play an extremely important and decisive role.[34–36] According to this approach, the condensation of specific organic colloids is thought to be the primary process in calculogenesis.[37] The deposition of inorganic salts is then regarded as a secondary phenomenon. It is conceivable that the organic substances that have been detected in calculi act as a trigger for heterogeneous nucleation of stone salts, which are then adsorbed onto the matrix skeleton.

Although direct proof that active sites in the matrix induce formation of crystal nuclei or that matrix plays the suggested architectonic role has not as yet been presented, various ultrastructural studies have provided much evidence in support of matrix material actively involved in the primary stages of stone formation. In a recent SEM study of whewhellite stones,[26] the crystalline phase was shown to occur in oriented clusters within which the crystals were stacked with their broad faces parallel. Gaps between the crystals were shown by darkfield transmission electron microscopic (TEM) imaging to contain an amorphous phase, thus indicating that stone matrix is sandwiched between the crystals and may therefore be responsible for cohesion in these stones. Other SEM studies are in agreement with this observation.[38–40] For example, the cystine crystals in Figure 6-8 appear to be "glued" to one another by mucoid material. This aggregating mechanism is not unlike that shown in Figure 6-9, which was recorded during SEM investigation of a matrix stone. The micrograph shows struvite crystals entrapped in mucoid. Similarly, in Figure 6-10, apatite spherules are linked by mucoid strands and deposits.

The sequence of micrographs from Figures 6-11 to 6-14 provides further evidence of the role of the amorphous matrix. The first of these (Figure 6-11), shows a large struvite concrement intimately admixed with a colony of apatite deposits. Figures 6-12 and 6-13 show the distribution of calcium and magnesium, respectively, while Figure 6-14 repre-

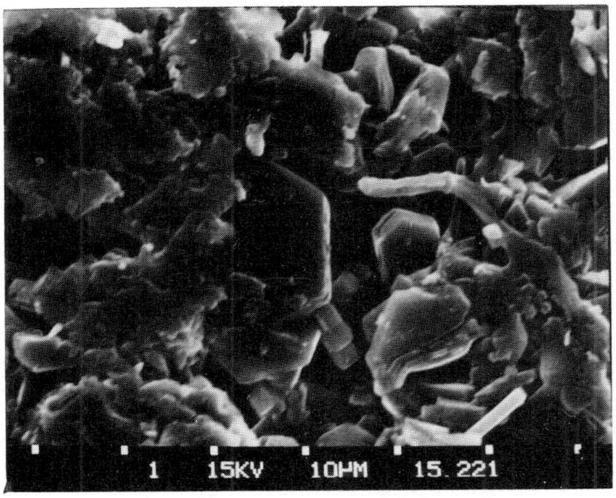

Fig. 6-8. Mucoid material "binding" cystine crystals in a urinary calculus (left-hand side of micrograph).

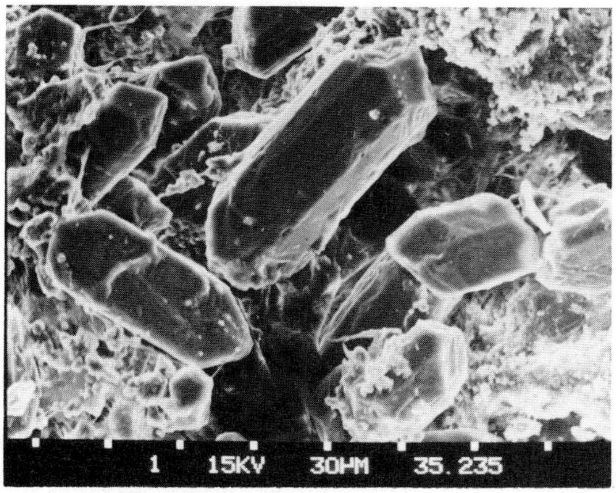

Fig. 6-9. Struvite crystals enmeshed in a matrix stone. (Note the nature of the material surrounding the crystals.)

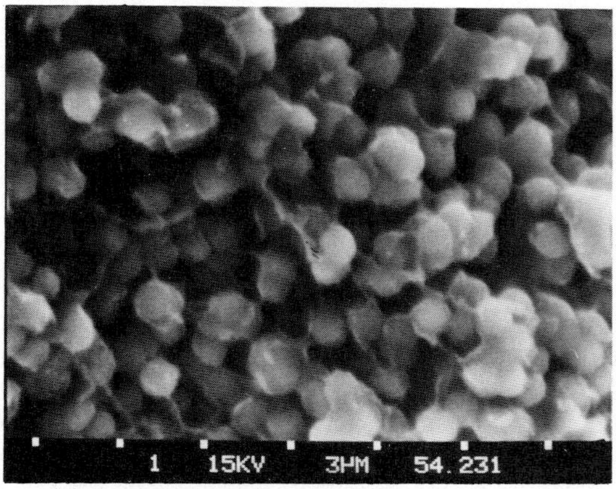

Fig. 6-10. Apatite spherules linked by mucoid material.

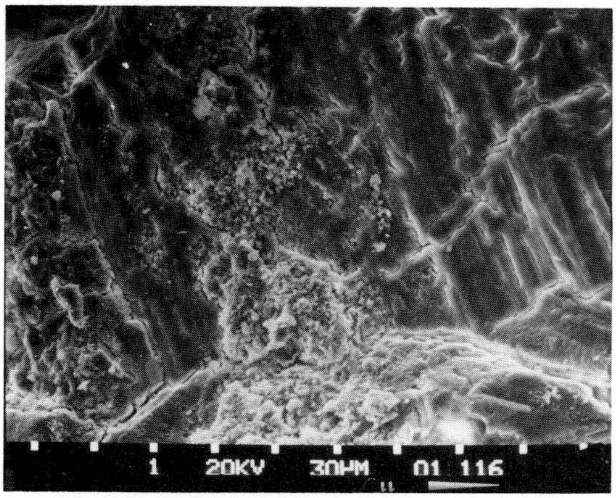

Fig. 6-11. Large struvite concrement intimately admixed with apatite deposits.

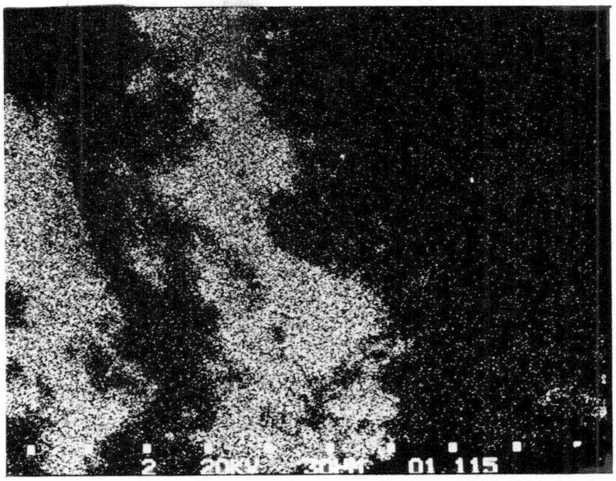

Fig. 6-12. X-ray elemental distribution map for calcium (viz., apatite) for the area shown in Figure 6-11. White dots correspond to presence of calcium.

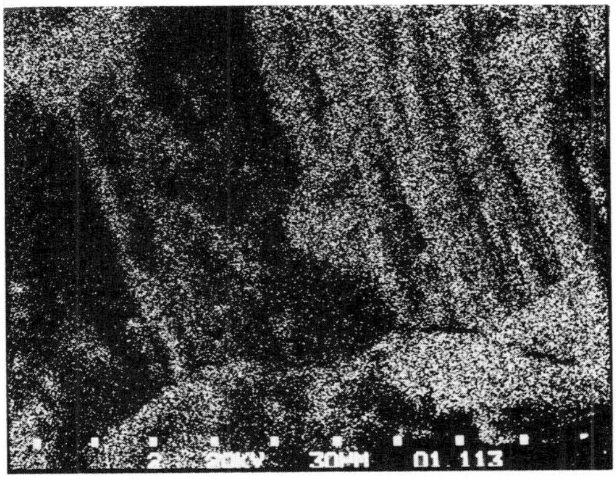

Fig. 6-13. X-ray elemental distribution map for magnesium (viz., struvite) for the area shown in Figure 6-11. White dots correspond to presence of magnesium.

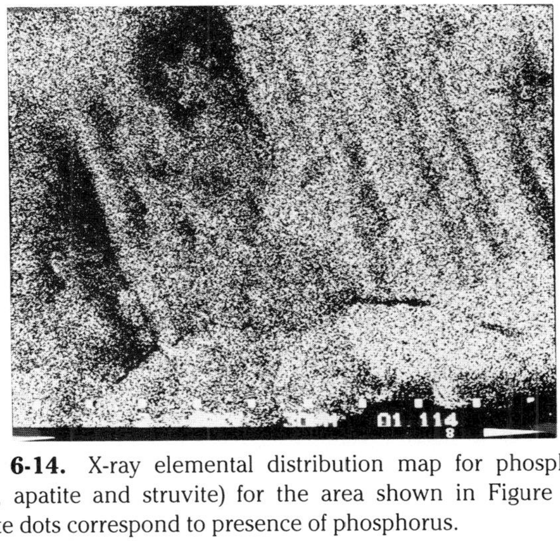

Fig. 6-14. X-ray elemental distribution map for phosphorus (viz., apatite and struvite) for the area shown in Figure 6-11. White dots correspond to presence of phosphorus.

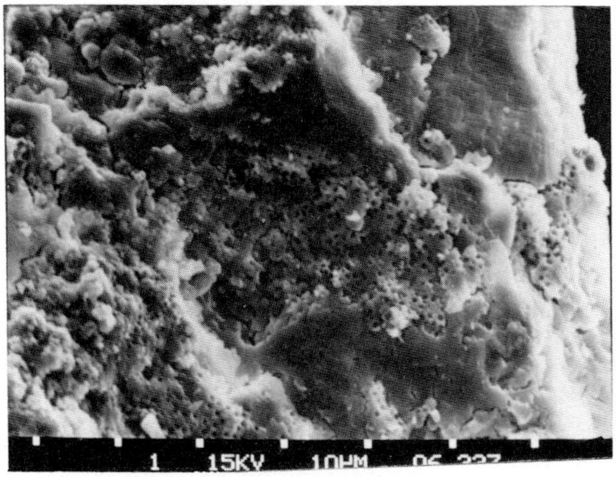

Fig. 6-15. Porous, spongelike appearance of apatite deposits (struvite also present). The holes are thought to be the sites from which calcified bacteria have been dislodged.

sents the phosphorus distribution. In this latter micrograph, the black areas correspond to the presence of matrix from which its "cementing" role can be reasonably envisaged.

Another ultrastructural pathogenic feature of stones is the appearance of small holes in apatite deposits. These have been previously reported for urinary and other calculi and are believed to arise from the dislodging of calcified bacteria.[23,33] An example is shown in Figure 6-15. A vein of apatite is seen within a large struvite substrate. Careful examination of the former clearly reveals a network of tiny holes—historical evidence of the presence of bacteria.

CRYSTALLIZATION EXPERIMENTS

An alternative approach that addresses the riddle of urinary stone morphogenesis (as opposed to pathogenesis) assumes that stone formation is governed and controlled mainly by crystallization phenomena, with the organic matrix as only a nonessential concomitance. According to this theory, supersaturation of urine is the most fundamental step in the formation of a concretion. Classical thermodynamics predicts that any supersaturated solution must eventually equilibrate by precipitation, a process that will cease only when the solution concerned is just (un)saturated. On one hand, kinetic factors might alter this precipitation process; on the other hand, metastable solutions might remain supersaturated until nucleation is induced by a seed crystal or other particle. In addition, the mechanisms of nucleation might be modified by the presence of surface-active inhibitors and epitaxially favorable nucleation sites. There are two further important steps in stone formation apart from supersaturation and nucleation: growth and aggregation of the formed crystals. As with nucleation, crystal growth might also be affected by inhibitors or promoters that may either retard or accelerate the growth of crystallites. Aggregation mechanisms such as polymeric bridging or aggregation by reduction of the zeta potential will be similarly influenced. The four main crystallization *real urine* *artificial urine*

STAGNANT SYSTEM

MSMPR CRYSTALLIZER

FAST EVAPORATOR

Fig. 6-16. Experimental arrangements used for the study of urinary crystallization characteristics.

approaches to the investigation of urinary stone formation thus involve examination of (1) the relationship between the concentrations of the precipitating substances in urine and their solubilities, (2) the role of nucleating substances, (3) crystal aggregation, and (4) the role of inhibitors of nucleation, crystal growth, and aggregation.[41]

Many different methods and experimental setups have been utilized to study the crystallization mechanisms of stone formation mentioned above (see Fig. 6-16). Some researchers have used a technique in which component ions are permitted to diffuse into a stagnant urine solution, causing encrustations to grow on fibers suspended in the medium.[42–44] Chemical supersaturation is reached by the gradual addition of ions. This may be achieved using a simple "paper wick technique"[45] or more sophisticated gel systems.[46–48] Others have examined the inhibitory effects of certain ions and compounds, again employing static supersaturated systems.[49–51] On the other hand, the concept of the urinary tract as a biologic analog of a sequence of continuous crystallizers has enjoyed much support since its initial description by Finlayson et al.[52,53] Many studies have been conducted in such mixed-suspension–mixed-product-removal (MSMPR) crystallizers.[54–57] Figure 6-17 depicts a typical continuous crystallization reaction chamber used for such studies.

The Coulter counter is another useful instrument for studying the qualitative and quantitative effect of inhibitors on nucleation and particle growth.[58,59] With the use of this instrument, ex vivo measurements of crystal distribution permit comparisons between the urines of stone formers and normal controls or examination of changes in standard synthetic urines after the addition of inhibiting substances.[60,61] Hallson and Rose employed yet another approach in which human urine samples were subjected to rapid

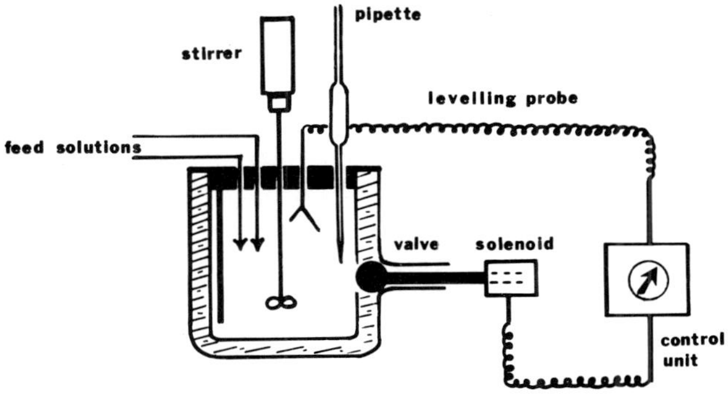

Fig. 6-17. Continuous crystallizer reaction chamber.

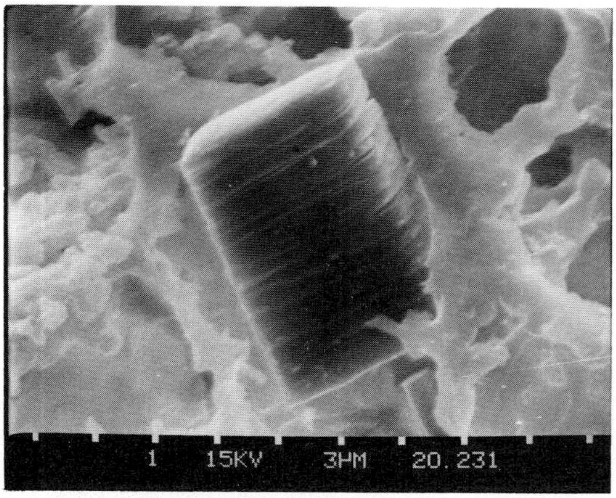

Fig. 6-18. Single crystal of calcium oxalate trihydrate obtained from a crystallization experiment using a synthetic urine in a rotary evaporator.

evaporation at 37 °C.[62,63] This process is thought to be analogous to the concentration of urine in the renal tubules, whereby water is removed and a state of supersaturation is maintained.

Much interesting data have been accumulated as a result of these different experimental approaches. The first concerns the role of the species calcium oxalate trihydrate (COT) (Fig. 6-18), which seldom, if ever, occurs in urine or calculi but frequently appears in crystallization experiments. Lyon and Vemeulen[42] and Gardner[64] have reported COT to be the initial phase precipitating from solutions supersaturated with respect to calcium oxalate. Indeed, it has been suggested that initially formed COT readily undergoes transformation to COM[65] and is a thermodynamically unstable precursor thereof.[66]

Although brushite has been found to precipitate at pH values as high as 7[67,68] and can also form in the pH range 7.0–7.4 under certain conditions,[69] it is seldom detected in urinary stones.[70,71] The observation, however, that brushite forms a thin surface layer around some apatite–brushite calculi[72] led to the suggestion that brushite may serve as the crystal nidus and precursor of calcium phosphate calculi.[73,74]

A role similar to that discussed above for brushite is thought to occur with octacalcium phosphate (OCP). There are a number of indications that OCP acts as a precursor to other solid phases, especially hydroxyapatite (HAP). Transformation of OCP to HAP has been observed, and both crystal structures have many similarities. It has been suggested that the transition layer between HAP and the aqueous phase consists of half a unit cell of OCP.[75] Both OCP and brushite are known to hydrolize to more basic calcium phosphates. Despite the fact that both compounds are more soluble than HAP,[76] they form under many different physiologic conditions. This is particularly the case with brushite. It has been suggested that the preferential formation of brushite (and OCP) is a kinetic phenomenon, yet the exact mechanisms allowing their precipitation are not yet known.[75] One reason might be that precipitation from aqueous solutions of hydrated compounds seems to be preferred for various reasons.[75]

It should be pointed out that tricalcium phosphate or whitlockite has also been proposed as a precursor of apatite formation.[77] It is apparently stabilized by magnesium ions and other small divalent cations that substitute for calcium in the crystal lattice.[78,79] In such cases, whitlockite might be even more stable than the microcrystalline apatite usually found in biologic concretions.

The role of apatite itself was demonstrated as early as 1932 by Schleede et al., who showed that all calcium phosphates will eventually transform into apatite when water is allowed to flush out excess phosphate radicals from the precursors' lattices.[80] This early observation might explain why apatite is usually the only calcium phosphate that is coprecipitated with struvite, since the latter captures most of the phosphate, leaving little for the formation of other calcium phosphates.

As far as uric acid and uric acid dihydrate (UAD) are concerned, it is interesting to note that the latter is seldom found in calculi. It has been suggested that this is due to its spontaneous dehydration to the thermodynamically more stable anhydrous acid.[81] Other workers have reported that it is mostly high molecular weight ($>$20,000) organic substances in urine that decrease the incidence of UAD in stones.

The role of urea in (calcium oxalate) stone formation is not clear. Miller et al. reported that the peptizing action of urea might be a factor in increasing the solubility of calcium oxalate in urine, causing a "supersolubility" of this compound in urine relative to water.[82] On the other hand, Finlayson et al. believe that the effect of urea on divalent ion activity is sufficiently small to justify its omission from first order considerations.[53] Further experiments are therefore needed to clarify the extent to which urea plays a role in calcium oxalate formation.

The role of macromolecules in stone morphogenesis is currently receiving much attention and has been extensively studied in a variety of crystallization experiments. Recently, isolated mucoproteins have been shown to promote precipitation of all the more important stone salts.[83,84] In contrast, other human urinary macromolecules are believed to have a protective (inhibitory) effect on the crystallization or agglomeration of stone salts.[85–87] Low-molecular-weight substances present in urine have also been shown to prevent calcification.[88,89] Amongst these are natural inhibitors such as citrate, pyrophosphate, and magnesium. Synthetic inhibitors such as diphosphonates are also very powerful in suppressing precipitation and aggregation of crystals.[90,91] Promotors and inhibitors of stone formation are thus thought to be another important factor in modifying urine crystallization parameters.

In concluding this section on crystallization experiments, the reader might very well wonder to what extent these experiments have yielded useful results. After all, dissolution of already existing calculi by a conservative medicinal treatment as well as prophylactic oral medication to prevent stone recurrence must clearly be the ultimate goals of such research. At the very simplest level it can be stated that, as a result of the studies previously described, current modes of therapy are mostly directed toward reducing urinary (super)saturation of stone-forming salts. If a state of undersaturation can be reached, existing stones should dissolve. The validity of this hypothesis has been demonstrated by local irrigation of calculi and their dissolution with (calcium) chelating agents.[92,93] Shifting of pH of urine to render it less congenial for stone formation is another approach to the dissolution of calculi based on crystallization theory. In this way, struvite stones in rats were dissolved by acidification of urine,[93a] while dissolution of uric acid calculi in humans was achieved by rigorously monitored alkalinization of urine.[94] In addition, moderately successful therapeutic regimens have been developed for all types of stones over the past 20 years.

ANIMAL MODELS

Extensive research involving the use of animal models, in particular the rat, has provided a wealth of meaningful data with respect to the pathogenesis of urinary calculi in humans. In contrast to humans, spontaneous urolithiasis is quite rare in rats, especially the calcium oxalate type; however, oxalate metabolism is virtually identical.[95] This together with the fact that the rat is the most readily available and commonly used laboratory animal, has resulted in numerous studies of calcium oxalate urolithiasis involving this species. An excellent review of the topic has recently been published.[95]

The disease is experimentally induced in rats by rendering the subjects hyperoxaluric. Several different methods have been employed in this regard. The main mechanism is via the addition of oxalate[96] or a precursor thereof[97,98] to the diet or by intraperitoneal injection.[99,100] It can also be induced by other dietary protocols such as pyridoxine-deficient diets[101] and low-phosphate diets.[102] Some examples follow.

Gregory et al. fed their rats diets that were supplemented with sodium or ammonium oxalate and calcium or ammonium chloride.[96] Sodium oxalate induced crystals of triple phosphate in the urine, while ammonium oxalate caused renal or bladder stones. Supplementation with calcium or ammonium chloride resulted in lower pH values, while the former also caused a lowering of urinary oxalate.

Studies utilizing intraperitoneal injections of sodium oxalate have permitted investigation of the kinetics of calcium oxalate nephrolithiasis[103] as well as the early phases of calcium oxalate formation in the rat kidney.[104] Histologic studies revealed that calcium oxalate crystals initially formed within the lumen or proximal tubules. Related ultrastructural studies described cellular debris and membranous and fibrillar material closely associated with intratubular calcium oxalate crystals.[105] More recently, damage of tubular epithelium from proximal tubule to the collecting ducts was shown to occur.[106]

Gershoff and Andrus administered vitamin B_6–deficient diets to investigate various metabolic parameters associated with calcium oxalate formation in rat kidneys.[107,108] Roberts and Finlayson later described the histologic changes associated with intrarenal crystal formation in stump-tailed monkeys administered ethylene glycol (a metabolic precursor of oxalic acid) and reported the presence of calcium oxalate crystals in proximal and distal tubules.[109]

One metabolic parameter that has received attention in numerous experimental and clinical studies has been urinary magnesium. Many studies have demonstrated that renal tubular calcium phosphate deposits can be produced by magnesium depletion in animals.[110,111] In a recent study magnesium deficiency was found to markedly enhance calcium oxalate renal tubular crystal deposits in rats on hyperoxaluric diets involving ethylene glycol administration over a period of several weeks.[98,112] These studies confirmed the early results of Gershoff and Andrus, who had suggested that magnesium deficiency might enhance renal tubular calcium oxalate formation in hyperoxaluric rats.[108] Related clinical investigations have reported low magnesium:calcium ratios in the urine of recurrent calcium oxalate stone formers[113] and have found magnesium hydroxide therapy to be effective in the treatment of individuals with renal stone disease.[114]

More recent studies using the rat model have shown that calcium oxalate monohydrate crystals predominate in the urines of hyperoxaluric and hypomagnesuric subjects while dihydrate crystals are the primary constituent of urines from rats administered ethylene glycol alone.[115] Since clinical studies of crystalluria have noted that the dihydrate predominates in the urine of controls and stone formers, the identification of COM

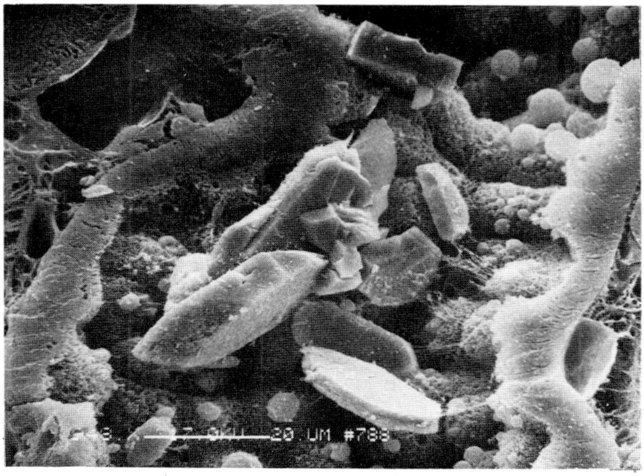

Fig. 6-19. Calcium oxalate crystals in the renal tube of a rat maintained on a hyperoxaluric–hypomagnesuric protocol.[112] Strandlike material appears to contribute to the adherence of the crystals to the luminal surface.

in the rat kidney is an important indicator of intranephronic calcium oxalate formation and the propensity toward stone formation. A similar correlation between monohydrate crystalluria and the propensity toward stone formation is also suggested by clinical data that show greater amounts of monohydrate in the crystalluria of stone formers than in the urines of non-stone-forming individuals.[116]

The role of matrix has also been demonstrated in many studies using animal models. Rushton et al., for example, reported that epithelium lining tubular lumina containing crystals frequently displayed a mucoid material emanating from their surfaces and adsorbed to both calcium oxalate and apatite deposits[112] (Figs. 6-19, and 6-20). This study showed that the mucoid material appears to be attaching crystal aggregates to the tubular

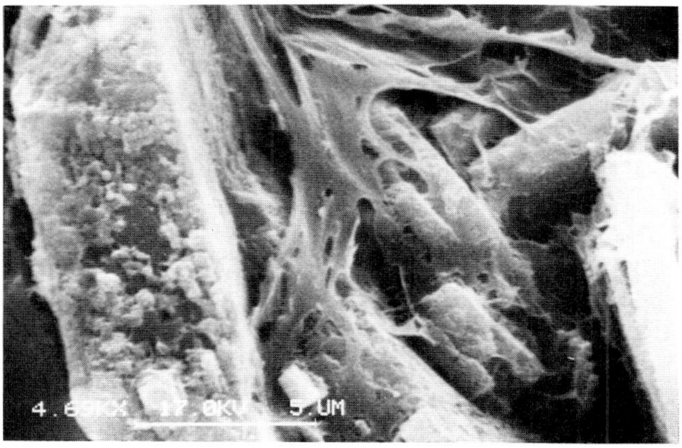

Fig. 6-20. Sheetlike mucoid substance on the surface of calcium oxalate crystals in rats in the same experiment as in Fig. 6-19.

walls. In some cases the matrix was strandlike in nature (Fig. 6-19) while in others it had a sheet or filmlike appearance (Fig. 6-20). It also occurred between individual platelike crystals (Fig. 6-20). In another study the mucoid material was observed as having a cementing action.[115] It is of some interest to note that cemented calcium oxalate monohydrate crystals have been observed in the nidi of renal stones induced in rats,[112] substantiating the hypothesis that the mucoid matrix plays a role in stone pathogenesis. That the above observations are a good model for gaining insight into the role of matrix in human urolithiasis is provided by the results of a study by Ogbuji and Finlayson.[26] They found that in human COM calculi, the matrix is sandwiched between the crystals and suggest that this could be responsible for cohesion in these stones.

Transmission electron microscopy of the renal tubules of rats on hyperoxaluric and hypomagnesuric protocols recently revealed for the first time the presence of crystals within cells (Figs. 6-21A and 6-21B), (unpublished results of the authors and A. W. Fogle). These crystals had profiles consistent in appearance with calcium oxalate. Intracellular crystals have gone previously unrecognized for a number of reasons. Conventional light-microscope embedding and sectioning procedures are inadequate for clear identification. In addition, identification of intracellular crystals is often obscured by tubular destruction from intraluminal crystal deposits. Preservation of crystalline material during preparation and thin sectioning of specimens for TEM is difficult. Our recent results were obtained by employing special techniques to preserve the tissue for study by light microscopy and TEM.

While the tubular reabsorption of calcium is well documented, until recently little has been known about the renal handling of oxalate. Studies in rat kidneys show that oxalate is not only secreted by tubular cells, but also is simultaneously filtered at the glomerulus and reabsorbed by proximal tubular cells. Investigation of the renal handling of calcium and oxalate thus suggests that conditions conducive to calcium oxalate crystallization could exist intracellularly. These findings suggest the following as a mechanism of renal stone genesis. Hyperoxaluria induces an environment conducive to the formation of calcium oxalate crystals inside the cells as well as within the lumina of renal tubules. Intracellular crystal size and number increase until cellular degeneration and destruction occur. Disruption and subsequent sloughing of the tubular cells introduce calcium oxalate crystals and cell debris into the tubular lumen. Cellular debris and other amorphous substances that coat the crystals aid in their retention to luminal walls. Fixed within the tubule, crystals undergo further growth and aggregation. Some aggregates become freed from the tubule and reach the renal pelvis, where they serve as the nidus of a renal stone.

"Is calcium oxalate urolithiasis in the rat a model for human stone disease?" is the question posed by Khan and Hackett in their excellent review.[95] They conclude that in a number of respects, it is. To begin with, these workers make the point that study of the two key processes in stone formation, that of nucleation and growth, is possible by use of the rat model. Their view shows that virtually all in vivo experimentations carried out in the past have utilized hyperoxaluria as the pathogenic factor. In human stone formation various physicochemical studies have revealed that hyperoxaluric conditions favor calcium oxalate crystalluria more than do hypercalciuric factors.[117,118] Khan and Hackett thus conclude that the hyperoxaluric rat has been, and still is, a valuable model for calcium oxalate stone disease.[95]

Utilization of this model has permitted investigation of the interaction between deposited crystals and renal or urothelial tissues and has provided much useful data for

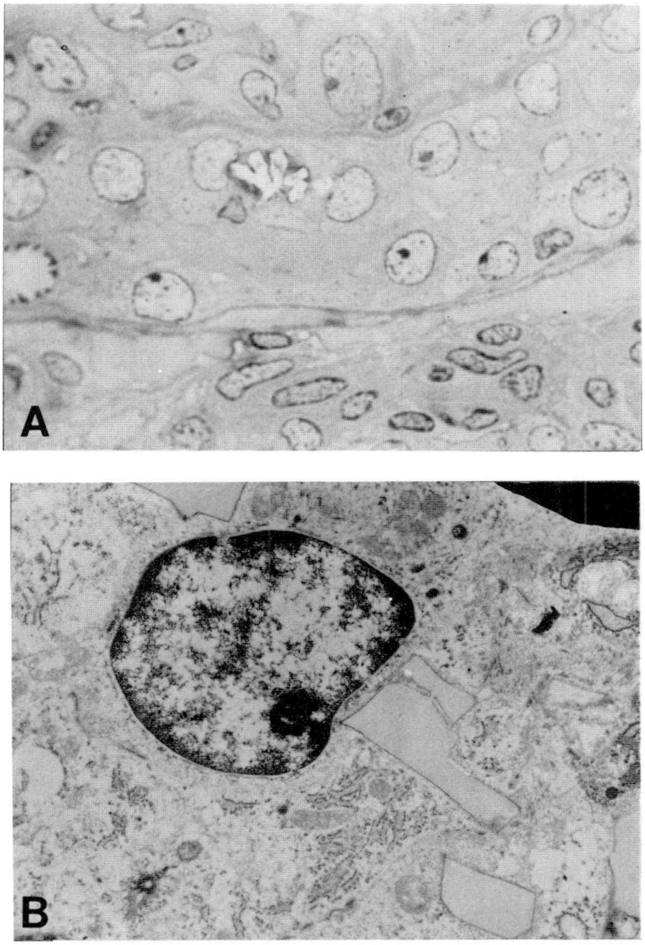

Fig. 6-21. Light microscopy (*A*, original magnification 1125×) and TEM (*B*, original magnification 9450×) of crystallites within renal tubular cells in rats after 9 weeks in a hyperoxaluric regimen.

the understanding of crystal entrapment.[119] Cell injury has been a common feature in renal crystal deposition experiments.[98,104,115,120] Such experiments have shown that crystals are often associated with cell debris similar to that observed in human urinary calculi. Exposure of the basement membrane as a result of sloughing of epithelial cells might provide sites at which crystals could become trapped.[106] Renal tubular damage has also been identified in human urolithiasis in the form of matrix substance A (MSA) and Tamm-Horsfall mucoprotein (THM), both of which are associated with renal injury and occur in stones and in high concentrations in the urine of stone formers.[37,104,121,122] Khan and Hackett draw attention to other experimental data that point to renal tubular damage.[95] These include the urinary enzyme patterns of stone patients[123] and morphologic evidence in papillectomy specimens from a stone patient.[124]

The precise role played by renal injury in the evolution of stone disease is as yet unresolved. The questions that have to be addressed are somewhat similar to those pertaining to the role of matrix, specifically, whether renal injury (or matrix) is a primary initiating factor or is secondary. If, indeed, it is the latter, is it capable of promoting increased crystallization or is it in fact inactive with no role whatsoever?

As far as matrix is concerned, the experimental rat model evidence strongly suggests a binding or cementing role for the mucoid material.[98,115] All experimentally induced or spontaneously formed calcium oxalate crystals appear to have an organic coating[95] similar to that observed in human calculi.

From the aforegoing it may be reasonably concluded that animal studies, in particular those involving the rat, have afforded researchers much useful data and have extended their understanding of the development mechanisms of stone morphogenesis.

CONCLUDING COMMENTS

While the different scientific approaches have yielded a wealth of meaningful data that have spawned theories concerning stone morphogenesis and pathogenesis, it should be pointed out that a few of the more popular hypotheses have failed to impress some of the most respected workers in this field. Thus it is, for example, that Finlayson et al. write concerning the role of epitaxy that it is "unfortunate that Lonsdale was so well respected because many times a stake has been driven through the chest of that idea and a silver cross hung on its gravestone, only to find the idea living and well in some remote and unaccessible region of an unorganized thought process." Finlayson and coworkers argue that good two-dimensional matches do not guarantee a three-dimensional match and that strain energy arising from lattice distortion while "forcing" such a match is the primary consideration.

The same workers also suggest that the species COT is not an important factor in urinary stone disease.[31] They cite in vitro crystallization experiments that show that the uninhibited transformation of COT to COM has a relaxation time of a few hours. In real urine there are many substances that inhibit this transformation thereby lengthening the relaxation time.

The concept of polycrystalline aggregation also leaves Finlayson et al. somewhat "uncomfortable."[31] They maintain that many stones grow, at least in part, by defect growth and that this appears to be more so the case when crystallite size is large.

Despite these "disagreements" with theories that are popular in many quarters, Finlayson et al. suggest that stone formation mechanisms are characterized by several distinct physical phenomena.[31] These are nucleation, crystal growth, aggregation, adsorption (of material from urine onto crystal surfaces thereby affecting mass acquisition kinetics), and matrix involvement. They further hypothesize that cellular injury is a preliminary to stone disease. The suggested sequence of events involves the establishment of a "receptive encrustation platform" at the site of the dystrophic mineralization.

While there are several areas of stone morphogenesis and pathogenesis that remain controversial and unresolved, certain basic physicochemical principles thus dictate the general pathways along which scientific and clinical research must be directed. The subtleties of the intricate mechanisms are beginning to emerge as a result of enormous input from several disciplines. In the final analysis, this kind of multidisciplinary approach, in which clinicians of different specialties pool their impressive resources and brain power, is necessary for the riddle of stone morphogenesis and pathogenesis to ultimately be solved.

REFERENCES

1. Lonsdale K: Human stones. Science 195:1199–1297, 1968
2. Lonsdale K: Human Stones. Sci Am 104–111, 1968
3. Rodgers AL, Spector M: Human stones. Endeavors 5:119–126, 1981
4. Butt AJ: Historical survey of etiologic factors in renal lithiasis, in Butt AJ (ed): Etiologic Factors in Renal Lithiasis. Springfield, IL, Thomas, 1956, pp 3–47
5. Clarke ES: Renal calculi—a history of the stone. Hops Med 2:1054–1057, 1968
6. Modlin M: A history of urinary stone. S Afr Med J 58:652–655, 1980
7. Hesse A, Hickurg W, Vahlensieck W: Harsteinanalyse und ihre diagnostische bedeuturg. GIT Labor-Med 4:19–27, 1981
8. Hesse A, Vahlensieck W: Indizienbeweise durch die harnesteinstruktur. Forsch Mitteill Dtsch Forchungsgem 2:6–8, 1983
9. Pak CYC: Disorders of stone formation, in Bremmer B, Rector F (eds): The Kidney, Vol 11. Philadelphia, WB Saunders, 1976, pp 1326–1354
10. Blacklock NJ: Epidemiology of urolithiasis, in Williams DI, Chisholm GD (eds): Scientific Foundations of Urology. London, William Heinemann Medical Books, 1982, pp 235–243
11. Robertson WG, Peacock M, Heyburn PJ, et al: Should recurrent calcium oxalate stone formers eat less animal protein? in Smith LH, Robertson WG, Finlayson B (eds): Urolithiasis: Clinical and Basic Research. New York, Plenum Press, 1981, pp 901–906
12. Sutor DJ: Crystallographic studies on the formation of renal calculi. Biochem J 122:6–7, 1971
13. Prien EL: The riddle of urinary stone disease. JAMA, 216:503–507, 1971
14. Kleeman CR, Coburn JW, Brickman AS, et al: Kidney stones. West J Med 132:313–332, 1980
15. Finlayson B: Physicochemical aspects of urolithiasis. Kidney Internatl 13:344–360, 1978
16. Nancollas GH: The mechanisms of formation of renal stone crystals. Proc Ear Dial Transplant Assoc 20:386–397, 1983
17. Vermeulen CW, Ellis JE, Te-Chin H: Experimental observations on the pathogenesis of urinary calculi. J Urol 95:681–690, 1960
18. Nancollas GH: The kinetics of crystal growth and renal stone formation. Urolithiasis Res Proc Internatl Symp 3d, 1976, pp 5–23
19. Finlayson B: Calcium stones: Some physical and clinical aspects, in David DS (ed): Calcium Metabolism in Renal Failure and Nephrolithiasis. New York, Wiley, 1977, pp 337–383
20. Hesse A, Lange P, Berg W, et al: Scanning electron microscope and microprobe investigations of phosphate phases in uroliths. Urol Internatl 34:81–94, 1979
21. Hesse A, Berg W, Bothor C: Scanning electron microscope investigations on the morphology and phase conversions of uroliths. Internatl Urol Nephrol 11:11–20, 1979
22. Kim KM: X-ray analysis of pathological calcifications including urinary stones. Scan Electron Microsc II:739–744, 1979
23. Leusunann DB: Routine analysis of urinary calculi by scanning electron microscopy, Scan Electron Microsc I:387–396, 1983
24. Leusunann DB: Texture analysis of urinary concrements by SEM, in Ryall R, Brokis G, Marshall V, et al (eds): Urinary Stone. Edinburgh, Churchill Livingstone, 1984, pp 343–348
25. Meyer AS, Finlayson B, DuBois L: Direct observation of urinary stone ultrastructure, Br J Urol 43:154–163, 1971
26. Ogbuji LU, Finlayson B: Crystal morphologies in whewhellite stones: Electron microscopy. Invest Urol 19:182–186, 1981
27. Santos M, Gonzales-Diaz PF: Ultrastructural study of apatites in urinary calculi. Calcif Tiss Internatl 31:93–108, 1980
28. Spector M, Garden N, Rous S: Ultrastructural features of human urinary calculi, in Fleisch H, Robertson WG, Smith LH (eds): Urolithiasis Research. New York, Plenum Press, 1976, pp 355–359

29. Spector M, Garden N, Rous SN: Ultrastructure and pathogenesis of human urinary calculi. Br J Urol 50:12–15, 1978
30. Spector M, Jamieson L: Scanning electron microscopy of urinary calculi. Scan Electron Microsc II:307–314, 1976
31. Finlayson B, Khan SR, Hackett RL: Mechanisms of stone formation—an overview. Scan Electron Microsc III:1419–1425, 1984
32. Lonsdale K: Epitaxy as a growth factor in urinary calculi and gallstones. Nature 217:56–58, 1968
33. Rodgers AL: Common ultrastructural features in human calculi. Micron Microscopic Acta 14:219–226, 1983
34. Boyce WH, Garvey FK, Norfleet CM: Ion-bonding properties of electrophoretically homogeneous patients with renal calculus disease. J Urol 72:1019–1031, 1954
35. Boyce WH, Garvey FK, Norfleet CM: The metal chelate compounds of urine. Am J Med 19:87–95, 1955
36. Boyce WH, Garvey FK: The amount and nature of the organic matarix in urinary calculi: Review. J Urol 76:213–227, 1956
37. Boyce WH, King JS: Present concepts concerning the origin of matrix and stones. Ann NY Acad Sci 104:563–578, 1963
38. Cheng PT: Heterogeneity of renal stones from patients on continuous ambulatory peritoneal dialysis, in Ryall R, Brockis J, Marshall V, et al: (eds): Urinary Stone: Edinburgh, Churchill Livingstone, 1984, pp 318–323
39. Cheng PT, Reid AD, Pritzker KP: Ultrastructural studies of crystal–organic matrix relations in renal stones. Scan Electron Microsc I:201–207, 1985
40. Rodgers AL: The application of physico-chemical procedures in the analysis or urinary calculi. Scan Electron Microsc II:745–758, 1985
41. Fleisch H, Russell RG: Experimental and clinical studies with pyrophosphonate and diphosphonates, in David D (ed): Calcium Metabolism in Renal Failure and Nephrolithiasis. New York, Wiley, 1977, pp 293–336
42. Lyon ES, Vermeulen CW: Crystallization concepts and calculogenesis: Observations on artificial oxalate concretions. Invest Urol 3:309–320, 1965
43. Sutor DJ: Growth studies of calcium oxalate in the presence of various ions and compounds. Br J Urol 41:171–178, 1969
44. Welshman S, McGeown M: A quantitative investigation of the effects on the growth of calcium oxalate crystals on potential inhibitors. Br J Urol 44:677–680, 1972
45. Vermeulen CW, Lyon ES, Gill WB: Artificial urinary concretions. Invest Urol 1:370–386, 1964
46. Bisaillon S, Tawashi R: Growth of calcium oxalate in gel systems. J Pharm Sci 64:458–460, 1975
47. Bisaillon S, Tawashi R: Retardation of dissolution and growth of calcium oxalate monohydrate. J Pharm Sci 65:222–225, 1976
48. Phaneuf-Mimeault F, Tawashi R: Scanning electron microscopic study of calcium oxalate concretions grown in gel systems and calcium oxalate stones. Eur Urol 3:171–175, 1977
49. Meyer JL, Smith LH: Growth of calcium oxalate crystals. Invest Urol 13:31–35, 1975
50. Robertson WG, Peacock M, Nordin BEC: Inhibitors of the growth and aggregation of calcium oxalate crystals. Clin Chim Acta 43:31–37, 1973
51. Sutor DJ: Experiments on the nucleation and growth of calcium oxalate in normal and stone formers' urine. Urinary Calculi Proc Internatl Symp, 1973, pp 313–317
52. Finlayson B: The concept of a continuous crystallizer. Invest Urol 9:258–263, 1972
53. Finlayson B, DuBois L: Kinetics of calcium oxalate deposition in vitro. Invest Urol 10:429–433, 1973
54. Drach GW, Randolph AD, Miller JD: Inhibition of calcium oxalate dihydrate crystallization by chemical modifiers: I. Pyrophosphate and methylene blue. J Urol 119:99–103, 1978
55. Drach GW, Thomson S, Randolph A: Effects of urinary organic macromolecules on crystallization of calcium oxalate: Enhancement of nucleation. J Urol 123:519–523, 1980

56. Rodgers AL, Garsidi J: The nucleation and growth kinetics of calcium oxalate in the presence of some synthetic urine constituents. Invest Urol 18:484–488, 1981
57. Drach GW, Sprungman K, Gottung B, et al: Effects of human urine on the aggregation of calcium oxalate crystals: Normal persons versus stone-formers, in Schwille P, Smith L, Robertson W, et al (eds): Urolithiasis and Related Clinical Research. New York, Plenum Press, 1985, pp 875–878
58. Desmans JF, Tawashi R: Dissolution and growth of calcium oxalate monohydrate. I. Effect of magnesium and pH. Biochim Biophys Acta 313:256–267, 1973
59. Desjardins A, Tawashi R: Growth retardation of calcium oxalate by sodium copper cholorphyllium. Eur Urol 4:294–297, 1978
60. Robertson WG, Peacock M, Nordin B: Inhibitors of the growth and aggregation of calcium oxalate crystals. Clin Chim Acta 43:31–37, 1973
61. Ryall R, Bagley C, Marshall V: Independent assessment of the growth and aggregation of calcium oxalate crystals using the Coulter counter. Invest Urol 18:401–405, 1981
62. Hallson PC, Rose GA: A new urinary test for stone activity. Br J Urol 50:442–448, 1978
63. Hallson PC, Rose GA: The additive effects of magnesium and tartrate upon inhibition of calcium oxalate crystal formation in whole urine, in Schwille P, Smith L, Robertson W, et al (eds): Urolithiasis and Related Clinical Research. New York, Plenum Press, 1985, pp 847–850
64. Gardner GL: Nucleation and crystal growth of calcium oxalate trihydrate. J Cryst Growth 30:158–168, 1975
65. Gardner GL: Kinetics of the dehydration of calcium oxalate trihydrate crystals in aqueous solution. J Colloid Interface Sci 54:298–310, 1976
66. Tomazic BB, Nancollas GH: A study of the phase transformation of calcium oxalate trihydrate-monohydrate. Invest Urol 16:329–335, 1979
67. Newman WF, Newman MW: The Chemical Dynamics of Bone Mineral. University of Chicago Press, 1958, p 29
68. Francis MD, Webb NC: Hydroxyapatite formation from a hydrated calcium monohydrogen phosphate precursor. Calcif Tiss Res 6:335–342, 1971
69. Furedi-Milhofer H, Purgaric B, Brecevic L, et al: Precipitation of calcium phosphates from electrolyte solutions. 1. A study of the precipitates in the physiological pH region, Calcif Tiss Res 8:142–153, 1971
70. Herring LC: Observations on the analysis of ten thousand urinary calculi. J Urol 88:545–562, 1962
71. Morriss RH, Beeler MF: X-ray diffraction analysis of 464 urinary calculi. Ann J Clin Pathol 48:413–417, 1967
72. Lagergren C: Biophysical investigations of urinary calculi. Acta Radiol Suppl 133:1–71, 1956
73. Pak C, Eanes E, Ruskin B: Spontaneous precipitation of brushite in urine: Evidence that brushite is the nidus of renal stones originating as calcium phosphate. Proc Natl Acad Sci (USA) 68:1456–1460, 1971
74. Pak C, Chu S: A simple technique for the determination of urinary state of saturation with respect to brushite. Invest Urol 11:211–215, 1973
75. Young RA, Brown WE: Structures of biological minerals, in Nancollas G (ed): Biological Mineralization and Demineralization. Berlin, Springer, 1982, pp 101–141
76. Nancollas GH: Phase transformation during precipitation of calcium salts, in Nancollas G (ed): Biological Mineralization and Demineralization. Berlin, Springer, 1982, pp 79–99
77. Francis MD, Webb NC: Hydroxyapatite formation from a hydrated calcium monohydrogen phosphate precursor. Calcif Tiss Res 6:335–342, 1971
78. Altschuler ZS: The weathering of phosphate deposits-geochemical and environmental aspects, in Griffith E, Beeton A (eds): Environmental Phosphorus Handbook. New York, Wiley, 1973, pp 33–96
79. Trautz OR, Zapanta RR: Effect of magnesium on various calcium phosphates. J Dent Res 41:28, 1962

80. Schleede A, Schmidt W, Kindt H: Zur Kenntnis der calcium phosphate und apatite. Z Elektrochem 33:633–641, 1932
81. Hesse A, Schneider H, Berg W, et al: Uric acid dihydrate as urinary calculus component. Invest Urol 12:405–409, 1975
82. Miller GH, Vermeulen CW, Moore JD: Calcium oxalate solubility in urine. Experimental urolithiasis XIV. J Urol 79:607, 1958
83. Hallson PC, Rose GA: Uromucoids and urinary stone formation. Lancet 1:1000–1002, 1979
84. Paternain JL, Bershtam J, Pinto B: Isolation of a mucoprotein processing mineral nucleating activity. Invest Urol 18:119–122, 1980
85. Gill WB, Karesh JW: Demonstration of protective (inhibitory) effects of urinary macromolecules on the crystallization of calcium oxalate. Urolithiasis Res Proc Internatl Symp 3d, 1976, pp 227–280
86. Leal JJ, Finlayson B: Adsorption of naturally occurring polymers onto calcium oxalate crystal surfaces. Invest Urol 14:278–283, 1977
87. Robertson WG, Knowles F, Peacock M: Urinary acid mucopolysaccharide inhibitors of calcium oxalate crystallization. Urolithiasis Res Proc Internatl Symp 3d, 1976, pp 331–334
88. Barber LM, Howard JE: Simple synthetic and natural urines have equivalent anticalcifying properties. Invest Urol 12:79–81, 1974
89. Finlayson B: Renal lithiasis in review. Urol Clin N Am 1:181–212, 1974
90. Fleisch H: Inhibitors and promotors of stone formation. Kidney Internatl 13:361–371, 1978
91. Pak C, Ohata M, Holt K: Effect of diphosphonate on crystallization of calcium oxalate in vitro. Kidney Internatl 7:154–160, 1975
92. Mulvaney WP, Henning DC: Solvent treatment of urinary calculi: Refinements in technique. J Urol 88:145–149, 1962
93. Zvolkowski F, Perrin D: Dissolution of urinary stones by calcium-chelating agents. Invest Urol 15:208–211, 1977
93a. Vermeulen CW, Ragins HD, Grove WJ, et al: Experimental urolithiasis III—prevention and dissolution of calculi by alteration of urinary pH. J Urol 66:1–5, 1951
94. Vermeulen CW, Lyons ES, Fried FA: On the nature of the stone forming process. J Urol 94:176–186, 1965
95. Khan SR, Hackett RL: Calcium oxalate urolithiasis in the rat: Is it a model for human stone disease? Scan Electron Microsc II:759–774, 1985
96. Gregory JG, Park KY, Burns T: The interaction of urinary oxalate, calcium and pH in renal calculus formation as demonstrated in a rat model, in Ryall R, Brockis J, Marshall V, et al (eds): Urinary Stone. New York, Churchill Livingstone, 1984, pp 355–362
97. Lyon ES, Borden TA, Vermeulen CW: Experimental oxalate lithiasis produced with ethylene glycol. Invest Urol 4:143–151, 1966
98. Rushton HG, Spector M, Rodger AL, et al: Crystal deposition in the renal tubules of hyperoxaluric and hypomagnesemic rats. Scan Electron Microsc III:387–398, 1980
99. Khan SR, Finlayson B, Hackett R: Experimental induction of crystalluria in rats using urine osmotic pumps. Urol Res 11:199–205, 1983
100. Tawashi R, Cousineau M, Sharkawi M: Calcium oxalate crystal formation in the kidneys of rats injected with 4-hydroxy-L-proline. Urol Res 8:121–127, 1980
101. Gershoff SN: Production of urinary calculi in vitamin B_6 deficient male, female, and castrated male rat. J Nutr 100:117–122, 1970
102. Werness PG, Knox FG, Smith LH: Low phosphate diet in rats: A model for calcium oxalate urolithiasis, in Smith L, Robertson W, Finlayson B (eds): Urolithiasis, Clinical and basic Research. New York Plenum Press, 1981, pp 731–734
103. Jordan WR, Finlayson B, Luxenberg M: Kinetics of early time calcium oxalate nephrolithiasis. Invest Urol 15:465–468, 1978
104. Khan SR, Finlayson B, Hackett RL: Histological study of the early events in oxalate induced intranephronic calculosis. Invest Urol 17:199–202, 1979

105. Dykstra MJ, Hackett RL: Ultrastructural events in early calcium oxalate crystal formation in rats. Kidney Internatl 15:64, 1975
106. Khan SR, Finlayson B, Hackett RL: Experimental calcium oxalate nephrolithiasis in the rat, role of renal papilla. Am J Pathol 107:59–69, 1982
107. Gershoff SN, Andrus SB: Dietary magnesium calcium and vitamin B_6 and experimental nephropathies in rats: Calcium oxalate calculi, apatite nephrocalcinosis. J Nutr 73:308–316, 1961
108. Gershoff SN, Andrus SB: Effect of vitamin B_6 and magnesium on renal deposition of calcium oxalate induced by ethylene glycol. Proc Soc Exp Biol 109:99, 1962
109. Roberts JA, Finlayson B: Oxalate nephrocalcinosis from ethylene glycol in monkeys, in Finlayson B, Thomas W (eds): Colloquium 5th Renal Lithiasis. Gainesville, University Press of Florida, 1976, pp 157–167
110. Whang R, Welt L: Observations in experimental magnesium depletion. J Clin Invest 42:305–313, 1963
111. Oliver J, Macdowell M, Whang R: The renal lesions of electrolyte imbalance. IV. The intranephronic calculosis of experimental magnesium depletion. J Exp Med 124:263–265, 1966
112. Rushton HG, Spector M, Rodgers AL, et al: Developmental aspects of calcium oxalate tubular deposits and calculi induced in rat kidneys. Invest Urol 19:52–57, 1981
113. Evans RA, Forbes MA, Sutton R, et al: Urinary excretion of calcium and magnesium in patients with calcium-containing renal stones. Lancet 4:958, 1957
114. Johanson G, Backman U, Ljungall S: Biochemical and clinical effects of the prophylactic treatment of renal calcium stones with magnesium hydroxide. J Urol 124:770, 1980
115. Rushton HG, Spector M: Effects of magnesium deficiency on intratubular calcium oxalate formation and crystalluria in hyperoxaluric rats. J Urol 127:598–604, 1982
116. Elliot JS, Rabinowitz IN: Calcium oxalate crystalluria: Crystal size in urine. J Urol 123:324–327, 1980
117. Finlayson B: Physicochemical aspects of urolithiasis. Kidney Internatl 13:334–360, 1978
118. Robertson WG, Nordin BE: Physicochemical factors governing stone formation, in Williams D, Chisholm G (eds): Scientific Foundations of Urology. London, Heinemann, 1976, pp 254–267
119. Finlayson B, Reid F: The expectation of free and fixed particles in urinary stone disease. Invest Urol 15:442–448, 1978
120. McIntosh GH, Belling GB, Bulman FH: Experimental oxalate urolith formation in rats. Aust J Exp Biol Med Sci 57:251–259, 1979
121. King JS: Currents in renal stone research. Clin Chem 17:971–982, 1971
122. Thorne I, Resnick M: Urinary macromolecules and renal lithiasis. World J Urol 1:138–145, 1983
123. Baggio B, Gambaro G, Ossi E, et al: Increased urinary excretion of renal enzymes in idiopathic calcium oxalate nephrolithiasis. J Urol 129:1161–1162, 1983
124. Khan SR, Finlayson B, Hackett RL: Renal papillary changes in patient with calcium oxalate lithiasis. Urology 23:194–199, 1984

PART II

Medical Treatment and Management of the Urolithiasis Patient

Stephen B. Erickson

7

Idiopathic Nephrolithiasis

Urolithiasis is a common affliction in the Western world. Most of these stones form in the upper urinary tract and are calcareous in nature. The causes of calcium nephrolithiasis are multiple—that is, formation of calcium-containing renal stones is the final common pathway for a diverse range of dietary, metabolic, and anatomic disorders. These next three chapters will consider the epidemiology, etiology, diagnosis, treatment, and follow-up of the most common calcium stone-forming states.

EPIDEMIOLOGY

Some of our best demographic data have been gathered from Olmsted County in southeastern Minnesota during the years 1950 to 1974.[11] This is the county that contains the city of Rochester and the Mayo Clinic. Because the local residents seldom go outside of this county for medical care, excellent records exist for calculation of demographic data. Prevalence data show that 12 percent of men and 5 percent of women over age 70 have experienced stones at some point in their lives. Furthermore, the incidence of stones is increasing among men, to 124 per 100,000 population; the incidence among women is stable at 36 per 100,000.

The Stone Analysis Laboratory of the Mayo Clinic analyzes nearly all stones from Olmsted County residents as well as from patients who live throughout much of the Upper Midwest. Approximately 60 percent of all stones analyzed are calcium oxalate or phosphate. Olmsted County data show that 77.5 percent of stone formers are men.[11] Men are 4 to 5 times more likely than women to form idiopathic calcium stones. Idiopathic calcium-stone formation is rare in children.

In several countries, the effect of life-style on stone formation has been studied. Those who are sedentary are more prone to form stones.[33] Those living in large urban areas seem to be more susceptible.[19] How much of this difference may be ascribed to diet,

STONE DISEASE: DIAGNOSIS AND MANAGEMENT

ISBN 0-8089-1873-7

as opposed to occupation, is unknown. Occupation does appear to have a role in stone formation. In some studies, white collar workers are more disposed to stone formation;[12,34] however, those in occupations associated with heat exposure also are at high risk.[9,35] Major contributing factors in these jobs are probably excessive fluid losses through perspiration and infrequent opportunities to drink fluid. Either situation would lead to a low urine volume and a urine more saturated in stone-forming salts.

Geography also seems to influence stone formation. In Israel and throughout the Middle East, stone formation is common. The United States purportedly has a "stone belt" in the Southeast, although supporting data are weak. Climate no doubt plays a role. Water composition may contribute; however, studies are inconclusive, some showing soft-water areas to predominate in stone prevalence and others showing no difference between hard- and soft-water areas.[3,6,7,28,29]

Regional dietary preferences certainly would be expected to alter urinary composition—for example, the high prevalence of stones in Olmsted County may reflect its location in the dairy belt. Genetics may be important—for example, it is known that absorptive hypercalciuria may be familial and presumably is inherited in a dominant pattern with a preference for males. A family history positive for stones is common in calcareous stone formers.

Blacks seldom form idiopathic calcium-containing stones. The discovery of a calcium oxalate or phosphate stone in a person of pure black ancestry should prompt a search for a secondary cause. Unfortunately, blacks are not so protected from other types of stone formation.

Stone recurrence is common. Olmsted County data document that, by 5 years after the passage of the first stone, 25 percent of the patients had experienced recurrence; by 10 years the proportion is about 35 percent.[11]

CAUSATIVE FACTORS FOR CALCIUM OXALATE OR PHOSPHATE STONES IN NORMOCALCEMIC NORMOCALCIURIC PATIENTS

Some calcium-containing stones have well-defined causes. Primary hyperparathyroidism, distal renal tubular acidosis, enteric hyperoxaluria, and sarcoidosis are a few examples. (These are covered in other chapters.) Most calcium stones are not signs of another disease as such; however, risk factors for stone formation abound. Hypercalciuria is the best known, although probably not the most important, risk factor. (It is discussed in a later chapter.) Other risk factors include low urine volume, hyperoxaluria, hypocitraturia, hyperuricosuria, and lack of inhibitors of crystallization. Even in view of these risk factors, there remains a group of calcium stone formers who have no identified abnormality. These constitute 19 percent of our stone-forming population,[32] and we call them *idiopathic stone formers.*

We have hypothesized that idiopathic stone formers have the same risk factors as do the other subgroups of normocalcemic normocalciuric stone formers but that we simply have not looked for the factors in the right way. Traditionally, the risk factors mentioned above have been assessed in 24-hour urine specimens. It is possible that fluxes in urine mineral content occur, especially postprandially, so that the supersaturation levels required to form stones are exceeded transiently. When averaged over 24 hours, these fluxes may disappear. We have published preliminary evidence supporting this view.[8]

In this study, patients given calcitriol orally were fed a physiologic breakfast. Postprandially, urine crystal counts and supersaturation for calcium salts were transiently elevated to a significant degree compared with control values. Data from our stone clinic show that patients with idiopathic urolithiasis differ from normal controls on the same diet in regard to postprandial urine composition. Preliminary studies show that changes favorable for stone formation occur in urine composition, crystalluria, and supersaturation for the major calcium crystal systems.[32]

Low Urine Volume

Low urine volume is one of the strongest risk factors in stone formation.[26] Excessive fluid loss is part of the problem. Copious perspiration occurs in warm climates, and diarrhea is a common affliction in certain locales. If fluid losses were replaced, there would be no problem; however, in these areas of the world, water supplies are often limited. Even more commonly, people do not drink much water even when it is freely available. Those who drink much fluid may do it episodically, with many "dry" hours between times of fluid consumption. To excrete an isotonic urine, the average adult must have a daily urine volume of 2 liters. In our area, the average urine volume is 1.0–1.4 liters daily. There is a subgroup of stone formers who excrete only 0.6–0.9 liter/day. These people, typically women, have great difficulty in drinking enough fluid to make a substantial improvement in their urine volume. Bloating is their most frequent complaint. In a group of idiopathic calcium stone formers, we found that those who could increase their urine output to just 0.5 liter above their baseline value formed many fewer stones—without preventive medication—than did a similar group who failed to increase their urine volume.[10]

Hyperoxaluria

Primary and enteric hyperoxaluria are covered elsewhere in this book. There also is an "idiopathic" hyperoxaluria. Characteristically, the urinary oxalate increases are mild. Many of these patients are thought to be consuming excessive amounts of oxalate or one of its precursors such as vitamin C. Another possible mechanism has been demonstrated. When people decrease their dietary consumption of calcium in an attempt to avoid stones but do not restrict dietary oxalate, an excess of uncomplexed oxalate ("free" oxalate) occurs in the intestinal lumen. This unbound oxalate is readily absorbed into the circulation and is excreted in the urine in abnormally large amounts.[1,17]

Another group of patients has been described. These stone formers have both hyperoxaluria and increased urinary levels of glycollate, suggesting a metabolic origin.[13] Primary hyperoxaluria is excluded by the mild increase in urinary oxalate, well-preserved renal function, and occurrence later in life. Prolonged responses to small doses of pyridoxine have occurred. Other metabolic abnormalities may exist. Recently, a group of stone formers with normal 24-hour urinary oxalate excretion was discovered to have high rates of oxalate transport across the erythrocyte membrane.[2] The importance of small changes in urine oxalate concentrations deserves emphasis. On a molar basis, an increase in urinary oxalate excretion is strongly associated with increased stone formation rate; an increase in urinary calcium is not.[25] Idiopathic hyperoxaluria alone accounts for 16 percent of our calcium stone formers.[32]

Hypocitraturia

Urine citrate excretion and its importance in inhibiting crystallization was suspected over 50 years ago.[18] Citrate, an organic acid produced by the renal tubular cells, is excreted into the urine in large quantities during intracellular alkalosis. This excretion nearly ceases during intracellular acidosis, when citrate is used via the Krebs cycle for cellular adenosine triphosphate (ATP) production. Urinary citrate complexes with cations such as calcium and magnesium. Citrate deficiency allows more calcium to exist ionized and to bind to oxalate. Hypocitraturia thus may be a risk factor for stone formation. It has been found in association with multiple subgroups of stone formers. Nineteen percent of our stone formers have only hypocitraturia.

Any condition that causes intracellular acidosis, such as renal tubular acidosis, can result in hypocitraturia. Hypocitraturia can occur when no acidosis is present. Multiple factors influence citrate excretion, including electrolyte fluxes (potassium, lithium, calcium, magnesium), organic acids (malate, fumarate, succinate), metabolic inhibitors (fluorocitrate, malonate, maleate), and hormones (calcitonin, vitamin D, estrogen).[30]

Hyperuricosuria

Hyperuricosuria is a common condition in calcium stone formers. Thirty-eight percent of our idiopathic stone formers have this risk factor.[32] Coe has estimated that about 40 percent of his male and 20 percent of his female recurrent calcium stone formers are hyperuricosuric.[5] This condition may result from hyperexcretion of uric acid, either as a primary condition or in response to uricosuric drugs such as aspirin in high doses, probenecid, or sulfinpyrazone. More commonly, hyperuricosuria results from excessive uric acid production. Gluttony of dietary protein results in large intakes of purine, the precursor of uric acid. The trend in Western countries has been an increase in protein intake, especially among men. In our experience, obese males are the most common hyperuricosurics.

Heterogeneous nucleation is a process in which one crystal, such as calcium oxalate, crystallizes with less thermodynamic energy on the nidus of a different crystal such as sodium urate. Coe has popularized the clinical aspects of this theory by showing that reduction of hyperuricosuria decreases the frequency of calcium stone formation.[4] This theory is not universally accepted, however; sodium urate crystals are seldom seen in urine. An even less popular theory suggests that uric acid precipitates naturally occuring inhibitors of calcium crystallization.[24] Nevertheless, hyperuricosuria is generally regarded as a risk factor for stone formation.

Lack of Inhibitors of Crystallization

Only calcium oxalate and calcium phosphate crystal systems are known to have inhibitors of crystal formation. Many inhibitors are known, and doubtless others are yet to be discovered. Calcium phosphate inhibitors include pyrophosphate, citrate, and magnesium. Some calcium oxalate inhibitors are glycosaminoglycans, acidic glycopeptides, RNA fragments, and heparinlike substances. Robertson et al. found that combining an index of urinary supersaturation with one of inhibition gave the best prediction of activity in calcium stone formers. An assay for inhibitors of crystallization is not available through most clinical laboratories. Even when looked for carefully, only 22 percent of patients in our practice had deficient levels of inhibitors.[32]

DIAGNOSIS

Most new calcium stones come to attention precipitously with severe ureteral colic. Others are discovered serendipitously during urography or even during radiographic examination of the back or abdomen. For stones that are passed, the most precise way to determine their composition is stone analysis. Several laboratories in the United States have the ability to perform infrared (IR) or x-ray diffraction crystallography. These methods are preferable to standard wet chemical analyses because of their accuracy, especially with small specimens. Calcium oxalate is usually reported as the monohydrate (whewellite) or the dihydrate form (wedellite), although the clinical significance of these data is unknown. Likewise, calcium phosphate is reported as apatite, brushite, or one of its less common habits. Pure calcium carbonate stone (limestone) should be suspected as factitial; however, carbonate-apatite stones are often produced in alkaline urine such as is found during infection with urea-splitting organisms.

If a stone is not available for analysis, the radiographic appearance on a KUB film may be helpful. Calcium metabolic stones are dense and often multiple. They do not form a true staghorn shape or have laminations. We have not found computed tomographic scanning to offer information on stone composition beyond that in a simple KUB film. Radionuclide scans and magnetic resonance imaging have little or no role in diagnosis of calcium stones. Excretory urography, ultrasonography, or retrograde pyelography may be of great help if obstruction is suspected or if one is not sure whether a calcification is in the urinary tract. Plain-film tomography is valuable in visualizing small stones, especially when gas or stool obscures the view.

The causes of calcium oxalate or calcium phosphate stones are determined by analyses of blood and urine. Although we cannot recommend any one approach, blood studies, including determination of creatinine, calcium, phosphorus, and uric acid concentrations, are helpful. Determinations of urinary creatinine, calcium, cystine, oxalate, uric acid, citrate, phosphate, total volume, and sodium are often performed. More detailed testing to confirm the presence of a suspected stone-forming process may be indicated. Such investigations are beyond the scope of this chapter and are covered in the appropriate sections.

THERAPY

Therapy can be considered in two broad forms. One form is the removal of offending stones. This topic is discussed in a separate section. The second form of therapy is prevention. Prevention includes inhibition of growth of existing stones as well as avoidance of production of new stones or the passage of gravel. This type of treatment is considered in the remainder of this chapter. This introduces the concept of metabolic stone activity, which has proved to be extremely valuable in assessing the efficacy of treatment. We define as *metabolically active* the stone former who has radiographic evidence of existing stone growth or new stone formation within the past year. Documented passage of gravel within the past year also signifies metabolic activity. *Metabolic inactivity* is the situation in which radiographs document no new stones or growth of old stones within the past year, no gravel has passed, and any stone passed had been present on earlier radiographs. Stone passage per se does not indicate metabolic activity. The situation in which the available data do not permit a determination, a common experience, is called *indeterminate metabolic activity.*

Our approach to treatment of idiopathic calcium oxalate or calcium phosphate nephrolithiasis begins with determination of metabolic activity. A metabolically inactive patient needs no additional treatment. We believe that all metabolically active or metabolically indeterminate stone formers should be offered treatment. Any program of prevention begins with advice concerning appropriate dietary and fluid consumption. This advice must be based on a carefully taken diet history because urine composition is highly dependent on diet—that is, the idiopathic stone former has considerable control over the concentration of urinary components known to influence urine supersaturation. By manipulating diet, and thus supersaturation, the stone former can make the urine less lithogenic. My colleagues and I routinely advise restriction of dietary calcium to 800–1200 mg/day in adults. This strikes a reasonable compromise between too little calcium with the risk of osteoporosis on one hand and too much calcium with the risk of stone formation on the other hand. In practice, this advice translates to one or two daily servings of dairy products (milk, cheese, ice cream, yogurt) in addition to the calcium content of nondairy foods in the diet. We advise the patient to restrict oxalate-containing foods and we provide a list of the relative oxalate content of common foods. A high protein intake is interdicted because it will contribute to excessive urinary excretion of acid, uric acid, calcium, and oxalate.[16] Sodium excesses are calciuric,[14,20,21] as are carbohydrates,[15] and are to be avoided; thus, the watchword is moderation and dietary balance.

Excesses are encouraged, however, when it comes to fluid intake. A urine output of 2 liters/day should be considered a minimum. Depending on insensible fluid losses, at least 2.5 liters must be consumed daily to achieve this goal; if sweating or diarrhea occurs, appropriate replacement volumes must be added. We often recommend consumption of 8 ounces of fluid hourly while awake and again at night if the patient is up to void. At least half of this intake should be water.

Finally, harmful "medications" should be stopped. Large amounts of vitamin C can be converted to oxalate. Vitamins A and D can cause hypercalcemia. Absorbable antacids alter urine pH and also may contain large amounts of calcium. Calcium supplements sometimes are used to excess. Laxative or emetic abuse by people with eating disorders will cause low urine volume. Some food supplements (e.g., wheat germ) are high in purines.

Often this "conservative" program alone is successful in bringing about metabolic inactivity. This phenomenon has been noted by many others and is dubbed the "stone clinic effect."[10] With essentially nothing more than the advice described above, conversion to metabolic inactivity will occur in 30 percent or more of idiopathic stone formers, making control groups mandatory in any stone prevention drug trial.

If a patient with idiopathic calcium stone formation does not become metabolically inactive on a conservative program, drug intervention should be considered. If hypocitraturia is noted, specific treatment for correction exists in the form of alkali—sodium bicarbonate or citrate, especially potassium citrate. These medications work by increasing intracellular pH and thus citrate production; they do not add citrate directly to the urine. An average dose is 25–30 mEq of base 3 times daily. Repeated urine citrate measurements are used to titrate the dose. Common side effects may be gastric gas (with sodium bicarbonate) or gastrointestinal distress and unpleasant taste (with citrate salts). All are quickly reversible on discontinuation of treatment. Complications are few. If the urine becomes too alkaline, calcium phosphate salts may precipitate. Sodium excess can aggravate hypertension, edema, or heart failure. Hyperkalemia can occur if renal insufficiency is present. Short-term results appear to be good. Pak et al. have reported a remission rate of almost 80 percent in hypocitraturic stone formers, from various causes, treated with potassium citrate.[22] Long-term results are not yet available for this rather new treatment approach.

If hyperuricosuria is present, allopurinol may be considered for returning uric acid excretion to normal; the standard dose for adults is 300 mg once daily. A proportional dose reduction must be made for patients with renal insufficiency. Side effects and complications include skin rash (occasionally exfoliating), hepatic toxicity, vasculitis, and hypersensitivity nephritis. Short-term effects are favorable. Coe reported a marked reduction ($P < 0.001$) in calcium stone formation in patients who had hyperuricosuria as their sole metabolic abnormality.[4] Again, long-term studies of efficacy are lacking. Recently, potassium citrate has been found to decrease the rate of stone formation in this condition.[23]

If no abnormality is found or if the problem seems to be lack of inhibitors, treatment with orthophosphates may give an excellent response. Orthophosphates are inorganic neutral pH sodium potassium hydrogen phosphate compounds (brand names are K-Phos Neutral [tablet, Beach Pharmaceuticals, Tampa, FL] or Neutra-Phos [liquid, Willen Co., Baltimore, MD]). When taken in adequate amounts (1500–2000 mg of elemental phosphorus per day) divided in four doses, these substances are excreted in the urine and form pyrophosphate. This compound has mild calcium-binding properties but, more important, inhibits calcium phosphate and calcium oxalate crystallization. Urine citrate levels increase after administration of neutral phosphates. Ionized calcium level in the urine decreases as phosphate increases. The only side effect of note is diarrhea. Those patients with a tendency toward constipation are pleased with the result. Those with normal stool consistency can tolerate the medication, but the dose may need to be increased gradually. Diarrhea-prone patients seldom can tolerate adequate doses. Acid phosphates exist but are less efficacious. Alkaline phosphates may precipitate phosphate-containing stones. Like the citric acid salts, orthophosphates can cause sodium or potassium excess. Smith et al. reported excellent long-term results.[31] With treatment for a median of 3 years in 150 patients, 91 percent experienced inactivation of stone formation.

Some success with magnesium and pyridoxine in the treatment of idiopathic calcium stone disease has been reported by others. We cannot recommend this program because it seems less effective and more cathartic than others we have tried.

FOLLOWUP

Followup is essential in the treatment of a stone former. Metabolic activity must be reexamined on a regular basis. This will require serial KUB films, often with tomograms. Diet, fluid, and drug compliance must be evaluated. Especially because stone growth (in contrast to passage) is painless and programs requiring alteration of long-standing dietary habits are difficult, these patients must be given much encouragement. The physician must inquire into drug side effects or complications that would make compliance difficult or hazardous. Dosage adjustments may be indicated on the basis of radiographs or 24-hour urine chemistry data. The frequency of followup depends on multiple factors including the suspected degree of metabolic activity and the complexity or potential morbidity of the treatment program. Stone formers with a high probability of metabolic inactivity usually do not need to be seen more often than once yearly.

ACKNOWLEDGMENT

The author wishes to thank his colleague, Dr. Lynwood H. Smith, for his critical review of this manuscript.

REFERENCES

1. Archer HE, Dormer AE, Scowen EF, et al: Primary hyperoxaluria. Lancet 2:320–322, 1957
2. Baggio B, Gambaro G, Marchini F, et al: An inheritable anomaly of red-cell oxalate transport in "primary" calcium nephrolithiasis correctable with diuretics. New Engl J Med 314:599–604, 1986
3. Bo G, Maida A, Muresu E, et al: Epidemiology of urinary calculosis in the Sassari province. Eur Urol 4:431–432, 1978
4. Coe FL: Treated and untreated recurrent calcium nephrolithiasis in patients with idiopathic hypercalciuria, hyperuricosuria, or no metabolic disorder. Ann Intern Med 87:404–410, 1977
5. Coe FL: Hyperuricosuric calcium oxalate nephrolithiasis. Kidney Internatl 13:418–426, 1978
6. Derezic D, Zebec M, Cecuk LJ, et al: Different rate of nephrolithiasis in coastal and inland part of Croatia and possible relation to water hardness, in XVIII Congrès de la Sociètè Internationale d'Urologie, Paris, 1979
7. Donaldson D, Pryce JD, Rose GA, et al: Tap water calcium and its relationship to renal calculi and 24 h urinary calcium output in Great Britain. Urol Res 7:273–276, 1979
8. Erickson SB, Cooper K, Broadus AE, et al: Oxalate absorption and postprandial urine supersaturation in an experimental human model of absorptive hypercalciuria. Clin Sci 67:131–138, 1984
9. Frank D, Schneider H-J, Hesse A: Untersuchungen zum Harnsteinleiden bei Hitzearbeitern. Dtsch Gesundheitswes 30:716–720, 1975
10. Hosking DH, Erickson SB, Van Den Berg CJ, et al: The stone clinic effect in patients with idiopathic calcium urolithiasis. J Urol 130:1115–1118, 1983
11. Johnson CM, Wilson DM, O'Fallon WM, et al: Renal stone epidemiology: A 25-year study in Rochester, Minnesota. Kidney Internatl 16:624–631, 1979
12. Joost J, Egger G, Hohlbrugger G, et al: Epidemiologie des Nierensteinleidens in Tirol. Oesterreichische Ärtezeitung 35:1016–1020, 1980
13. Kasidas GP, Rose GA: Metabolic hyperoxaluria and its response to pyridoxine, in Ryall R, Brockis JG, Marshall VR, et al (eds): Urinary Stone. Melbourne, Churchill Livingstone, 1984, pp 138–147
14. Kleeman CR, Bohannan J, Bernstein D, et al: Effect of variations in sodium intake on calcium excretion in normal humans. Proc Soc Exp Biol Med 115:29–32, 1964
15. Lemann J Jr, Piering WF, Lennon EJ: Possible role of carbohydrate-induced calciuria in calcium oxalate kidney-stone formation. New Engl J Med 280:232–237, 1969

16. Linkswiler HM, Joyce CL, Anand CR: Calcium retention of young adult males as affected by level of protein and of calcium intake. Trans NY Acad Sci 36:333–340, 1974
17. Marshall RW, Cochran M, Hodgkinson A: Relationships between calcium and oxalic acid intake in the diet and their excretion in the urine of normal and renal-stone-forming subjects. Clin Sci 43:91–99, 1972
18. Mårtensson J: On the citric acid metabolism in mammals. Acta Physiol Scand Suppl 2:1–96, 1940
19. Mates J: External factors in the genesis of urolithiasis, in Hodgkinson A, Nordin BEC (eds): Proceedings of the Renal Stone Research Symposium. London, J & A Churchill, 1969, pp 59–64
20. Meyer WJ III, Transbol I, Bartter FC, et al: Control of calcium absorption: Effect of sodium chloride loading and depletion. Metbolism 25:989–993, 1976
21. Modlin M: The interrelation of urinary calcium and sodium in normal adults. Invest Urol 4:180–189, 1966
22. Pak CY, Fuller C, Sakhaee K, et al: Long-term treatment of calcium nephrolithiasis with potassium citrate. J Urol 134:11–19, 1985
23. Pak CYC, Peterson R: Successful treatment of hyperuricosuric calcium oxalate nephrolithiasis with potassium citrate. Arch Intern Med 146:863–867, 1986
24. Robertson WG, Knowles F, Peacock M: Urinary acid mucopolysaccharide inhibitors of calcium oxalate crystallisation, in Fleisch H, Robertson WG, Smith LH, et al (eds): Urolithiasis Research. London, Plenum Press, 1976, pp 331–334
25. Robertson WG, Peacock M: The cause of idiopathic calcium stone disease: Hypercalciuria or hyperoxaluria? Nephron 26:105–110, 1980
26. Robertson WG, Peacock M, Heyburn PJ, et al: Risk factors in calcium stone disease, in Brockis JG, Finlayson B (eds): Urinary Calculus. Littleton, MA, PSG Publishing Company, 1981, pp 265–273
27. Robertson WG, Peacock M, Marshall RW, et al: Saturation-inhibition index as measure of the risk of calcium oxalate stone formation in the urinary tract. New Engl J Med 294:249–252, 1976
28. Rose GA, Westbury EJ: The influence of calcium content of water, intake of vegetables and fruit and other food factors upon the incidence of renal calculi. Urol Res 3:61–66, 1975
29. Sierakowski R, Finlayson B, Landes R: Stone incidence as related to water hardness in different geographical regions of the United States. Urol Res 7:157–160, 1979
30. Simpson DP: Citrate excretion: A window on renal metabolism. Am J Physiol 244F: 223–234, 1983
31. Smith LH, Thomas WC Jr, Arnaud CD: Orthophosphate therapy in calcium renal lithiasis, in Cifuentes Delatte L, Rapado A, Hodgkinson A (eds): Urinary Calculi: Recent Advances in Aetiology, Stone Structure and Treatment. Basel, S Karger, 1973, pp 188–197
32. Smith LH, Werness PG, Erickson SD, et al: Postprandial response to a normal diet in patients with idiopathic calcium urolithiasis, in Ryall RL, Brockis JG, Marshall VR, et al (eds): Urinary Stone. Melbourne, Churchill Livingstone, 1984, pp 47–56
33. Steg A, Landier JF, Teyssier P, et al: in XVIII Congrès de la Sociètè International d'Urologie, Paris, Kongrebbericht, Tome 1, 1979, pp S163–S178
34. Vahlensieck W, Hesse A, Bach D: Zur Prävalenz des Harnsteinleidens in der Bundesrepublik Deutschland. Urologe [B] 20:273–276, 1980
35. Zielinski J: Epidemiologie und klinisch-chemische Zusammenhänge des Harnsteinleidens in Oberschlesien, in II Jenaer Harnsteinsymposium (Wissenschaftliche Beiträge der Friedrich-Schiller-Universität). Jena, Friedrich-Schiller-Universität, 1972, pp S100–102

Stephen B. Erickson

8

Hypercalciuric Nephrolithiasis

Idiopathic hypercalciuria was first described in 1939 in a classic article by Flocks.[12] Since then, studies of hypercalciuric stone formation have been confounded by the difficulty of defining the problem. As yet, there is no single well-accepted definition. Probably the most common definition is 24-hour urinary calcium excretion greater than 250 mg in women or 300 mg in men on an ad lib. diet.[14]

This definition suffers from the fact that dietary calcium intake may vary enormously and depends particularly on the amount of dairy foods in the diet because these sources are high in calcium that is bioavailable and so they increase the urinary calcium excretion. To avoid the variations introduced by dietary factors, hypercalciuria has also been defined with a diet specified. One common definition of hypercalciuria is the excretion of greater than 200 mg of calcium daily during intake of a low-calcium diet (400 mg/day).[27]

Another problem is that these definitions do not take body size into account. Urinary excretion of 4 mg of calcium per kilogram of body weight per day (on an unrestricted diet) is generally accepted as normal[6] and allows studies to be done on children. Another approach is to express calcium excretion per gram of urinary creatinine, an index of body mass. Hypercalciuria thus may be defined as more than 0.11 mg of calcium per milligram of creatinine in the fasting state or more than 0.20 mg of calcium per milligram of creatinine after a 1-g oral calcium load.[26]

Still another idea is to define hypercalciuria on the basis of percentages of absorption of increasingly large oral loads, to represent mass transfer of calcium across the intestinal mucosa. In this line of reasoning, normal is a plot of intake versus excretion that has a slope of less than 7 percent.[15,28] This definition is too cumbersome to be practical, although it is attractive theoretically.

Given the variability of definitions, it is not surprising that values reported for frequency and incidence of hypercalciuria also vary considerably. There are important differences between studies that often make comparison impossible. Diet is a major

STONE DISEASE: DIAGNOSIS AND MANAGEMENT
ISBN 0-8089-1873-7

feature. Many factors affect calcium excretion. Calcium content is primary: the more calcium in the diet, the more calcium in the urine. Protein intake has been well studied; the fixed acid metabolites of protein induce a metabolic acidosis that promotes calcium excretion.[1,17,18] Sodium excretion is correlated with calcium excretion in the urine;[19,31] thus, dietary salt must be controlled in a study of calcium homeostasis. Likewise, glucose and alcohol ingestion have at least transient hypercalciuric effects.[16] Although dietary phosphate has no effect within a wide range, hypercalciuria will occur when intake is extremely low. In fact, it has long been known that dietary phosphate deprivation is an excellent way to induce stone formation in otherwise normally fed rats.[32]

To diagnose hypercalciuria, multiple data are helpful, such as body weight, sex, diet history, 24-hour urinary calcium excretion on an ad lib. diet, 24-hour urinary calcium excretion on a 400-mg/day calcium and 100-mEq/day sodium intake, fasting urine calcium, urine calcium after a 1-g oral calcium load, and serum parathyroid hormone concentration or some index of parathyroid function such as serum calcium or urinary cyclic AMP. It is helpful to know the patient's 1,25-$(OH)_2$-vitamin D status because this is a major factor in absorption of calcium in the gut.[13]

A "fast-and-load" study is sometimes used to subdivide the hypercalciuric states into those caused by excessive absorption of dietary calcium from the gut (absorptive) and those caused by inappropriate excretion of calcium by the kidney (renal leak). There are two basic ways to perform a fast-and-load study. In the first method, the patient collects a 24-hour urine specimen on an ad lib. diet. If hypercalciuria is detected, the patient fasts overnight (16 hours) and then, while fasting, collects the urine excreted between 1000 (10:00 A.M.) and 1200 (12:00 noon) hours the next morning. Excretion of less than 20 mg of calcium indicates absorptive hypercalciuria; excretion of more than 30 mg of calcium indicates renal leak hypercalciuria. Intermediate values are indeterminate. We prefer this method because the calcium load is in the initial phase of the study, when hypercalciuria is defined. Prolonged pretest preparation and a second load are thus avoided.

The more popular (and lengthy) method involves definition of hypercalciuria by standard criteria. The patient then consumes a diet that provides 400 mg of calcium (no dairy products) per day for 1 week. After an overnight fast from 9:00 P.M. to 7:00 A.M., 600 ml of distilled water is ingested and a 2-hour fasting urine specimen is collected. At 9:00 A.M., a 1-g oral calcium load is administered in 300 ml of water. Urine collection continues from 9:00 A.M. to 1:00 P.M.; 300 ml of distilled water is ingested at 11:00 A.M.. Absorptive hypercalciuria is defined as excretion of more than 0.2 mg of calcium per milligram of urinary creatinine in the 4-hour postload collection. Renal leak hypercalciuria is defined as excretion of more than 0.11 mg of calcium per milligram of urinary creatinine in the 2-hour fasting urine specimen.[26]

In either type of study there are a large number of patients who do not fit precisely into either the absorptive or renal leak category. Although the overlap may represent defects in the testing protocol, it may also signify that the two populations are not separate entities. Some authors think that the hypercalciurias represent a physiologic continuum with artificially defined absorptive and renal leak types at the extremes.[8]

CLASSIFICATION

With the information given in the preceding paragraphs, hypercalciuria may be classified into five subtypes, although only the last three are of major clinical interest.

Dietary Excess Hypercalciuria

In some parts of the United States, consumption of one or more 8-ounce glasses of milk at each meal may be baseline, along with ingestion of cheese, ice cream, or yogurt. Diets providing more than 2 g of calcium daily abound. Although the body tightly controls production of the active form of vitamin D, 1,25-$(OH)_2$-vitamin D, there is a non-vitamin-D-dependent intestinal calcium transport mechanism in the jejunum.[22] Calcium transport is passive. A large oral calcium load thus produces a large urinary excretion.[2,5] Diagnosis is by diet history.

Noncomplexation Hypercalciuria

Normally, much of the dietary calcium is bound within the gut. This may occur as calcium oxalate, calcium citrate, calcium phosphate, or other calcium salts. Bound calcium is assumed to be unavailable for absorption and is excreted in the feces. When the concentration of ionized calcium is increased in the intestinal lumen, hyperabsorption of calcium may occur.[11] This situation may arise when less-soluble salts, such as oxalates, are replaced by more soluble ones. In general, this mechanism is not considered to be clinically important.

Resorptive Hypercalciuria

The term *resorptive hypercalciuria* refers to the situation in which the excess urinary calcium derives from bone. Clinically, this condition is caused by hyperparathyroidism or immobilization,[34] especially after multiple fractures in young people or in older patients with Paget's disease of bone. In other conditions, such as myeloma, bone metastasis, or humoral hypercalcemia of malignancy, hypercalciuria also derives from bone, but the patient usually dies before nephrolithiasis is manifested.

The mechanism of hypercalciuria in hyperparathyroidism is complex. Parathyroid hormone concentration is almost always increased, but 1,25-$(OH)_2$-vitamin D concentration is variably increased in hyperparathyroid patients.[3] The obvious factors causing hypercalciuria are bone resorption mediated by 1,25-$(OH)_2$-vitamin D- and parathyroid hormone-dependent osteoclast activation. 1,25-$(OH)_2$-Vitamin D also increases calcium absorption in the gut. The resultant hypercalcemia thus increases the filtered load while suppressing renal tubular resorption. These effects are opposed by net enhancement of tubular calcium absorption by parathyroid hormone. The end result may be normal or mildly increased urinary calcium excretion. Severe hypercalciuria (more than 600 mg/day) rarely is present in primary hyperparathyroidism.

Absorptive Hypercalciuria

The absorptive hypercalciurias represent a major form of hypercalciuria. They are characterized by normal serum calcium, hypercalciuria, normal or suppressed parathyroid hormone or cyclic AMP values, and high or normal 1,25-$(OH)_2$-vitamin D levels. There is a male predominance and often a family history of stones.[9] It should be noted that, although the absorptive defect is primary, there must be a secondary renal "leak" to maintain homeostasis. Differentiation of the absorptive type from the renal leak type thus rests on the response to fasting and the parathyroid hormone assay. Three well-defined subtypes have been identified.[24]

Type I—normal serum phosphorus and hypercalciuria (>0.2 g of calcium/24 hours) on a low-calcium (400-mg) diet. During the 4 hours after an oral load of 1 g of calcium, the urine calcium exceeds 0.2 mg/mg of creatinine.

Type II—identical to type I except that hypercalciuria is not observed on a low-calcium diet but is on a high-calcium (1000-mg) diet. This is true even when the diet is controlled for sodium. It should be noted that, although the calciuric response to a low-sodium diet is within the normal range, it is higher than in non-stone-forming controls. The magnitude of the response to the high-calcium diet in type II cannot be differentiated from that in type I. The cause of the exaggerated response to a high-calcium diet is unknown. The site affected is probably in the jejunum, but whether it is vitamin D-dependent or -independent is also unknown.

Type III—patients also are hypophosphatemic. The serum phosphate level seems to depend on the dietary phosphate intake: the higher the intake, the lower the tubular maximum reabsorption in the kidney. Type III patients thus must be diagnosed under standardized phosphate intake (800 mg/day) to avoid the confusion induced by a high phosphate intake.

Renal Leak Hypercalciuria

This disorder is characterized by excessive renal calcium loss through the kidney. The diagnosis is made by urine calcium measurements under conditions of fasting, usually for 12 hours or more. If the urine calcium exceeds 0.1 mg/100 ml of glomerular filtrate, the diagnosis is secure. As the result of ongoing renal losses, serum ionized and total calcium are slightly lower than in matched controls, although not absolutely low. Parathyroid hormone and cyclic AMP values are slightly higher than normal. 1,25-$(OH)_2$-Vitamin D levels are stimulated by parathyroid hormone; thus, hyperabsorption is also a feature but is secondary, not primary.

Most authors find that the absorptive types of hypercalciuria outnumber the nonabsorptive types.[21,27,29] Other studies disagree, however, having found that the majority of hypercalciurics have a primary defect in renal calcium conservation.[7,20] Differentiation between absorptive and renal leak hypercalciurias may be difficult, especially when fasting urinary calcium excretion is high, suggesting a renal leak, but the parathyroid hormone concentration is low, suggesting hyperabsorption. Sometimes this results from too short a fast[25] or a diet too high in calcium or sodium. The standard dietary recommendations are 400 mg of calcium and 100 mEq of sodium per day for 1 week before the test. In these circumstances the interference is from residual calcium in the intestine. Other problems often result from use of inaccurate or insensitive parathyroid hormone assays.

THERAPY

Therapy for the hypercalciuric calcium oxalate–calcium phosphate stone-former begins with the same approach as does therapy for idiopathic normocalciuric stone formers; that is, one does not need to proceed directly to drug intervention if hypercalciuria is noted. Adjustments of diet and fluid intake have a good chance of success in these disorders if the instructions are followed conscientiously. First, one must pay attention to fluid intake. A large volume of urine can hold a large amount of calcium in solution. The patient must be instructed in detail to drink 8 ounces of fluid hourly throughout the day and whenever up to void at night. The admonition "drink a lot" is inadequate and gets inadequate results. The concept of drinking when not thirsty will require reinforcement over several visits if it is to be followed.

The calcium content of the diet must be addressed next. Calcium gluttony (calcium intake disproportionate to oxalate intake) and type II absorptive hypercalciuria will respond to appropriate dietary calcium restriction. The resorptive and renal leak hypercalciurias will not respond to dietary calcium restriction. The level of calcium restriction is currently undergoing reevalution. In the past, conventional wisdom suggested that the lower the dietary calcium, the lower the urinary calcium; hence low-calcium diets (approximately 400 mg of calcium daily) were in vogue. There are two problems with such a vigorous restriction: (1) with little calcium in the intestinal lumen to bind to, oxalate tends to be hyperabsorbed[30]—what is gained by urinary calcium deficit is lost to urinary oxalate surfeit; and (2) osteoporosis seems to be aggravated by failure to ingest adequate amounts of calcium throughout life, especially in women. The necessary amount of daily calcium is debatable. Currently, 1200–1500 mg/day seems popular, and it is surprising how aware patients have become of this potential problem. Because the normal American diet without dairy products is estimated to contain about 400 mg of calcium per day, the addition of 400–800 mg of calcium daily in the form of dairy products is recommended for stone formers. This constitutes one to two 6-ounce glasses of milk, 2–4 ounces of cheese, or two to four cups of ice cream, coupled with liberal amounts of water.

Finally, the oxalate component of the diet must be brought into accord with the calcium portion. The oxalate content of foods has not been well studied, and most oxalate assays clinically available are inaccurate. Common foods are simply divided into "low," "moderate," and "high" oxalate categories; even this may exceed the limits of significance at times. The patient is instructed to avoid high-oxalate foods, moderate the intake of moderate-oxalate foods, and consume generous amounts of low-oxalate foods. Such an approach should not require the expense of a dietitian except in unusual circumstances.

Thiazides

Thiazides are a valuable adjunct in the treatment of hypercalciurias. There can be no question that therapeutic doses decrease urinary calcium excretion by one-third to one-half. In most studies that have evaluated the efficacy of this change on the rate of stone formation, the results have been favorable; however, these studies have been statistically flawed by small numbers of patients, lack of control groups, and short treatment periods. When the studies are lumped together, the therapeutic benefit does not reach statistical significance according to Churchill.[4] Most clinicians, including the author, believe that thiazides are effective, on the basis of their own experience. The use of thiazides is extensive, extending nearly two decades from the work of Yendt.[36] Safety is well documented. Common side effects include hypokalemia, hypercalcemia (which may cause confusion with hyperparathyroidism during reevaluations), hyperuricosuria, and hyperglycemia. These biochemical changes usually are mild and well tolerated and seldom require discontinuation of treatment. Impotence, experienced by a minority of men, requires cessation of this treatment; potency should return promptly. Urinary excretion of citrate will diminish in patients who are taking thiazides. This change may partially negate the beneficial effect of thiazides on hypercalciuria. The thiazides also may exert a beneficial side effect. Obviously, a major decrease in urinary calcium excretion changes other aspects of calcium metabolism. Although intestinal absorption decreases, some short-term evidence suggests that there is additional calcium deposition in bone.[35] Long-term studies are yet to be done. If augmentation of bone calcium can be shown, this would be a boon not only to osteoporotics but also to patients who have slowly lost bone calcium over the years because of renal leakage.

The dosages are as follows: hydrochlorothiazide, 25–50 mg once or twice daily; chlorthalidone, 25–50 mg once daily; or trichlormethiazide, 2–4 mg once or twice daily. The last thiazide is reputed to be more hypocalciuric than other thiazides, but evidence is lacking on this point.

One would expect thiazides to be used principally in the treatment of renal leak hypercalciurias. In this situation, thiazides are pharmacologically ideal in that they reverse the renal tubular leak.[10] Thiazides work equally well in absorptive hypercalciurias by secondarily lowering intestinal calcium absorption, thus addressing the root of the problem, even if not directly.

It becomes apparent from this information that fast-and-load metabolic studies are not of great importance in clinical practice although they may be of use in research. If a trial of moderate calcium restriction does not reduce hypercalciuria and stop stone formation, one simply adds thiazide treatment. The argument against this approach is that a mild renal leak hypercalciuria may be missed and the calcium restriction might intensify bone mineral loss. The rebuttal to this line of thinking is that calcium restriction, often complete avoidance of dairy products, has been practiced for years—long before mechanisms of hypercalciuria began to be worked out—and whatever bone disease occurred as the result was not enough to be noticed. Formal studies are lacking.

Orthophosphate

Another treatment option is orthophosphate. In addition to the inhibition of crystal formation noted in Chapter 7, phosphate has a mild binding affinity for calcium in both the intestinal contents and the urine, which is of additional therapeutic benefit. The short- and long-term effects of this treatment on a purely hypercalciuric group of stone formers have not been well studied, although it appears to be effective in combined normocalciuric and hypercalciuric subjects.[33]

Sodium Cellulose Phosphate

Sodium cellulose phosphate has been promoted by Pak for treatment of absorptive hypercalciuria.[23] Of theoretical interest, its mechanism of action is basically flawed. Cellulose phosphate complexes dietary calcium in the gut when taken with meals. Unfortunately, this leaves excess unbound oxalate that is hyperabsorbed and hyperexcreted into the urine. Also, dietary magnesium is indiscriminately bound, reducing urinary magnesium, an inhibitor of calcium crystallization. Although these disadvantages may be circumvented by use of a low-oxalate diet and magnesium supplements, when combined with high cost and every-meal compliance problems, use of this product is not attractive. The long-term effect of cellulose phosphate's restriction of calcium absorption on bones has not been evaluated.

FOLLOWUP

Close followup is mandatory, as discussed in Chapter 7. The same guidelines are used. It must be noted that urinary calcium excretion is not predictive of metabolic stone activity and should be followed only to assess biochemical response to dietary or drug therapy.

ACKNOWLEDGMENT

The author wishes to thank his colleague, Dr. Lynwood H. Smith, for his critical review of this manuscript.

REFERENCES

1. Adams ND, Gray RW, Lemann J Jr: The calciuria of increased fixed acid production in humans: Evidence against a role for parathyroid hormone and 1,25$(OH)_2$-vitamin D. Calcif Tissue Internatl 28:233–238, 1979
2. Adams ND, Gray RW, Lemann J Jr: The effects of oral $CaCO_3$ loading and dietary calcium deprivation on plasma 1,25-dihydroxyvitamin D concentrations in healthy adults. J Clin Endocrinol Metab 48:1008–1016, 1979
3. Broadus AE, Horst RL, Lang R, et al: The importance of circulating 1,25-dihydroxyvitamin D in the pathogenesis of hypercalciuria and renal-stone formation in primary hyperparathyroidism. New Engl J Med 302:421–426, 1980
4. Churchill DN: Appraisal of methodology in studies of either thiazide or orthophosphate therapy for recurrent calcium urolithiasis, in Schwille PO, Smith LH, Robertson WG, et al (eds): Urolithiasis and Related Clinical Research. New York, Plenum Press, 1985, pp 479–481
5. Clarkson EM, McDonald SJ, de Wardener HE: The effect of a high intake of calcium carbonate in normal subjects and patients with chronic renal failure. Clin Sci 30:425–438, 1966
6. Coe FL: Nephrolithiasis: Pathogenesis and Treatment. Chicago, Year Book Medical Publishers, 1978, p 72
7. Coe FL, Canterbury JM, Firpo JJ, et al: Evidence for secondary hyperparathyroidism in idiopathic hypercalciuria. J Clin Invest 52:134–142, 1973
8. Coe FL, Favus MJ, Crockett T, et al: Effects of low-calcium diet on urine calcium excretion, parathyroid function and serum 1,25$(OH)_2D_3$ levels in patients with idiopathic hypercalciuria and in normal subjects. Am J Med 72:25–32, 1982
9. Coe FL, Parks JH, Moore ES: Familial idiopathic hypercalciuria. N Engl J Med 300:337–340, 1979
10. Costanzo LS, Windhager EE: *In vivo* microperfusion study of calcium (Ca) and sodium (Na) transport in the distal convoluted tubule (abstract). Kidney Internatl 12:456, 1977
11. Favus MJ: Intestinal calcium transport, in Coe FL (ed): Hypercalciuric States: Pathogenesis, Consequences, and Treatment. Orlando, FL, Grune & Stratton, 1984, pp 37–63
12. Flocks RH: Calcium and phosphorus excretion in the urine of patients with renal or ureteral calculi. JAMA 113:1466–1471, 1939
13. Haussler MR, McCain TA: Basic and clinical concepts related to vitamin D metabolism and action. New Engl J Med 297:974–983; 1041–1050, 1977
14. Hodgkinson A, Pyrah LN: The urinary excretion of calcium and inorganic phosphate in 344 patients with calcium stone of renal origin. Br J Surg 46:10–18, 1958
15. Lemann J Jr, Adams ND, Gray RW: Urinary calcium excretion in human beings. New Engl J Med 301:535–541, 1979

16. Lemann J Jr, Piering WF, Lennon EJ: Possible role of carbohydrate-induced calciuria in calcium oxalate kidney-stone formation. New Engl J Med 280:232–237, 1969
17. Lemann J Jr, Relman AS, Connors HP: The relation of sulfur metabolism to acid-base balance and electrolyte excretion: The effects of DL-methionine in normal man. J Clin Invest 38:2215–2223, 1959
18. Linkswiler HM, Joyce CL, Anand CR: Calcium retention of young adult males as affected by level of protein and of calcium intake. Trans NY Acad Sci 36:333–340, 1974
19. McCarronn DA, Luft F, Rankin L, et al: The response of PTH and Ca^{++} to progressive volume expansion in man (abstract). Clin Res 27:47a, 1979
20. Muldowney FP, Freaney R, Ryan JG: The pathogenesis of idiopathic hypercalciuria: Evidence for renal tubular calcium leak. Quart J Med 49:87–94, 1980
21. Nordin BEC: Hypercalciuria. Clin Sci Molec Med 52:1–8, 1977
22. Nordin BEC, Peacock M, Wilkinson R: Hypercalciuria and calcium stone disease. Clin Endocrinol Metab 1:169–183, March 1972
23. Pak CYC: Calcium Urolithiasis: Pathogenesis, Diagnosis, and Management. New York, Plenum Press, 1978, p 56
24. Pak CYC: Pathogenesis of idiopathic hypercalciuria, in Coe FL (ed): Hypercalciuric States: Pathogenesis, Consequences, and Treatment. Orlando, FL, Grune & Stratton, 1984, pp 205–220
25. Pak CYC, Galosy RA: Fasting urinary calcium and adenosine 3',5'-monophosphate: A discriminant analysis for the identification of renal and absorptive hypercalciurias. J Clin Endocrinol Metab 48:260–265, 1979
26. Pak CYC, Kaplan R, Bone H, et al: A simple test for the diagnosis of absorptive, resorptive and renal hypercalciurias. N Engl J Med 292:497–500, 1975
27. Pak CYC, Ohata M, Lawrence EC, et al: The hypercalciurias: Causes, parathyroid functions, and diagnostic criteria. J Clin Invest 54:387–400, 1974
28. Peacock M, Hodgkinson A, Nordin BEC: Importance of dietary calcium in the definition of hypercalciuria. Br Med J 3:469–471, 1967
29. Peacock M, Knowles F, Nordin BEC: Effect of calcium administration and deprivation on serum and urine calcium in stone-forming and control subjects. Br Med J 2:729–731, 1968
30. Robertson WG, Peacock M: The cause of idiopathic calcium stone disease: Hypercalciuria or hyperoxaluria? (editorial). Nephron 26:105–110, 1980
31. Sabto J, Powell MJ, Breidahl MJ, et al: Influence of urinary sodium on calcium excretion in normal individuals. Med J Aust 140:354–356, 1984
32. Schneider H, Steenbock H: Calcium citrate uroliths on a low phosphorus diet. J Urol 43:339–344, 1940
33. Smith LH, Thomas WC Jr, Arnaud CD: Orthophosphate therapy in calcium renal lithiasis, in Cifuentes DeLatte L, Rapado A, Hodgkinson A (eds): Urinary Calculi: Recent Advances in Aetiology, Stone Structure and treatment. New York, S Karger, 1973, pp 188–197
34. Stewart AF, Adler M, Byers CM, et al: Calcium homeostasis in immobilization: An example of resorptive hypercalciuria. New Engl J Med 306:1136–1140, 1982
35. Wasnich RD, Benfante RJ, Yano K, et al: Thiazide effect on the mineral content of bone. New Engl J Med 309:344–347, 1983
36. Yendt ER: Renal calculi. Can Med Assoc J 102:479–489, 1970

Stephen B. Erickson

9

Hypercalcemic Nephrolithiasis

Hypercalcemia is uncommon among stone formers. When present, a secondary cause for urolithiasis almost always exists and must be found. Hypercalcemic stone formers usually can be cured by treatment appropriate to their underlying disease.

By far the most common hypercalcemic stone-forming state is primary hyperparathyroidism. Less common causes include sarcoidosis, chronic vitamin D intoxication, milk-alkali abuse, and Cushing's syndrome (including exogenous steroid use). Hypercalcemia can occur in other disease states. In the hypercalcemia of malignancy the patient does not live long enough for stones to develop; this is also true with multiple myeloma or osseous metastasis. Granulomatous disease other than sarcoidosis, such as tuberculosis or beryl-liosis, can cause hypercalcemia but rarely is a cause of stones. Endocrinopathies such as Addison's disease or thyrotoxicosis also can cause hypercalcemia but seldom cause stones. Thiazide diuretics commonly cause hypercalcemia but actually are used to prevent stones by virtue of their ability to increase renal tubular calcium resorption. Patients with familial hypercalcemic hypocalciuria do not form stones, presumably because the concentration of calcium in their urine is low.

PRIMARY HYPERPARATHYROIDISM

Although once considered a rare disease, primary hyperparathyroidism has been found more frequently with the advent of automated analysis of blood, which discloses asymptomatic mild hypercalcemia. In the days before automated analysis, hyperparathyroidism was mostly diagnosed in its symptomatic state—either bone or stone disease. Then, about 50 percent of hyperparathyroidism patients had stones. Now, only about 5–15 percent do.[14] The age-adjusted incidence of primary hyperparathyroidism in Olmsted County, Minnesota, is now estimated to be 42 per 100,000.[14] In persons over 40 years of age, the incidence may rise to more than 1 per 1000.[6,9] The disease is most common in the middle years of life, but infants and elderly people may be affected. It is more

STONE DISEASE: DIAGNOSIS AND MANAGEMENT
ISBN 0-8089-1873-7

common in women than in men. Familial occurrence has been reported.[13] The chance of hyperparathyroidism developing increases in persons who had been exposed to head and neck irradiation when they were children.[27] (Irradiation was once used for acne, tonsillitis, and thymus enlargement but has been abandoned.) Although the normal person has four parathyroid glands (rarely, five), usually only one is affected. If only the adenomatous gland is removed, the other three remain normal in almost all cases. Less than 2 percent of hyperfunctional parathyroid glands are malignant.[2]

Diagnosis

Hyperparathyroidism may be subtle and difficult to diagnose. Only a minority of stone formers with hyperparathryoidism are florid stone producers. Searching extensively for hyperparathyroidism in *all* florid stone formers is as erroneous as failing to look for it at all in a solitary stone former. Some clues suggest the possibility of hyperparathyroidism. For example, the onset of idiopathic calcium stone disease in a middle-aged person—especially a woman—is unusual. Idiopathic stone disease usually starts in the third to fifth decades of life. The incidence of primary hyperparathyroidism begins to increase after the fifth decade.[1] A predominantly calcium phosphate (apatite) stone is unusual in idiopathic urolithiasis; however, calcium phosphate stones are common in primary hyperparathryoidism[16,19] and may reflect the relatively alkaline urine pH that hyperparathryoidism may produce through its bicarbonaturic effect on the renal tubules.[3,15,26]

Mild hypercalcemia is also a clue. Often the serum calcium value will be 10.2–10.5 mg/dl. In many laboratories in which the calcium analysis is not rigorously standardized, such values would be called "normal," placing the clinician at a disadvantage in diagnosis. Many patients diagnosed as having "normocalcemic" hyperparathyroidism actually would be found to be mildly hypercalcemic if a more rigorous assay were used. A marked increase in serum calcium in response to a thiazide diuretic is another clue.[18,34] The hypercalcemia caused by thiazides alone is mild, nearly always less than 11.0 mg/dl at my institution. The "thiazide challenge" is not sensitive.

Once the possibility of primary hyperparathryoidism has been raised, there are many ways of establishing the diagnosis. At the Mayo Clinic, we rely heavily on the total serum calcium value and our immunoreactive parathyroid hormone (iPTH) assay. A word of caution about parathyroid hormone assays is in order. There are many different assays. Some measure the molecule's carboxy-terminal (COOH-terminal) fragments, others measure amino-terminal (NH_2-terminal) fragments, and still others measure fragments from various sites in the middle region. Some assays measure only biologically active hormone; most measure inactive fragments as well. The caveat is that one must know the properties of the assay being used.

A low serum phosphorus value is a helpful clue, if present, but is not sensitive. In renal failure, a normal serum phosphorus value may be a consequence of excessive phosphaturia such as occurs in hyperparathyroidism. Normally, serum phosphorus is increased in renal failure. The 24-hour urinary calcium excretion may be normal (due to parathyroid hormone–mediated renal tubular calcium absorption) or mildly high due to an increased filtered load and hypercalcemic suppression of renal tubular calcium absorption. Severe hypercalciuria (more than 600 mg/day) is rarely seen in hyperparathyroidism.

Some have used ionized calcium, ultrafiltered calcium, cyclic AMP, nephrogenous cyclic AMP, or thyroid vein parathyroid hormone (by selective catheterization) values in making the diagnosis of primary hyperparathyroidism. My colleagues and I rarely use these procedures, placing our confidence in our total serum calcium and parathyroid hormone assays. Tubular reabsorption of phosphorus is no longer used in the diagnosis of hyperparathyroidism.

A real-time ultrasonographic examination of the neck may localize the adenoma preoperatively if it is as large as 1 cm;[28] many adenomas are too small to be visualized, however. Computed tomography of the chest may locate an aberrant gland. Magnetic resonance imaging has not been of any additional advantage. Magnified views of the hand bones on industrial film may reveal osteitis fibrosa cystica, the typical finding of parathyroid bone disease.[12] Some authors emphasize the discordance between parathyroid hormone–induced bone and stone disease,[1,10,20] but they often occur together.[25]

Treatment

Although there is controversy regarding how to manage asymptomatic hyperparathyroidism, there is consensus about the need for surgical treatment for the calcium stone former who has hyperparathyroidism. It is important that the neck exploration be done by a surgeon experienced in the vagaries of hyperparathyroidism. Adenomas frequently occur in unusual locations such as within the thyroid, within the carotid sheath, or behind the jugular vein. It is most important that the adenoma(s) be found and excised during the initial operation because subsequent procedures are much more difficult due to scarring and distortion of the anatomy. If there is concern that the vascular supply to all parathyroids has been disrupted, normal parathyroid tissue may be frozen for subsequent autotransplantation.[35]

Medical treatment of hyperparathyroidism has been sought. At present, these approaches remain experimental. Estrogen has proved successful in decreasing serum calcium in postmenopausal women with primary hyperparathyroidism.[11,21,29] Cimetidine has been reported to lower parathyroid hormone levels in both primary and tertiary hyperparathyroidism.[17,30,32] Even propranolol has been tried and has given biochemical improvement.[7] Corticosteroids have no place in the treatment of hyperparathyroidism.

Followup

Long-term results of parathyroidectomy are excellent. Recurrent adenoma is rare. Nearly all stone formers become metabolically inactive, although they often continue to pass preformed stones. The major surgical complications are vocal cord paralysis and hypoparathyroidism. Serum calcium should be assessed postoperatively and then at yearly intervals.

SARCOIDOSIS

Less than 15 percent of the patients with sarcoidosis are hypercalcemic,[22,31] and even fewer form stones. The cause of the hypercalcemia probably lies in the granulomatous tissue. The blood level of calcitriol (1,25-$[OH]_2$-vitamin D_3), the most active form of vitamin D, increases when hypercalcemia develops.[5,24] Although the 1α hydroxylation of the precursor 25-(OH)-vitamin D normally occurs only in the kidney, high levels of calcitriol were found in an anephric patient with sarcoidosis.[4] This suggests that the granulomatous tissue itself may produce calcitriol. Sarcoidosis-related stone formation thus actually represents a type of endogenous vitamin D intoxication.

Acuity is helpful in diagnosis. A chest radiograph that shows hilar adenopathy or infiltrates often is the signal to proceed with the evaluation. Another clue is an extraordinarily high urinary calcium excretion (>700 mg/24 hours). The effect of parathyroid hormone on renal tubular calcium absorption is inconsistent with such high values. In hypercalcemic sarcoidosis, there is no stimulus for the large filtered load of calcium to be resorbed by the renal tubules. Increased values for calcitriol or serum angiotensin-converting enzyme inhibitor are strong clues also. The diagnosis is proved by tissue biopsy, usually of scalene or mediastinal nodes, which shows noncaseating granulomas.

Sarcoidosis may resolve spontaneously. When stones are forming, rapid resolution of the hypercalcemia is necessary. This is accomplished with prednisone, beginning with a moderate dose, about 20–40 mg/day.[4,8,24] Although the steroids themselves may cause hypercalciuria from bone resorption, it is usually milder than that caused by the sarcoidosis. This treatment has worked well in a small group of patients.

The short-term emphasis is on getting the sarcoidosis into remission and documenting metabolic stone inactivation and reversal of hypercalcemia. Long-term considerations focus on attempts to taper the steroid therapy without reactivation of the sarcoidosis. It may be necessary to continue the steroid therapy indefinitely on a low-dose alternate-day regimen to prevent disease reactivation.

VITAMIN D TOXICITY

This toxicity may be self-induced, although the patient may deny vitamin D use through either ignorance or embarrassment. Also, patients seldom consider vitamins to be medications, and one must inquire specifically about them. The vitamin abuse and consequent hypercalcemia may have occurred in the past, or sporadically, and may not be evident at the time of evaluation. The mechanisms of hypercalcemia are hyperabsorption of dietary calcium and some resorption of bone calcium.

Apart from the patient's history and hypercalcemia, vitamin D level is the only useful diagnostic study. As in sarcoidosis, 24-hour urinary calcium excretion may be high.

Patient education and discontinuation of the vitamin use are obvious treatment steps. In the case of "plain" vitamin D overdose (as opposed to dihydrotachysterol or dihydroxyvitamin D), the hypercalcemia and hypercalciuria may last for several months. In such cases, a short course of oral corticosteroid therapy, as given in sarcoidosis, will be of benefit.

CUSHING'S SYNDROME

Whether caused by endogenous or exogenous corticosteroid excess, this condition may predispose to urolithiasis. Typically, if hypercalcemia is present, it is mild. Hypercalciuria is also mild to moderate. Only a small percentage of patients with Cushing's syndrome form stones.

With exogenous steroid use, the diagnosis is made on the basis of history. One may have to ask specifically, especially if the patient is no longer taking the drug. The presence of lupus erythematosus, rheumatoid arthritis, vasculitis, or some other illness often treated with long-term steroid intake may be a clue. Physical findings are helpful. Patients with Cushing's syndrome tend to be obese in a truncal distribution. The face is rounded (moon facies), and there is a fat pad over the upper dorsal spine ("buffalo hump"). The abdomen may have purplish striae. The skin is thin, and ecchymoses may be prominent. Women may appear hirsute. Morning and afternoon plasma cortisol values are high and do not show the usual diurnal variation. The plasma cortisol level is not suppressed by a 2-mg dose of dexamethasone. The 24-hour urinary excretion of 17-hydroxysteroids and ketosteroids usually is increased, except that it is low when exogenous steroids have been given.

Oral steroid therapy should be tapered or stopped in the stone former, if possible. If not, treatment is as outlined for idiopathic hypercalciuria. For Cushing's syndrome due to excessive ACTH production by the pituitary, transsphenoidal removal of the adenoma is the treatment of choice. Radiation therapy to the pituitary adenoma or adrenalectomy may also succeed. For Cushing's syndrome due to adrenal adenoma or carcinoma, surgical removal of the adrenal is the treatment of choice. The first choice for chemotherapy of metastatic disease is *o,p′*-DDD (mitotane, Lysodren; Bristol-Myers Oncology, Syracuse, NY). Patients with ACTH-producing malignancies such as bronchogenic carcinoma seldom live long enough to develop stones.

MILK-ALKALI SYNDROME

This interesting process is seldom seen at present. It occurs in patients who consume large amounts of calcium and absorbable alkali, such as were used in the Sippy regimen for treatment of peptic ulcer.[33] Absorption of alkali promotes calcium absorption and decreases calcium excretion. The resulting hypercalcemia produces alkalosis—a double positive feedback cycle.[23] The chronic form of this condition (Burnett's syndrome) has long been known to cause nephrocalcinosis and renal failure. Modern equivalents still occur in people who self-medicate ulcers or during pregnancy when extra calcium is prescribed by the obstetrician and the patient also uses absorbable alkali (Tums, Rolaids, baking soda) for relief of heartburn.

The history is vital in making this diagnosis. In the absence of hypercalcemia, a high index of suspicion is also necessary. As in vitamin D toxicity, many patients do not consider antacids to be medication and must be specifically asked.

Discontinuation of the alkali intake breaks the positive feedback cycle and is the correct treatment. One of the many nonabsorbable magnesium-containing antacids or even a histamine H_2 receptor antagonist (cimetidine or ranitidine) may be substituted.

OTHER ENDOCRINOPATHIES

Thyrotoxicosis and hypoadrenalism (Addison's disease) have been reported to cause hypercalcemia and, in very rare cases, stones. The experience at any one center is insufficient for characterization of the peculiarities of such stone formers. Diagnosis is based on observation of characteristic symptoms and signs and is confirmed by appropriate endocrinologic testing. Treatment for the stones is the treatment required for the endocrinopathy.

ACKNOWLEDGMENT

The author wishes to thank his colleague, Dr. Lynwood H. Smith, for his critical review of this manuscript.

REFERENCES

1. Albright F: A page out of the history of hyperparathyroidism. J Clin Endocrinol 8:637–657, 1948
2. Arnaud CD, Strewler GJ: Parathyroid hormone and primary hyperparathyroidism, in Coe FL (ed): Hypercalciuric States: Pathogenesis, Consequences, and Treatment. Orlando, FL, Grune & Stratton, 1984, pp 275–312
3. Bank N, Aynedjian HS: A micropuncture study of the effect of parathyroid hormone on renal bicarbonate reabsorption. J Clin Invest 58:336–344, 1976
4. Barbour GL, Coburn JW, Slatopolsky E, et al: Hypercalcemia in an anephric patient with sarcoidosis: Evidence for extrarenal generation of 1,25-dihydroxyvitamin D. New Engl J Med 305:440–443, 1981
5. Bell NH, Stern PH, Pantzer E, et al: Evidence that increased circulating 1α,25-dihydroxyvitamin D is the probable cause for abnormal calcium metabolism in sarcoidosis. J Clin Invest 64:218–225, 1979
6. Boonstra CE, Jackson CE: Hyperparathyroidism detected by routine serum calcium analysis: Prevalence in a clinic population. Ann Intern Med 63:468–474, 1965
7. Caro JF, Castro JH, Glennon JA: Effect of long-term propranolol administration on parathyroid hormone and calcium concentration in primary hyperparathyroidism. Ann Intern Med 91:740–741, 1979
8. Chesney RW, Hamstra AJ, DeLuca HF, et al: Elevated serum 1,25-dihydroxyvitamin D concentrations in the hypercalcemia of sarcoidosis: Correction by glucocorticoid therapy. J Pediatr 98:919–922, 1981
9. Christensson T, Hellström K, Wengle B, et al: Prevalence of hypercalcaemia in a health screening in Stockholm. Acta Med Scand 200:131–137, 1976
10. Dent CE: Some problems of hyperparathyroidism. Br Med J 2:1419–1425; 1495–1500, 1962
11. Gallagher JC, Nordon BEC: Treatment with oestrogens of primary hyperparathyroidism in post-menopausal women. Lancet 1:503–507, 1972
12. Genant HK, Heck LL, Lanzl LH, et al: Primary hyperparathyroidism: A comprehensive study of clinical, biochemical and radiographic manifestations. Radiology 109:513–524, 1973
13. Goldsmith RE, Sizemore GW, Chen I-W, et al: Familial hyperparathyroidism: Description of a large kindred with physiologic observations and a review of the literature. Ann Intern Med 84:36–43, 1976
14. Heath H III, Hodgson SF, Kennedy MA: Primary hyperparathyroidism: incidence, morbidity, and potential economic impact in a community. New Engl J Med 302:189–193, 1980
15. Hellman DE, Au WYW, Bartter FC: Evidence for a direct effect of parathyroid hormone on urinary acidification. Am J Physiol 209:643–650, 1965
16. Hodgkinson A, Peacock M, Nicholson M: Quantitative analysis of calcium-containing urinary calculi, in Hodgkinson A, Nordin BEC (eds): Renal Stone Research Symposium. London, J & A Churchill, 1969, pp 113–122
17. Jacob AI, Lanier D Jr, Canterbury J, et al: Reduction by cimetidine of serum parathyroid hormone levels in uremic patients. New Engl J Med 302:671–674, 1980

18. Jørgensen FS, Transbøl I, Binder C: The effect of bendroflumethiazide on total, ultrafiltrable and ionized calcium in serum in normocalcaemic renal stone formers and in hyperparathyroidism. Acta Med Scand 194:323–326, 1973
19. Lagergren C, Öhrling H: Urinary calculi composed of pure calcium phosphate: Roentgen crystallographic analysis and its diagnostic value. Acta Chir Scand 117:335–341, 1959
20. Lloyd HM: Primary hyperparathyroidism: An analysis of the role of the parathyroid tumor. Medicine (Baltimore) 47:53–71, 1968
21. Marcus R, Madvig P, Crim M, et al: Conjugated estrogens in the treatment of postmenopausal women with hyperparathyroidism. Ann Intern Med 100:633–640, 1984
22. Mayock RL, Bertrand P, Morrison CE, et al: Manifestations of sarcoidosis: Analysis of 145 patients, with a review of nine series selected from the literature. Am J Med 35:67–89, 1963
23. Orwoll ES: The milk-alkali syndrome: Current concepts. Ann Intern Med 97:242–248, 1982
24. Papapoulos SE, Clemens TL, Fraher LJ, et al: 1,25-Dihydroxycholecalciferol in the pathogenesis of the hypercalcaemia of sarcoidosis. Lancet 1:627–630, 1979
25. Purnell DC, Smith LH, Scholz DA, et al: Primary hyperparathyroidism: A prospective clinical study. Am J Med 50:670–678, 1971
26. Puschett JB, Zurbach P: Acute effects of parathyroid hormone on proximal bicarbonate transport in the dog. Kidney Internatl 9:501–510, 1976
27. Rao SD, Frame B, Miller MJ, et al: Hyperparathyroidism following head and neck irradiation. Arch Intern Med 140:205–207, 1980
28. Reading CC, Charboneau JW, James EM, et al: High-resolution parathyroid sonography. Am J Roentgenology 139:539–546, 1982
29. Selby PL, Peacock M: Ethinyl estradiol and norethindrone in the treatment of primary hyperparathyroidism in postmenopausal women. New Engl J Med 314:1481–1485, 1986
30. Sherwood J, Reinhard D, Garcia M: Does cimetidine inhibit parathyroid hormone secretion? (letter to the editor) New Engl J Med 300:200–201, 1979
31. Siltzbach LE, James DG, Neville E, et al: Course and prognosis of sarcoidosis around the world (editorial). Am J Med 57:847–852, 1974
32. Simon B, Stiehl A, Feurle G, et al: Erfolgreiche Ulkusbehandlung mit Cimetidin bei einem Patienten mit primärem Hyperparathyreoidismus. Med Klin 73:1513–1516, 1978
33. Sippy BW: Gastric and duodenal ulcer: Medical cure by an efficient removal of gastric juice corrosion. JAMA 64:1625–1630, 1915
34. Sode J, Sabol JJ, Meloni CR, et al: Thiazide challenge in primary hyperparathyroidism (abstract). Clin Res 17:550, 1969
35. Wells SA Jr, Ellis GJ, Gunnells JC, et al: Parathyroid autotransplantation in primary parathyroid hyperplasia. New Engl J Med 295:57–62, 1976

David M. Wilson

10

Uric Acid Lithiasis

Uric acid and its salts are sparingly soluble, resulting in precipitation of crystals and stones in the urinary tract. Uric acid stones account for 5–10 percent of all renal stones in the United States. This is true in a series at the Mayo Clinic and also those series reported by Herring,[15] and Prien.[23] The incidence of uric acid stones seems to vary from country to country. Atsmo̊n et al. reported 75 percent of the stones in Israel were uric acid.[3] In another study in the Sudan, 57 percent of stones contained uric acid.[16]

Although the prevalence of uric acid stones in the United States is about 0.01 percent based on Boyce's survey, certain patient subgroups have a much higher prevalence of uric acid stones, such as post ileostomy patients where 80 percent of stones are uric acid. In patients with gout it has been reported that 479 of 2038 patients (23 percent) had a history of renal calculi. In a study by Yu, 80 percent of stones were uric acid, whereas 10 percent were calcium-oxalate and 2–3 percent were calcium-phosphate.[32] In patients who have hyperuricemia without gout, the risk of urolithiasis seems somewhat less. Gouty patients have 1 stone per 114 patients. Those with hyperuricemia have approximately 1 stone per 295 patients per year, compared with 1 stone in 852 patients per year in a normal uricemic control population.[12] Yu and Gutman have shown that in patients with gout the risk of forming uric acid stones is related to the uric acid excretion levels.[31] Of those patients excreting over 1000 mg per 24-hour period, 50 percent have stones; over 900 mg, 38 percent; over 700 mg, 34 percent; and over 500 mg, 21 percent.

Uric Acid Chemistry

Uric acid is the end product of purine ribonucleotide metabolism that originates from either nuclear degradation or nucleic acid content of the diet. Nucleic acids break down to hypoxanthine, and in the presence of xanthine oxidase convert to xanthine, which in the presence of xanthine oxidase converts to uric acid. The average adult consumes about 2 mg of purine per kilogram of body weight, which results in 200–300 mg of urine

STONE DISEASE: DIAGNOSIS AND MANAGEMENT

ISBN 0-8089-1873-7

Table 10-1
Solubility of Uric Acid and Urate

Effect of pH on uric acid solubility			
	Total uric acid solubility		*Ratio of Na urate/free uric acid*
pH 5.0	8 mg/100 ml		0.23
pH 7.0	158 mg/100 ml		23.0
Effect of salt on urate solubility (pH 7.4)*			
		Solubility of urate salts in water	
Sodium	(6 mEq/l)	140 mg/100 ml	
Sodium	(140 mEq/l)	6.4 mg/100 ml	
Potassium	(12 mEq/l)	248 mg/100 ml	
Ammonium	(3 mEq/l)	54 mg/100 ml	
Solubility of uric acid relative to other compounds			
	Urine pH 5.0†	*Urine pH 7.0*†	*Cold water*‡
Uric acid	15 mg/100 ml	200 mg/100 ml	6.7 mg/100 ml
Hypoxanthine	140 mg/100 ml	150 mg/100 ml	—
Xanthine	5 mg/100 ml	13 mg/100 ml	—
Allantoin	—	—	526 mg/100 ml

Reprinted from Holmes EW, Jr, Kelley WN: Renal pathophysiology of gout, in Kurtzman NA (ed): Pathophysiology of the Kidney. Courtesy of Charles C Thomas, Publisher, Springfield, 1977.

*Data from Peters JP, Van Slyke KK: Quantitative Clinical Chemistry, 2nd ed, Vol. 1. Baltimore, Williams and Wilkins, 1946, p 937.

†Data from Klinenberg JR, Goldfinger S, Miller J, et al: The effectiveness of a xanthine oxidase inhibitor on the treatment of gout. Ann Intern Med: 62–639, 1965.

‡Data from Stecher PG (ed): The Merck Index. Rahway, NJ, Merck, 1968.

uric acid daily. Endogenous production is also about 300 mg/day. Total uric acid excretion is about 600 mg/day for an average person. Excretion of xanthine and hypoxanthine is normally in the range of 10–50 mg per 24-hour period.

Since the large majority of uric acid stones are composed of uric acid itself, the characteristics of the solubility of total uric acid in urine are of prime importance in understanding uric acid calculi. As seen in Table 10-1, the primary determinant of uric acid solubility is the pH of the urine. At a pH of 5, uric acid solubility is 8 mg/dl; at a pH of 7.0, it is 158 mg/dl. The pK_a of uric acid is variously quoted as being 5.35–5.75. Figure 10-1 shows the urine pH on the abscissa, the percent of total uric acid as free uric acid on the ordinant, and a pK_a of 5.57. At this point 50 percent of the total uric acid is free uric acid. The solubility of free uric acid in urine is somewhat different than in water because of the modulating effect of other cations. At a pH of 5.0 in urine, therefore, the solubility of free uric acid is approximately 15 mg/dl, while at a pH of 7.0 the solubility is 200 mg/dl. Figure 10-2 is a nomogram showing how much total uric acid will provide enough free uric acid to saturate the urine assuming a solubility of 100 mg/liter. It shows that at a solubility limit of 100 mg/dl, at a pH of 4.5, saturation would occur at about 105 mg/liter of total uric acid, whereas at a pH of 7.0, a total uric acid excretion of 1000 mEq/liter would be just saturated.

Table 10-1 also shows that increasing the sodium concentration from 6 to 140 mEq/L results in a twentyfold reduction in the solubility of sodium urate. These other salts of

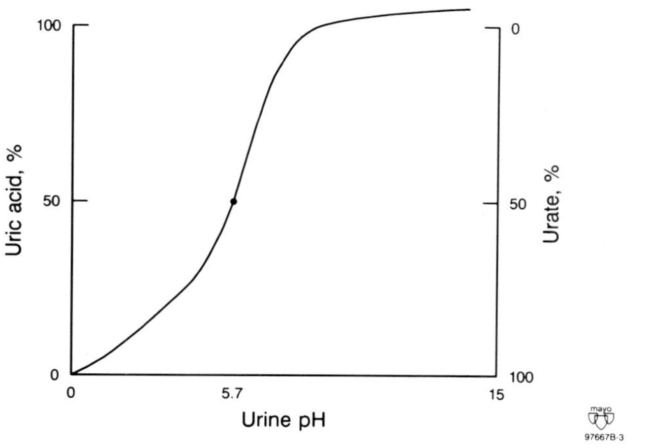

Fig. 10-1. Dissociation curve for uric acid versus sodium urate (using the Henderson-Hasselbach equation and a pK_a of 5.7).

uric acid may rarely precipitate and form stones in urine under certain circumstances. Sodium urate may precipitate in the presence of high urate, an alkaline urine pH, and high sodium content. Only occasionally does this precipitation result in sodium urate stones, and this usually occurs in patients receiving large sodium and alkali loads with diuretic administration. Ammonium urate is also sparingly soluble, and it is less soluble in an alkaline urine. Ammonium urate stones usually form in conditions of high ammonia and urate excretion, such as in urines infected with urea splitting bacteria. Occasionally these salts may precipitate in patients with extremely high acid and ammonia

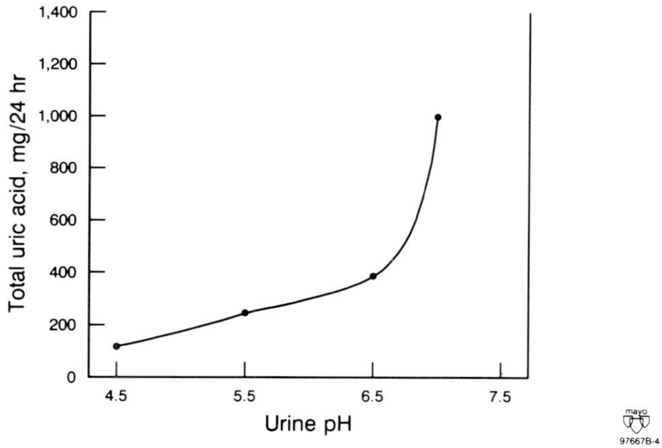

Fig. 10-2. Uric acid solubility. Assuming a solubility of 100 mg/liter of free uric acid, the total uric acid necessary to cause saturation of free uric acid is plotted against urinary pH (using a pK_a of 5.7 for uric acid).

excretion in an acid urine pH if urine flows are low enough. Note that the solubility of ammonium urate is only 5.4 mg/dl at a pH of 7.4.

At an average uric acid excretion of 600 mg/per 24-hour period and an average urine volume of 1.5 liters/day, 400 mg/liter total uric acid is excreted. At a pH of 5.5 this would be 200 mg/liter of free uric acid, which is supersaturated. This urine would be supersaturated with respect to free uric acid at any pH less than 6.4 (Fig. 10-2).

Urinary pH

The American diet usually produces an excess of 70–100 mEq of hydrogen ion daily; therefore, the pH of the urine is usually acidic. The exact pH depends on the amount of acid excreted, the amount of phosphate and other titratable acids available to buffer it, and the rate of ammonia production and excretion. Normally about two-thirds of net acid is excreted in the form of NH_4^+, and one-third as titratable acids, primarily phosphate. Ammonium excretion can be, and usually is, modified over a wide range to buffer the net acid load that must be excreted. The exact controls for NH_3 production are not clear, but they may relate to the cellular pH, which controls entry of glutamine into mitochondria for conversion to ammonia.

After an acid load the urine pH becomes more acid. The percentage of phosphate present as H_2PO_4 rather than $NaHPO_4$ increases. Acid excretion is also raised by increasing ammonium buffer production and/or lowering the urine pH. Patients in whom uric acid stones form characteristically have an inordinately acid urinary pH most of the time. Gutman and Yu reviewed urinary pH data on 233 patients.[14] After a 12-hour fast, the first morning specimen showed a pH range of less than 4.8 to 5.0 in about one-third of the patients, under 5.4 in 70 percent, and 6.0 or more in 4 percent. After the same overnight fast, 15 percent of normals showed a pH of under 5, 60 percent were between 5.1 and 5.6, and about 26 percent were over 5.7. This change has been described in cases of idiopathic uric acid calculi as well.

Studies concerning the pathogenesis of persistently acid urine in gout and other uric acid stone patients have led to controversial results. It is known that urine ammonia excretion rates are often low in uric acid stone formers. Since titratable acid excretion is limited by the number of buffers available, this leads directly to abnormally low urinary pHs. The low ammonia excretion rate is not ascribed to age, depressed renal function, or any known specific metabolic lesion. Acid loading with ammonium chloride normally provokes a large increase in ammonia production and excretion in normals. It does not increase as much in uric acid stone formers as in normal persons.[21] Patients with gout also do not get a normal urinary alkaline tide after meals. The alkaline tide is related to the secretion of hydrogen ions into the stomach, which results in increased bicarbonate reabsorption. This bicarbonate is normally excreted by the kidney, increasing urinary pHs. This same phenomenon is not seen in patients with gout. The urine pH drops even lower during the evening hours in those with gout and hyperuricemia than in controls. Nighttime is a high-risk time for uric acid stone formers.

The exact reasons for low ammonia excretion levels in gout or nongouty uric acid stone formers are not known. It is proposed that there is a disturbance of glutamine deamination, which would result in deficient ammonia production and lower available ammonia in the tubular fluid in the distal nephron. It is postulated that the loss of the alkaline tide results from a mild metabolic acidosis in these patients, which leads to the lower urine pHs. The decrease in ammonia excretion is normally about 30 percent, which would decrease total acid excretion by about 15–20 percent. This could be overcome by an increase in titratable acid of about 40–50 percent. Studies have revealed that there is increased phosphate and titratable acid in these patients. Consequently, net acid excretion is normal over a 24-hour period, but at the expense of lower urinary pHs.

Dietary Factors

Many patients with uric acid stones ingest excess animal protein. The amount of acid excreted each day would obligate a more acid urine even if the ability to produce ammonium were normal. In a like number of patients with ileostomies, which are associated with a bicarbonate loss, a continuously acid urine compensates for the bowel loss of alkali.

Animal protein consumption contributes to uric acid stone formation for at least three reasons: (1) the sulfur-containing amino acids and phospholipids are the chief source of nonvolatile acid, (2) glandular meats are particularly high in purine derivatives that are converted to excess uric acid, and (3) protein or amino acid loading is uricosuric in and of itself by increasing renal tubular secretion.[19]

Potential Risk Factors For Stone Formation

Three major conditions control the potential for uric acid calculi: the quantitative excretion of uric acid, the volume of urine as it affects the urinary concentration of uric acid, and the urinary pH. There is also some question of a nondialyzable substance in the urine of idiopathic uric acid stone formers. Most investigators, however, feel that there are no inhibitors for uric acid, and that the supersaturation of uric acid is the critical issue.

There are a number of clinical conditions associated with increased urine uric acid excretion. Uricosuric drugs such as probenecid, sulfinpyrazone, and salicylates produce an increase in uric acid excretion that predisposes to stone formation. The importance of this phenomenon to long-term stone formation is unclear. These drugs lead to only a transient increase in uric acid excretion until a new balance between filtration and reabsorption of uric acid is established. Then uric acid excretion often returns to baseline levels, but at a lower plasma urate level. Yu did report an increase of uric acid stone formation after the introduction of probenecid in their gouty patients.[32] Fessel was unable to document any difference between the incidence of stones in patients treated with allopurinol versus probenecid.[12]

Increased ingestion of a diet high in purine content as outlined above will increase urinary uric acid. An increase from 2 mg/kg to 4 mg/kg of animal protein will increase uric acid excretion by about 300 mg per 24-hour period into a range that is clearly hyperuricosuric.

Enzyme defects in purine biosynthesis may lead to increased uric acid excretion. Inosinic acid (IMP) is the parent purine compound and is formed through two primary paths: (1) the enzymatic addition of small amino acids, such as glutamine, glycine, and formate to phosphoribosylprophosphate (PRPP); and (2) the synthesis of ribonucleotides from free purine bases, specifically, adenylic acid, xanthylic acid, and guanylic acid. Reutilization of these products are of major importance in purine metabolism as has been shown in those patients who have a deficiency of hypoxanthine–guanine phosphoribosyltransferase (HGPRTase) (Figure 10-3).

The three purine bases are reutilized in the formation of their respective mononucle-

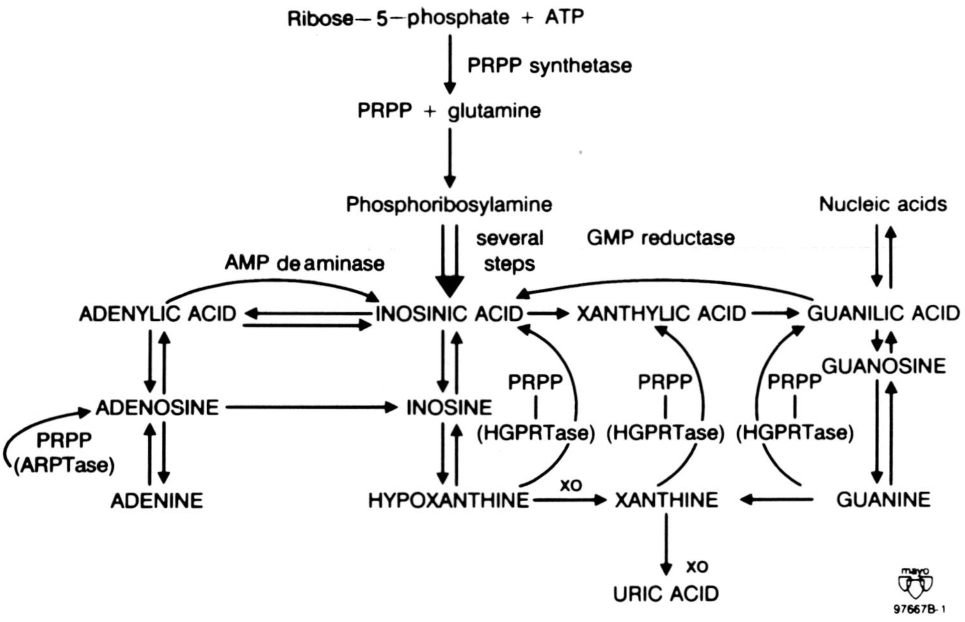

Fig. 10-3. A simplified scheme of uric acid metabolism indicating the major sources of uric acid, the rescue pathways for nucleotides, and the enzymes that control those reactions. See text for explanation.

otides. The HGPRTase enzyme transfers the ribose-5-phosphate (PRPP) to hypoxanthine and guanine to "rescue" them and form IMP and GMP, respectively. A separate enzyme, ARPTase, converts adenine to AMP. Xanthine is also sparingly reutilized by a reaction catalyzed by HGPRTase. These reutilization reactions are alternate pathways of purine ribonucleotide formation. The rates for both de novo purine formation and reutilization are reciprocally controlled by competition for a common substrate (PRPP) and are inhibited by the same end products. The degradation of AMP and GMP to IMP and ammonia is catalyzed by the enzymes AMP deaminase and GMP reductase. Analyses of alterations in various steps of this process resulting in hyperuricemia have been undertaken. It is estimated that 1–10 percent of the hyperuricemic population may have an enzyme defect in one of these steps.

A common defect is associated with the increased presence of PRPP synthetase. At least two families have been described in which structural alterations of PRPP synthetase have resulted in excessive uric acid production and gout.[4]

Hyperuricemia occurs in patients with type I glycogen storage disease. These patients lack glucose-6-phosphatase activity. The elevated levels of lactic acid and beta-hydroxybutyrate in these patients inhibit renal tubular excretion of uric acid, which increases serum uric acid. In addition, these patients have an increased production of uric acid.[1]

A deficiency of HGPRTase was initially described in 1964. This was reported as a familial disorder in patients who had a central nervous system (CNS) dysfunction, mutilating behavior, choreoathetosis, mental retardation, and/or cerebral palsy. These patients develop severe hyperuricemia and profound hyperuricosuria. Uric acid production is increased to 5–6 times normal. The lack of HGPRTase activity prevents reutilization of hypoxanthine, accounting for the predominance of hypoxanthine over xanthine in the urine.

The deficiency is sex-linked, and the disorder is found only in males. Examination of amniotic fluid cells allows identification of affected male offspring in utero.[10] The onset of gouty arthritis and uric acid nephrolithiasis usually occurs in adolescents and young adults. Stones often are seen in patients with only partial deficiency of HGPRTase as reflected by intermediate levels of the cellular enzyme.

Screening for other biochemical defects in purine metabolism has lead to the discovery of APRTase deficiency. This is inherited as an autosomal dominant trait, and there is overproduction of uric acid in the families in which this has been found; however, PRPP values are normal.[17]

Van Acker, et al. have also reported a patient with homozygote deficiency for APRTase.[28] This patient had recurrent stones that were composed of 2,8-dihydroxyadinine. The urinary excretion of 2,8-dihydroxyadinine was increased in the patient and in an asymptomatic older brother. Allopurinol decreased stone formation.[28]

In 25 percent of patients with primary gout there is overproduction of purine and, therefore, uric acid.[26] The mechanism responsible for the overproduction is poorly understood other than the small minority of cases outlined above. Gutman and Yu have proposed that a large fraction of glutamine is diverted from ammonia production to purine synthesis in the kidney due to an abnormality of renal glutaminase.[14] Direct measurement of this enzyme, however, has not substantiated any decrease in renal glutaminase. Increased uric acid production is seen in patients with increased protein intake, obesity, and in individuals with excessive ethanol consumption.[13]

The majority of patients with gout do not have increased purine production, but rather an abnormally low renal excretion for uric acid that results in hyperuricicemia and a subsequently higher than normal filtered urate. Since 75 percent of the patients with gout do not have overproduction of uric acid, increased excretion of uric acid cannot explain the increased incidence of stones in the majority of gouty patients.

The renal handling of uric acid has been exceedingly difficult to evaluate in patients with gout. Uric acid is initially filtered at the glomerulus, and 90–95 percent of the filtered urate is reabsorbed proximally. There is subsequently a proximal tubular secretory component for uric acid secretion. A fourth step involves the reabsorption of the secreted uric acid just distal to the secretory site.[5,22,29]

Gouty patients with decreased excretion of uric acid were studied by a combination of benzbromarone, which blocks urate reabsorption, and pyrazinamide, which blocks the secretory component of uric acid secretion. In the presence of pyrazinamide the uricosuric response to benzbromarone was less than in the normals, suggesting that a deficient secretory apparatus explains the hyperuricemia in these patients with gout.

Uric acid excretion is markedly elevated in patients with myeloproliferative disorders. Yu and Gutman have reported that the prevalence of uric acid calculi is twice as high as in patients with primary gout and 4000 times as high as the general population.[31] It is their observation that the major difference between these patients, and those with primary gout, or those with lead nephropathy is the quantity of uric acid excreted.

The effect of urine volume seems obvious, and there are several clinical experiments confirming that urine volume is particularly important in uric acid stone formation. The studies by de Vries et al. in Israel have indicated that the first generation Jews transplanted to Israel had extremely low urine volumes, presumably because of preformed drinking habits that did not change on arrival in Israel.[3] This is thought to explain the extremely high incidence of uric acid stones in this population. Uric acid excretion rates actually fell in these patients, but uric acid concentrations rose because of the marked decrease in urinary volumes. A second group of patients with low urine volumes known to be at high risk for uric acid stones include those with small bowel diseases, colon disease, and postileostomy patients. Presumably this is due to the low volume acid urines these patients exhibit.

Uric Acid Calculi: Diagnosis

The differential diagnosis of uric acid calculi is often the differential diagnosis of a filling defect on the intravenous pyleogram (IVP). In the 1940s Muellner concluded that most nonopaque stones contain uric acid,[20] but there was no infallible method for demonstration of the presence, nature, size, or location of a nonopaque stone. In the 1950s the Bucky tomographic modification of a KUB improved the resolution of these filling defects since larger uric acid calculi were shown to have a miniscule amount of opaqueness that helped to differentiate them from tumors, blood clots, and other lesions. In the 1970s ultrasonic evaluation of radiolucent defects in the kidney was developed. With this technique, uric acid calculi caused a negative shadow not seen by clots and tumors that improved the differentiation between them. Computed tomography (CT) clearly differentiates uric acid stones from nonopaque masses.[11] The density of uric acid stones is 350–400 Hounsfield units on a ± 1000 scale. This is similar to xanthine stones but different from cystine at 585 Hounsfield units and calcium-oxalate at 510 Hounsfield units.[24] For the first time precise definition of these radiolucent stones is made possible by CT scanning.

Uric Acid Calculi: Management

The management of patients with uric acid calculi is most effective when the pathogenesis of the stone disease is understood. To ascertain that a lucent defect or stone is actually a uric acid calculi is critical to this approach. The diagnosis of uric acid calculi is most firmly based when the stone has been analyzed. The differential diagnosis of lucent stones, in addition to uric acid, includes sodium urate stones, ammonium urate stones, xanthine stones (all of which have different treatments and solubilities), and the rare 2,8-dihydroxyadinine stones that have been reported. Occasionally cystine stones are sufficiently lucent to be confusing. They are usually more dense on KUB than uric acid stones. Xanthine stones are lucent and are almost always found in the presence of a low serum uric acid and low to absent uric acid excretion. Most of these are associated with large doses of allopurinol or in patients with primary xanthinuria. The presence of 2,8-dihydroxyadinine stones rarely is suspected but may be diagnosed by x-ray difraction or infrared spectroscopy of the stone and also suggested by the absence of adenine phosphoribosyltransferase activity in erythrocytes. Stones that are refractory to usual therapy for uric acid stones often come to extraction or surgical procedures, so that stone analysis is carried out and often leads to the discovery of the unusual lucent stones such as xanthine, urate, and 2,8-dihydroxyadinine stones. Both surgical and medical management of uric acid stones need to be individualized.

Uric Acid Calculi: Surgical Management

The role for surgical management of uric acid stones may be critical in certain instances. A surgical approach to a uric acid stone may be indicated in the presence of high-grade obstruction, persistent pain, or sepsis. Prior to the advent of percutaneous ultrasonic lithotripsy (PUL) and extracorporeal shock-wave lithotripsy (ESWL), uretero-lithotomy and/or pylelolithotomy occasionally were necessary. Current technology using ureteroscopy, placement of double-J stents around an obstructing uric acid stone and the availability of a urologist or a radiologist for percutaneous treatment has virtually eliminated the need for surgical intervention for uric acid stones. Infected or mixed uric acid/struvite stones may require pelviolithotomy if PUL is not successful. Since ESWL is often disappointing in the complete removal of struvite, it has been our practice to consider ultrasonic lithotripsy in the presence of struvite stones. Occasionally the combination of ESWL and PUL is necessary. Percutaneous ultrasonic lithotripsy has been performed in over 20 Mayo Clinic patients with uric acid stones and extracoporeal lithotripsy in a like number. Although uric acid stones are quite hard with respect to PUL, it is possible to break them up and extract them, and/or manipulate the stones. Extracorporeal shock-wave lithotripsy has also been successful in breaking up uric acid stones. This technique is complicated by the necessity for using intravenous pyelographic dye or retrograde dye in order to localize the stone prior to the ESWL.

The dissolution kinetics of uric acid calculi has been described by Burns, et al.[8] The effect of tromethamine for injection (THAM) and sodium bicarbonate in vitro was explored with the idea that these solutions could be used to irrigate uric acid calculi. A 1-cm uric acid stone could theoretically be dissolved in 4.4 days at a pH of 7.0 with THAM, but the effect of sodium bicarbonate was somewhat slower. Kursh and Resnick showed that it is possible to dissolve uric stones in a period of 5–7 days with intravenous administration of 40–50 ml/hour of $^1/_6$-molar lactate.[18] In Kursh and Resnick's study, 8 of 10 stones were successfully dissolved, and the 2 that failed were composed of a mixture of uric acid and sodium acid urate. This approach might be appropriate in those few circumstances in which other procedures are contraindicated.

Uric Acid Calculi: Medical Management

Table 10-2 outlines the therapeutic steps in the management of uric acid stones based on (1) the assessment of urinary volume status, (2) identification of urinary pH profiles, and (3) identification of disorders leading to excessive urate production or excretion.

Urinary volume status is determined clinically by reviewing oral intake of fluids and correlating this with the 24-hour urine volumes which the patient obtains under local ambient conditions. Discrepancies between the intakes and outputs are usually caused by dietary, occupational, environmental, or medical problems. Patients with high uric acid excretion rates due to obesity also perspire heavily, resulting in low urine volumes. Often the patient's surroundings, in either occupational or recreational settings, play an important role in urine volumes. For example, patients who perform manual labor in hot climates, or those who have avocations such as jogging, often have low urine volumes. Patients with bowel disorders not only have bicarbonate loss from their stools, but often large volume losses that are difficult to control.

Table 10-2
Physiologic Parameters in the Evaluation of Patients with Radiolucent Stones

Excretory Urogram (EXU; also IVP) ultrasound, CT scan: to establish presence of stone
Blood studies
Uric acid
Creatinine (BUN)
Bicarbonate
Urinary studies
24-hour urine volume
Urinalysis
First morning urine pH
Random urinary pHs (multiple)
Uric acid
Sodium
Xanthine (if uric acid <200)
Uric acid production (excretion after 72 h, purine-free diet)
Special studies: when indicated
HGPRTase—tissue level
ARPTase—tissue level
G-6-PD—tissue level
PRPP—tissue level
Stone analysis: x-ray diffraction or infrared analysis
Xanthine
Sodium Urate
NH_4 Urate
2,8-Dihydroxadenine

Urinary pH data are critical. In addition to assessing the first morning urine pH on a urinalysis, we often have the patient check multiple voidings with nitrazine paper to determine whether there are persistently acid urines as have been described for the gouty and hyperuricosuric patients.

Uric acid excretion is an important element in the evaluation of patients with uric acid stones. Only 25 percent of patients with uric acid stones have hyperuricemia or hyperuricosuria. Rational therapy for uric acid lithiasis depends on identifying those patients with hyperuricosuria since treatment may well be altered. Uric acid excretion may be dietary dependent since many people in the United States have a high protein intake. Cultural factors may be identified such as in body builders or weight lifters who often ingest large amounts of powdered protein supplements. Treatment for overproduction of uric acid requires allopurinol, while increased intake of uric acid may respond to dietary protein restriction. Overproduction can be adduced clinically by placing the patient on a meat-free diet for 72 hours and assessing uric acid excretion rates.

In patients with excessive uric acid excretion one should identify patients with malignancies and myeloproliferative or lymphoproliferative disorders and consider the inherited enzymatic abnormalities outlined previously.

An adequate fluid output is critical for the treatment of uric acid stones as it is for other forms of nephrolithiasis. Current recommendations are that patients attempt to excrete 2500 ml of urine on a daily basis. For most patients this involves the intake of about 3 liters, or twelve 8-ounce glasses of fluid daily. The patients are carefully counseled about the effect of extra fluid on lifestyle. A single discussion usually is insufficient. Repeated reminders must be given since behavior modification is required.

Patients with bowel disease are of special concern. Many patients with ileostomies or bowel disorders have increased bowel motility and decreased urine volumes. More frequent but smaller amounts of fluid for these patients are stressed. Patients are encouraged to increase intake and calculate net urine losses, even if there is some increase in stool or ileostomy volumes. Lomotil (diphenoxylate hydrochloride with atropine sulfate; Searle, San Juan, PR) or other opiate-type drugs are not usually effective in reducing bowel fluid losses; however, these should be tried. Patients with high stool fat losses often decrease stool volumes with dietary fat restriction.

For hyperuricemia it is our practice to use allopurinol during the early phase of therapy while attempting to dissolve current stones. It is important to maximize the use of all the parameters available during this phase.

Although the literature is not clear in its suggestion that probenecid causes stones, gouty patients on Benemid may be at risk for more stones at the onset of treatment.[31] Fessel's data, however, suggest that on a long-term basis it is not a major risk factor for stones,[12] and Boger and Strickland reported only 17 cases of stones in 2500 cases of gout treated with probenecid.[6] Most authors feel that allopurinol is the drug of choice in the setting of overproduction of uric acid.[2,9,30] It is the authors' experience that a 300-mg dose of allopurinol in a patient will reduce urinary uric acid by about 300 mg per 24-hour period. Several other investigators have shown a much greater reduction of urinary uric acid, for example, from 1500 mg down to 600 mg in some patients.[30]

Theoretically the decrease in uric acid excretion would be matched by a similar increase in xanthine or hypoxanthine in the urine, both of which have sparing solubility. It is apparent from the metabolic data, however, that the hypoxanthine and xanthine are reclaimed and rescued for further purine synthesis; therefore, there are only modest rises in xanthine and hypoxanthine. There have been very few xanthine or hypoxanthine stones reported as a complication of uric acid therapy except in patients who have severe overproduction and/or exceedingly high allopurinol doses such as 600–900 mg per 24-hour period.[7,27]

Physiologic information available about urate solubility and pH make it clear that the urinary pH is of primary importance in the dissolution and undersaturation of uric acid in urine. Alteration of the urine pH is the primary mode of therapy in patients with uric acid stone disease.

The PK_a of uric acid in urine is 5.5; thus, maintenance of urinary pH at 6.5 assures that 90 percent of the urate measured in the urine is in the form of urate and 10 percent is uric acid. If urine pH can be maintained at that level, and uric acid excretion were constant at 800 mg/day throughout the day, urine could remain undersaturated in as little as 800 ml/day, assuming the solubility product to be 100 mg/dl. At a urine pH of 4.5, only 10 percent of the measured urate is sodium urate and 90 percent is free uric acid. Consequently, 720 mg of the 800-mg excretion rate described above would be in the form of free uric acid, and a daily output of over 7.2 liters would be necessary to maintain the urine undersaturated. The addition of allopurinol could reduce excretion to about 500 mg per 24-hour period, necessitating 5 liters of fluid daily at a pH of 4.5 in order to maintain the urine at the same level of saturation. The manipulation of urinary pH is much more efficacious than either allopurinol or urinary volume manipulations in dealing with uric acid stones.

Persistently acid urines in patients with uric acid stones are sometimes refractory to therapy. Patients with ileostomies and persistently acid urines secondary to bicarbonate loss in the stool may require large amounts of alkali to maintain the urine pH at 6.5. Large amounts of alkaline salts may promote diarrhea in this setting. It is difficult to assess urine pHs in patients who have ileal conduits. The conduit itself modulates the pH of the urine so that one is not certain of the pH in the renal pelvis.

Patients who do not have metabolic abnormalities causing bicarbonate wasting or excess acid production will remain alkaline if the dietary acid intake is neutralized with approximately 1 mEq/kg base daily. Potassium hydrogen sodium citrate has a long half-life, and the metabolic conversion of the citrate to bicarbonate promotes a smooth prolonged increase in the urinary pH. Sodium bicarbonate (10 tablets daily = 75 mEq) is an alternative but is absorbed and excreted rapidly, causing peaks and valleys in the urinary pH. Many patients complain of gas and eructation. The theoretical advantage of using a potassium salt over a sodium salt has been reported by Sakhaee et al.[25] The urine becomes undersaturated with respect to uric acid with both potassium and sodium salts, but the sodium citrate salt causes relative supersaturation for monosodiumurate. More importantly, because there is no drop in calcium excretion with the sodium salt, the activity product ratio is higher for calcium oxalate, brushite, and the formation product ratio is lower for sodium citrate than for potassium citrate. Consequently, the treatment of uric acid stones could be complicated by the precipitation of both calcium oxalate and brushite during the therapy of uric acid stones with sodium alkalai salts.

Complications of Therapy and Secondary Evaluations

Experience has shown that the success rate for dissolution of uric acid stones is about 90 percent when medical therapy is undertaken. There are several reasons for the failure of medical therapy in the other 10 percent.

Mixed calcium oxalate–uric acid stones are poorly dissolved by the therapies mentioned above. Uric acid stones that contain more than a very minimal amount of calcium are quite refractory to dissolution. Current policy in these cases is to attempt dissolution with alkali, volume, and allopurinol for a period of 2–3 months before making a decision concerning intervention.

The two forms of urate stones are rare but are particularly troublesome with respect to medical therapy. Sodium urate stones occasionally form in the presence of high sodium content. At 140 mEq/liter of sodium, the solubility of sodium urate is only 6.4 mg/dl. This level is occasionally exceeded if there are high sodium and uric acid excretion rates (Table 10-1). Resolution can sometimes be effected by the use of a potassium citrate solution.

Ammonium urate stones have been seen in two settings. Patients with infected urine with urea-splitting organisms have alkaline urines and high ammonia excretion rates. About 3.0 mEq/liter of ammonia will reduce the solubility of the urate salt in this setting (Table 10-1). An additional setting in which we have begun to recognize formation of ammonia urate stones is in patients who are extremely aciduric, often laxative abusers with very low urine volumes. These patients can produce sufficient ammonia so that, with their very low urine volumes, the ammonium urate solubility product is exceeded despite the acidity of their urine. Ammonium urate stones are usually more soluble in acid urine than in alkaline urine. Many of these patients are also hypokalemic, which promotes increased ammonia production (personal communication William Dick, M.D.).

Treatment for these patients involves counseling relative to increased urinary volume and correction of the hypokalemia.

Prophylaxis

Long-term prophylaxis for uric acid stones is dependent on pathophysiologic parameters identified in a given patient. Current therapeutic programs include the following:

1. Sufficient fluid intake to provide 2500 ml urinary output on a regular basis throughout the day and evening.
2. Alkali therapy, preferably with potassium or mixed alkali salt. Monitor urinary pHs with nitrazine paper, and alter the alkali dose to provide appropriate pH (pH 6–7 80 percent of the time). Nighttime pH values are particularly critical since this is when the urine is most acid. Initially urine pH should be monitored throughout the night, and, if necessary, sufficient alkali should be taken at bedtime to prevent acid urines on arising in the morning. Patients taking sodium bicarbonate are encouraged to take a longer acting form of alkali at bedtime. The use of Diamox (acetazolamide; Lederle, Wayne, NJ) at bedtime should probably be avoided since it has been noted that calcified rims may develop easily on uric acid stones in this setting. The calcified rims are presumably as a result of the extremely low urinary citrates that develop.
3. Patients with increased uric acid excretion are initially counseled to reduce their meat intake to about 80 g/day and their purine intake to a range of 2 mg/kg. Normally, allopurinol therapy is instituted for long-term prophylaxis only in those patients who continue to have metabolically active stone formation despite fluid and alkali therapy. Allopurinol is used in uric acid stone-forming patients, using the same criteria that are used in non-stone-forming gouty patients with respect to the serum uric acid. There is little justification for the use of allopurinol in asymptomatic women with serum uric acids under 10 mg/dl or in men with serum uric acid levels below 12 mg/dl.

In summary, uric acid lithiasis is an example of a disorder in which the physiology and pathophysiology of the stone formation is quite well understood. The major physiologic principles governing uric acid solubility and supersaturation include the concentration of uric acid, pH of the urine, and the accompanying monovalent anions and cations in the urine. In the vast majority of patients, attention to modulation of these factors using diet, volume, and pH manipulation will prevent and/or dissolve their stones. The refractory cases include patients in whom some of these parameters are uncontrollable or circumstances in which the theraputic maneuvers promote epitaxy or alternate stone forms such as sodium urate, ammonium urate, and xanthine. Analysis of medical treatment failures through application of physiologic principles can lead to satisfactory medical management of most clinical problems.

REFERENCES

1. Alepa FP, Howell RR, Klinenberg JR, et al: Relationships between glycogen storage disease and Tophaceous gout. Am J Med 42:58–66, 1967
2. Anderson EE, Rundles RW, Silberman HR, et al.: Allopurinol control of hyperuricosuria: A new concept in the prevention of uric acid stones. J Urol 97:344–347, 1967
3. Atsmon A, de Vries A, Frank M: Uric acid lithiasis. Amsterdam, Elsevier, 1963, p 6

4. Becker, Meyer LJ, Seegmiller JE: Gout with purine overproduction due to increased phosphoribosylpyrophospate synthetase activity. Am J Med 55:232–242, 1973
5. Bennett JS, Bond J, Singer I, et al.: Hypouricemia in Hodgkins disease. Ann Intern Med 76:751–756, 1972
6. Boger WP, Strickland SC: Probenecid (Benemid). Its uses and side-effects in 2,502 patients. Arch Intern Med 95:83–92, 1955
7. Brock WA, Golden J, Kaplan GW: Xanthine calculi in the Lesch-Nyhan syndrome. J Urol 130:157–159, 1983
8. Burns JR, Gauthier JF, Finlayson B: Dissolution kinetics of uric acid calculi. J Urol 131:708–711, 1984
9. De Vries A, Frank M, Liberman UA, et al.: Allopurinol in the prophylaxis of uric acid stones. Ann Rheumat Dis 25:691–693, 1966
10. DeMars R, Sarto C, Felix SS, et al: Lesch-Nyhan mutation: Prenatal detection with amniotic fluid cells. Sciences 164:1303–1305, 1969
11. Federle MP, McAninch JW, Kaiser JA, et al: Computed tomography of urinary calculi. Am J Roentgenology 136:255–258, 1981
12. Fessel WJ: Renal outcomes of gout and hyperuricemia. Am J Med 67:74–82, 1979
13. Grunst J, Dietze G, Wicklmayr M: Effect of ethanol on uric acid production of human liver. Nutr Metab 21:138(382)–141(385), 1977
14. Gutman A, Yu TF: Urinary ammonium excretion in primary gout. J Clin Invest 44:1474–1481, 1965
15. Herring LC: Observations in the analysis of ten thousand urinary calculi. J Urol 88:545–562, 1962
16. Ibrahim A, Zein M, Beleil O: Uric acid lithiasis in the Sudan. J Trop Med Hyg 80:173–176, 1977
17. Kelley WN, Levy RI, Rosenbloom FM, et al: Adenine phosphoribosyltransferase deficiency: A previously undescribed genetic defect in man. J Clin Invest 47:2281–2284, 1968
18. Kursh ED, Resnick MI: Dissolution of uric acid calculi systemic alkalization. J Urol 132:286–287, 1984
19. Matzkies F, Berg G: The uricosuric action of amino acids in man. Adv Exp Med Biol 76B:36–40, 1977
20. Muellner SR, Sears B: The problem of the nonopaque urinary tract stone. J Urol 67:832–836, 1952
21. Plante GE, Durivage J, Lemieux G: Renal excretion of hydrogen in primary gout. Metabolism 17:377–385, 1968
22. Praetorius E, Kirk JE: Hypouricemia: With evidence for tubular elimination of uric acid. J Lab Clin Med 35:865–868, 1950
23. Prien EL: Crystallographic analysis of urinary calculi: A 23 year survey study. J Urol 89:917–924, 1963
24. Resnick MI, Kursh ED, Cohen AM: Use of computerized tomography in the delineation of uric acid calculi. J Urol 131:9–10, 1984
25. Sakhaee K, Nicar M, Hill K, et al: Contrasting effects of potassium citrate and sodium citrate therapies on urinary chemistries and crystallization of stone-forming salts. Kidney Internatl 24:348–352, 1983
26. Seegmiller JE, Grayzel AI, Laster L, et al: Uric acid production in gout. J Clin Invest 40:1304–1314, 1961
27. Stote RM, Smith LH, Dubb JW, et al: Oxypurinol nephrolithiasis in regional enteritis secondary to allopurinol therapy. Ann Inter Med 92:384–385, 1980
28. van Acker KJ, Simonds AJ, Cammeron JS: Complete deficiency of phosphoribosyltransferase (APRT): Report of a family. J Clin Chem Biochem 14:227–332, 1976

29. Wilson DM, Goldstein NP: Renal urate excretion in patients with Wilson's disease. Kidney Internatl 4:331–336, 1973
30. Yu TF, Gutman AB: Effect of allopurinol in relation to purine biosynthesis. Ann Rheum Dis 25:601–607, 1966
31. Yu TF, Gutman AB: Uric acid nephrolithiasis in gout. Ann Intern Med 67:1133–1148, 1967
32. Yu TF: Urolithiasis in hyperuricemia and gout. J Urol 81:424–430, 1981

Christian J. Van Den Berg

11

Cystinuria

Cystinuria is an inherited disorder characterized by abnormalities in the renal and intestinal cell transport for basic amino acids: cystine, ornithine, lysine, and arginine (COLA). If it were not for the relative insolubility of cystine in urine resulting in the formation of cystine calculi, this disorder would be only a metabolic curiosity. Cystinuria is inherited as an autosomal recessive trait, and the incidence of heterozygotes in the population is estimated at 1:200 to 1:600. From a practical standpoint, heterozygotes usually excrete less than 400 mg cystine daily and seldom form cystine calculi. People with homozygous cystinuria usually excrete more than 400 mg cystine daily and may form cystine calculi. Increased urinary excretion of ornithine, lysine, and arginine is also present; however, this does not present a practical problem as these amino acids remain soluble in urine. Initial cystine calculi may form at any age; however, the diagnosis is especially suggested by the finding of a homogeneous radiodense calculus in a young patient who has a family history of nephrolithiasis. Typically, cystine calculi are moderately opaque on x-ray and, if not contaminated with calcium salts, appear homogeneous with a ground-glass appearance. While solitary stones are common, cystine calculi may assume the configuration of the renal pelvis and calyces, forming a staghorn calculus that, if associated with multiple smaller, more peripheral calculi, results in a KUB x-ray very typical for cystine urolithiasis (Fig. 11-1).

The diagnosis of cystinuria is not difficult and is made by an analysis of a cystine stone and the finding of increased urinary excretion of cystine. Cystine crystalluria with typical hexagonal "benzine ring" crystals may be present and is a valuable clue to the diagnosis (Fig. 11-2). The cyanide nitroprusside test for the presence of cystine in urine is positive if the urinary concentration of cystine exceeds 75 mg/g of creatinine. This qualitative test is useful in screening all patients with renal calculi in order to detect those who may have homozygous cystinuria; however, it is not sufficiently sensitive to detect heterozygotes who have only a small increase in the urinary excretion of cystine. A quantitative determination of the urinary excretion of cystine is necessary for family studies and if the screening test is positive.

STONE DISEASE: DIAGNOSIS AND MANAGEMENT

ISBN 0-8089-1873-7

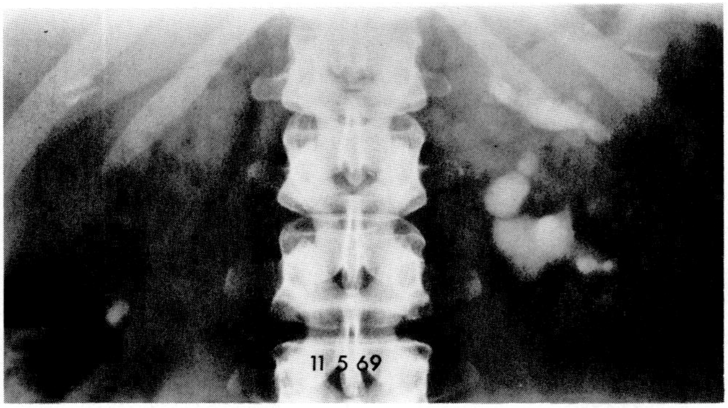

Fig. 11-1. Cystine urolithiasis. (From Van Den Berg CJ: Urolithiasis, in Spittell JA Jr (ed): Clinical Medicine. Philadelphia, Harper & Row, 1981, p 9. With permission.)

Treatment is designed to decrease the level of urinary cystine saturation by increasing the solubility of cystine and decreasing the urinary concentration of cystine. Solubility increases as the urine pH increases. It is possible to dissolve approximately 300 mg of cystine in 1 liter of urine at a pH of less than 7.0. By increasing the urine pH to 7.5, the capacity of urine to accept cystine in solution is more than doubled. It should be noted that the solubility curve for cystine dictates a clinically significant increase in solubility only as the urine pH increases above 7.0. This is at the upper end of the pH range of urine and requires vigorous alkalinization of the urine to a pH greater than 7.5 throughout a 24-hour period if this is to be helpful in preventing cystine crystal formation. Oral alkali usually is started in a dose of 1 mEq/kg daily in divided doses. Although sodium bicarbonate may be used, it must be administered frequently because of its short duration

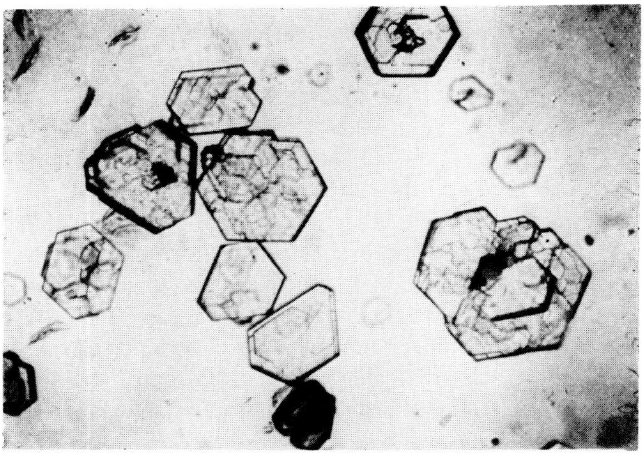

Fig. 11-2. Cystine crystalluria. (From Van Den Berg CJ: Urolithiasis, in Spittell JA Jr (ed): Clinical Medicine. Philadelphia, Harper & Row, 1981, p 9. With permission.)

of action and often causes gaseous gastrointestinal complaints. For these reasons, a citrate solution is usually recommended. Citrate is metabolized to bicarbonate equivalents and usually is free of adverse effects. Sodium, potassium, or combined sodium-potassium preparations are available. Care must be taken in providing potassium to people with severely impaired renal function, and any additional sodium must be considered in situations such as hypertension or states of fluid retention where sodium restriction is required. The dose and administration schedule is adjusted on the basis of results of testing the urine pH in the morning and in the evening. If the urine pH is below 7.0 on a first morning voided urine, the evening dose is increased. Similarly, if the urine pH is below 7.0 during the afternoon or evening, the daytime doses are increased. If there is persistent difficulty in maintaining the first morning urine pH equal to or greater than 7.5, the addition of a carbonic anhydrase inhibitor at night may be helpful. The urine concentration of cystine is decreased by increasing the urine volume and the use of d-penicillamine. Patients are requested to increase their oral fluids adequate to ensure at least 3 liters of urine daily. We ask our patients to periodically collect a 24-hour urine sample to monitor the volume of their urine output in order to ensure that this remains as directed despite changes in activity or climate. If the patient awakens during the night to void, this opportunity should be used for an extra glass or two of water and a dose of alkali if appropriate. Indeed, many of our patients with cystinuria are encouraged to awake at night for extra oral fluids. The urinary excretion of cystine is reduced (40–80 percent) in proportion to the dose of oral d-penicillamine. d-Penicillamine and cystine undergo a disulfide reaction resulting in a mixed disulfide (cysteine-penicillamine) which has greater solubility in urine than cystine. It is not clear whether this disulfide exchange occurs in the blood, the urine, or both. Unfortunately, d-penicillamine is not an innocuous drug. Adverse reactions occur in approximately one-half of our patients who take d-penicillamine and include serum sickness–type hypersensitivity reactions, bone marrow depression, high-grade proteinuria with frank nephrotic syndrome (membranous glomerulonephritis), abnormalities in taste, skin lesions, and gastrointestinal complaints. For minor problems such as changes in taste, arthralgias, and mild gastrointestinal upset, d-penicillamine may usually be continued. For the more serious adverse reactions such as agranulocytosis, nephrotic syndrome, and serum sickness–type reactions. It usually is necessary to discontinue d-penicillamine. In rare instances where continued cystine stone formation threatens the loss of remaining renal function and all other measures have failed, d-penicillamine has been successfully restarted under the cover of corticosteroids after an initial adverse reaction. In instances of d-penicillamine-related nephrotic syndrome, the drug has been continued without loss of renal function. d-Penicillamine is started carefully, beginning with 250 mg daily, and the dose is increased by 250 mg/day each week until the usual adult dose of 1.5–2.0 g/day is reached. Absorption from the gastrointestinal tract is facilitated if d-penicillamine is ingested on an empty stomach. The hemoglobin, white blood cell count, platelets, blood enzymes, and the urinalysis, with particular reference to proteinuria, should be monitored during d-penicillamine therapy. Initially, these parameters should be checked monthly for 3 months followed by quarterly evaluations. It is important to persist in monitoring these laboratory parameters as adverse reactions may occur at any time while taking d-penicillamine.

α-Mercaptopropionylglycine shares similar chemical properties with d-penicillamine and in urine preferentially forms a soluble mixed disulfide between α-mercaptopropionylglycine and cystine. Several investigators in Europe and Japan have reported that this drug decreases the urinary excretion of cystine, dissolves existing cystine stones, and prevents recurrent cystine calculi. They report less frequent and less serious adverse reactions than with the use of d-penicillamine. Our experience with α-mercaptopropionylglycine suggests that this drug has a similar range of adverse reactions with similar severity as compared to adverse reactions associated with d-penicillamine. Patients who react adversely to d-penicillamine may, however, tolerate α-mercaptopropionylglycine. If α-mercaptopropionylglycine becomes available for routine clinical use in the United States, its primary usefulness may well be an alternate therapy for patients who have experienced an adverse reaction to d-penicillamine.

The correct mix of treatment options, including increased oral fluids, alkalinization of the urine, and d-penicillamine therapy, must be individualized according to the patient's peculiar situation. d-Penicillamine usually is required to dissolve existing stones. Four-fifths of our patients who have existing cystine calculi and are treated with increased oral fluids and urine alkalinization alone continue to manifest x-ray evidence of persistent stone growth. By contrast, three-fourths of our patients with cystine calculi treated with increased oral fluids, urine alkalinization, and d-penicillamine show x-ray evidence of decreasing stone mass, usually leading to a stone-free state. Among the patients who fail to become stone-free on this regimen, the reason for failure usually is clinically apparent. The most common reason for failure is an inadequate decrease in the urinary excretion of cystine. The response to d-penicillamine may be assessed by periodically monitoring the 24-hour urinary excretion of cystine, and the dose of d-penicillamine should be adjusted to achieve a 24-hour urinary excretion of cystine of approximately 200 mg/day. The occurrence of calcium salts within a cystine stone is another common problem limiting success with this regimen. One should remember that patients with cystinuria may also have abnormalities of calcium metabolism, and we have experienced difficulties in dissolving "cystine" stones in patients who have both cystinuria and primary hyperparathyroidism or idiopathic hypercalciuria. The resultant cystine-calcium stone is resistant to dissolution. It is also important to note that it is unusual for a moderate-sized cystine stone to require 6–12 months before it will dissolve. During this time, aggressive alkalinization of the urine may result in the precipitation of a calcium-containing shell surrounding the cystine stone, thus hindering further dissolution. This is a very real problem in the dissolution of large cystine calculi, and for this reason it is reasonable to attempt stone dissolution simply by increasing oral fluids and using d-penicillamine as required to decrease the urinary excretion of cystine to approximately 200 mg per 24-hour period and avoid aggressive alkalinization of the urine. Maintenance of a stone-free state after existing calculi have been dissolved or surgically removed may be accomplished without the use of d-penicillamine. Approximately one-half of our patients who begin stone-free and are treated with increased oral fluids and urine alkalinization remain stone-free on this program. In view of this information and recognizing the potential dangers of d-penicillamine therapy, once existing calculi are dissolved or surgically removed, d-penicillamine may be discontinued and the patient followed on a more conservative program of increased oral fluids and urine alkalinization. If stone formation recurs, d-penicillamine is restarted and continued at the lowest dose required to maintain a stone-free state. Treatment of cystinuria is, by necessity, lifelong. Good fluid drinking habits must be emphasized and reemphasized and the alternating administration of urine alkalinization and d-penicillamine is used as the clinical situation dictates. The stone formation situation is usually followed by periodic KUB x-rays. In general, we would suggest a KUB x-ray 6 months after stone removal or stone dissolution followed by an annual KUB x-ray if there is no evidence of continued stone formation.

The medical therapy of cystinuria must now be decided in the context of newer surgical procedures that will successfully remove cystine calculi without a major flank incision and pelviolithotomy. Extracorporeal shock-wave lithotripsy has been disappointing because of its inability to adequately pulverize cystine stones. Cystine calculi in the renal pelvis are, however, nicely removed by the percutaneous ultrasonic lithotripsy technique. This procedure is generally well tolerated with low morbidity and should be considered as a very reasonable alternative to many months of treatment with a potentially dangerous drug (d-penicillamine) for patients who have large cystine stones. This technique is the treatment of choice for patients who have mixed calcium-cystine calculi or patients who have experienced a severe adverse reaction to d-penicillamine.

In summary, early diagnosis, aggressive medical therapy, and opportune urologic intervention make it unlikely for a person to lose significant renal function as a result of cystine urolithiasis.

REFERENCES

1. Dahlberg PJ, Van Den Berg CJ, Kurtz SB, et al: Clinical features and management of cystinuria. Mayo Clin Proc 52:533–542, 1977
2. Van Den Berg CJ: Urolithiasis, in Spittell JA Jr (ed): Clinical Medicine. Philadelphia, Harper & Row, 1981, pp 1–15

Christian J. Van Den Berg

12

Renal Tubular Acidosis and Urolithiasis

Renal tubular acidosis is a syndrome of metabolic acidosis resulting from renal tubular abnormalities. Classic clinical presentations include episodic muscle weakness, metabolic bone disease (osteomalacia), and, not infrequently, renal lithiasis. In one of our reviews, approximately 70 percent of patients with renal tubular acidosis (RTA) had x-ray evidence of renal lithiasis.[1] Symptoms referable to renal lithiasis were the presenting manifestation of RTA in approximately 50 percent of our patients. In every instance, the calculi were multiple and, with one exception, bilateral (Fig. 12-1). Evidence for extensive renal parenchymal calcification is frequently noted (Fig. 12-2). Renal lithiasis is thought to accompany type I, or "distal," RTA. In this disorder, systemic acidosis results from the inability of the nephron to maintain a hydrogen ion gradient between the lumen of the renal tubule and the peritubular fluid. As a consequence of this, the urine pH remains relatively alkaline despite the presence of systemic acidemia. Type II, or "proximal," RTA is caused by impaired absorption of filtered bicarbonate in the proximal nephron and resultant loss of bicarbonate in the urine. Renal lithiasis is not an expected consequence of proximal RTA unless it is accompanied by type I or distal RTA. Type I RTA may be familial as an autosomal dominant character but is more frequently sporadic or concomitant with systemic diseases such as Wilson's disease, galactosemia, hereditary fructose intolerance, Fanconi's syndrome, primary biliary cirrhosis, hypercalcemic states, dysproteinemias, and various drugs. All of these conditions in some way result in interference with the transport of hydrogen ion from the systemic circulation into tubular urine. The onset of RTA may be insidious, manifested by few, if any, symptoms. Usually when symptoms develop, they are related to musculoskeletal problems or nephrolithiasis.

The diagnosis of type I RTA is not difficult. The essential prerequisite for the diagnosis is an inappropriately high urine pH ($pH > 5.50$) in the presence of a systemic acidemia (serum bicarbonate < 20 mEq/liter). The metabolic acidosis in this situation is a "hyperchloremic" acidosis with an increased serum concentration of chloride replacing anion lost by a decrease in the serum concentration of bicarbonate. Incomplete forms of type I RTA are quite common and are also associated with renal stone formation. In this

STONE DISEASE: DIAGNOSIS AND MANAGEMENT
ISBN 0-8089-1873-7

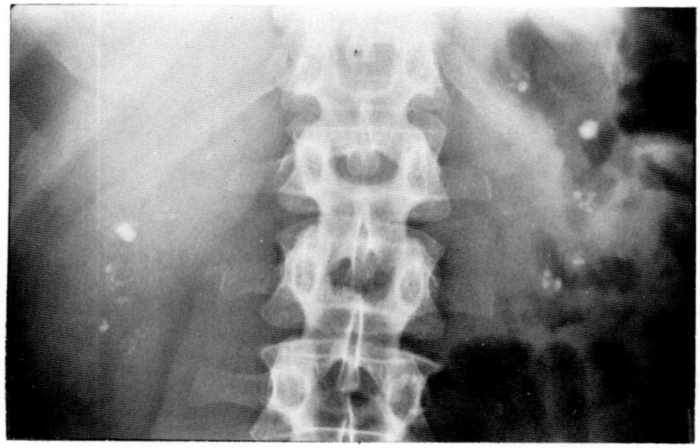

Fig. 12-1. Multiple, bilateral calculi in a person with renal tubular acidosis. (From Van Den Berg CJ: Urolithiasis, in Spittell JA, Jr (ed): Clinical Medicine. Philadelphia, Harper & Row, 1981. With permission.)

situation, the patient is not frankly acidemic. The urine pH, however, remains inappropriately high after the patient is challenged with an acid load. For screening purposes, the best time to obtain urine with a pH less than 5.5 (which usually eliminates the possibility of type I RTA) is on the first morning fasting void. The urine must be free of infection with urea-splitting bacteria. If the urine pH is greater than 5.5, RTA is always a possibility, and if this is coincident with a definite systemic acidemia, the diagnosis of RTA is confirmed. In the absence of acidemia, the possibility of incomplete RTA remains and the diagnosis is confirmed by documenting a urine pH above 5.5 coincident with systemic acidemia induced by ammonium chloride. Oral ammonium chloride (100 mg/kg as a 10 percent solution) is taken at bedtime and the urine pH is repeated on the first morning fasting urine. The urine pH should be less than 5.5. If at that time the urine pH remains above 5.5 and a blood sample indicates presence of a systemic acidemia, the diagnosis of

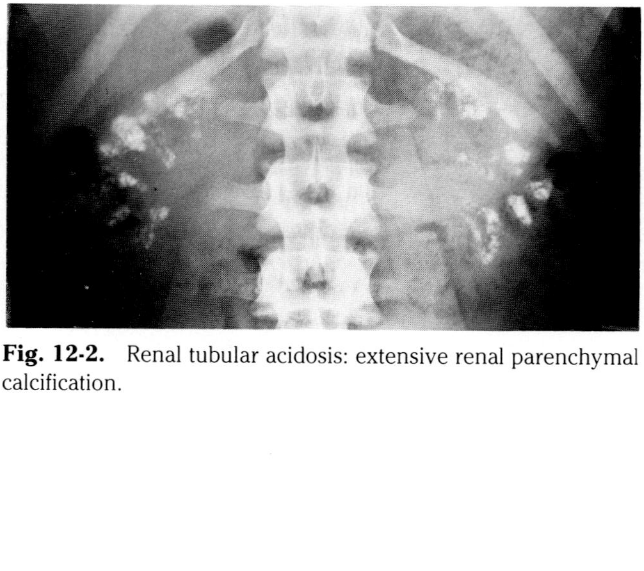

Fig. 12-2. Renal tubular acidosis: extensive renal parenchymal calcification.

incomplete RTA is confirmed. If a systemic acidemia is not present on this testing, it is possible that the ammonium chloride was not absorbed or not taken, and the oral ammonium chloride is repeated, followed by sequential testing of the urine pH and serum bicarbonate over the following few hours. More recently, the urinary excretion of citrate has been used as a convenient marker for both complete and incomplete type I RTA. Citrate is freely filtered at the glomerulus, and its absorption along the nephron is dependent on renal tubular cell pH. Even minor degrees of cellular acidemia result in increased renal tubular absorption of citrate and a very low urinary excretion of citrate. In type I RTA, the urinary excretion of citrate is very low, usually less than 50 mg per 24-hour period. This is a very helpful test in screening for RTA, and we routinely measure citrate in the same 24-hour urine sample obtained as part of an etiologic urolithiasis evaluation: a 24-hour urine collection obtained under conditions of usual activity and diet. If the urinary excretion of citrate under these conditions is within the normal range (400–600 mg/24 h), the person does not have type I (distal) RTA and it is not necessary to perform the tedious ammonium chloride loading test even if the urine pH on the screening urinalysis is greater than 5.5. In patients with type II, proximal, RTA, the urinary excretion of citrate may be normal as the underlying problem is one of impaired absorption of anion in the proximal tubule, resulting not only in bicarbonaturia but also inappropriately high urinary excretion of citrate despite a systemic acidemia.

Calcium phosphate is the most frequent renal calculus associated with RTA. Several pathophysiologic explanations have been proposed including decreased solubility of calcium phosphate in alkaline urine and hypercalciuria accompanying chronic systemic acidemia. In our experience, hypercalciuria is not a predominant feature in patients with RTA, and the urine pH actually increases during treatment of RTA with systemic base coincident with cessation of renal stone formation. These observations make it unlikely that these two explanations are primarily responsible for calcium stone formation in people with RTA. More recently, decreased urinary excretion of citrate has been highlighted in the etiology of renal calculi associated with RTA. Citrate is a natural inhibitor of calcium crystal formation in the urine. This is accomplished by citrate complexing with calcium ions and effectively limiting calcium ions available for calcium phosphate or calcium oxalate crystal formation. In addition, there is evidence to suggest that citrate acts on the surface of calcium crystals to inhibit further crystal growth. In this context, the very low urinary excretion of citrate in type I RTA may be the most important alteration in urine favoring calcium stone formation. It is interesting to speculate that the apparent absence of renal lithiasis in patients with proximal RTA may be related to the fact that the urinary excretion of citrate is not markedly decreased in this disorder.

Treatment of type I RTA is likewise very easy. Oral base in a dose of one mEq/kg of body weight daily in divided doses usually is adequate. Oral citrate solution as a sodium and potassium salt usually is well tolerated. If hypokalemia is present in combination with systemic acidemia, care must be taken to avoid a further decrease in the serum concentration of potassium as the serum pH increases with base therapy. This complication of therapy is avoided by using the potassium salt of citrate for initial base replacement, changing to a mixed sodium–potassium citrate preparation after acidemia has been corrected and the serum potassium is within the normal range. Stone formation usually ceases with adequate treatment. Essentially all of our patients who are compliant with therapy show x-ray evidence that continued stone growth and new stone formation have ceased during many years of followup examinations. The cessation of stone growth and the absence of new stone formation is the final arbiter as to the effectiveness and adequacy of stone prevention therapy. This radiographic determination, however, may take years to ascertain. More recently, the urinary excretion of citrate has been used as a marker for adequacy of therapy and is useful as an interim guide as to the proper dose of oral base. Adequate base is given to ensure that the urinary excretion of citrate is in the range of 400–600 mg daily. The stone situation is followed by periodic KUB x-rays, the first study taken in 3–6 months, and if there is no evidence of increased stone growth or new stone formation, a KUB x-ray is checked annually. If there is evidence of continued stone growth and base replacement is adequate as assessed by the urinary excretion of citrate and good compliance, the patient should be evaluated for other causes of calcium renal lithiasis.

Carbonic anhydrase inhibitors induce a functional RTA that may be associated with renal lithiasis. The ideal treatment, if possible, is to discontinue this medication. If this is not possible, as in the case of some patients with glaucoma, oral base replacement could be tried with the intent of increasing the urinary excretion of citrate. Intraocular pressures should be monitored carefully during this trial to ensure that base replacement does not interfere with the intended effect on intraocular pressure.

REFERENCES

1. Harrington TM, Bunch TW, Van Den Berg CJ: Renal tubular acidosis. Mayo Clin Proc 58:354–360, 1983

Edmund R. Yendt

13

Medullary Sponge Kidney and Urolithiasis

Medullary sponge kidney (MSK), a disorder characterized by the presence of dilated collecting ducts and tubules in one or more renal papillae, was first described in 1938,[22] but the clinical, radiographic, and morphologic features of the disease were not established until 1949.[2]

The reported incidence of MSK in patients with nephrolithiasis varies widely. Some reports suggest a fairly low incidence of 2.6–3.6 percent.[21,28,37] In 1981, however, we reported that 21 percent of 400 consecutive patients with nephrolithiasis had MSK if milder degrees of the condition frequently missed by routine intravenous urography were included.[41] Subsequently, Sage et al. found evidence of MSK in 17 percent of 200 randomly selected patients with nephrolithiasis,[34] and Parks et al. found the disorder in 12 percent of 624 male patients and 33 percent of 175 female patients with nephrolithiasis.[32] The incidence of the disorder in unselected patients undergoing excretory urography is approximately 0.5 percent.[27,30] The true incidence of the disorder is unknown because it is asymptomatic unless complicated by nephrolithiasis, hematuria, or urinary infection. A systematic examination of kidneys at autopsy to determine the incidence of the condition has not been reported.

PATHOLOGY AND PATHOGENESIS

The pathologic changes are confined to the medullary portions of the kidney, especially to their inner papillary portions.[7,23] One or more renal papillae contain dilated collecting ducts and tubules associated with multiple small cysts. The affected pyramids and the associated calyces often are enlarged,[23] and there may be generalized renal enlargement when numerous papillae are involved. The renal cortex, columns of Bertin, calyces, and pelvis appear normal unless affected by complications of the disease such as pyelonephritis or obstruction.

MSK is probably a developmental anomaly. Evidence supporting this includes the histologic appearance of the lesions, the lack of progression of the lesions for many years

STONE DISEASE: DIAGNOSIS AND MANAGEMENT
ISBN 0-8089-1873-7

(in the absence of complications),[20] and the occasional presence of embryonal tissue.[7] Coexistent anomalies of the urinary tract are frequent,[7] and there are numerous reports of association with other developmental abnormalities, especially congenital hemihypertrophy, which has been reported in as many as 25 percent of patients.[11] Familial cases have been described in a pattern consistent with autosomal dominant inheritance in a minority of patients with this disorder.[19,20] It has been suggested that a hereditary basis for the disorder is unlikely in most families,[26] but this report must be interpreted with caution because of the frequent difficulty in making the diagnosis by radiographic means.

Pathogenesis of Urolithiasis in Medullary Sponge Kidney

Several factors probably contribute to the formation of the intrapapillary concretions. Urinary stasis within the ectatic lesions is undoubtedly a major factor, but increased pH of the tubular fluid resulting from impaired acidification (see section on renal function) might also be important. Acidification could be impaired within ectatic ducts even when the final urinary pH is normal if the majority of the collecting ducts were unaffected. Increased pH diminishes the solubility of apatite, which has been shown to be the major component of the concretions.[7] The frequent occurrence of hypercalciuria in MSK also favors supersaturation of urine with apatite, although stone formation occurs in normocalciuric patients as well. It is also possible that the calcium concentration of the tubular fluid in the ectatic lesions could be higher than that of the unaffected collecting ducts. Intracavitary hyaline material and cellular debris noted in many cases may also act as a matrix for stone formation.[7] Urinary infection, particularly with urease-producing organisms, is occasionally an important secondary factor, but stone formation occurs in the absence of infection in the majority of patients.

Although the intrapapillary concretions in 10 patients with MSK were found to be composed of pure apatite in 70 percent of the cases and an admixture of apatite and calcium oxalate in the remaining 30 percent,[7] the passage of pure apatite stones in this disorder is rare. In the absence of infection, approximately 50 percent of the stones passed by our patients consist of an admixture of calcium oxalate and apatite when examined by optical crystallography, and the remainder are composed entirely of calcium oxalate. It is likely that some of the papillary concretions find their way into the renal collecting systems, probably by erosion through cyst walls, but before they are finally passed, the superimposition of calcium oxalate crystals seems to be an almost universal event. The initial site of formation of stones composed entirely of calcium oxalate and their pathogenesis is uncertain.

CLINICAL FEATURES

MSK is asymptomatic unless complicated by nephrolithiasis, hematuria, or urinary infection. The possibility of this disorder should always be considered in patients presenting with these problems. The onset of symptoms frequently occurs within the second and third decades of life, but the onset occasionally is delayed to the sixth decade. Onset during childhood has been documented occasionally, and the sexes are equally involved.[20]

The clinical manifestations of nephrolithiasis in patients with MSK are similar to those of stone patients who do not have the disorder. The numbers of stones present within the kidneys at the time of initial presentation to our clinic has been significantly greater in the patients with MSK than in those who do not have this disorder, however, even when patients with widespread nephrocalcinosis are excluded.[41] The frequency of stone passage is also greater in patients with medullary sponge kidney.[32] Urinary tract infection is a frequent complication of MSK either in the presence or absence of nephrocalcinosis and nephrolithiasis.

RENAL FUNCTION

In the absence of complications, urinalysis, glomerular filtration rate, and renal plasma flow are normal;[6,10,14] however, urinary concentration is often diminished,[6,10,14,20] although urinary dilution remains normal.[10,14]

Urinary acidification is impaired in about 40 percent of patients associated with reduced excretion of titratable acid but normal ammonium excretion.[6,14] Since the terminal portion of the collecting duct has the ability to generate steep pH gradients between tubular fluid and interstitial fluid in acidosis,[9] the impairment of urinary acidification seen in patients with MSK is consistent with the anatomic site of the lesions. Although the acidification defect is not accompanied by systemic acidosis and is of no clinical consequence in most patients, a few cases of systemic acidosis have been described,[5,7,10,20,26] one of whom presented with hypokalemic paralysis due to renal potassium wasting.[17]

Most of the reported renal function studies in MSK probably have involved patients with bilateral florid disease, although information regarding the extent of renal involvement is not provided in some of the reports. In one patient with segmental disease and one with unilateral disease, urinary concentration was impaired but acidification was normal.[15]

HYPERCALCIURIA IN MEDULLARY SPONGE KIDNEY

The reported incidence of hypercalciuria in patients with MSK is about 40–50 percent.[7,12,32,38] In our patients the incidence of hypercalciuria was 30 percent of 140 patients overall, with 45 percent of the 74 males, and 26 percent of the 66 females.

Idiopathic hypercalciuria in women with nephrolithiasis is uncommon in the experience of ourselves and others.[12] In women with MSK, however, hypercalciuria is frequent; the incidence is 26 percent in our patients, 30 percent in the experience of Harrison and Rose,[12] and 51 percent in the experience of Parks et al.[32] Hypercalciuria in a female stone patient thus is a strong indication for a search for an underlying disorder such as MSK, although primary hyperparathyroidism with normal or borderline total serum calcium levels is another strong possibility.[39] Many of our female patients with MSK had been previously misdiagnosed as having idiopathic hypercalciuria.

The cause of hypercalciuria in patients with MSK is uncertain. In view of the fact that net calcium reabsorption has been demonstrated to occur along the inner medullary collecting duct of the rat,[1] it is possible that the hypercalciuria may be yet another manifestation of abnormal function of the terminal nephron, but as yet this has not been conclusively demonstrated. A primary renal tubular calcium leak could produce parathyroid stimulation, which, in turn, could lead to hypophosphatemia; prolonged parathyroid stimulation might also give rise to an increased incidence of hyperparathyroidism. However, fasting serum phosphate levels in our patients with MSK have not been significantly lower than in other groups of stone patients. The reported data regarding parathyroid hormone secretion in patients with MSK are as yet inconclusive. Until recently, the question has been difficult to resolve because of the unreliability of many of the available immunoassays used for the measurement of parathyroid hormone. These immunoassays lacked the precision and sensitivity to detect variations within the normal range, and some of them frequently failed to detect elevated values in patients with proven parathyroid adenomas. In our experience, measurement of total urinary cyclic AMP excretion also lacks the sensitivity required to detect slight hypersecretion of parathyroid hormone; we have found normal values in most patients with surgically proven hyperparathyroidism when the degree of hypercalcemia was slight and when parathyroid adenomas weighed less than one gram.

When the hypercalciuria of 10 patients with MSK was investigated, a renal calcium leak was found in 8 and intestinal calcium hyperabsorption in 2,[25] but this report is at variance with another in which the hypercalciuria of 15 patients was classified as absorptive in 10, renal in 3 and unclassified in 2.[28] Our own data regarding parathyroid function in MSK are inconclusive. Until recently, the immunoassays employed in our laboratory to measure serum parathyroid hormone levels lacked the sensitivity to detect mild degrees of parathyroid hyperfunction. Urinary cyclic AMP excretion was within the normal range in all of the 30 patients studied by us under standardized dietary conditions.

Four of our patients have had overt hyperparathyroidism corrected by surgical removal of parathyroid adenomas. There are isolated reports of more than 20 other such patients in the literature,[20,25] and it has been suggested that the hyperparathyroidism resulted from prolonged parathyroid stimulation due to a primary renal tubular calcium leak.[30] These reports, however, do not provide proof that there is a higher incidence of hyperparathyroidism in patients with MSK than in stone patients who do not have this disorder. The only report of an abnormally high incidence of hyperparathyroidism in MSK is that of Maschio et al., who found seven cases with surgically proven hyperparathyroidism (single adenomas in six patients, hyperplasia in one) during the investigation of 28 patients with MSK.[25]

DIAGNOSIS*

The diagnosis of MSK is made by excretory urography.[7,20,23] Dilated collecting tubules, when opacified by the contrast medium, are seem as linear striations that impart a characteristic brushlike pattern to the renal papillae (Fig. 13-1) or as spherical cystic lesions (Fig. 13-2). The appearance of the latter has often been likened to that of "bouquets of flowers" or "bunches of grapes." During retrograde pyelography, the dilated tubules or cysts either do not fill with contrast medium, or they fill incompletely. The cystic lesions may be the first structures to be opacified and the last to empty during excretory urography, but the linear streaking of the papillae indicative of dilated collecting ducts and tubules may be an evanescent phenomenon. The affected renal papillae and their corresponding calyces may be enlarged. Enlarged papillae have been described

*Excerpts from this section are reprinted from Yendt ER: Medullary Sponge Kidney, in Schrier R, Gottschalk C (eds): Diseases of the Kidney, 4th ed. Boston, copyright © 1987 by Little Brown & Company, Chapter 17. With permission.

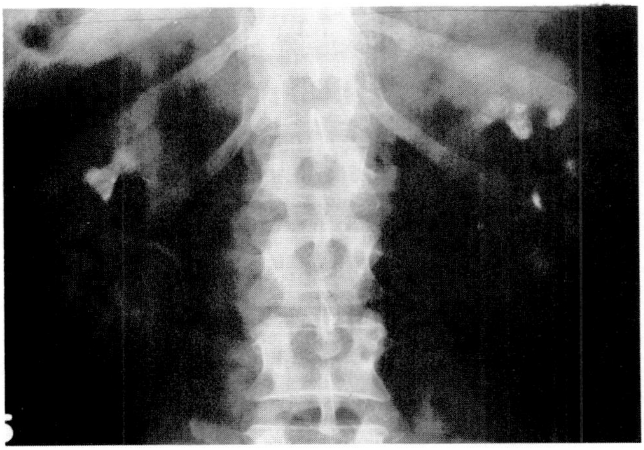

Fig. 13-1. Excretory urogram of a patient with medullary sponge kidney showing diffuse linear streaking of the renal papillae due to contrast medium in dilated collecting ducts and tubules.

in parts of the kidney where no ectatic tubules were visible on urography, and histologic examination of the papillae in such cases has shown the typical changes of medullary sponge kidney.[7,23] On the preliminary x-ray film, dense papillary spherical concretions often occurring in clusters are frequently seen (Fig. 13-3), and radiopaque stones situated within the renal collecting system may also be present. After the injection of the contrast medium, additional radiopacities should be evident and the papillary concretions are usually surrounded by the contrast medium. Unilateral enlargement of the innominate bone of the pelvis indicative of hemihypertrophy may be evident. Ultrasonography, arteriography, and computed tomography have little, if any, role in diagnosis.

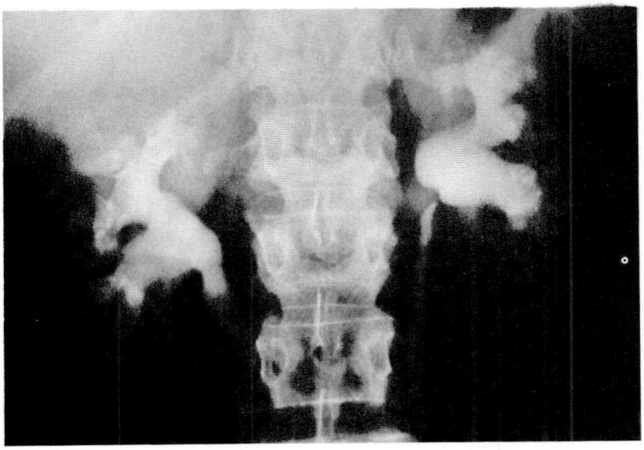

Fig. 13-2. Excretory urogram of a patient with medullary sponge kidney showing widespread cystic dilatations of medullary ducts and tubules. (Reproduced from Yendt ER: Medullary sponge kidney. In Schrier R, Gottschalk C [eds]: Diseases of the Kidney, 4th ed., Boston, copyright © 1987 by Little, Brown & Company, Chapter 17. With permission.)

Radiologic diagnosis of the disorder is relatively easy in florid cases when virtually all papillae of both kidneys are involved. When the disease is less extensive, however, the ectatic lesions may not be apparent unless the excretory urogram is of high quality. A satisfactory excretory urogram must clearly opacify the collecting systems, including each calyx and its infundibulum, detail must not be obscured by overlying bowel contents, and urinary tract obstruction must not be present. We have found that the excretory urograms performed in most patients with nephrolithiasis do not fulfill these criteria[41] (only 3 of 53 excretory urograms performed in 25 consecutive patients with nephrolithiasis were of satisfactory quality). Another problem concerning diagnosis is that the lesser degrees of MSK are frequently not recognized or commented on by radiologists and urologists. In our 74 male patients with MSK, the diagnosis had been established in only 16 (22 percent) prior to referral to our clinic: in 37 of the remaining patients, the diagnosis was apparent when the excretory urograms performed previously were reviewed. In 21 patients, the available x-rays were of such poor quality that the diagnosis could not be made until satisfactory excretory urograms were obtained. It is now standard practice in our stone clinic to review all available excretory urograms with our radiologists. If the quality of the available x-rays is inadequate, we have attempted to obtain a satisfactory examination whenever feasible, often by utilizing the technique of high dose drip infusion nephrotomography and an x-ray apparatus with a small focal spot. In the absence of a satisfactory excretory urogram, the diagnosis of "idiopathic calcium nephrolithiasis" or "idiopathic hypercalciuria" is unjustified.

Isolated lesions simulating those seen in MSK are occasionally seen during routine excretory urography. We found that one or two such lesions occurred in one or two renal papillae in 6 to 8 percent of excretory urograms performed in patients who did not have nephrolithiasis,[41] whereas lesions in three or more renal papillae were present in only 2 percent of these patients, most of whom did not have the classic widespread form of the disease. This raises the question as to when the urographic changes justify a diagnosis of MSK. At the present time, there is no firm evidence on which a definitive resolution of this problem could be based. When only a few lesions are present, we do not diagnose

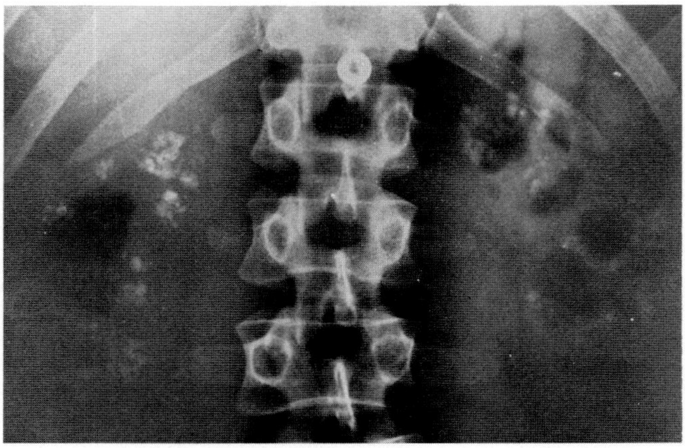

Fig.13-3. Preliminary film of a patient with medullary sponge kidney showing clusters of papillary concretions. (Reproduced from Yendt ER: Medullary sponge kidney. In Schrier R, Gottschalk C [eds]: Diseases of the Kidney, 4th ed. Boston, copyright © 1987 by Little, Brown & Company, Chapter 17. With permission.)

MSK unless three or more renal papillae are involved; however, the diagnosis is justified if numerous characteristic lesions are identified in only one or two renal papillae. Future experience may necessitate revision of these criteria.

Another problem concerning the radiographic diagnosis of MSK relates to the significance of opacification or "blushing" of the renal pyramids during excretory urography (Fig. 13-4). On reviewing 2465 excretory urograms, Palubinskas noted papillary blushing in the absence of other evidence of MSK in 21 cases, an incidence of less than 1 percent.[31] He also found that the radiographic changes noted in different papillae of individual cases of MSK ranged all the way from a pyramidal haze, through a few distinguishable dilated tubules combined with pyramidal haze, to the classic appearance of multiple cystic lesions occurring within a papilla. The characteristic dilated collecting tubules of MSK were found on pathologic examination of papillae that demonstrated only a papillary blush[31] or pyramidal enlargement[7] on excretory urography. The technique of direct magnification excretory urography[13] has demonstrated individually dilated tubules in renal pyramids that showed only a pyramidal blush on conventional films. In view of these findings, it is probable that many instances of papillary blush represent minor degrees of

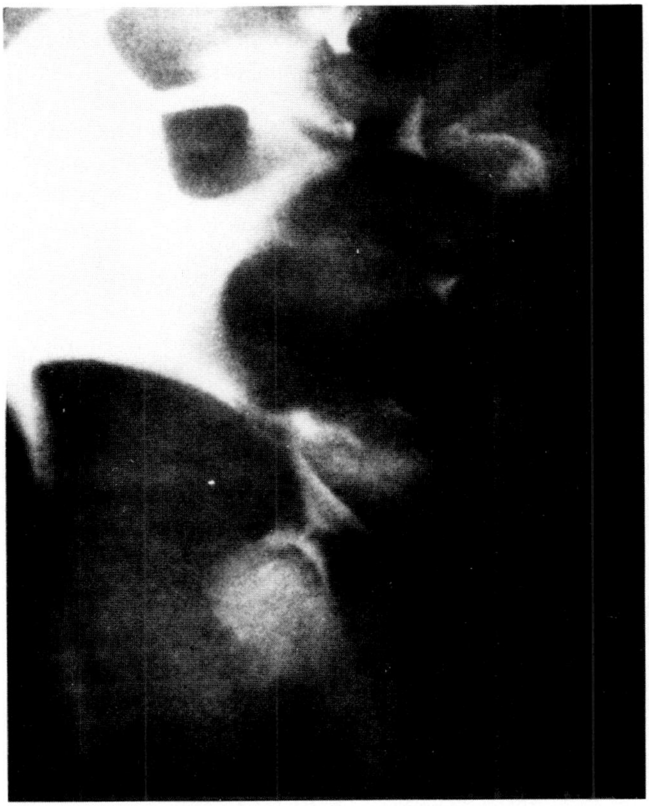

Fig. 13-4. Excretory urogram of a patient with diffuse papillary blushing. This figure shows at least one discrete dilated tubule in the lowermost papilla of the left kidney. Similar changes present in a few other papillae justify a diagnosis of medullary sponge kidney. Minor changes such as these are not detected unless the quality of the excretory urogram is excellent.

MSK, although there is still disagreement among clinicians and radiologists as to the significance of these changes.[35] In our clinic, a firm diagnosis of MSK is not made when papillary blushing is the sole radiographic abnormality, although a strong suspicion of the disease is entertained in such cases. Kuiper states that pyramidal blushing is diagnostic of MSK when it is diffuse, persistent in successive examinations, and present on early and delayed films without the use of compression, especially if accompanied by pyramidal enlargement, intraductular papillary concretions, or linear or cystic dilatations within one or more pyramids.[20]

Differential Diagnosis

When the changes of MSK are extensive, there is little difficulty with diagnosis. Where the changes are minimal and involve a single pyramid or only a few pyramids, however, the disorder must be differentiated from calyceal diverticula, renal tuberculosis, renal papillary necrosis, and other causes of nephrocalcinosis.

MSK must also be distinguished from pyelotubular stasis, a fine brushlike opacification of the renal pyramids that may result from the application of excessive ureteric pressure during excretory urography. No cystic lesions are present, however, and repeat examination without ureteral compression does not reproduce the findings. Pyelovenous backflow is a lacy dye pattern over the renal papillae produced by disruption of the calyceal fornices by raised intrapelvic pressure. This may be due to excessive injection pressure in the renal pelvis during retrograde pyelography, in which case the changes are not reproducible during excretory urography. Pyelovenous backflow may also be demonstrated during excretory urography when stones produce acute ureteric occlusion. Microcalyces may also produce peculiar opacifications around the calyces, which can simulate the lesions of sponge kidney.[33]

TREATMENT

The management of nephrocalcinosis, nephrolithiasis, and urinary tract infection associated with MSK is basically the same as when these complications occur in the absence of the disorder. Active and progressive stone formation can nearly always be arrested by the use of thiazides,[40,42] which have been proven effective in preventing calcium stones in randomized controlled clinical trials.[8,38] In our experience, thiazides are just as effective in patients with MSK as in those who do not have this disorder.

The original rationale for the use of thiazides to prevent calcium stones was their now well-known hypocalciuric action, an effect that is unique to thiazides and related diuretics such as chlorthalidine and metolazone, which act at the same site in the distal nephron. The magnitude of the reduction in urine calcium induced by thiazides is variable, but with 50 mg of hydrochlorothiazide administered twice daily, the mean reduction is 150 mg/day. Occasionally the hypocalciuric effect is much less pronounced, and in the occasional normal subject or stone patient, there is little discernible effect. Thiazides may prove effective, however, even when the hypocalciuric effect is minimal because there are other thiazide-induced changes in urinary composition that probably contribute to their remarkable efficacy[43] such as the reduction in urine oxalate excretion that occurs in the majority of thiazide treated patients.[4] This effect is delayed and rarely is evident during the first year of thiazide therapy.

Although it has been suggested that the use of thiazides should be restricted to hypercalciuric patients, we[40,43] and others[24] have observed that these agents are just as effective in normocalciuric patients. In our clinic no attempt is made to select patients suitable for thiazides on the basis of metabolic studies designed to distinguish between "absorptive" and "renal" hypercalciuria as advocated by Pak et al.[29] There is no evidence that overall results are improved by such selective therapy and the investigation required to categorize patients in this fashion is expensive and unnecessary in the average urologic and nephrologic practice; moreover, the validity of the categorization of patients in this manner is debatable. Although the administration of allopurinol along with a thiazide has been advocated for hypercalciuric patients who also have hyperuricosuria,[3] we administer thiazides alone in such patients, and allopurinol is added to the regimen only if and when thiazide-induced gout supervenes.

The preparations and doses of thiazides used by various authors have varied considerably. In our initial trials, we used hydrochlorothiazide at the upper end of the therapeutic dose range (i.e., 50 mg twice daily), whereas others have tended to use smaller equivalent doses of the various benzothiadiazides.[42] We now use smaller doses of hydrochlorothiazide (25 mg twice daily) in women and normocalciuric men but continue to use 50 mg twice daily for hypercalciuric men. If the larger doses are not well tolerated, the dose is reduced to 25 mg twice daily. Some patients may continue to form stones on the smaller dose but cease to do so on the larger dose. As yet there is no evidence that one form of thiazide is more effective than another. It is important to realize that the doses of thiazides used in the various clinical trials reported to date are not equivalent.[42,43]

Hydrochlorothiazide and bendroflumethiazide are short-acting drugs that should be given in two divided doses per day, whereas the longer-acting trichlormethiazide and related diuretics such as chlorthalidone and metolazone need be administered only once per day. When the shorter-acting thiazides are used, the evening dose should be administered no later than 6:00 P.M. to minimize nocturia, which causes insomnia in some patients. If nocturia proves troublesome despite this precaution, switching to a long-acting drug administered in the morning may alleviate the problem. The use of a longer-acting agent may also be helpful in patients whose compliance is poor and who often neglect to take the evening dose of medication.

It has not been our practice to restrict the dietary intake of calcium, oxalate, or sodium chloride in thiazide-treated patients unless the intake of these substances is excessive. Before thiazides are started, the radiologic status of the patient should be determined as precisely as possible in order to determine whether stone incidents occurring at a later date are due to newly formed stones or to stones that had formed prior to starting treatment. The routine plain film of the abdomen frequently is of such poor quality that the presence or absence of stones or the exact number of stones cannot be established with certainty, and for this reason renal tomography is usually advisable at this stage.

The incidence of side effects in patients treated with 50 mg of hydrochlorothiazide twice daily is 30–35 percent. These tend to be most troublesome during the initial phases of therapy and often disappear or lessen with the passage of time. They usually are mild, but in 7 percent of patients they are of sufficient severity to necessitate stopping treatment. The most common side effects are lassitude, diminished energy, and an increased need for sleep, and these effects may persist despite the correction of hypokalemia. Other side effects include headaches, constipation, impotence, and depression. Some patients develop thiazide-induced gout, in which case allopurinol 300 mg/day is prescribed in addition to the hydrochlorothiazide. A gradual decline in serum magnesium levels often occurs during long-term thiazide therapy; we have not observed any clinical disturbances associated with this biochemical abnormality, but nonetheless the provision of magnesium supplements occasionally may be advisable. To minimize the incidence and severity of thiazide side effects, which tend to be more troublesome during the first few weeks of treatment, we no longer initiate therapy with the full dose of hydrochlorothiazide but start with 25 mg/day and increase the daily dose by 25 mg/day at weekly intervals until the maintenance dose has been achieved.

Most patients who take 50 mg of hydrochlorothiazide twice daily (without potassium supplements) develop hypokalemia; if serum potassium levels remain normal, poor compliance should be suspected. Although there is no need to prescribe potassium supplements routinely for all patients treated with thiazides, they are prescribed for (1) patients with side effects, (2) patients with a history of angina pectoris or myocardial infarction and those receiving digitalis, (3) diabetic patients, and (4) asymptomatic patients with serum potassium levels below 3.0 mEq/liter. An alternative to the provision of potassium supplements is the addition of a potassium-sparing diuretic.

In our experience the most common cause of apparent failure of thiazides to prevent stones is poor compliance. This is sometimes extremely difficult to detect. The second most common cause of apparent thiazide failure is inadequate dosage; even a dose of 50 mg of hydrochlorothiazide twice daily occasionally is insufficient, and the possibility of insufficient dosage is considerably greater with the smaller doses of thiazides used by others. Inadequate dosage is most apt to occur in the patient who is free of side effects and who remains normokalemic and hypercalciuric while taking thiazides. The next step in the management of the apparently thiazide-resistant patient is to review the diagnosis. It should be emphasized that the ability to detect minimal hypercalcemia is essential for the diagnosis of primary hyperparathyroidism. Other undiagnosed disorders such as hyperoxaluria, anatomic abnormalities such as a caliectatic sac in the lower pole of a kidney, and unrecognized urinary tract infection may be present in patients resistant to thiazides. The significance of infection with coagulase-negative staphylococci with colony counts less than 100,000/ ml urine is especially apt to be unrecognized.

If the above-mentioned causes of thiazide resistance have been ruled out, we recommend the combined use of thiazides and inorganic phosphates as the next step in therapy. In our experience the need for such combined therapy is very infrequent, but Klein and Griffith found that combination treatment gave excellent results in eight patients who continued to form stones on thiazides alone.[18] It has been suggested that combined therapy with thiazides and phosphates is contraindicated because of the danger of renal damage;[16] however, these experimental observations are of dubious relevance to the treatment of renal lithiasis in humans.[42] We have used combined thiazide-phosphate therapy in one patient for 10 years without adverse effects of any sort, and no ill effects were observed in the patients treated by Klein and Griffith.

Inorganic phosphate used alone has also been reported to be effective in arresting progression of stone disease in patients with MSK.[36] Because of the proven efficacy, convenience, and low cost of thiazides, it has been our policy to use thiazides as the agent of first choice, but if thiazides are contraindicated or poorly tolerated, the use of inorganic phosphates is well worth a try. However, inorganic phosphates should not be administered to patients with urinary infection because of the danger of producing struvite stones.

When nephrolithiasis is accompanied by urinary tract infection, appropriate antibacterial therapy is essential. There is a tendency for the infections to recur after antibacterial therapy is discontinued, and long-term therapy may be necessary.[12] The combination of MSK with urinary infection (especially with urease-producing coagulase-negative staphylococci) occasionally may lead to an explosive progression of the stone disease; thus careful monitoring of patients with frequent cultures and prompt treatment of urinary infection is of utmost importance.

When the complications of MSK are managed properly, the long-term prognosis is excellent and the development of serious renal damage is uncommon.[12]

REFERENCES

1. Bengele HH, Alexander EA, Lechene CP: Calcium and magnesium transport along the inner medullary collecting duct of the rat. Am J Physiol 239:F24–F29, 1980
2. Cacchi R, Ricci V: Sur une rare maladie kystique multiple des pyramides renales, le "rein en eponge." J Urol Nephrol (Paris) 55:497–519, 1949
3. Coe FL: Treated and untreated recurrent calcium nephrolithiasis in patients with hypercalciuria, hyperuricosuria or no metabolic disorder. Ann Intern Med 87:404–410, 1977
4. Cohanim M, Yendt ER: Reduction of urine oxalate during long term thiazide therapy in patients with calcium urolithiasis. Invest Urol 18:170–173, 1980
5. Deck MDF: Medullary sponge kidney with renal tubular acidosis. A report of 3 cases. J Urol 94:330–335, 1965
6. Defronzo RA, Thier SO: Functional abnormalities in renal cystic diseases, in KD Gardner (ed): Cystic Diseases of the Kidney. New York, Wiley, 1976, pp 65–81.
7. Ekstrom T, Engfeldt B, Lagergren C, et al: Medullary Sponge Kidney. Stockholm, Almqvist and Wiksell, 1959
8. Ettinger B, Citron J, Tang A: Controlled studies in stone prophylaxis: Comparison of placebo versus allopurinol/chlorthalidone/magnesium hydroxide. Urol Res 12:491, 1984
9. Graber ML, Bengele HH, Schwartz JH, et al: pH and P CO2 profiles of the rat inner medulla. Am J Physiol 241:F659–F668, 1981
10. Granberg PO, Lagergren C, Theve NO: Renal function studies in medullary sponge kidney. Scand J Urol Nephrol 5:177–180, 1971
11. Harris RE, Fuchs EF, Kaempf MJ: Medullary sponge kidney and congenital hemihypertrophy: Case report and literature review. J Urol 126:676–678, 1981
12. Harrison AR, Rose GA: Medullary sponge kidney. Urol Res 7:197–207, 1979
13. Hayt DB, Perez LA, Blatt CJ, et al: Direct magnification intravenous pyelography in the evaluation of medullary sponge kidney. Roentgenol Radium Ther Nucl Med 119:701–704, 1973
14. Higashihara E, Nutahara K, Tago K, et al: Medullary sponge kidney and renal acidification defect. Kidney Internatl 25:453–459, 1984
15. Higashihara E, Nutahara K, Tago K, et al: Unilateral and segmental medullary sponge kidney: Renal function and calcium excretion. J Urol 132:743–745, 1984
16. Holliday MA, Winters RW, Welt LG, et al: The renal lesions of electrolyte imbalance: The combined effect on renal architecture of phosphate loading and potassium depletion. J Exp Med 110:161–168, 1954
17. Jayasinghe KSA, Mendis BLJ, Mohideen R, et al: Medullary sponge kidney presenting with hypokalaemic paralysis. Postgrad Med J 60:303–304, 1984
18. Klein AS, Griffith DP: Neutral potassium phosphate and thiazide: Combined treatment in recurrent stone formers, in Smith LH, Robertson WG, Finlayson B (eds): Urolithiasis: Clinical and Basic Research. New York, Plenum Press, 1981, pp 253–258.

19. Kuiper JJ: Medullary sponge kidney in three generations. NY State J Med 71:2665–2669, 1971
20. Kuiper JJ: Medullary sponge kidney, in KD Gardner (ed): Cystic Diseases of the Kidney. New York, Wiley, 1976, pp 151–171
21. Lavan JN, Neale FC, Posen S: Urinary calculi: Clinical, biochemical and radiological studies in 619 patients. Med J Aust 2:1049–1061, 1971
22. Lenarduzzi G: Reperto pielograficco poco commune (dilatazione delle vie urinarie intrarenali). Radiol Med (Torino) 26:346–347, 1939
23. Lindvall N: Roentgenologic diagnosis of medullary sponge kidney. Acta Radiol 51:193–206, 1959
24. Ljunghall S, Backman V, Danielson BG, et al: Long term treatment with bendroflumethiazide for prevention of renal stones. Clinical experiences, in Smith LH, Robertson WG, Finlayson B (eds): Urolithiasis: Clinical and Basic Research. New York, Plenum Press, 1981, pp 241–244
25. Maschio G, Tessitore N, D'Angelo A, et al: Medullary sponge kidney and hyperparathyroidism . . . a puzzling association. Am J Nephrol 2:77–84, 1982
26. Morris RC, Yamauchi H, Palubinskas AJ, et al: Medullary sponge kidney. Am J Med 38:883–892, 1965
27. Myall GF: The incidence of medullary sponge kidney. Clin Radiol 21:171–174, 1970
28. O'Neill M, Breslau NA, Pak CYC: Metabolic evaluation of nephrolithiasis in patients with medullary sponge kidney. JAMA 245:1233–1236, 1981
29. Pak CYC, Peters P, Hart G, et al: Is selective therapy of recurrent nephrolithiasis possible? Am J Med 71:615–622, 1981
30. Palubinskas AJ: Medullary sponge kidney. Radiology 76:911–918, 1961
31. Palubinskas AJ: Renal pyramidal structure opacification in excretory urography and its relation to medullary sponge kidney. Radiology 81:963–970, 1963
32. Parks JH, Coe FL, Strauss AL: Calcium nephrolithiasis and medullary sponge kidney in women. New Engl J Med 306:1088–1091, 1982
33. Pollack HM: Some limitations and pitfalls of excretory urography. J Urol 116:537–543, 1976
34. Sage MR, Lawson AD, Marshall VR, et al: Medullary sponge kidney and urolithiasis. Clin Radiol 33:435–438, 1982
35. Talner LB: Functional aspects of uroradiology. Contrib Nephrol 5:3, 1977
36. Thomas WC Jr: Use of phosphates in patients with calcareous renal calculi. Kidney Internatl 13:390–396, 1978
37. Wikstrom B, Backman U, Danielson BG, et al: Ambulatory diagnostic evaluation of 389 recurrent renal stone formers. A proposal for clinical classification and investigation. Klin Wochenschr 61:85–90, 1983
38. Wilson DR, Strauss AL, Manuel MA: Comparison of medical treatments for the prevention of recurrent calcium nephrolithiasis. Urol Res 12:39, 1984
39. Yendt ER, Gagne RJA: Detection of primary hyperparathyroidism with special reference to its occurrence in hypercalciuric females with normal or borderline serum calcium. Can Med Assoc J 98:331–336, 1968
40. Yendt ER, Cohanim M: Prevention of calcium stones with thiazides. Kidney Internatl 13:397–409, 1978
41. Yendt ER, Jarzylo S, Finnis W, et al: Medullary sponge kidney (tubular ectasia) in calcium urolithiasis, in Smith LH, Robertson WG, Finlayson B (eds): Urolithiasis: Clinical and Basic Research. New York, Plenum Press, 1981, pp 105–112
42. Yendt ER, Cohanim M: Experience with thiazide diuretics in calcium oxalate urolithiasis. World J Urol 1:176–179, 1983
43. Yendt ER, Cohanim M: The prevention of calcium stones with thiazides, in Schwille PO, Smith LH, Robertson WG, et al (eds): Urolithiasis and Related Clinical Research. New York, Plenum Press, 1985, pp 463–470

David M. Wilson

14

Gastrointestinal Disorders and Urolithiasis

The coexistence of renal stones and gastrointestinal (GI) disease was initially emphasized by Gelzayd et al. in 1968.[11] Prior to that time renal lithiasis had been recognized primarily in patients with peptic ulcer disease treated with absorbable alkali and primary hyperparathyroidism associated with peptic ulcer disease and in those who had undergone an ileostomy.[19] Gelzayd et al. reported that 7.2 percent of a series of 880 patients with inflammatory bowel disease had stones. That initial study revealed that in patients with ulcerative colitis about 80 percent of the stones were calcium and 10 percent uric acid. In patients with regional enteritis or ileocolitis, the distribution was about the same. The unraveling of the reasons for the increased incidence of stone disease in these patients is one of the more interesting chapters in the elucidation of a pathophysiologic phenomenon and clearly has clinicotherapeutic implications. This chapter will review some of the studies of the pathophysiologic phenomena that have led to our understanding of this disorder and the resultant potential treatment modalities.

ENTERIC HYPEROXALURIA AND OTHER HYPEROXALURIC STATES

Most of the renal stones reported over the last 20 years, in all types of stone disease, contain calcium oxalate. Of all stones from the urinary tract, 65–80 percent contain calcium oxalate. The vast majority of these stones contain pure calcium oxalate, although Breslau and Pak suggested that calcium phosphate may be an important nucleating crystalite.[2] In any case, most stones in patients with bowel disease have a high percentage of calcium oxalate.

Much of the physiologic and pathophysiologic data relate to the increased excretion of oxalate in many bowel disease patients, particularly those with small bowel disease or resection. A brief review of oxalate metabolism would seem appropriate for further understanding stones in these groups.

Calcium oxalate solubility is extremely low, about 7 mg per 100 ml of water, which is almost always exceeded even in urine from normal persons without stones. It is now

STONE DISEASE: DIAGNOSIS AND MANAGEMENT
ISBN 0-8089-1873-7

known that other urinary constituents have a major influence on calcium oxalate solubility. Robertson and Nordine were able to demonstrate that the role of oxalate is more pronounced in altering the ion activity product of calcium oxalate than changes in calcium concentration. They also showed that an oral load of oxalate, even in normal individuals, results in a much higher volume of calcium oxalate crystals than a calcium load.[20,21] Finlayson also studied this phenomenon and suggested that oxalate was approximately 15 times greater on a milligram per milliliter basis than calcium in changing the relative supersaturation of calcium oxalate.[9] The normal mean excretion of oxalate is 20–40 mg per 24-hour period for normal subjects and 30–45 mg per 24-hour period in stone formers.

A diurnal variation in the urinary excretion of oxalate has been reported by Tiselius and Almgård[25] and Zarembski and Hodgkinson.[28] The source of urinary oxalate for excretion is multifactorial, but in normal individuals the endogenous production of oxalate accounts for 90 percent of the oxalate present in urine. The absorption of preformed oxalate from the diet produces the remaining 10 percent.

The metabolic pathways producing oxalate, as seen in Figure 14-1, include the conversion of vitamin C to oxalate. About 35–40 percent of oxalate is normally derived from ascorbic acid.[15] Other sources include the conversion of glycolate to glyoxalate and then to oxalate. Glycolate is in part recycled or "rescued" by conversion to glycine and serine in the presence of vitamin B_6. Vitamin B_6 deficiency has been proposed as a cause of renal stone disease and there are controversial papers in the literature suggesting that the increased oxalate in idiopathic stone formers may relate to vitamin B_6 deficiency. Tiselius et al. were unable to correlate vitamin B_6 levels with hyperoxaluria in a group of idiopathic stone formers.[26] Harrison and Rose and others have reported that in a percentage of those patients with idiopathic renal lithiasis and mild hyperoxaluria, there may be a significant decrease in oxalate excretion with either physiologic or pharmacologic doses of vitamin B_6.[16]

The reaction that converts glyoxalate to oxalate is affected by several enzymes, including xanthine oxidase, LDH, and glyoxalate oxidase. Some studies suggest that oxalate excretion can be suppressed with xanthine oxidase inhibitors such as allopurinol. This has not been widely confirmed. Tiselius has reviewed the substances known to increase urinary oxalate excretion, which include glycine, glutamic acid, purines, and salycilates. Several toxic substances such as ethyleneglycol and methoxyflurane can also increase oxalate production and excretion.

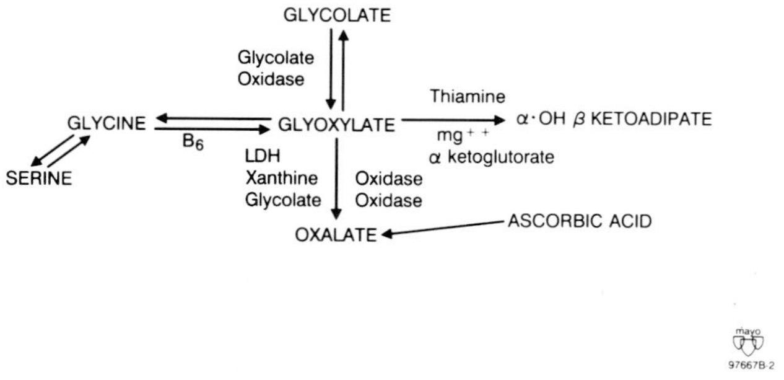

Fig. 14-1. Major pathways in glyoxylate metabolism with pertinent enzymes and cofactors affecting oxalate production.

Primary oxaluria is a hereditary disorder of the metabolism of oxalate.[27] Two different forms of this disorder are known with enzyme defects at different metabolic stages. In one of these, designated type I because it was the first discovered, glycolic acid is overexcreted along with oxalate. In the second, type II, L-glyceric acid, a substance that we have not yet discussed, is overexcreted with oxalate, but glycolate excretion is normal. In these patients the urinary excretion of oxalate is in the range of 140–150 mg per 24-hour period, generally higher than in patients with enteric hyperoxaluria. The onset of stone disease is severe and early in life.

DIETARY OXALATE

Although the source of urinary oxalate is primarily metabolic in normal individuals, dietary oxalate is of primary importance in patients with bowel disease and stones. Evaluation of the mechanisms for oxalate absorption is hampered by a lack of understanding of the form of oxalate in foods. Oxalate is absorbed at different rates from different foodstuffs with the apparent same content. It is thought that some foods have a soluble form of oxalate and others a more insoluble form. Although there is some uncertainty about our measurements of total oxalate content of foods, the oxalate content in typical diets is thought to range between 130 and 900 mg per 24-hour period. Table 14-1 outlines our general knowledge of the total oxalate content of foods that are high and moderately high in oxalate.

The intestinal absorption of dietary oxalate in healthy patients ranges from 2.3 to 7.5 percent.[7] If the oxalate load is given during fasting, however, a much higher percentage of an administered dose given as ^{14}C oxalate appears in the urine in normal subjects.[8] It is absorbed by a passive diffusion process throughout the intestinal tract.[3] The rate of absorption of oxalate decreases from the colon to the duodenum. Several factors determine the amount of oxalate absorbed. These relate primarily to the solubility of the salt of oxalate, which, in turn, is dependent on the ionic content of the gut with respect to the cations. Consequently, the gut concentrations of calcium, magnesium, zinc, and similar metallic elements are important to oxalate absorption. For example, it has been shown by several authors that when dietary calcium is low in relationship to oxalate in the intestine, the proportional absorption of oxalate is increased and conversely, that when the oral calcium is high, oxalate absorption and excretion are low.

URINARY OXALATE MEASUREMENT

There are widely discrepant results in the measurement of urinary oxalate. Many of the methods that are available are subject to large errors, are tedious, and are not easily available for clinical studies. This has resulted in a major problem in the study of oxalate metabolism. Several of the methodologies have been compared by Zerwekh et al.[29] These workers studied the enzymatic method modified by Hodgkinson and mass spectroscopy, gaschromatographic, ionchromatographic, and high-pressure liquid chromatographic methods. All of these methods had large coefficients of variation within (5–58 percent) and between (15–88 percent) assays. The analytical recovery by most of the assays was more than 100 percent of the added oxalate, ranging from 86 to 237 percent. Crawford et al. evaluated the measurement of urinary oxalate in the presence of ascorbic acid.[5] In

Table 14-1
Compendium of Oxalate Content of Foodstuffs as Collated by Mayo Clinic Dietetic Department

	Food Oxalate		
	High-Oxalate Foods	Moderate-Oxalate Foods	Low- or No-Oxalate Foods
Beverages	Draft beer, ovaltine, and other beverage mixes; tea; cocoa	Coffee (limited to 8 oz daily)	Beer—bottled; carbonated cola (limited to 12 oz per day); distilled alcohol; lemonade or limeade without peel; wine—red, rose, white (≤2 cups/day recommended);
Milk			buttermilk; low-fat or skim milk; yogurt made with allowed fruits
Meat and substitutes	Baked beans canned in tomato sauce, peanut butter, soybean curd (tofu)	Sardines	Eggs, cheese, beef, lamb or pork, poultry, fish and shellfish
Vegetables	Beans—green, wax, dried; beets—tops, roots, greens; celery; chives; collards; dandelion greens; eggplant; escarole; kale; leeks; mustard greens; okra; parsely; peppers—green, pokeweed potatoes–sweet; rutabagas; spinach; summer squash; swiss chard; watercress	Asparagus; broccoli; carrots; corn—sweet white, sweet yellow; cucumber—peeled; green peas—canned; lettuce, lima beans; parsnips; tomato—1 small or juice (4 oz); turnips	Avocado, brussels sprouts, cauliflower, cabbage, mushrooms, onions, peas, green (fresh or frozen) potatoes—white, radishes
Fruits and juices	Blackberries; blueberries; currants—red, dewberries, fruit cocktail, grapes—purple, gooseberries, lemon peel, lime peel, orange peel, raspberries, rhubarb, strawberries, tangerines, juices made from the above fruits	Apples; apricots; black currants; cherries—red, sour; cranberry juice (4 oz); grape juice (4 oz); orange—fruit and juice (4 oz); peaches; pears; pineapple; plums—purple; prunes	Apple juice; banana; bing cherries; grapefruit—fruit and juice; grapes—green; mangoes; melons—cantaloupe, casaba, watermelon; nectarines; peaches, pineapple juice; plums—green or yellow
Bread and starches	Fruit cake; grits—white, soybean cracker; wheat germ	Cornbread, sponge cake, spaghetti canned in tomato sauce	Breakfast cereals, macaroni, noodles, rice, spaghetti, bread
Nuts	Almond, pecans, cashews, peanuts, walnuts		
Fats and oils			Bacon, mayonnaise, salad dressing, vegetable oils, butter, margarine
Miscellaneous	Chocolate—cocoa, vegetable soup, tomato soup, marmalade	Chicken noodle soup—dehydrated	Jelly or preserves (made with allowed fruits), lemon and lime juice, salt, pepper (limit to 1 tsp/day), soups with allowed ingredients, sugar, coconut

Modified from Dietetic Staff of Mayo Clinic: Low Oxalate Diet Brochure. Rochester, MN, Rochester Methodist Hospital and Saint Mary's Hospital, copyright © 1986, Mayo Foundation. With permission.

most methods used, ascorbate alters the quantitative measurement of oxalate. It is now appreciated that under alkaline conditions ascorbic acid autooxidizes to produce oxalate while standing in the urine, even in the bladder. Consequently, any urine collection that is not acidified may have an artificially elevated oxalate content because of this conversion. Further, any methodology that includes a step in which the urine is alkalinized is subject to the conversion of varying amounts of ascorbic acid to oxalate during the procedure unless this reaction is prevented. Recent methods have used ferric chloride in hydrochloric acid to stablize the ascorbic acid and prevent this conversion. Nevertheless, some authors have reported interference with very large doses (>2.5 mmol) of ascorbic acid. In summary, the methodologies for urinary oxalate are not yet settled. Many clinical studies are difficult to interpret because of these methodologic problems for the measurement of urinary oxalate. It is also possible that the apparent increase in urinary oxalate in patients taking ascorbic acid may be related to conversion in the bladder and not a clinically relevant problem in renal stone formation.

The urinary excretion of oxalate in normal adults ranges from 15–50 mg per 24-hour period with a mean of 35 mg. There are no apparent differences in the excretion levels between the sexes, although there does seem to be an increase with size, and some authors correct the oxalate excretion for creatinine excretion.

INTESTINAL DISORDERS WITH STONES

Table 14-2 outlines the GI disorders that are associated with renal lithiasis. In 1970 the association of hyperoxaluria and calcium oxalate urolithiasis after small bowel resection was noted by Smith, et al.[23]

A disturbance of intestinal absorption of oxalate has been identified in the disorders listed in Table 14-2 with the exception of category III, which includes chronic ulcerative

Table 14-2
Gastrointestinal Disorders Associated with Stones and Hyperoxaluria

Primary GI diseases
Regional enteritis
Nontropical sprue
Chronic pancreatitis
Blind loop syndrome
Bacterial overgrowth
Biliary tract disease
Postsurgical causes
Small-bowel resection
Small-bowel bypass for obesity
Gastric plication for obesity
Nonhyperoxaluria syndromes
Chronic ulcerative colitis
Peptic ulcer disease
Dumping syndrome
Chronic diarrhea (unspecified)
Ileostomy

colitis (CUC), ileostomy, and GI water losses (diarrheal syndromes). Although hyperoxaluria is a major predisposing factor for stones, it is clear that the renal lithiasis is not entirely attributable to the hyperoxaluria. Multiple etiologic factors have now been identified that promote the formation of urinary calculi in these patients.

HYPEROXALURIA

Several mechanisms have been identified that account for the increased oxalate excretion in patients with bowel disorders. The proposed mechanism for the increased oxalate absorption relates to the availability of more oxalate for absorption. With bowel disease and/or resection, steatorrhea often results from malabsorption of fat. The unabsorbed fatty acids bind calcium in the gut, decreasing the calcium content of the intestine available to complex the oxalate.[8] Steatorrhea may also increase the permeability of the colon to oxalate. Bile acid malabsorption, which occurs in varying degrees because of the interruption of enteral hepatic cycle for bile acid absorption in the ileum, results in delivery of these bile acid salts to the colon. Chadwick et al. showed that bile acids increase the permeability of the colon, but not other portions of the intestine, to oxalate absorption.[4] The increase in oxalate absorption from the normal 5–7 percent of the ingested intake to as high as 50 percent of the ingested intake of oxalate has been reported in these patients. Patients with resection of the large intestine in general do not have hyperoxaluria.

Initial studies concerning the pathogenesis of the hyperoxaluria suggested that glycine conjugated bile acids increase relative to taurine, and it was thought that the increased glycine could be converted to oxalate. Subsequent studies using choleoglycine 1-^{14}C administered orally to patients with enteric hyperoxaluria did *not* show that the administered isotope was converted to urinary ^{14}C oxalate.[17] It remains to be seen whether bile acid metabolism is playing any additional role since hyperoxaluria cannot be entirely explained by either fat malabsorption or increased colon permeability in all patients. Hofmann et al. showed that high urinary oxalate excretion persisted, averaging 38 mg/day, despite ingestion of a low-oxalate (6-mg/day) diet. They suggested that the diet contained oxalogenic substances other than preformed dietary oxalate, which contributed to the dietary oxalate in these patients.[18] Their study suggested that protein-rich foods were the source of this oxalate production and that creatinine may be converted by the enteric bacteria to glyoxalate, a precursor of oxalate. It is possible that other amino acids such as glycine could be promoting oxalate production.

To summarize, the etiologic factors promoting oxalate absorption in the gut include the following: (1) bile acid malabsorption increases the permeability of the colon to oxalate, (2) fatty acid malabsorption decreases the intestinal calcium content that normally binds oxalate, and (3) fatty acids increase colon permeability to oxalate absorption. Any maneuver that would alleviate these factors might be helpful in limiting hyperoxaluria.

Hyperoxaluria is not the only abnormality promoting stones in these patients. Many patients with intestinal disorders and stones have no hyperoxaluria; furthermore, virtually all patients with bowel bypass for obesity have hyperoxaluria. The incidence of stones in those patients is only 10–40 percent.

Alterations in the state of saturation or in crystal growth inhibitors caused by bowel problems or malabsorption may well be etiologic agents for stone formation in many of these patients. The state of saturation of a potential crystal, such as calcium oxalate, is determined by the relative supersaturation of that crystal system, that is, the free calcium ion activity times the free oxalate ion activity in a given solution. The free ion activity is determined by the ionic strength of the solution, the pH, complexation by other chemicals in solution, and the ion concentrations of calcium and oxalate.

Urinary constituents and abnormalities that affect the state of saturation for calcium oxalate crystal system have been reported by Smith and are reproduced in Table 14-3.[24] This table was generated by evaluating patients in a clinical study unit on a diet that was calculated to be identical with their home diets in terms of calcium, oxalate, and protein intake as determined by a research dietician. A review of the major alterations leads to an understanding of the problems involved.

Disturbances of intestinal absorption result in increased water loss in the stool, resulting in a decreased urine volume and increased concentration of many constituents, without change in the total excretion rate. Because of losses of sodium, potassium, and bicarbonate in the stool, however, there is urinary conservation of these ions, which results in decrease in the ionic strength of urine as well as the solubility of calcium and oxalate. Stool bicarbonate losses result in a metabolic acidosis and a consistently acid

Table 14-3
Urinary Abnormalities that Affect the State of Saturation in Patients with Enteric Hyperoxaluria

	I Normal Subjects ($n = 16$)	II Enteric Hyperoxaluria ($n = 20$)	III Primary Hyperoxaluria ($n = 10$)
Ion content (mg/g creatinine)			
Oxalate	25 ± 1*	61 ± 8	114 ± 10
Calcium	98 ± 8	84 ± 13	107 ± 22
Magnesium	96 ± 6	39 ± 6	106 ± 9
Phosphate	640 ± 53	477 ± 28	713 ± 89
Sulfate	350 ± 26	183 ± 25	311 ± 51
Citrate	427 ± 49	128 ± 31	457 ± 119
CO_2 content	366 ± 61	141 ± 38	237 ± 46
Ionic Ca ($\times 10^{-3}$ *M*)	1.00 ± 0.1	1.10 ± 0.2	0.74 ± 0.2
Total Ca ($\times 10^{-3}$ *M*)	2.21 ± 0.2	1.82 ± 0.3	1.58 ± 0.4
Percent ionic Ca	46 ± 2	62 ± 2	50 ± 4
Ionic C_2O_4 ($\times 10^{-3}$ *M*)	0.11 ± 0.01	0.30 ± 0.03	0.40 ± 0.04
Total C_2O_4 ($\times 10^{-3}$ *M*)	0.24 ± 0.03	0.59 ± 0.07	0.81 ± 0.08
Percent ionic C_2O_4	47 ± 1	53 ± 2	49 ± 2
Activity products			
C_2O_4 ($\times 10^{-9}$)	12 ± 2	37 ± 5	32 ± 4
CaP ($\times 10^{-7}$)	3.5 ± 0.6	2.2 ± 0.5	1.6 ± 0.4
Supersaturation†			
C_2O_4	+2.3 ± 0.5	+9.1 ± 1	+7.7 ± 1
CaP	+0.6 ± 0.3	−0.01 ± 0.2	−0.3 ± 0.2

Modified from Smith LH: Enteric hyperoxaluria and other hyperoxaluria states, in Coe FL, Benner BM, Stein JH (eds): Nephrolithiasis, Contemporary Issues in Nephrology. New York, Churchill Livingstone, 1980.

**M* = ±.

†Saturation equals zero: positive numbers represent supersaturation; negative numbers represent undersaturation.

urine, which has a deleterious effect on stone formation through the following several mechanisms. The urinary excretion of citrate is dependent on the state of acid–base balance in the body. Any stress promoting an acidosis will reduce urinary citrate. Citrate is an important complexor of calcium in urine and also acts as an inhibitor of the calcium phosphate crystal growth system. Gregory has emphasized the deleterious effect of an acid urinary pH.[13] He points out that at a urinary pH of 5, all the calcium salts except calcium oxalate have a much lower stability constant than at a pH of 8. For example, citrate, phosphate, bicarbonate, and sulfate salts of calcium are all much more stable in an alkaline urine and, therefore, suppress the formation of calcium oxalate even though the stability of calcium oxalate itself is not particularly affected because of its exceedingly low p*K*. It has also been reported that oral phosphates and pyrophosphate are more effective inhibitors at an alkaline pH than acid pH. Magnesium absorption is also reduced in bowel disease. It normally has a role in the complexation of urinary oxalate. Magnesium depletion would favor calcium oxalate precipitation.

Patients with bowel disorders may have protein malabsorption, which decreases urinary sulfate and phosphate, as is emphasized in Table 14-3. The reduction of available phosphate results in a decrease in the urinary excretion of pyrophosphate, an inhibitor of the crystal growth of calcium salts. Both phosphate and sulfate are important in complexing calcium, depending on the urine pH. A review of Table 14-3 reveals that the total calcium concentration is low in enteric hyperoxaluric patients at 1.82 mmol/liter, compared with 2.21 mmol/liter in normal subjects. Free ionic calcium, however, is actually elevated at 1.1 mmol/liter, and the percent of total calcium that is ionized has risen from 46 to 62 percent. The same pattern is seen with the urinary oxalate. Not only is total oxalate increased but also the percent of ionized oxalate has increased in these patients. This has resulted in an increase in supersaturation, from about 2.3 times supersaturated to 9 times supersaturated, which is highly significant. The supersaturation for calcium oxalate is even higher than that seen in the primary hyperoxaluria patients, even though the urinary oxalate is usually much lower in the enteric hyperoxaluric patients than those with primary hyperoxaluria. The possibility that there is epitaxial formation of oxalate crystals on uric acid crystals is also promoted since the urine of these patients is extremely acid, and uric acid excretion is not reduced.

SMALL-BOWEL BYPASS FOR OBESITY

Bowel bypass for obesity has been successful in controlling morbid obesity but has been associated with a high incidence of urolithiasis and has resulted in a physiologic model for studying the problem of enteric hyperoxaluria.

Gregory reported 681 patients who had undergone a small-bowel bypass procedure for morbid obesity.[13] The stone formation rate in this group was 16.4 percent. Of the 86 patients who passed stones, two-thirds passed only 1 stone. The incidence of recurrent stones was about 57 percent in the first year, 18 percent in the second year, 18 percent in the third year, and 7 percent after 3 years. Most patients have cyrstalluria of the oxalate variety in freshly voided urine. Additional renal complications in this group included progressive renal insufficiency with oxalosis and acquired renal tubular dysfunction of type I, or distal, renal tubular acidosis (RTA).

Bachman et al. have shown that the incidence of kidney stones after intestinal bypass operations may vary depending on the type of bypass procedure.[1] In their study, at a 2-year follow-up, those patients who had received an end-to-end jejunoiliostomy with ileocecostomy had a stone incidence of 89 percent, whereas an end-to-side anastomosis had an incidence of only 48 percent. The end-to-end jejunoileostomy showed the highest incidence of stones. Griffen et al. noted that there was higher fecal fat loss after the end-to-end operation that is associated with higher oxalate excretions and could explain the high incidence of stones after that procedure.[14]

Griffen et al. compared gastric and jejunoileal bypass procedures for morbid obesity (90 percent gastric exclusion with a Roux-en-Y reconstitution).[14] Although they found a 10 percent incidence of stones in the ileal bypass group, none of their 32 patients with gastric bypass developed stones at the time of followup. Although this would seem to be a remarkable difference, it is a very small group and this author has seen patients with gastric bypass who have developed urolithiasis.

NONHYPEROXALURIC DISORDERS

Fukushima et al. reported a 7 percent incidence of stones in patients with ulcerative colitis.[10] The mean period of time between the onset of the colitis and the initial stones was about 5 years. Virtually all of Fukushima's patients had calcium oxalate stones. Those disorders of the GI tract that are not associated with hyperoxaluria, such as CUC and postileostomy patients, have a marked increase in the incidence of both oxalate and uric acid stones. An increased calcium:magnesium ratio may explain the increased incidence of stones in these patients. Urinary output and urinary pH are low. Patients with ileostomies often have uric acid urolithiasis, which is somewhat more common than calcium urolithiasis. This is presumably because of the extremely acid urines that are a result of the intestinal bicarbonate wasting from the ileostomy. There is a normal uric acid excretion rate, which results in an increased uric acid concentration. The solubility of uric acid is decreased in the acid urine. At a urine pH of 4.5, 90 percent of all urate is in the form of uric acid, and the solubility is only 100 mg/liter.

CLINICAL EVALUATION

The clinical evaluation of patients with bowel disease and stones is somewhat more complex than in other types of stone patients because of the wide array of physiologic factors which promote stone growth. They should be evaluated for the several pathophysiologic disturbances as outlined in Table 14-4. A diet history is extremely important. It may be helpful to have the diet evaluated by a dietician, particularly with respect to oxalate intake, fat intake, and calcium intake.

TREATMENT MODALITIES

There are many potential therapeutic modalities for these patients. Unfortunately, a systematic analysis of the comparison of the various treatment modalities is not available at this time. A review of an unselected group of 32 patients referred to our renal stone clinic because of Crohn's disease and hyperoxaluria indicated that we were able to reduce or abolish stone formation in those patients shown to be metabolically active in

Table 14-4
Physiologic Parameters in the Clinical Evaluation of Bowel Disease and Stones

Blood studies
Acid–base balance
Electrolytes
Magnesium
Serum protein electrophoresis
Creatinine
Calcium
Phosphorus
Uric acid
Urinary studies
24-hour urine volume
Urinalysis for pH and osmolality
Urine culture
24-hour urine for calcium, phosphorus, uric acid, sodium, potassium, magnesium, and citrate
Stone analysis
Renal x-rays: KUB, tomograms
Stool studies
Stool collection for fat and volume

90 percent of the cases. Our experience with the bowel bypass for obesity has not been as favorable, and in 6 of 30 patients the bypass was reversed to prevent stones or renal failure.

Gregory studied one patient who had persistent, severe oxalate stone formation and crystalluria with a series of therapeutic modalities in an attempt to gauge the effect of various treatment programs.[12] It is instructive to evaluate the range of treatment modalities that he used and their effect in this particular patient who had a small-bowel bypass for obesity with hyperoxaluria. Gregory initially started the patient on a low-oxalate, low-fat diet. The diet did not alter the 24-hour urine oxalate excretion. Cholestyramine, magnesium oxide, calcium gluconate, and calcium carbonate were then added one at a time. None had any influence on the number of stones per week, which averaged about three to four stones. When the patient was placed on a no-oxalate diet, urinary oxalate and stone formation were reduced. A no-fruit or no-vegetable diet slightly moderated the stone formation. Nevertheless, specific instances of response to each of these modalities have resulted in reduced stone formation in some patients. Specific evaluation of each of these therapies has been undertaken.

Earnest et al. have shown that a reduction in steatorrhea is associated with a reduction in urinary oxalate.[8] Rudman et al. showed that patients with GI malabsorption had hypocitraturia that responded to an oral citrate supplement.[22] Correction of the hypomagnesemia and hypomagnesuria was important in these patients as it further increased urinary citrate excretion as well as urinary magnesium excretion. It is thought that the magnesium supplements reduced the cellular acid content promoting increased citrate excretion from the kidney.

A low-oxalate diet is critical in limiting increased oxalate absorption. This type of diet can be designed by reviewing the foods containing high oxalate shown in Table 14-1.

However, many foods containing oxalate are obscure and are difficult to eliminate from the diet. As outlined earlier, it is exceedingly difficult to establish a good low-oxalate diet, but known oxalate containing foods should definitely be avoided.

Restriction of dietary fat intake should limit steatorrhea and be of help in preventing oxalate absorption. A 60-g fat diet may be unacceptable in view of the difficulty of providing an appropriate number of calories to these patients. Medium-chain triglycerides can be substituted if necessary, since medium-chain fatty acids do not increase the permeability of the colon to oxalate and do not bind calcium to form soaps.[6]

The administration of a base such as sodium bicarbonate or polycitra will decrease systemic acidemia and improve citrate excretion. Polycitra is preferred because it is somewhat better tolerated with less eructation and gas formation. Bowel disease patients may be intolerant of this form of therapy, however, since it may be poorly absorbed and increases water excretion via the bowel.

The administration of calcium is somewhat controversial. Initial studies revealed that calcium will bind oxalate in the gut and reduce urinary oxalate excretion. Subsequent studies have suggested that the urinary calcium excretion usually rises as oxalate decreases. The result is no change in the activity product for calcium oxalate. Calcium supplements are important for other problems however; for example, many patients have calcium depletion and a tendency toward osteomalacia that needs to be treated whenever possible.

The administration of cholestyramine can be helpful in some settings. As an anion binding agent, cholestyramine binds oxalate as well as bile acids. This results in decreased permeability of the colon to oxalate as well as a decrease in oxalate availability. This treatment, however, may actually worsen the steatorrhea in some patients with severe steatorrhea. Cholestyramine has a limited role because it is not well tolerated by most patients on a long-term basis. With the exception of patients with a primary bile acid malabsorption problem, it is wise to delay the use of cholestyramine until other therapies have been tried.

Magnesium supplements may be useful if the urinary magnesium or the serum magnesium is low. The supplements help to increase the excretion of both citrate and magnesium, both of which decrease the free ion activity for calcium. Magnesium may be a competitive inhibitor at the crystal face also. Most patients cannot tolerate magnesium oxide or magnesium hydroxide orally since these agents promote diarrhea. When indicated, 1 g of magnesium sulfate intramuscularly (IM) can be given on a weekly basis. Protein may be oxalogenic as reported by Hofmann, but we have not utilized protein restriction in this group of patients.

Patients with persistent, recurrent stones following bowel bypass for obesity may require reconstruction of their intestine to prevent further stone formation. We have carried this out in six such patients with relief of their stone disease.

In those patients in whom hyperoxaluria is not an issue, the primary therapeutic maneuver includes an increase in the urinary volume. Although patients with GI disorders have a limited capability for increasing urinary volume, it is an extremely important parameter and should be encouraged. Most patients do much better if the fluid intake is divided into small amounts and taken on a frequent basis to allow for increased absorption. The recommended approach is to slowly increase the volume of fluid until it is clear that the stool output of fluid is becoming burdensome and/or that it is not increasing urinary output.

Polycitra, bicitra, or Shohl's solution are primary choices for increasing urinary citrate excretion, although an occasional patient prefers sodium bicarbonate. Polycitra is usually given at a starting dose of 1 tablespoon tid and increased as necessary to bring urinary citrate into normal range (above 400 mg/24 hours) for calcium stone disease or the urinary pH into the desired range for uric acid stone disease (^{U}pH 6.5–7.0). Monitoring is done with nitrazine paper. A poor response warrants evaluation and/or treatment for magnesium depletion, which inhibits citrate excretion.

Dietary alterations of fat and/or oxalate usually are difficult therapeutic maneuvers. We employ a registered dietician to help with this program. Many patients rely on oxalate containing foods particularly fluids, such as Coca-Cola, for their major source of calories. Restriction of these, without appropriate substitution of calories, can lead to severe malnutrition. Patients with excess fat excretion (> 15 g/day) are treated with dietary fat restriction. If it is not demonstrated that there is fat excess, it may be detrimental to restrict fat since it limits caloric intake unnecessarily.

Allopurinol, 300 mg/day, can be used for patients with uric acid stones or in suspected cases of epitaxial growth of oxalate on uric acid crystals. Finally, with bile acid diarrhea, cholestyramine 4 g qid or taurine 3 g tid may be helpful. For patients whose high volume output is not due to steatorrhea, it may be helpful to use nonspecific measures, such as Lomotil (diphenoxylate hydrochloride; Searle) or opiates to reduce bowel motility.

Increased stones in patients with peptic ulcer disease are often associated with the milk-alkali syndrome. In these cases there is a high dietary intake of absorbable alkali as well as dairy foods. There often is a mild to moderate renal insufficiency that prevents calcium excretion and leads to nephrocalcinosis and stones. In general, absorbable alkali should be limited when excessive calcium is present.

REFERENCES

1. Bachman L, Nordenvall B, Hallberg D: Difference in kidney stone incidence after three types of intestinal bypass operations. Scand J Urol Nephrol 53S:149–157, 1980
2. Breslau NA, Pak CYC: Urinary saturation, hetergenous nucleation, and crystallization inhibitors in nephrolithiasis, in Coe F, Brenner BM, Stein, JH (eds): Nephrolithiasis, Contemporaray Issues in Nephrology. New York, Churchill Livingstone, 1980, pp 13–36
3. Caspary WF: Intestinal oxalate absorption. I. Absorption in vitro. Res Exp Med 171:13–24, 1977
4. Chadwick VS, Phillips SF, Hofmann AF: Measurements of intestinal permeability using low molecular weight polyethylene glycols (PEG 400). II. Application to normal and abnormal permeability states in man and animals. Gastroenterology 73:247–251, 1977
5. Crawford GA, Mahony JF, Györy AZ: Measurement of urinary oxalate in the presence of ascorbic acid. Clin Chem Acta 147:51–57, 1985
6. Dobbins JW, Binder HJ.: Effect of bile salts and fatty acids on the colonic absorption of oxalate. Gastroenterology 70:1096–1100, 1976
7. Dowling RH, Rose GA, Sutor DJ: Hyperoxaluria and renal calculi in ileal disease. Lancet 1:1103–1106, 1971
8. Earnest DL, Johnson G, Williams HE, et al: Hyperoxaluria in patients with ileal resection: An abnormality in dietary oxalate absorption. Gastroenterology 66:1114–1122, 1974
9. Finlayson B. Renal lithiasis in review. Urol Clin N Am 1:181, 1974
10. Fukushima T, Ishiguro N, Matsuda Y, et al: Clinical and urinary characteristics of urolithiasis in ulcerative colitis. Am J Gastroenterol 77:238–242, 1982
11. Gelzayd EA, Breuer RI, Kirsner JB: Nephrolithiasis in inflammatory bowel disease. Am J Digest Dis 13:1027–1033, 1968

12. Gregory JG, Park KY, Schoenberg HW: Oxalate stone disease after intestinal resection. J Urol 117:631–634, 1977
13. Gregory JG: Hyperoxaluria and stone disease in the gastrointestinal bypass patient. Urol Clin N Am 8:331–351, 1981
14. Griffen WO, Young VL, Stevenson CC: A prospective comparison of gastric and jejunoileal bypass procedures for morbid obesity. Ann Surg 186:500–509, 1977
15. Hagler L, Herman RH: Oxalate metabolism. Am J Clin Nutr 26:758–765, 1973
16. Harrison AR, Kasidas GP, Rose GA: Hyperoxaluria and recurrent stone formation apparently cured by short courses of pyridoxine. Br Med J (Clin Res) 282:2097–2098, 1981
17. Hofmann AF, Tacker MM, Fromm H, et al: Acquired hyperoxaluria and intestinal disease: Evidence that bile acid glycine is not a precusor of oxalate. Mayo Clin Proc 48:35–42, 1973
18. Hofmann AF, Laker MF, Dharmsathaphorn K, et al: Complex pathogenesis of hyperoxaluria after jejunoileal bypass surgery. Gastroenterology 84:293–300, 1983
19. Maratka Z, Nedbal J: Urolithiasis as a complication of the surgical treatment of ulcerative colitis. Gut 5:214–217, 1964
20. Robertson WG, Nordine BEC: Activity products in urine, in Hodgkinson A, Nordine BEC (eds): Renal Stone Research Symposium: London, Churchill, 1969, pp 221–232
21. Robertson WG, Peacock M, Nordine BEC: Crystalluria, in Finlayson B, Hench LL, Smith LH (eds): Urolithiasis—Physical Aspects. National Academy of Sciences, Washington, DC, 1972, pp 243–254
22. Rudman D, Debonis JL, Fountain MT, et al: Hypocitraturia in patients with gastrointestinal malabsorption. New Engl J Med 303:657–661, 1980
23. Smith LH, Fromm H, Hofmann AF: Acquired hyperoxaluria, nephrolithiasis and intestinal disease: Description of a syndrome. New Engl J Med 286:1371–1375, 1972
24. Smith LH: Enteric hyperoxaluria and other hyperoxaluria states, in Coe FL, Brenner BM, Stein JH (eds): Nephrolithiasis, Contemporary Issues in Nephrology. New York, Churchill Livingstone, 1980
25. Tiselius HG, Almgård LE: The diurnal urinary excretion of oxalate and the effect of pyridoxine and ascorbate on oxalate excretion. Eur Urol 3:41–46, 1977
26. Tiselius HG: Excretion of 4-pyridoxic acid and oxalic acid in patients with urinary calculi. Invest Urol 15:5–8, 1977
27. Williams HE, Smith LH: Disorders of oxalate metabolism. Am J Med 45:715–735, 1968
28. Zarembski P, Hodgkinson A: Some factors influencing the urinary excretion of oxalic acid in man. Clin Chim Acta 25:1–10, 1969
29. Zerwekh JE, Drake E, Gregory JG, et al: Assay of urinary oxalate: Six methodologies compared. Clin Chem 29/11:1977–1980, 1983

Robert Campbell
Donald P. Griffith

15

Infected (Struvite) Calculi

Struvite urinary stones occurred in antiquity; bladder stones composed of struvite ($MgNH_4PO_4 \cdot 6H_2O$) have been recovered from a 5000-year-old Egyptian mummy.

The term *struvite* derives from a Prussian naturalist, Baron Von Struve. The mineral—$MgNH_4PO_4 \cdot 6H_2O$—was first identified in bat guano by one of Von Struve's students, who named the mineral in honor of his mentor.

The terms *infectious stones* and *triple-phosphate stones* are synonymous with *struvite stones*. The term *triple-phosphate* derives from the coexistence of struvite and carbonate apatite [$Ca_{10}(PO_4)_6CO_3$], thereby leading to the presence of three cations [Ca^{2+}, Mg^{2+}, and NH_4^+] and one predominant anion [PO_4^{3-}].

Extensive experimental and clinical investigations demonstrate that in humans the bacterial enzyme urease is the basis for struvite and carbonate apatite calculogenesis.[29]

INCIDENCE

Struvite stones account for 15–28 percent of all stones in various series.[32,58] The exact incidence is unknown, since many metabolic stones pass spontaneously and are not included in the data from reference laboratories analyzing large numbers of stones. The female population is at higher risk, constituting 60–80 percent of struvite stone formers.[58,60] This is probably related to the overall increased susceptibility of females to urinary infections.

Other high-risk groups have also been identified. Patients on long-term antimicrobial therapy may develop urinary infection with resistant urease-producing organisms such as *Proteus* or *Pseudomonas*. Patients with neuropathic bladders or spinal cord injuries[5] on intermittent catheterization regimens or with indwelling catheters, and patients with vesical or supravesical diversion (ileal conduits, nephrostomy tubes, suprapubic drainage)[13] are prone to infectious stones. Eight percent of patients with spinal cord injuries developed struvite stones in Comarr's series.[7]

STONE DISEASE: DIAGNOSIS AND MANAGEMENT
ISBN 0-8089-1873-7

CLINICAL MANIFESTATION

Four principal types of infectious stones are generally recognized.

Staghorn or Branched Calculi

Staghorn renal calculi are commonly, although not always, of infectious origin. They are often asymptomatic; typically a female patient presents with chronic, recurrent bacteriuria and symptomatic cystitis. Colicky symptoms are rare; only 8 percent of struvite stones pass spontaneously.

Bladder Stones

Bladder calculi that form in sterile urine as a consequence of bladder outlet obstruction are most often composed of calcium oxalate and uric acid. Struvite bladder stones typically form around indwelling urethral and suprapubic catheters and are invariably associated with urinary infection.[12]

Matrix Concretions

Matrix concretions[2,72] are soft, mucoid mixtures of mucopolysaccharides, inflammatory cells, protein debris, and scattered crystals of struvite.[73] They may contain glycosaminoglycans. The aggregation of organic molecules, epithelial cell debris, and crystals increases supersaturation at local sites and promotes stone formation. Matrix concretions are radiolucent initially but become radiopaque as they mineralize.

Secondary Stones

Metabolic stones that become infected with subsequent growth of struvite on to the primary stone are known as *secondary stones.* As much as 50 percent of struvite stones may contain a primary nidus of calcium oxalate, hydroxyapatite, cystine, or uric acid.[61]

PATHOPHYSIOLOGY

Microbiology

Numerous clinical and experimental reports implicate urea-splitting infections with calculogenesis.[30,39] Infrequent reports of non-urea-splitting bacteria associated with stones[69] likely represent infection with urease-producing *Mycoplasma* or anaerobic species not routinely isolated on standard culture media. Struvite stone formation in humans requires the presence of a urease-producing organism in the urine.[3,27–29,53,71]

Many species of gram-negative and gram-positive bacteria produce urease. *Staphylococcus* is the most common gram-positive species. *Proteus* is the number one gram-negative pathogen. Greater than 90 percent of *Proteus* isolates in one series were urease-positive. *Klebsiella* and *Pseudomonas* are also common urinary pathogens involved in stone formation and were found to contain urease in 64 and 33 percent of isolates, respectively. In the same series no *Escherichia coli* isolates contained urease.[30] *Streptococcus faecalis, Corynebacterium* group D2, and *Ureaplasma urealyticum* have also been implicated.

Urease

Urease is one of the largest, most potent, and most specific enzymes known. It was the first enzyme crystallized,[65] for which Sumner received the Nobel Prize in 1946. It has a wide distribution in nature and is found in bacteria, invertebrates, and certain flowering plants. It is absent in vertebrates.[8,47] The gastrointestinal (GI) tracts of animals harbor urease-containing bacterial flora that hydrolyze dietary urea into ammonia.[9] Most of the ammonium ion in blood comes from this intestinal source.

The plant enzyme has a molecular weight of about 500,000[66] and probably is composed of six identical subunits.[4,24] Although highly specific for urea, four additional substrates have been unequivocably identified, including dihydroxyurea,[21] semicarbazide,[26] hydroxyurea,[20] and foramide.[23] There are kinetic differences between plant and bacterial urease.[38,45,48] Bacterial urease has half the molecular weight of the plant enzyme,[25] suggesting that it may be a trimer.

Jack bean and bacterial urease[10,22] contain nickel, an essential structural and catalytic component of the enzyme. The affinity of urease inhibitors to bind to urease may be related to the nickel atoms in the enzyme.[52]

Urease catalyzes the hydrolysis of urea to ammonia and CO_2 by the following reaction:

$$H_2N-\overset{\overset{\displaystyle O}{\|}}{C}-NH_2 \xrightarrow[H_2O\ (Ni)]{\text{Urease}} \underset{\text{ammonia}}{2NH_3} + CO_2 \qquad (15\text{-}1)$$

Ammonia is subsequently converted to ammonium by further hydrolysis:

$$NH_3 + H_2O \rightleftharpoons NH_4^+ + OH^- \qquad (15\text{-}2)$$

Ureolysis and Struvite Formation

The end result of the reactions in equations 15-1 and 15-2 is production of high urinary ammonium levels and elevation of urinary pH. Virtually all authorities concur in the belief that urine must be supersaturated for crystallization to occur.[19,56] Hyperammonuria and urinary alkalinization create conditions favorable for supersaturation and precipitation of struvite and carbonate apatite.[29]

Pharmacologic alkalinization of urine with sodium bicarbonate does not result in struvite formation because it induces little or no ammonium in urine.[54] Under physiologic conditions, urinary ammonia increases in response to induced acidity, not alkalosis. Urinary alkalinization and hyperammonuria must both be present for urine to become supersaturated with respect to struvite.[15,16,28,29,56] These conditions occur only in the presence of ureolysis. Several studies have revealed that sterile urine is invariably undersaturated with respect to struvite.[15,56] In fact, experimental investigations have shown that sterile urine may dissolve struvite stones.[3,16,28,46,70] Elliot[14] and Stamey[63] have reported the dissolution of human renal calculi that were presumed to be struvite.

Carbonate-Apatite Formation

Three types of calcium phosphate stones occur clinically. These include brushite ($CaHPO_4$), hydroxyapatite [$Ca_{10}(PO_4)_6 \cdot (OH_2)$], and carbonate-apatite [$Ca_{10}(PO_4)_6 \cdot CO_3$]. Human "infection stones" are a mixture of struvite and carbonate-apatite.

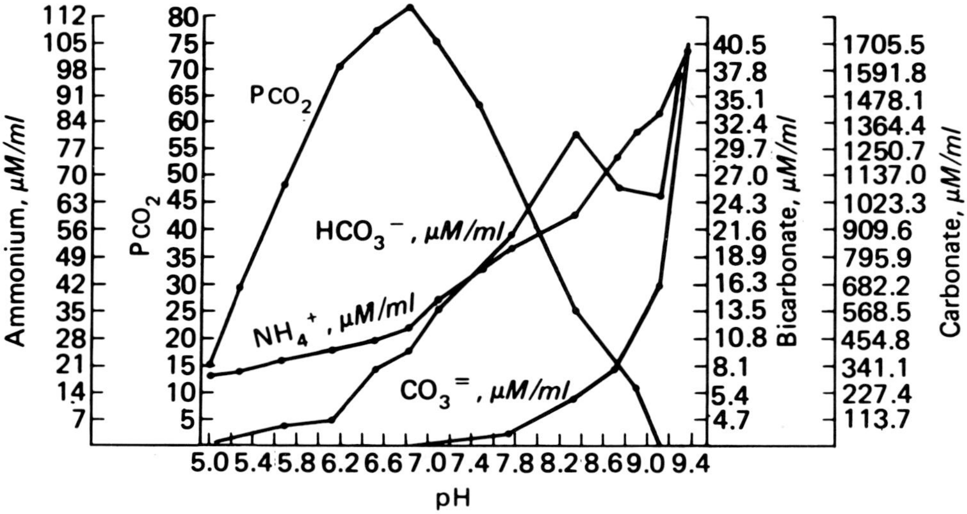

Fig. 15-1. The biochemical changes occurring during a 2-hour period following the addition of urease to normal human urine. (From Griffith DP: Struvite Stones. Kidney Internatl 13:374, 1978. Reprinted from Kidney International with permission.)

Physiologic urine is intermittently supersaturated with respect to calcium phosphate.[36] If bicarbonaturia is induced by pharmacologic alkalinization, the likelihood of calcium phosphate formation (as brushite or hydroxyapatite) increases. In the clinical setting, hydroxyapatite crystalluria (either pure or mixed with calcium oxalate) occurs commonly in sterile urine, especially under conditions of increased alkalinity.

The carbonate ions in carbonate-apatite result from the high concentrations of CO_2 generated by ureolysis. Bicarbonate is subsequently converted to carbonate ion under the highly alkaline conditions produced by ureolysis, according to the following reaction:

$$H_2O + CO_2 \rightleftharpoons H_2CO_3 \rightleftharpoons H^+ + HCO_3^- \rightleftharpoons CO_3^{2-} \qquad (15\text{-}3)$$

Under physiologic and sterile pathologic conditions, the urinary excretion of bicarbonate and/or carbonate is low or nonexistent—too low to result in the formation of carbonate-apatite. Concentrations of bicarbonate and carbonate-apatite and alkalinity sufficient to bring about crystallization of carbonate-apatite occur only in the presence of ureolysis (Fig. 15-1).

UREASE INHIBITORS

The hydroxamic acids have been known to chemists for nearly 200 years. Kobashi et al. first noted the inhibitory effect of these compounds on urease.[40] The general structure of hydroxamic acids is shown in Figure 15-2 (where the R substituent may represent a hydrogen atom, an alkyl group, or an aromatic residue; R^2 may equal R except when R is hydrogen).

The primary hydroxamates (Fig. 15-2) are potent urease inhibitors. Substitution on the nitrogen with carbon chains yields secondary hydroxamic acids.

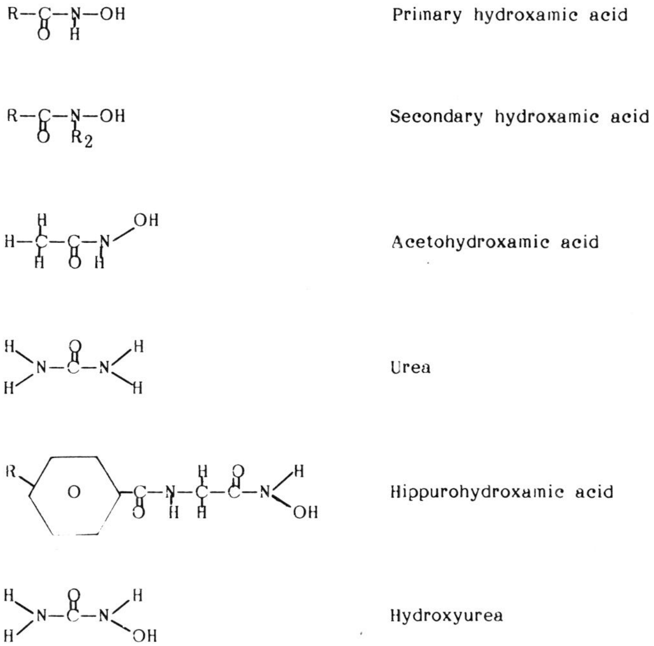

Fig. 15-2. Molecular structure of primary and secondary hydroxamic acids. (Reproduced from Griffith DP: Struvite stones. Kidney Internatl 13:374, 1978. With permission.)

A number of experimental investigations have considered the structure-activity-toxicity relationships for a series of hydroxamate analogs.[41,42,44] These studies may be briefly summarized as showing: (1) the inhibition by aliphatic hydroxamates reaches maximum effect as the carbon chain reaches 7–9, (2) toxicity increases as the carbon chain lengthens; and (3) the addition of charged groups to the chain usually decreases inhibition.

Kobashi and coworkers' recent work[67] suggests that aromatic hydroxamates may be potent urease inhibitors. Their study compares the inhibitory power and urinary excretion of various hydroxamic acid derivatives of hippuric acid with several other hydroxamic acid derivatives. The dosage levels of I_{50} (at which 50 percent inhibition of urease occurred) for the various drugs were determined for both jack bean urease and for intact *Proteus* cell suspensions. Percent urinary recovery was also determined. The effective index (EI) for each drug was then calculated by the formula:

$$EI = \frac{\text{recovery }\%}{I_{50}\ (\mu M)}$$

The data are summarized in Table 15-1.

Acetohydroxamic acid (AHA) has a very high I_{50}, but this disadvantage is offset somewhat by the high urinary excretion of the drug, giving an effective index of 1.17 in the intact cell suspension. The highest effective index values were obtained for *p*-methoxyhippuro- and *m*-nitrohippurohydroxamic acid. The next most effective drug, *m*-methoxyhippurohydroxamic acid (UCD II), has an EI of 1.77 in the *Proteus* cell suspen-

Table 15-1
Urease Inhibition and Urinary Excretion of Hippurohydroxamic Acid Derivatives

	I_{50} (μM)		Urinary Excretion (%)			Effective Index*	
Hydroxamic Acid	Jack Bean Urease	Proteus Mirabilis Intact cell	0–6 h	6–24 h	Total	Jack Bean Urease	*Proteus mirabilis* Intact Cell
Hippuro-	0.77	—†	3.7	0.3	4.0	5.19	—
o-Chloro-hippuro-	0.50	2.65	3.7	0.2	3.9	7.80	1.47
m-Chloro-hippuro-	0.74	7.3	4.1	0.2	4.3	5.81	0.59
p-Chloro-hippuro-	1.00	2.1	1.7	0.4	2.1	2.10	1.00
o-Methoxy-hippuro-	1.3	31.0	3.0	0.1	3.1	2.38	0.10
m-Methoxy-hippuro-	1.2	8.8	15.0	0.6	15.6	13.00	1.77
p-Methoxy-hippuro-	1.7	3.2	16.0	0.3	16.3	9.59	5.09
m-Nitro-hippuro-	1.2	3.6	14.6	0.3	14.9	12.40	4.14
Aceto-	10.0	26.0	28.0	2.53	30.5	3.05	1.17
Nicotino-	2.15	—	0.98	0.10	1.08	0.56	—
Caprylo-	0.97	—	0.61	0.39	1.00	1.03	—
Benzo-	3.9	—	0.4	0.19	0.59	0.15	—

Reproduced from Takeuchi H, Kobashi K, Yoshida O: Prevention of infected urinary stones in rats by urease inhibitor. A new hydroxamic acid derivative. Invest Urol 18:102, 1980. Copyright © 1980 by Williams & Wilkins. With permission.

*Effective index: excretion %/I_{50} (μM).

†Not determined.

sion. The higher I_{50} values for urease inhibition of the *Proteus* cell suspensions compared with jack bean urease is related to the permeability of the drug across the bacterial cell membrane. Work with whole cells provides a situation closer to in vivo conditions.[57] Rats treated with UCD II had a statistically significant reduction in bladder stone formation after implantation of *Proteus* infected disks. Clinical application of UCD II and other hydroxamic derivatives awaits clinical evaluation of efficacy and toxicity. It is noteworthy that AHA and *p*-methoxyhippuro- and *m*-nitrohippurohydroxamic acid are mutagenic in high doses.

There have been several studies reporting that hydroxamic acids potentiate the antibacterial effect of antibiotics.[3,51] A new hydroxamic acid, *N*-(pivaroyl) glycinohydroxamic acid (P-GHA), in combination with cephalexin, prevented bladder stone formation in rats, while separate therapy with either agent alone was ineffective against stone formation and bacterial growth.[68] This effect was felt to be secondary to potentiation of the permeability of the bacterial cell wall to P-GHA by cephalexin.

The pharmacokinetic parameters of acetohydroxamic acid were evaluated by Griffith and Feldman in patients with staghorn renal calculi.[55] Acetohydroxamic acid is rapidly absorbed from the GI tract with peak drug levels occurring approximately 1 hour after administration. Acetamide and CO_2 are identified as the two major metabolites in humans. Carbon dioxide is eliminated via the lungs and accounted for 20–45 percent of the administered dose, while acetamide is eliminated in the urine and accounted for only 9–14 percent of a given dose. The remaining 9–48 percent was eliminated as intact AHA in the urine.

The half-life of AHA in normal subjects is 3.5–5 hours.[18] The half-life is considerably longer in patients with decreased renal function (~ 15–24 hours)[55] when compared to

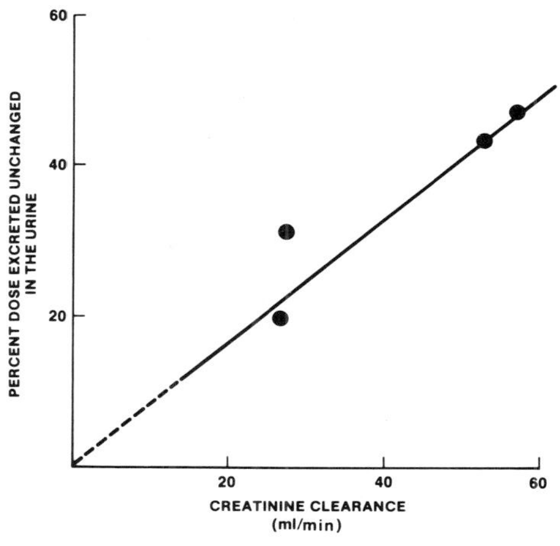

Fig. 15-3. Plot of the percent of AHA dose excreted unchanged in the urine as a function of creatinine clearance in the four patients studied. (Reproduced from Putcha L, Griffith DP, Feldman S: Pharmacokinetics of acetohydroxamic acid in patients with staghorn renal calculi. Eur J Clin Pharm 28:442, 1985. With permission.)

normal subjects and patients with cirrhosis (~9–13 hours).[64] This is in agreement with previously recorded data in another study population where the half-life ranged from 7.5 to 17.5 hours.[18] Total-body clearance and renal clearance of AHA are thus considerably lower in patients with compromised renal function and clearly show a linear relationship between AHA half-life and creatinine clearance[55] (Fig. 15-3).

The effectiveness of AHA depends on the concentration achieved in the urine.[31] In patients with impaired renal function, extrarenal elimination accounts for a considerable portion of the drug's disposition.[74] When the serum creatinine exceeds 2 mg/dl, full therapeutic concentrations of AHA in the urine are unachievable. The dose should not be increased in these patients because high doses increase urinary acetamide and increase the incidence of toxic reactions and side effects. Acetamide in high doses poses some risk of carcinogenesis[37] and teratogenesis.[43]

DIAGNOSIS AND TREATMENT

The treatment of struvite stones involves eradication of infection and elimination of all calculi. Consideration must also be directed toward appropriate management of any underlying metabolic disorder. The adjunctive use of urease inhibitors such as acetohydroxamic acid and hydroxyurea is beneficial in cases where urea-splitting infection persists. Successful treatment is evidenced by radiographic absence of stones and multiple negative urine cultures in the absence of antibiotics. This is often difficult to achieve, since incomplete stone removal is common. Residual stone fragments harbor residual infection, leading to further stone growth. The urine may become sterile while the patient is maintained on antibiotics, but when antimicrobials are discontinued, recrudescence is virtually assured if residual foreign bodies (stones) are present. Bacteria locked in the interstices of the stone are resistant to eradication by even the most potent antimicrobial agents.

Infection stones are particularly amenable to elimination by lithotripsy because the stones are typically soft and crumbly. However, the extensive staghorn size and configuration leads to a relatively high incidence of residual fragments following percutaneous and/or extracorporeal shock-wave lithotripsy (ESWL).

Approximately 40 percent of patients treated conventionally (with surgery and antibiotics) will have persistent urinary infection, with 60 percent of these developing recurrent stones.[30] This amounts to an overall recurrence rate of approximately 25 percent. The recurrence rates in patients treated with percutaneous and/or shock-wave lithotripsy have not yet been reported. Even among patients with complete eradication of stone at the time of surgery, there is a 15 percent rate of stone recurrence. If stone removal is incomplete, 70 percent of patients will exhibit new stone formation or an increase in stone size.[60] Patients with staghorn struvite stones who receive no treatment have a 50 percent chance of losing the kidney.[59,75] There is a 25 percent 5-year mortality for bilateral, untreated struvite stones.[75] Fifty percent of World War II and Korean War veterans with spinal cord injuries died of stone-related problems.[11]

Diagnostic evaluation of the patient with infectious urinary stones should include: (1) appropriate biochemical evaluation of blood and urine to ascertain the presence of an associated metabolic abnormality; (2) bacteriologic evaluation of the urine and extracted stone material with identification of the organism involved and the antimicrobial sensitivities; (3) pre- and postoperative determination of size, number, and location of stones; and (4) radiographic documentation of any anatomic abnormalities.

MEDICAL TREATMENT

Antimicrobials

Short-term antimicrobial therapy virtually never eliminates infection when a foreign body harbors the infection. Antimicrobial therapy may yield sterile urine during the course of treatment, and, in rare instances, stone dissolution has occurred during such therapy.[31,63] A good theoretical argument can be made for antimicrobial therapy that reduces the bacterial density (i.e., drugs that reduce bacterial colonies from 10^7/ml to 10^5/ml have eliminated 99 percent of the bacteria and thereby 99 percent of the urease). However, long-term antimicrobial treatment usually results in the appearance of new, more resistant organisms.

Use of culture-specific antimicrobial drugs is superior to broad-spectrum agents such as sulfonamides, nitrofurantoins, and methenamine. Methenamine salts are particularly unsuited in the upper urinary tract because their retention time in the pyelocaliceal system is usually less than 3 minutes, and the generation time for the conversion of methenamine into formaldehyde exceeds 1 hour, even in the most acidic urine.[34,35,50] Methenamine salts thus are clearly inappropriate in the alkaline environment of a urease-producing bacterium.

Penicillin or ampicillin have been particularly effective in achieving sterile urine in patients with stones and infection with *Proteus mirabilis*. One study revealed that 93 percent of *P. mirabilis* strains were inhibited by concentrations of less than 20 μg/ml of either drug. Sterile urine was obtained in 80 percent of cases thus treated, and stone dissolution was noted in two cases.[17] Standard doses of oral penicillin (500 mg q6h) or ampicillin (250 mg q6h) were shown to produce urinary levels of 150 and 300 μg/ml of urine, respectively.[63] Penicillins, thus, are the drugs of choice in patients with infection due to *P. mirabilis*.

Urease Inhibitors

Substantial clinical experience with the urease inhibitors AHA and hydroxyurea (HU) over the past 12 years has demonstrated their efficacy in preventing new stone formation and in decelerating progression of disease when infection is incurable or incompletely suppressible.[1,6,31,49,62,74] Both agents effectively reduce urinary alkalinity and ammonia levels[31,74] in virtually every patient studied. Of the two drugs, AHA is the more potent urease inhibitor and has fewer toxic side effects.

Martelli et al. compared the effects of AHA and HU in 41 patients with struvite stones and chronic infections after surgical stone removal, treated concurrently with culture-specific antibiotics.[49] Figure 15-4 characterizes the changes in urinary ammonia levels in their patients. Ammonia reduction was clearly greater in patients treated with AHA. Increased doses of HU (1 g/day) resulted in a corresponding reduction of ammonia levels; however, side effects were observed more commonly in the HU-treated patients (Fig. 15-5), requiring reduction of dosage or elimination of therapy. Reduction of ammonia levels was seen in the AHA-treated group in both the presence and the absence of renal stones (Fig. 15-6).

Carmignani et al. found no toxic side effects in 15 patients treated with HU and antibiotics for 5–9 months.[6] Urinary acidification was rapidly achieved in all 10 patients without stones at a dose of 500 mg of HU per day (Fig. 15-7). Two of the five patients with stones required an increase in the dose of HU to 1 g/day to produce urinary acidification (Fig. 15-8).

Stone recurrence at 1 year in Martelli's study was markedly reduced (18 percent) when AHA or HU were used,[49] compared to a comparable group of historical controls in

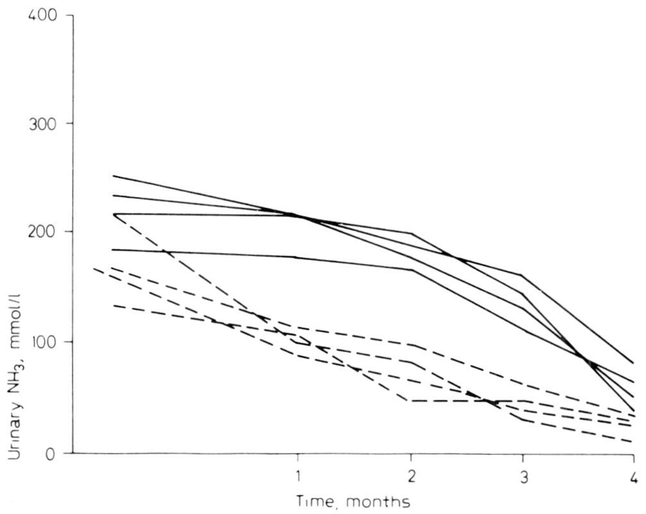

Fig. 15-4. Urinary ammonia concentration during treatment with AHA (----; 500 mg/day) and HU (—; 500 mg/day). (Reproduced from Martelli A, Buli P, Cortecchia V: Urease inhibitor therapy in infected renal stones. Eur Urol 7:292, 1981. With the permission of S. Karger AG, Basel.)

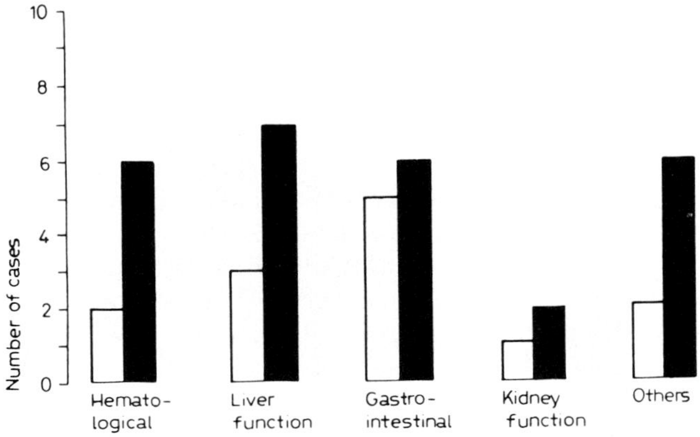

Fig. 15-5. Side effects of therapy with AHA (□; 28 cases) and HU (■; 13 cases). (Reproduced from Martelli A, Buli P, Cortecchia V: Urease inhibitory therapy in infected renal stones. Eur Urol 7:292, 1981. With the permission of S. Karger AG, Basel.)

whom recurrence ranged from 37 to 45 percent. Similar inhibitory effects on stone growth were noted by Williams et al. in a randomized, double-blind study comparing AHA to placebo in the treatment of struvite nephrolithiasis.[74] Of 19 placebo-treated patients, 7 had a 100 percent or greater increase in stone size during the study, and 10 of 19 patients had stone growth greater than 20 percent over baseline. By comparison, no AHA-treated patient had a 100 percent increase in stone size, and only 4 had 20 percent measured stone growth.

In another double-blind study of 94 patients, stone growth occurred in 8 of 45 patients (17 percent) of the AHA group and 23 of 46 patients (50 percent) of the placebo group. According to the "odds ratio" statistic, there was a four times greater risk of stone growth in the placebo than for the treatment group.[33] Table 15-2 lists the toxic reactions and side effects that occurred in this clinical trial. In the table, a given patient commonly had more than one complaint, so that the number of symptoms exceeds the number of patients; 10 (22 percent) AHA patients and 25 (51 percent) placebo patients had no side

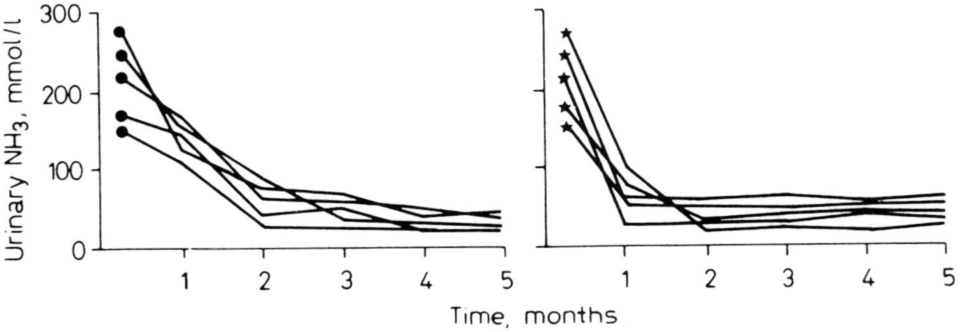

Fig. 15-6. Urinary ammonia concentration in patients with (*a*) and without (*b*) renal stones treated with AHA. (Reproduced from Martelli A, Buli P, Cortecchia V: Urease inhibitor therapy in infected renal stones. Eur Urol 7:292, 1981. With the permission of S. Karger AG, Basel.)

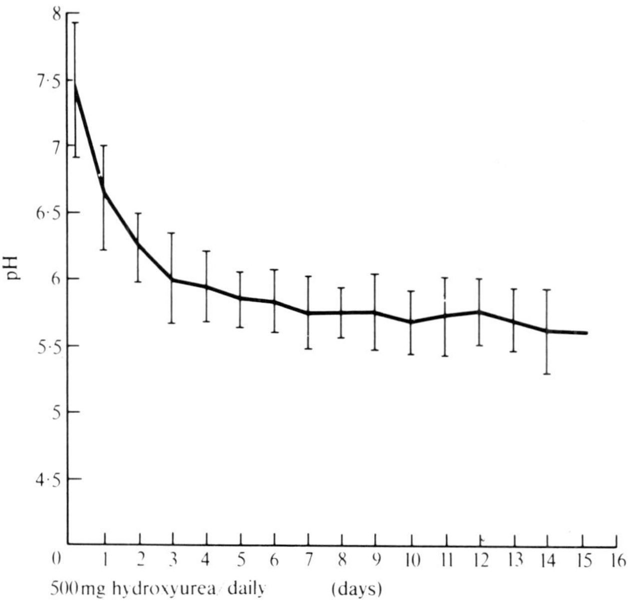

Fig. 15-7. Mean urinary pH modification during administration of hydroxyurea (patients without stones). (Reproduced from Carmignani G, Belgrano E, Puppo P, et al: Hydroxyurea in the management of chronic urea-splitting urinary infections. Br J Urol 52:318, 1980. With permission.)

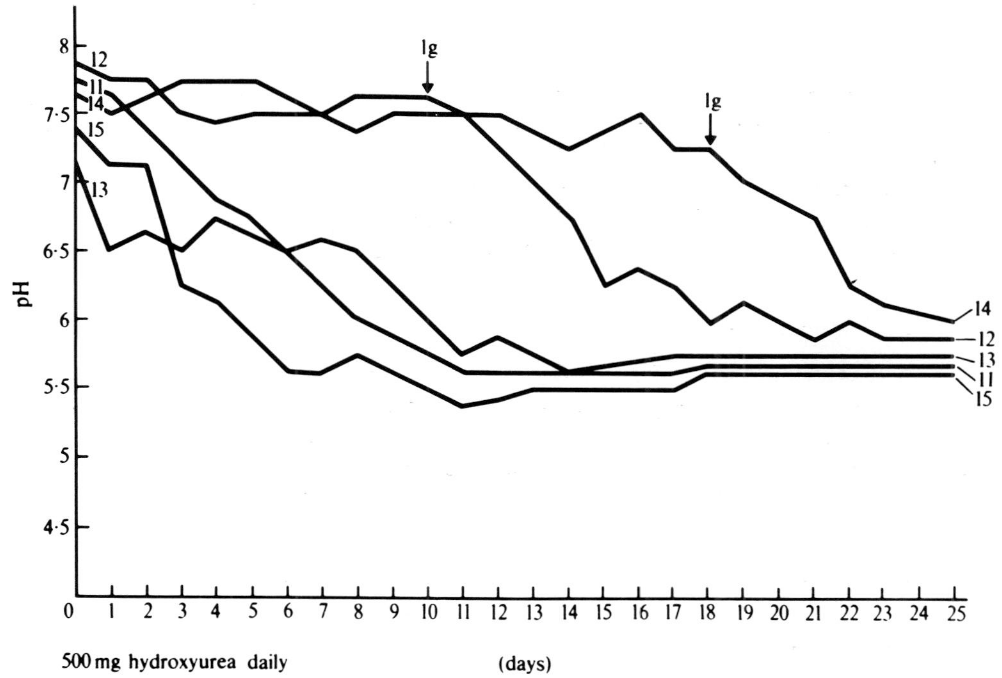

Fig. 15-8. Mean urinary pH modification during administration of hydroxyurea (patients with renal stones). (Reproduced from Carmignani G, Belgrano E, Puppo P, et al: Hydroxyurea in the management of chronic urea-splitting urinary infections. Br J Urol 52:318, 1980. With permission.)

Table 15-2
Patient complaints (both tolerable [Tol.] and intolerable [Intol.]) by organ system

	AHA: $N = 45$			Placebo: $N = 49$		
	Tol.	Intol.	Total	Tol.	Intol.	Total
Psychoneurologic symptoms						
(Number of patients)	14	6	20	13	2	15
Headache	8(17.8)	4(8.9)		12	2(4.1)	
Malaise	5(11.1)	1(2.2)		1	2(4.1)	
Nervousness	5(11.1)	1(2.2)		0	0(0.0)	
Tremulousness	4(8.9)	3(6.7)		0	1(2.0)	
Gastrointestinal symptoms						
(Number of patients)	6	3	9	12	1	13
Anorexia	2(4.4)	1(2.2)		2(4.1)	0(0.0)	
Diarrhea	3(6.7)	1(2.2)		8(16.3)	0(0.0)	
Nausea	3(6.7)	1(2.2)		6(12.2)	1(2.0)	
Vomiting	2(4.4)	0(0.0)		4(8.2)	1(2.0)	
Dermatologic and muscular symptoms						
(Number of patients)	9	7	16	6	2	8
Alopecia	1(2.2)	4(8.9)		2(4.1)	1(2.0)	
Leg pain	1(2.2)	0(0.0)		0(0.0)	1(2.0)	
Muscle ache	2(4.4)	1(2.2)		0(0.0)	0(0.0)	
Rash	3(6.7)	1(2.2)		4(8.2)	0(0.0)	
Swelling of legs	4(8.9)	0(0.0)		0(0.0)	1(2.0)	

effects. Side effects and toxicity are dose-related and reversible. At therapeutic doses of AHA, reticulocytosis is prevalent, but anemia occurred in less than 5 percent of patients. Phlebitis was observed in 2 percent of patients in this study,[33] although 15 percent of the AHA-treated patients in Williams's study[74] had phlebitis.

Acetohydroxamic acid is a teratogen in high doses; therefore, female subjects should be counseled extensively and should be strongly encouraged to utilize contraception.

Clinical Management

Clinical management of the patient with struvite stones must be individualized. Curative therapy is realistic only when all the calculous material has been eliminated. Palliative treatment with antimicrobials and concomitantly with urease inhibitors is appropriate in patients who are not operative candidates and patients who have failed operative treatment and continue to harbor chronic urea-splitting urinary infection.

REFERENCES

1. Akers HA: Urease inhibition by hydroxamic acids. Experientia 37:229, 1981
2. Allen TD, Spence HM: Matrix stones. J Urol 95:284, 1966
3. Andersen JH: Benureastat, a urease inhibitor for the therapy of infected ureolysis. Invest Urol 12:381, 1975
4. Bailey CJ, Boulter D: The subunit structure of jack bean. Biochem J 113:669, 1969

5. Burr RG: Urinary calculi composition in patients with spinal cord lesions. Arch Phys Rehab 59:84, 1978
6. Carmignani G, Belgrano E, Puppo P, et al: Hydroxyurea in the management of chronic urea-splitting urinary infections. Br J Urol 52:316, 1986
7. Comarr AE, Kawaichi GK, Bors E: Renal calculosis of patients with traumatic cord lesions. J Urol 87:647, 1962
8. Delluva HM, Markley K, Davies RE: The absence of gastric urease in germ-free animals. Biochim Biophys Acta 151:646, 1968
9. Dintzis RZ, Hastings HB: Effect of antibiotics on urea breakdown in mice. Proc Natl Acad Sci (USA) 39:571, 1953
10. Dixon NE, Gazzola C, Blakeley RL, et al: Jack bean urease (EC 3.5.1.5): A metalloenzyme. A simple biological rule for nickel? J Am Chem Soc 97:4131, 1975
11. Donnelly J, Hackler RH: Present urologic status of the WW II paraplegic. J Urol 108:508, 1972
12. Drach GW: Urinary lithiasis, in Walsh PC, Gittes RF, Perlmutter AD, et al (eds): Campbell's Urology, 5th ed. Philadelphia, Saunders, 1986, pp 1094–1172
13. Dretter SP: The pathogenesis of urinary tract calculi occurring after ileal conduit diversion. I. Clinical study. II. Conduit study. III. Prevention. J Urol 109:204, 1973
14. Elliot JS: Spontaneous dissolution of renal calculi. J Urol 72:331, 1954
15. Elliot JS, Quaide WL, Sharp RF, et al: Mineralogic studies of urine: The relationship of apatite, brushite and struvite to urinary pH. J Urol 80:269, 1958
16. Elliot JS, Sharp RF, Lewis L: The solubility of struvite in urine. J Urol 81:366, 1959
17. Feit RM, Fair WR: The treatment of infection stones with penicillin. J Urol 122:592, 1979
18. Feldman S, Putcha L, Griffith DP: Pharmokinetics of acetohydroxamic acid. Preliminary investigations. Invest Urol 15:498, 1978
19. Finlayson B: Renal lithiasis in review. Urol Clin N Am 1:181, 1974
20. Fishbein WN, Winter TS, Davidson JD: Urease catalysis. I. Stoichiometry, specificity and kinetics of a second substrate: Hydroxyurea. J Biol Chem 240:2402, 1965
21. Fishbein WN: Urease catalysis. III. Stoichiometry, kinetics, and inhibitory properties of a third substrate: Dihydroxyurea. J Biol Chem 244:1188, 1969
22. Fishbein WN, Smith MJ, Nagarjan K, et al: The first natural nickel metalloenzyme: Urease. Fed Proc 35:1680, 1976
23. Fishbein WN: Foramide: The minimum-structure substrate for urease. Biochim Biophys Acta 484:433, 1977
24. Fishbein WN, Engler WF, Griffin JL, et al: Electron microscopy of negatively stained jack bean urease at three levels of quarternary structure, and comparison with hydrodynamic studies. Eur J Biochem 73:185, 1977
25. Friedrich B, Magasarik B: Urease of *Klebsiella aerogenes:* Control of its synthesis by glutamine synthetase. J Bacteriol 131:446, 1977
26. Gazzola C, Blakely RL, Zerner B: On the substrate specificity of jack bean urease (urea amidohydrolase, EC 3.5.1.5). Can J Biochem 51:1325, 1973
27. Griffith DP, Musher DM: Prevention of infected urinary stones by urease inhibition. Invest Urol 11:228, 1973
28. Griffith DP, Musher DM: Pathogenesis of infection stones, in Finlayson B, Thomas WC (eds): Proceedings of the International Colloquium on Urinary Stones. Gainesville, University of Florida Press, 1976, p 54
29. Griffith DP, Musher DM, Itin C: Urease: The primary cause of infection-induced urinary stones. Invest Urol 13:346, 1976
30. Griffith DP: Struvite stones. Kidney Internatl 13:372, 1978
31. Griffith DP, Gibson JR, Clinton CW, et al: Acetohydroxamic acid: Clinical studies of a urease inhibitor in patients with staghorn renal calculi. J Urol 119:9, 1978
32. Griffith DP, Bruce RR, Fishbein WN: Infection (urease)-induced stones, in Coe FL, Brenner BM, Stein JH (eds): Nephrolithiasis. New York, Churchill Livingstone, 1980, pp 231–260

33. Griffith DP, Lee H, Longuet R, et al: Double-blind clinical trial of Lithostat™ (acetohydroxomie acid) in the palliative treatment of infection-induced urinary stones, unpublished data
34. Hamilton-Miller JMT, Brumfitt W: Methenamine and its salts as urinary tract antiseptics: Variables affecting the antibacterial activity of formaldehyde, mandelic acid and hippuric acid *in vitro*. Invest Urol 14:287, 1977
35. Heathcote RSA: Hexamine as a urinary antiseptic. I. Its rate of hydrolysis at different hydrogen ion concentrations. II. Its antiseptic power against various bacteria in urine. Br J Urol 7:9, 1935
36. Hodgkinson A, Marshall RW, Cochran M: Diurnal variation in calcium phosphate and calcium oxalate activity products in normal and stone-forming urines. Israel J Med Sci 7:1230, 1971
37. Jackson B, Dessau FI: Lower tumors in rats fed acetamide. Lab Invest 10:909, 1961
38. Kamel MY, Hamed RR: Aerobacter-aerogenes Pr L-R3 urease—purification and properties. Acta Biol Med 34:971, 1975
39. Klausner JS, Osborne CA, Griffith DP: Canine struvite urolithiasis. American Association of Pathologists 0002-9400/81/0313-0457
40. Kobashi K, Hase J, Uehara K: Specific inhibition of urease by hydroxamic acids. Biochim Biophys Acta 65:380, 1962
41. Kobashi K, Kumaki K, Hase J: Effect of acyl residues of hydroxamic acids on urease inhibition. Biochim Biophys Acta 227:429, 1971
42. Kobashi K, Takebe S, Tereshima N, et al: Inhibition of urease activity by hydroxamic acid derivatives of amino acids. J Biochem (Japan) 77:837, 1975
43. Kreybig T, Preussmann R, Schmidt W: Chemische constitution and teratogene wirkung beider ratte. Arznein Pub 18:645, 1968
44. Kumaki K, Tomioka S, Kobashi K, et al: Structure activity correlations between hydroxamic acids and their inhibitory powers on urease activity. I. A quantitative approach to the effect of hydrophobic character of acyl residue. Chem Pharm Bull 20:1599, 1972
45. Larson AD, Kallio RE: Purification and properties of bacterial urease. J Bacteriol 68:67, 1954
46. Leoschke WL, Elvehjem CA: Prevention of urinary calculi formation in mink by alteration of urinary pH. Proc Soc Exp Biol Med 84:42, 1954
47. Levenson SM, Crowley LV, Horowitz RE, et al: The metabolism of carbon-labeled urea in the germ-free rat. J Biol Chem 234:2061, 1959
48. Magana-Plaza I, Montes C, Ruiz-Herrera J: Purification and biological characteristics of urease from *Proteus rettgeri*. Biochim Biophys Acta 242:230, 1971
49. Martelli A, Buli P, Corechhia V: Urease inhibitor therapy in infected renal stones. Eur Urol 7:291, 1981
50. Miller H, Phillips E: Antibacterial correlates of urine drug levels of hexamethylenetetramine and formaldehyde. Invest Urol 8:21, 1970
51. Musher DM, Saenz C, Griffith DP: Interaction between acetohydroxamic acid and 12 antibiotics against 14 gram-negative pathogenic bacteria. Antimicrob Agents Chemother 5:106, 1974
52. Nagarajan K, Fishbein WN: Interaction of urease nickel atoms with thiols and the specific inhibitor, acetodroxamate: A circular dichroism study. Fed Proc 36:700, 1977
53. Nielsen IM: Urolithiasis in mink: Pathology, bacteriology and experimental production. J Urol 75:602, 1956
54. Pitts RF: Production and excretion of ammonia in relation to acid–base regulation, in Orloff J, Berlinger RW (eds): Renal Physiology. Washington, DC, American Physiological Society, 1973, p 455
55. Putcha L, Griffith DP, Feldman S: Pharmokinetics of acetohydroxamic acid in patients with staghorn renal calculi. Eur J Clin Pharmacol 28:439, 1985
56. Robertson WG, Peacock M: Calcium oxalate crystalluria and inhibitors of crystallization in recurrent renal stone-formers. Clin Sci 43:499, 1972
57. Rosenstein IJ, Hamilton-Miller JM, Brumfitt W: Role of urease in the formation of infection stones: Comparison of urease from different sources. Infect Immun 32:32, 1981

58. Rudman D, Affarah H, Tuttle EP, et al: Medical management of the patient with renal calculi. AUA Update Series, vol 11, lesson 9, 1983
59. Singh M, Chapman R, Tresidder GC, et al: The fate of the unoperated staghorn calculus. Br J Urol 45:581, 1973
60. Sleight MW, Wickham JEA: Long-term follow-up of 100 cases of renal calculi. Br J Urol 49:601, 1977
61. Smith LH: Medical evaluation of urolithiasis. Urol Clin North Am 1(2):241, 1974
62. Smith MJV: Hydroxyurea and infected stones. Urology 11:274, 1978
63. Stamey TA: Infection stones, in Stamey TA: Urinary Infections. Baltimore, Williams and Wilkins Company, 1972, p 213
64. Summerskill WHJ, Thorsell F, Feinberg HJ, et al: Effects of urease inhibition in hyperammonemia: Clinical and experimental studies with acetohydroxamic acid. Gastroenterology 54:20, 1967
65. Sumner JB: Isolation and crystallization of enzyme urease: Preliminary paper. J Biol Chem 69:434, 1926
66. Sumner JB, Gralen N, Eriksson-Quensel IB: The molecular weight of urease. J Biol Chem 125:37, 1938
67. Takeuchi H, Kobashi K, Yoshida O: Prevention of infected urinary stones in rats by urease inhibitor. Invest Urol 18(2):102, 1980
68. Takeuchi H, Okada Y, Kobashi K, et al: Treatment of infection urinary stones in rats by a new hydroxamic acid, *N*-(pivaroyl) glycinohydroxamic acid. Urol Res 10:217, 1982
69. Thompson RB, Stamey TA: Bacteriology of infected stones. Urology 2:627, 1973
70. Vermuelen CW, Ragans HD, Grove WJ, et al: Experimental urolithiasis. III. Prevention and dissolution of calculi by alteration of urinary pH. J Urol 66:1, 1951
71. Vermuelen CW, Goetz R: Experimental urolithiasis. IX. Influence of infection on stone growth in rats. J Urol 72:761, 1954
72. Wickham JEA: Matrix and the infective renal calculus. Br J Urol 47:726, 1976
73. Williams DI: Matrix calculi. Br J Urol 35:411, 1963
74. Williams JJ, Rodman JS, Peterson CM: A randomized double-blind study of acetohydroxamic acid in struvite nephrolithiasis. New Engl J Med 311:760, 1984
75. Wojewski A, Zajaczkowski T: The treatment of bilateral staghorn calculi of the kidneys. Internatl Urol Nephrol 5:249, 1974

G. Alan Rose
Colin T. Samuell

16

The Hyperoxaluric States

Many surveys in unselected populations have illustrated the rising incidence of upper urinary tract lithiasis, and the sheer magnitude of this problem is still emerging.[4,91,93,94,126,138] In the Western world the calcium oxalate containing stone is clearly the predominant form,[67,70,71] and the large number of patients presenting with this problem seems set to remain.

There has been much debate as to the role of hypercalciuria in the pathogenesis of calcium oxalate stone disease, but the frequency with which this abnormality is found has caused an enormous and perhaps disproportionate amount of effort to be directed toward attempts to classify its aetiology in the belief (perhaps misguided) that this might provide a basis for logical treatment.[21,45,72,103,108–110,122]

The role of urinary oxalate as a risk factor in these patients has become fully appreciated only recently,[114–116] and it must now be accepted that hyperoxaluria is a more directly important finding for urolithiasis than hypercalciuria in many patients. Indeed, as discussed later, the finding of hypercalciuria should provoke an immediate search for associated hyperoxaluria.

The awareness of the risk of calculus formation posed by even mild hyperoxaluria has led to urinary oxalate being measured much more frequently than hitherto, although the need for this approach has yet to be fully appreciated outside of specialist centers. Thus the clinician in the metabolic stone clinic is faced with an ever-increasing number of patients whose underlying problem is hyperoxaluria that needs to be documented, investigated, and successfully treated if stone recurrence is to be avoided. This chapter is an attempt to aid the clinician in this process.

LABORATORY TECHNIQUES AND PROBLEMS

Correct investigation and management of the hyperoxaluric patient will require ready access to a laboratory able to provide the appropriate specialist assays, many of which may not be available in general departments of clinical chemistry. The following

STONE DISEASE: DIAGNOSIS AND MANAGEMENT
ISBN 0-8089-1873-7

are considered to be essential in this context and some comment on potential problems is appropriate here.

Urinary Oxalate

The need for precise, accurate, and rapid assay of urinary oxalate is obvious. There have been many approaches to this measurement and the subject has been reviewed elsewhere;[70,118,119,157] however, it is worth emphasizing that many of the old precipitation procedures, while able to detect the very high levels found in primary hyperoxaluria, are totally inadequate for recognizing the small elevations in oxalate excretion that are important in many patients with calcium oxalate urolithiasis. Of the methods currently applicable to everyday use, the most popular are enzymatic and utilize the specific action of either oxalate decarboxylase[20,28,59] or oxalate oxidase.[11,17,88,105] Various modifications have been developed, and assay procedures based on both these enzymes are now available as commercial kits. Oxalate oxidase yields hydrogen peroxide as one of the products and since this compound lends itself to a number of proven sensitive detection systems,[12,55] methods based on this enzyme are more convenient. In the authors' laboratory an automated continuous-flow technique based on immobilized oxalate oxidase[84] has proved to be very successful in coping economically with a large workload. For smaller workloads the colorimetric kit marketed by Sigma Chemical Company Ltd. has obvious attractions and is probably the most popular method in the United Kingdom. Experience has shown, however, that the original Sigma procedure is not without its problems: (1) the color development period must be extended to at least 45 minutes to allow maximum reaction in all urines, and (2) it is necessary to remove preformed ascorbate that will undergo in vitro conversion to oxalate during the extraction procedure, as well as inhibiting the peroxidase-mediated chromogen development.[145,146] There is thus the potential for both negative and positive interference from ascorbate in this procedure.

The problem of ascorbate interference in the assay of oxalate is a major one and extends to any technique where the urine is subjected to an alkaline pH during the procedure. It was demonstrated in 1933[66] that an alkaline pH favors the conversion of L-ascorbate to oxalate, but only recently has this been appreciated in the context of oxalate assay.[17,83] Ascorbate removal prior to analysis therefore seems essential, and the two approaches adopted involve the use of either ferric chloride[83,105] or sodium nitrite,[84] both under acidic conditions. Ferric chloride treatment is currently the most popular approach, but work in this department suggests that its use may cause poor recovery in the Sigma procedure, and use of sodium nitrite is possibly more reliable.[84] The potential for in vitro oxalogenesis from ascorbate under alkaline conditions also reemphasizes the need for acid preservation of urine during collection and for care in the interpretation of oxalate levels in urine infected with urea-splitting organisms. The authors have seen factitious hyperoxaluria resulting from the combination of increased ascorbate ingestion and urine infection.

Even with the availability of enzymatic procedures it seems that the quality of results produced still leaves much to be desired in many laboratories. A recently instigated quality assurance scheme operating from the authors' laboratory indicates that the between-laboratory coefficient of variation for this assay is around 25 percent, even for an apparently well defined procedure such as the Sigma kit.

Plasma Oxalate

The reliable measurement of plasma oxalate presents a much greater analytical challenge than the assay in urine and as such is not so widely available. The reasons for this are probably twofold: (1) the normal plasma oxalate level is so low (approximately 2 μmol/liter) that a procedure of very high sensitivity is required; and (2) the potential for in vitro oxalogenesis is very great, as generation of oxalate from glyoxylate, ascorbate, and other precursors during sample storage and processing have all been demonstrated.[1,26,47] This latter problem almost certainly accounts for the massive discrepancy between plasma oxalate levels obtained from in vivo radioisotopic methods[27,73,111,148] and those produced by the earlier chemical or enzymatic techniques.[14,24,64,104,155]

In the authors' laboratory the continuous-flow oxalate oxidase procedure described above for urine has been successfully adapted to provide the necessary sensitivity for the routine assay of plasma samples.[85] Sample handling is critical if in vitro oxalogenesis is to be avoided; chilled centrifugation of blood is followed by acidification and ultrafiltration. Ascorbate is removed by sodium nitrite. Using this procedure the adult reference range is 1.3–3.1 μmol/liter, a figure in agreement with the in vivo isotopic procedures.

Knowledge of the plasma oxalate level, while important in certain special situations discussed elsewhere in this chapter, is not yet necessary for the assessment of the vast majority of oxalate urolithiasis patients.

Urinary Glycollate and Glycerate

Assay of these organic acids is necessary for distinguishing between the types of primary hyperoxaluria and urinary glycollate measurements find a more general application in differentiating metabolic from nonmetabolic causes of hyperoxaluria. The extreme rarity of type II primary hyperoxaluria means that the need for glycerate assay is very infrequent, and this is best satisfied by reference to a department with special expertise in organic acid profiling. Glycollate assays, however, do need to be readily available, and while such techniques as gas liquid chromatography are extremely useful here,[22,23] the enzymatic approach using glycollate oxidase (*S*-2-hydroxyacid oxidase; EC 1.1.3.15) may be more convenient. The hydrogen peroxide produced can easily be measured by using a standard peroxidase-linked color reaction. The commercially available enzyme is expensive, but in-house preparations can be made from spinach.[80] Ascorbate and other reducing substances must be removed prior to analysis as they inhibit color development, and the ability of the enzyme also to utilize lactate as a substrate means that lactate must either be removed by using lactate oxidase or that corrections must be made on the basis of a simultaneous lactate assay. Unfortunately, the enzyme does not appear to be stable in an immobilized form,[10] and so possible economies afforded by this approach cannot be realized. There does appear to be some variation in quoted normal values, and local assessment of the reference range would seem essential.

Attempts to assay glycollate in plasma by the same approach have not been completely successful in the authors' laboratory because of some inhibition of the glycollate oxidase and the higher lactate:glycollate ratio found in plasma. There is still a need for a reliable and simple assay for plasma glycollate since the measurement is useful in diagnosis of type I primary hyperoxaluria in situations where urine is difficult to collect or not available (e.g., anuric renal failure, neonatal patients).

Urinary 4-Pyridoxic Acid

Assay of this compound, the major urinary metabolite of vitamin B_6, is invaluable for checking compliance in those patients on pyridoxine therapy. The well-established fluorimetric procedure[153] is adequate here, although the time-consuming chromatographic isolation procedure can be shortened by the use of prepacked columns (e.g., Sep-Pak C_{18} cartridges from Waters Associates, Milford, Massachusetts). Nonspecific background fluorescence is minimized by the high urine predilution possible in patients taking high doses. In a research setting, and for measurements in the nonsupplemented patient, high-performance liquid chromatography (HPLC) is the current method of choice.[25,95]

Urinary Crystal Studies

Facilities for such studies in whole urine must be available since a knowledge of the severity and type of oxalate crystalluria forms an important aspect of the assessment of hyperoxaluric patients. This is particularly true when studying the effect of therapeutic maneuvers on the risk of stone formation. For a complete picture it is necessary to study the urine not only as voided but also after rapid concentration to 1200 mOsmol/kg by rotary evaporation.[61] It is important to recognize that valid data will be obtained only on urine maintained and studied at 37°C.

MECHANISMS OF HYPEROXALURIA

Sources of Urinary Oxalate

A very detailed review of oxalate metabolism is not necessary here, and indeed some of the pathways in humans are not completely understood. The major aspects are shown in Figure 16-1. There is no evidence for further metabolism or reutilization of oxalate, and once formed, it is excreted unchanged in the urine. Small amounts of oxalate may be secreted into the gut,[70] and this may increase further when body pools are high. However, as a significant route of excretion it can probably be ignored.

Urinary oxalate is derived from a combination of exogenous oxalate in the diet and endogenous metabolic production. The relative contributions of these two sources have been the subject of much controversy. Traditionally, it has been considered that the majority of the urinary oxalate arises endogenously from glycine and ascorbate[56,70,139,150] and that the absorption from the gastrointestinal tract is small. Absorption studies using both stable and ^{14}C-labeled oxalate have yielded figures ranging from 2 to 14 percent of the ingested dose;[7,136,156] the higher values are associated with the use of fasting subjects. Finch et al., however, showed that urinary oxalate fell to levels below 0.2 mmol per 24-hour period when normal subjects were placed on a constant low-oxalate diet,[42] suggesting that dietary sources must make a significant contribution when one considers the normal range for urinary oxalate is up to 0.45 mmol per 24-hour period (40 mg) in most laboratories.* These workers also showed that the absorption of oxalate from various oxalate-rich foods was very variable and rose to a mean of 22 percent when tea was used to supplement the low-oxalate diet. It is likely, therefore, that the diet is in fact a major

**Note:* Millimoles of oxalate can be converted to milligrams by multiplying by 88.

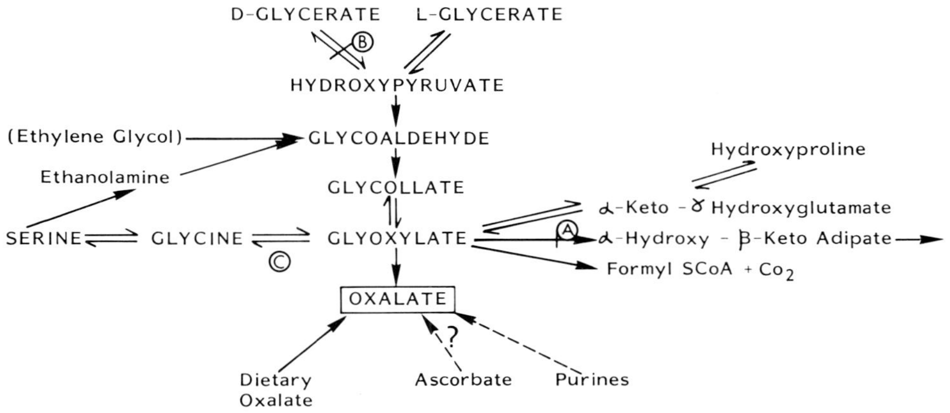

Fig. 16-1. Major pathways of oxalate metabolism. The postulated enzyme deficiencies in type I and type II primary hyperoxaluria are indicated by Ⓐ (2-oxoglutarate: glyoxylate carboligase) and Ⓑ (D-glycerate dehydrogenase), respectively; Ⓒ indicates the site of action of the vitamin-B_6-requiring enzyme, glyoxylate transaminase.

source of urinary oxalate in some individuals depending on the form in which the oxalate is ingested and on other dietary components that can affect its absorption such as calcium. Certainly a thorough dietary history is essential when one is confronted with a hyperoxaluric patient. In contrast to the above-mentioned debate, the increased oxalate absorption that occurs in certain gastrointestinal diseases is well documented and is discussed later.

The relationship between ascorbate ingestion and oxalate excretion is one that merits current reexamination to assess its importance. Ascorbate in humans is converted to oxalate, but there has always been doubt regarding the magnitude of this pathway.[8,18,70,90,135,150] In addition, a considerable variation between individuals has been shown, some apparently having a very high capacity for converting ascorbate to oxalate.[16] It should also be noted that secondary oxalosis has been described in a patient with acute renal failure receiving parenteral nutrition including high levels of ascorbate.[48] While accepting that this is a rather atypical situation since oxalate excretion is prevented, it is another aspect of the link between ascorbate and oxalate. Unfortunately, much of the data in this area was collected before the problem of in vitro conversion of ascorbate to oxalate referred to in the previous section was appreciated, so that how much of the urinary oxalate measured in these studies was derived from this mechanism cannot be judged. Hence the need to reevaluate the role of dietary ascorbate using modern analytical procedures. Of recent interest is a study comparing the effects of oral versus intravenous ascorbate on oxalate excretion.[21] These workers showed that the intravenous route had little effect on the urinary oxalate, suggesting that conversion in tissues was unlikely, while oral ascorbate did elevate the urinary oxalate, and this elevation was more marked in calcium stone formers. This indicates that the conversion of ascorbate to oxalate may occur in the gastrointestinal tract, and this concept is certainly worthy of further study. There is still a trend for megadose ascorbate therapy to be practiced by some individuals for dubious health reasons, and it is important that this area be clarified as soon as possible so that relevant advice can be given.

The influence of changes in purine intake on urinary oxalate seldom is appreciated.

High-purine diets have been shown to produce significant elevations in urine oxalate,[130,156] although the exact pathway involved is not clear, and reduction of purine catabolism by allopurinol therapy can reduce oxalate excretion.[137] Indeed, the benefits of giving allopurinol to the calcium stone former may well accrue from this mechanism rather than via any effect of reduced urine urate levels on calcium oxalate solubility and crystallization.

Causes of Hyperoxaluria

The causes of hyperoxaluria are summarized in Table 16-1.

Primary Hyperoxaluria

Primary hyperoxaluria is really a general term used to encompass two rare genetic disorders associated with increased endogenous oxalate synthesis. Urine oxalate excretion is thus markedly increased and levels are typically between 1.0 and 5.0 mmol per 24-hour period (88–440 mg), although higher figures can occur. On the basis of associated abnormalities in organic acid excretion the disease is classically divided into types I and II, as these are accompanied by increased excretion of glycollic and L-glyceric acid, respectively. Type I is by far the most common of the two forms. Of the 50 or so patients seen by the authors, only one appears to have the type II disorder and very few patients with this latter defect have in fact been described in the literature. Most of the experience in diagnosing and treating primary hyperoxaluria has thus been gained in relation to the type I form. It is interesting to note that although the mode of inheritance for both disorders is thought to be autosomal recessive, there does appear to be a preponderance of males in some reports[65] and certainly this is the authors' experience.[82,120] The finding that testosterone can increase oxalate synthesis in rat liver may be relevant here.[101]

The basis enzyme defect in type I hyperoxaluria has been considered a deficiency of the cytosolic form of 2-oxoglutarate:glyoxylate carboligase.[87] The impaired metabolism of glyoxylate results in excessive production and excretion of both oxalate and glycollate (Fig. 16-1). However, recent careful studies[29] have indicated that the so-called cytosolic

Table 16-1
The Causes of Hyperoxaluria

Primary hyperoxaluria
Type I (with glycollic aciduria)
Type II (with L-glyceric aciduria)
Secondary hyperoxaluria
Dietary oxalate excess
Hyperabsorption of oxalate: intestinal disease; lowered intestinal Ca^{2+} levels
Excess ascorbate intake (? mechanism)
Ethylene glycol ingestion (? diethylene glycol)
Methoxyflurane anesthesia
Aspergillosis
Glycine loading during TUR of prostate
Vitamin B_6 deficiency
Mild metabolic hyperoxaluria

form of this enzyme, claimed by earlier workers to be deficient in the type I disease, does not exist as such even in the normal liver and is probably an artifact caused by leakage of the mitochondrial form. A deficiency of D-glycerate dehydrogenase appears to be the underlying defect in the type II condition, and this abnormality has been demonstrated in the leukocytes of affected patients.[149] Diversion of hydroxypyruvate to L-glycerate accounts for the high excretion of this latter metabolite that is not detectable in normal urine. The mechanism by which oxalate synthesis is increased in this condition is not completely clear but is probably a combination of two effects: (1) hydroxypyruvate may be converted to glycollate and then directly to oxalate via glycollate acid oxidase;[92] (2) the increased NAD/NADH ratio produced by the reduction of hydroxypyruvate to L-glycerate favors the oxidation of glyoxylate to oxalate, as the reactions are coupled via lactate dehydrogenase.[57,150] However, the rarity of cases has severely limited the study of the type II disease.

It is fair to conclude that the underlying metabolic defect in both types I and II is still a very open question and our lack of understanding is further illustrated by the spectrum of response to pyridoxine therapy seen in patients with the type I disorder.[82,120] It is possible that this represents a single genetic defect with variable penetrance or that there are in fact a number of closely related defects at present grouped under the umbrella of primary hyperoxaluria. The classic clinical picture is one of recurrent calcium oxalate nephrolithiasis and progressive nephrocalcinosis in the early years of life leading to renal impairment. Unless treatment is successful (see later), a vicious circle is established with the rising plasma oxalate that accompanies failing renal function, leading to widespread deposition of oxalate crystals in the body (i.e., oxalosis). Deposition in the kidney further compromises renal function such that terminal renal failure by the third decade of life often is the natural history of this disease. Milder cases carrying a better prognosis do seem to occur however, and it is important to realize that primary hyperoxaluria is obviously a condition with marked differences in severity.

Secondary Hyperoxaluria

Of the causes shown in Table 16-1, only the first two, and possibly the third, occur commonly enough to warrant detailed discussion. In addition, the long duration of these causes makes them more likely to lead on to a recurrent nephrolithiasis problem.

Dietary oxalate excess. As stated earlier, the absorption of oxalate from foodstuffs is variable and can be influenced by other dietary components. Although the question as to whether idiopathic calcium stone formers absorb more ingested oxalate than do normals has not been resolved, there is evidence that as a group their mean urinary oxalate is higher than in normals.[9,117] Certain foods must be considered when assessing the hyperoxaluric patient, however, and rhubarb, spinach, nuts, beetroot, parsley, chocolate, and tea can all be regarded as high risk in this context. Studies in the authors' laboratory utilizing an enzymatic assay procedure applied to food analysis[81] not only confirm this but also indicate the low oxalate content of meat, dairy products, cereals, and tomatoes. Apart from tea- and chocolate-based drinks, no beverage was found to be high in oxalate. In contrast to earlier reports,[38] Coca-Cola and beer were found to be virtually oxalate free.

Hyperabsorption of oxalate. The hyperoxaluria and consequent nephrolithiasis associated with inflammatory bowel disease and with jejunoileal bypass surgery is well documented.[33,36,69] The reported incidence of oxalate calculi in these patients varies considerably, but figures of up to 30 percent have been reported in the bypass group. Three major mechanisms have been proposed to account for the hyperoxaluria, although the relative importance of each may differ in individual patients. First, the associated steatorrhea leads to increased binding of calcium ions by free fatty acids in the gut, thus leaving free oxalate ions in solution for absorption. A direct correlation has been shown between urinary oxalate and fecal fat in these patients,[5,39,100,133] and, indeed, oxalate excretion following an oral sodium oxalate load has been proposed as a screening test for steatorrhea,[112] although the reliability of this approach has recently been questioned.[46] The second explanation for the hyperoxaluria relates to the increased colonic permeability to oxalate, which can be induced by malabsorbed bile salts and free fatty acids.[34,41] The absence of hyperoxaluria in patients who have undergone an ileostomy, in contrast to the high incidence in the bypass group where virtually a whole intestine is unavailable for absorption, strongly suggests that the colon is the site of oxalate hyperabsorption. The third possible mechanism is reduced bacterial breakdown of oxalate in the colon.[3] It must be appreciated that any situation that lowers the concentration of free calcium ions in the gut, thereby reducing oxalate binding, is liable to lead to overabsorption of the free oxalate ion. The treatment of hypercalciuria with the binding agent sodium cellulose phosphate, while effectively lowering urinary calcium, thus can lead to a secondary rise in urinary oxalate.[58] One must also question the wisdom of using low-calcium diets to treat idiopathic hypercalciuria associated with calcium hyperabsorption, as increased oxalate excretion has been described in exactly this situation.[78] Both of these treatments thus require simultaneous restriction of dietary oxalate.

Other secondary causes. It is obviously important to document any excess ascorbate ingestion in a patient with an unexplained high urinary oxalate, but as stated earlier, the magnitude and mechanism of ascorbate induced hyperoxaluria is still very much in doubt. Of the remaining secondary causes, most are rare acute situations and, although of importance in their own right, are not encountered in the routine management of oxalate stone disease.

Ethylene glycol is widely used as an antifreeze, and acute poisoning following deliberate or accidental ingestion is well documented.[49] Acute hyperoxaluria and oxalate crystalluria are thus a feature of this condition; however, whether they are the sole cause of the acute renal failure commonly seen in these patients is not clear, as tubular damage by other metabolites possibly is equally important.[113] The recently reported practice of adulteration of wines with diethylene glycol as a sweetening agent raises the question as to whether a more chronic hyperoxaluria might be produced in regular wine drinkers. It has been stated that, unlike ethylene glycol, the diethylene derivative is not converted to oxalate, although there is evidence to the contrary,[43] and this matter urgently needs further investigation.

Use of the volatile anaesthetic methoxyflurane (1,1-difluoro-2, 2-dichlorethyl methyl ether) has been shown to result in a marked postoperative hyperoxaluria in some patients,[129,151] and this has been implicated as a cause of the acute renal dysfunction that can occur following administration of this agent. The metabolism of methoxyflurane leads not only to oxalate production but also to the release of inorganic fluoride,[70,139] however, and it is likely that both of these products contribute to the subsequent renal impairment.

It is known that certain fungi of the *Aspergillus* genus can produce oxalate when growing in animal tissues, and oxalosis with renal damage has been reported following infection with this agent,[102] although this is apparently a very rare complication.

The use of glycine solutions as a bladder and urethral irrigant during transurethral resection of the prostate is standard practice in many centers. Considerable absorption of such solutions can sometimes occur across the vascular bed during surgery and contributes to the acute electrolyte disturbance seen in the so-called TUR syndrome. The high glycine load received by such patients is partly metabolized to oxalate (see Fig. 16-1) and leads to a hyperoxaluria that can be sustained for up to 2 weeks.[44] However, the high urine volumes usually maintained during the postoperative period in these patients mean that nephrolithiasis and renal damage do not occur.

Examination of the pathways involved in oxalate production indicates that pyridoxine (vitamin B_6) deficiency can theoretically lead to impaired transamination of glyoxylate to glycine, resulting in overproduction of glycollate and oxalate. There have been reports of hyperoxaluria accompanying induced pyridoxine deficiency in humans[40,97] and animals.[50,51] Clinical pyridoxine deficiency is believed to be rare in developed countries where the vitamin is widely available in the diet; thus this association is rarely considered in the routine investigation of oxalate urolithiasis. Whether a state of pyridoxine dependency can occur with respect to the above mechanism, as is documented for a number of other metabolic abnormalities,[99,127] is not known, but the response to high-dose pyridoxine seen in patients with the mild metabolic form of hyperoxaluria detailed below suggests that such a situation might exist. It must also be remembered that certain drugs such as isonicotinic acid hydrazide[15,132] and penicillamine[75] can lead to an increased requirement for pyridoxine as may pregnancy and the use of oral contraceptives.[37] The entire role of pyridoxine and its metabolism in the pathogenesis and treatment of both primary and mild metabolic hyperoxaluria is not really understood, and this is further illustrated during the section on treatment later in this chapter.

Mild Metabolic Hyperoxaluria

This is the term used by the authors to describe an important condition that has emerged as a result of ensuring that urinary oxalate is measured on every patient presenting with calcium nephrolithiasis irrespective of whether a possible cause for their problem has already been documented. Such an approach clearly demands the use of a precise automated assay procedure such as described earlier. In addition, the differentiation from other causes requires the assay of urine glycollate to be available. Our early experience with this entity has been detailed elsewhere,[82,86,120] and the cardinal features are as follows:

1. Hyperoxaluria typically within the range of 0.5–0.8 mmol per 24-hour period (44–70 mg) although higher values have been found.
2. Raised urinary glycollate, indicating a metabolic cause for the hyperoxaluria and thereby excluding dietary excess or overabsorption of oxalate.
3. Variable age of onset with cases ranging from childhood to the sixth decade. No case so far has shown a family history, thus making a genetic basis rather unlikely.
4. As with primary hyperoxaluria, the condition seems to be more common in males than females.
5. A very variable response to pyridoxine therapy, although none of the patients has shown clinical or biochemical evidence of pyridoxine deficiency apart from hyperoxaluria.

A single factor connecting all the patients in this group seen by the authors has not yet been found; however, some points are common to several patients. One group had been on long-term cellulose phosphate therapy, but the raised urinary glycollate rules out, as the sole cause, the secondary hyperoxaluria usually associated with this drug. The possibility of binding of pyridoxine by cellulose phosphate in the gastrointestinal tract obviously arises, but no evidence of such binding could be found from in vitro studies. Some patients had coexisting distal renal tubular acidosis,[82] and there is a high incidence of other causes of calcigenous stones such as idiopathic hypercalciuria, medullary sponge kidney, and primary hyperparathyroidism.

DIAGNOSIS AND FURTHER INVESTIGATION

Documentation of Hyperoxaluria

In the authors' laboratory the quoted adult reference range for urinary oxalate is 0.10–0.46 mmol per 24-hour period (9–40 mg). However, values in excess of 0.40 mmol per 24-hour period (35 mg) are regarded as potentially significant in stone-forming patients and are carefully monitored.

It must be stressed that while severe and sustained increases in urinary oxalate such as usually occur in the genetic disorders are not difficult to recognize, lesser, but equally important, degrees of hyperoxaluria will be detected only if they are diligently searched for. In addition, the abnormality may be of an intermittent nature, particularly if it has a dietary basis. It is thus essential to measure the urinary oxalate on several occasions in all patients with calcium urolithiasis, and these studies should ideally be performed on an outpatient basis so that possible dietary and environmental factors are not excluded. The presence of an existing diagnosis relevant to the patient's stone problem such as idiopathic hypercalciuria should not prevent a thorough search for marginal hyperoxaluria since this may represent a more significant finding.

For the purposes of this section, it is assumed that the patient with calcium oxalate urolithiasis, ideally verified by quantitative stone analysis, has been subjected to the relevant battery of investigations, that hyperoxaluria has been documented, and the investigator is faced with the problem of defining the underlying etiology. The acute hyperoxaluric states will not be discussed.

Primary Hyperoxaluria

This diagnosis must be seriously considered in any child with recurrent oxalate urolithiasis, hematuria, and renal colic although urinary tract infection, and pyelonephritis, secondary to the presence of calculi, can occasionally be the presenting symptoms. Presentation under 5 years of age is common[150] and may occur in the first year of life; however, onset of symptoms can sometimes be delayed until the second or third decade.[65] Many cases will have renal impairment by the time the disease is manifest, in which case radiology will probably show the presence of multiple radiodense stones in one or both kidneys. A family history of calculous disease can often be elucidated.

Diagnosis is made by documenting gross elevation of the urinary oxalate. This is usually accompanied by severe oxalate crystalluria; the predominant crystal type often is the "dumbbell" of calcium oxalate monohydrate rather than the more common "envelope" of the dihydrate (Figs. 16-2*A* and 16-2*B*). To exclude completely a secondary hyperoxaluria, and to classify the primary type, assay of urinary glycollate is essential. In

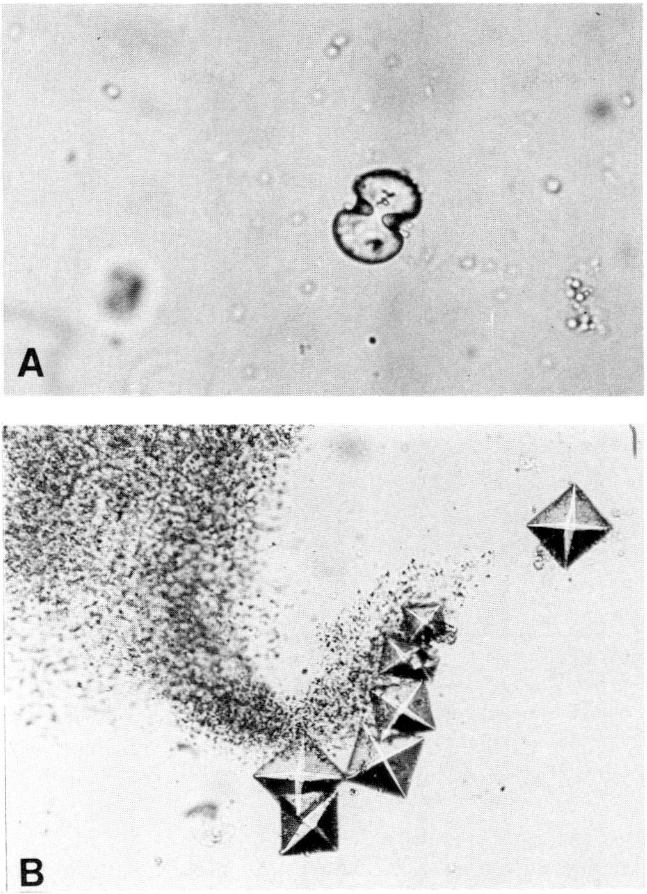

Fig. 16-2. (*A*) Typical dumbbell crystal of calcium oxalate monohydrate; (*B*) Envelope crystals of calcium oxalate dihydrate.

practice, assay of the L-glycerate is rarely needed. In most patients the daily oxalate excretion remains diagnostically elevated in the face of renal impairment, but eventually, in extreme renal failure, the falling glomerular filtration rate (GFR) will reduce levels to within the normal range. The urine oxalate:creatinine ratio, however, usually remains abnormal. In the presence of advanced renal failure the assay of plasma oxalate, if available, can be valuable in confirming the diagnosis. Plasma oxalate rises in renal failure from any cause, but in primary hyperoxaluria the levels are disproportionately elevated at any plasma creatinine level. Our early findings in this context are shown in Figure 16-3. Limited experience with the assay of plasma glycollate in this situation has indicated that this may also be a very useful index since, unlike plasma oxalate, levels are not significantly increased in renal failure,[79,98] thus making the test relatively specific for type I hyperoxaluria. Unfortunately, technical difficulties have prevented us gaining widespread experience with this assay.

Interpretation of urinary oxalate values in children is not without problems. There is some reference range data available for 3 years and upward,[70] and it is obviously sensible

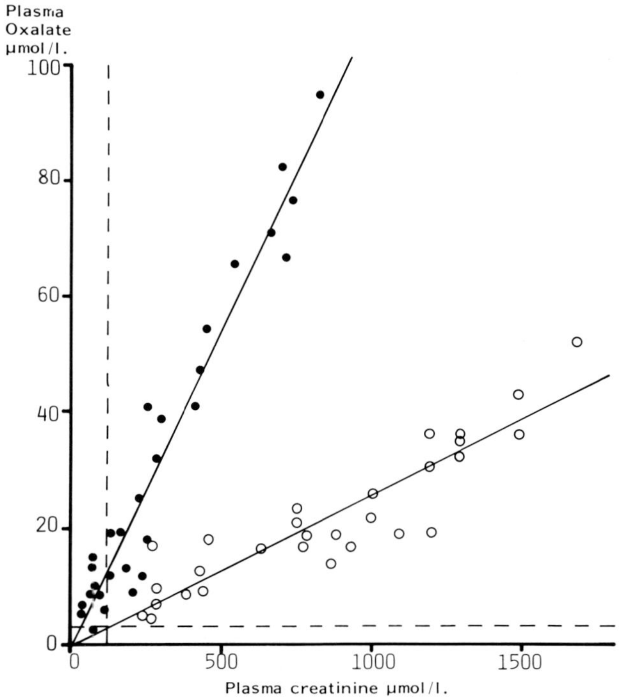

Fig. 16-3. Relationship between plasma oxalate and plasma creatinine in patients with primary hyperoxaluria (•) and in patients with renal failure from other causes (○). Upper limits of reference ranges are shown.

to correct to a body surface area of 1.73 m^2 in this group.[53] Unfortunately, little or no reliable data exist for oxalate excretion in the early weeks and months of life, making early diagnosis difficult in infants with a previously affected sibling. Measurement of plasma oxalate may well prove to be the most valuable investigation in this situation, but again there is a need for good reference range data produced by reliable techniques before this can be substantiated. The situation may be further complicated by the delay in appearance of the hyperoxaluria in affected infants, a phenomenon that the authors have seen and reported[121] (Fig. 16-4). In this case, the urine oxalate and glycollate were considered normal at 7 days of age but were grossly abnormal at 5 weeks when type I hyperoxaluria was diagnosed. Whether this represents delayed synthesis of oxalate as a result of hepatic immaturity in the early days of life or whether exposure to some dietary or environmental factor is necessary is not clear.

In spite of interpretive problems, it is, of course, essential that all siblings are investigated when a diagnosis of primary hyperoxaluria is made in a family. Normal radiology and lack of symptoms do not exclude the diagnosis, and urinary oxalate must always be measured. An early diagnosis may thus be made and treatment instituted before renal function has become severely compromised. A key question is whether it is possible to make a prenatal diagnosis of primary hyperoxaluria in families where an affected child has already been produced, thus permitting therapeutic abortion to be considered. In the case mentioned above, amniotic fluid oxalate was measured at 15 weeks' gestation in an attempt to answer this question. Oxalate was detectable at a

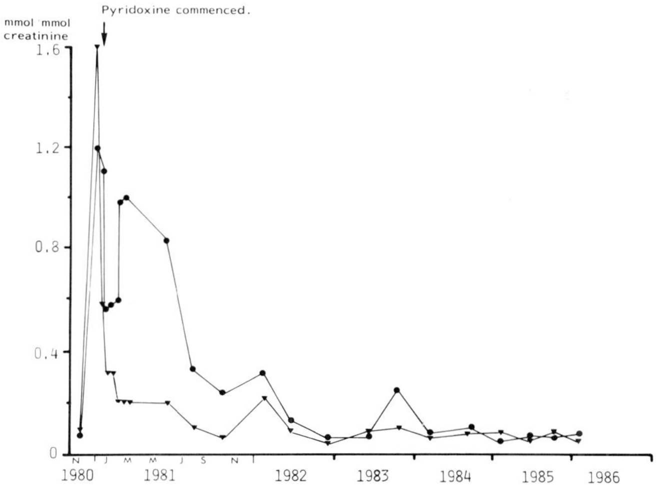

Fig. 16-4. Urinary oxalate and glycollate excretion (expressed in relation to creatinine output) in a child with type I primary hyperoxaluria (dob: 18.11.1980). Note the initial normal values and the delayed fall in oxalate in response to pyridoxine. The initial pyridoxine dose was 200 mg/day, increased to 400 mg/day after 1 month (• = oxalate); ▲ = glycollate).

concentration of 0.1 mmol/liter but was undetectable in fluid from six normal pregnancies at the same stage. It was also noted that the maternal urine oxalate was 0.44 mmol per 24-hour period while on a low oxalate diet, a figure that may have been significant. Similar studies have recently been made in a second family, but by use of a more sensitive procedure to measure the amniotic fluid oxalate level. The outcome of this pregnancy is not yet known. Whether the enzyme defect is expressed in cells shed into the amniotic fluid does not appear to have been investigated; however, until the defects are accurately defined in primary hyperoxaluria, this may not be a fruitful area to pursue.

Other Hyperoxalurias

Genetic errors will obviously account for only a small percentage of patients presenting with hyperoxaluria. In the majority the key problem will be to decide whether the hyperoxaluria is of the mild metabolic type associated with oxalate overproduction or whether it is a secondary consequence of dietary oxalate excess or overabsorption. The important differential test here is the simultaneous measurement of urine glycollate, and it is essential that this assay be readily available. As stated earlier, there is some discrepancy over normal ranges for urine glycollate, possibly related to method differences, but in the authors' department the adult reference range is regarded as 0.10–0.33 mmol per 24-hour period. Depending on the glycollate result, further assessment is made as follows.

Normal glycollate excretion. A persistently normal urine glycollate indicates a nonmetabolic cause for the hyperoxaluria. If there is obvious inflammatory bowel disease or a history of relevant gastrointestinal surgery, there may be little need to look further for the underlying problem. It should be noted that the urine of these patients often contains subnormal amounts of citrate and magnesium,[123] thus increasing the risk of stone formation, and these should also be measured. If there is no obvious gastrointestinal pathology, a careful search should still be made for any evidence of malabsorption, remembering that the absence of diarrhea does not preclude steatorrhea.

Dietary excess of oxalate is common, and a very thorough dietary history is absolutely essential in this group. The most important foods are mentioned earlier, but it must be realized that ingestion of these substances may be intermittent. For example, some patients may indulge in dietary excess of certain foods only at weekends, and this is not always reflected in urine levels if collections are made during the working week. Many of the high-oxalate foods are seasonal (at least in the United Kingdom), suggesting that dietary hyperoxaluria might be expected to occur more frequently during summer and autumn, and there is evidence to support this.[60] It must not be forgotten, however, that frozen foods and tea are always available, as are oxalate-rich derivatives such as peanut butter and some homemade wines, and all these need to be considered. There are, in addition, other aspects of the diet that must be documented. Some patients will have been advised to pursue a low-calcium diet for coexisting idiopathic hypercalciuria. There is increasing evidence that the excess absorption of calcium in these patients can lead to a secondary overabsorption of oxalate as described earlier, and this situation can be exacerbated by low-calcium diets and use of calcium binding agents. Patients should also be questioned concerning any excess ascorbate ingestion. For example, a high intake of fruit juices can lead to hyperoxaluria, although it is difficult to know whether the conversion from ascorbate is prerenal or is occurring in the kidneys or bladder. Very high purine intakes must also be noted.

Elevated glycollate excretion. A high urine glycollate puts the patient into the mild metabolic hyperoxaluria category; differentiation from the preceding group is important since first line treatment is then by pyridoxine. As stated previously, these are a heterogenous group at present with a high incidence of a second diagnosis, but it seems important to document any drug history and to look for renal tubular acidosis (RTA).

TREATMENT

Primary Hyperoxaluria

Type I

As type I is the more common of the two genetic disorders, virtually all the treatment experience has been gained with this condition, although type II is mentioned briefly later. The basic problem in this disease is gross overproduction of oxalate; therefore, the logical approach to treatment is to attempt by some means to reduce oxalate synthesis. A variety of drugs have been tested in this context, aimed mostly at reducing the formation of glyoxylate from its precursors and/or its subsequent oxidation to oxalate.[52,57,141] They include tyrosine, tryptophan, and thiamine, together with a group of compounds that are potential "aldehyde oxidase" inhibitors such as calcium carbimide, disulfiram, allopurinol and acetomenaphthone. Suffice it to say that none has been shown to cause a sustained and reproducible reduction in oxalate excretion in primary hyperoxaluria. Equally unrewarding in the long term have been attempts to reduce oxalogenesis from glycine by dietary protein restriction or by trapping of glycine as hippurate using sodium benzoate. Pyridoxine (vitamin B_6) is the one compound that is of established value in this context and thus will be the first aspect of treatment to be discussed in detail.

Pyridoxine. The early attempts to use pyridoxine in the treatment of primary hyperoxaluria stemmed from the observation that increased oxalate excretion was a consequence of deficiency of this vitamin in animals. They met with limited success possibly because of inadequate dosage regimes; however, successful responses in a percentage of patients have subsequently been reported by a number of groups.[54,82,120,147] The mechanism of action of pyridoxine in this disorder is not known. No evidence of pyridoxine deficiency has been clinically obvious in those patients who respond and biochemical studies have not supported any defect in vitamin B_6 metabolism.[54] Some have been tempted to speculate[30] that the vitamin may activate glyoxylate transaminase (see Fig. 16-1), which is known to utilize a pyridoxine derivative as a coenzyme. Glyoxylate thus would be increasingly diverted to glycine, preventing its conversion to glycollate and oxalate. This theory has not been proved, however, and other mechanisms of action may exist.

The first line of attack in treating a newly diagnosed patient must therefore be a sustained period of high-dose pyridoxine therapy to assess any responsiveness. It must be stressed that before accepting a negative response, the dose must have been high enough and given for a sufficiently long period. In adults the authors use a starting dose of 100 mg/day given for one month. If no fall in urinary oxalate is seen, the dose is doubled at monthly intervals until a response is seen or until a dose of 800 mg/day has been reached. Only when this maximum dose has been given for about 6 months with no significant reduction in oxalate excretion is the patient regarded as being completely nonresponsive to pyridoxine. For children the dose is reduced in proportion to body surface area, and 10 mg/day is used as the arbitrary starting dose in infants.

This dose regime has been used in a group of 34 patients with type I primary hyperoxaluria seen at the St. Peter's Hospitals in London. Ten patients (29.4 percent) have shown a clear response to pyridoxine with a sustained fall in urine oxalate and glycollate for as long as therapy was maintained at the appropriate dose, while 14 patients (41.2 percent) have shown no significant response. The behavior of the remaining 10 patients (29.4 percent) is interesting and illustrates the unpredictable variation in response to pyridoxine that is so typical of this disease. Within this latter group some patients have shown a partial response to pyridoxine, with only a small fall in oxalate excretion achieved, while others have given an erratic response, with intermittent hyperoxaluria while on a constant pyridoxine dose. In yet other patients an initial good response to pyridoxine, often sustained for several months, has been observed but followed by relapse with subsequent increases in dose having little further effect, with the patients apparently becoming resistant to pyridoxine. Delay in response to pyridoxine is another phenomenon that can occur, and the neonate referred to in the previous section in fact had 6 months of therapy before a clear response was obtained (see Fig. 16-4). These variable responses may well reflect subtle differences in the underlying genetic defect. Differences in response have been seen even within affected siblings, however.

The possibility of noncompliance during pyridoxine therapy must continually be borne in mind and has probably contributed to the debate over the success of the treatment in many reports. Compliance can be conveniently checked by measuring the simultaneous 4-pyridoxic acid excretion on all urines collected for oxalate assay, and this is routine practice in the authors' department. There is some variation in the percentage of a given oral pyridoxine dose that is excreted as pyridoxic acid (see Fig. 16-5), but it is still a very useful index. Experience has shown that values for pyridoxic acid that are less than 25 percent of the ingested dose on a milligram/milligram basis should raise the suspicion of noncompliance. If compliance is a problem during the initial trial of pyridoxine, it may be necessary to admit the patient to hospital for a period of supervised therapy to avoid incorrectly labeling that patient nonresponsive. It has also been suggested that an index of the effect of pyridoxine therapy in stimulating enzyme activity might be afforded by assaying erythrocyte aspartate transaminase levels since this is a vitamin-B_6-requiring enzyme that is readily amenable to study.[147] Certainly if differences in this parameter could be related to the degree of response, it might be a valuable tool, but the authors, albeit with limited experience, have not seen such a relationship. While preservation of renal function is obviously the goal of treatment, a particularly rewarding aspect of successful pyridoxine therapy is the ability to achieve occasionally an actual improvement in renal function as has been briefly described elsewhere.[106] Figure 16-6 shows the complete data relating to this 21-year-old male admitted with a view to assessment for hemodialysis and a plasma creatinine of 670 μmol/liter; however, treatment with a high pyridoxine dose successfully induced a fall in urine oxalate. This was followed by a steady reduction in plasma creatinine to a plateau of 250–300 μmol/liter, and this situation has remained stable for 8 years. It is presumed that the improvement in renal function was due to some reversal of the oxalosis related to a fall in plasma oxalate, although this could not be measured at the time.

It is clear, therefore, that if a sustained response to high dose pyridoxine can be achieved, this is obviously the treatment of choice. These patients must be made aware that pyridoxine does not represent a permanent cure for their condition and that failure to comply with the appropriate dose will result in a rapid return of their hyperoxaluria.[144] Caution must be exercized over the size of the pyridoxine dose used since a sensory neuropathy has recently been reported in nonhyperoxaluric adults taking 2–6 g/day for

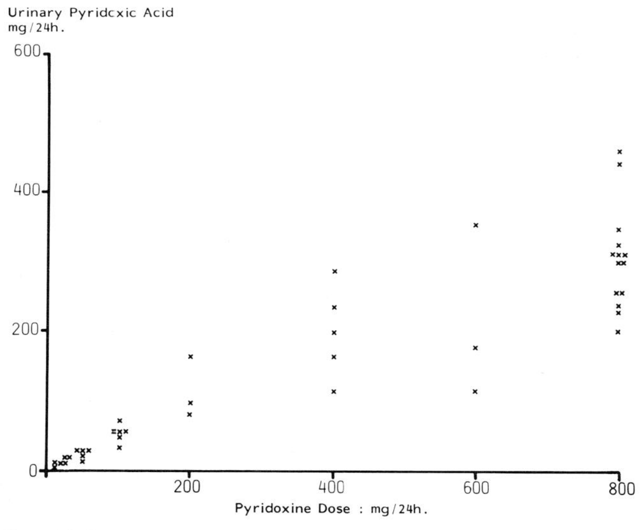

Fig. 16-5. Relationship between pyridoxine dose and urinary pyridoxic acid in hyperoxaluric patients.

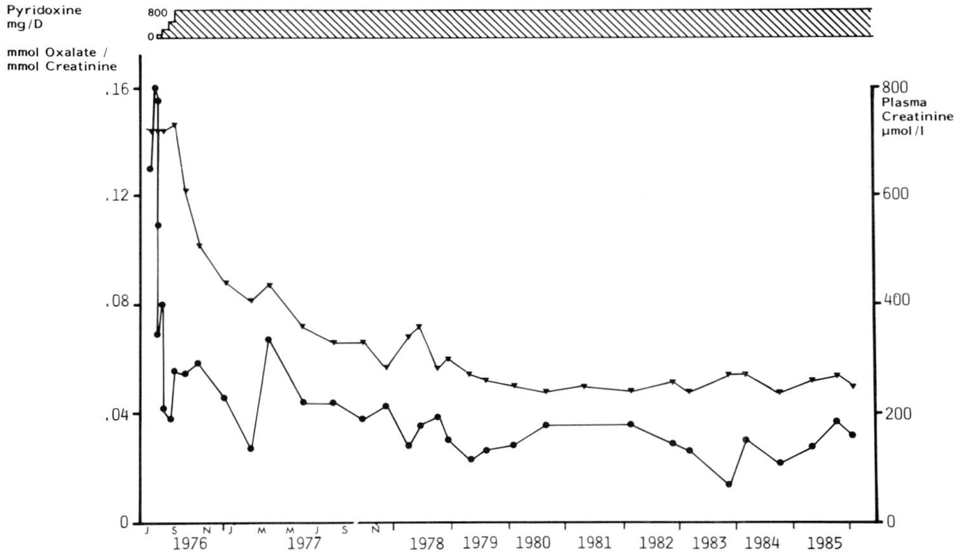

Fig. 16-6. Dramatic response to high dose pyridoxine therapy in a patient with type I primary hyperoxaluria. Note the steady improvement in renal function, possibly due to some regression of oxalosis (• = urinary oxalate: ▲ = plasma creatinine).

other purposes.[124] In addition, neuropathy and encephalopathy have been described in a hyperoxaluric infant given a dose of 1 g/day.[32] It would seem sensible to regard 1 g/day as the maximum dose in adults with the appropriate reduction in infants and children.

Why some patients fail to respond to high-dose pyridoxine therapy is not clear, but an abnormality in the further metabolism of pyridoxine might be suggested since conversion to pyridoxal phosphate and pyridoxamine phosphate is necessary for the vitamin to exert its coenzyme function.[13] Interestingly, some response to pyridoxal phosphate has been reported in vitamin-B_6-dependent anemia.[96] To test this hypothesis, two pyridoxine-resistant patients were given a 14-day course of pyridoxal phosphate (250 mg/day IV), while a third received pyridoxamine phosphate for 7 days (250 mg/day). Neither regime led to any reduction in oxalate excretion, and this approach has not been pursued further in this department.

Other medical aspects. A failure to respond to pyridoxine, and thereby reduce oxalate production and excretion, means that attention must be focused on other means of preventing further oxalate lithiasis. Attempts must therefore be made to modify the urine environment so as to minimize calcium oxalate precipitation. The following points, while relevant to all hyperoxaluric patients, are particularly important in the nonpyridoxine responsive group, where they represent the only hope of preventing further renal damage associated with the very high oxalate excretion. Simply reducing the urine oxalate concentration by increasing urinary volume to, say, 3 liters per 24-hour period, is essential, but many patients experience great difficulty in maintaining the high fluid intake necessary, since it is vital to produce a high urine flow rate throughout the entire 24 hours. It is also sensible to ensure that patients avoid high-oxalate foods and so do not add to their problems by this mechanism. The other important aspect is to utilize substances that have a nonspecific inhibitory action on calcium oxalate precipitation.

Magnesium and orthophosphate are relevant in this context,[31,62,128] and use should be made of them. Administered as milk of magnesia and neutral phosphate, respectively, both have laxative properties. To achieve the highest dose possible, it is therefore necessary to increase the dose gradually in each patient until the limit of tolerance is reached. Magnesium may be the preferred therapy in patients with renal impairment where phosphate retention is a risk; in addition, the sodium or potassium loads necessarily associated with phosphate administration may cause other problems including hypertension. For these reasons magnesia has been the preferred treatment in the authors' experience. The combination of high fluid intake and magnesium supplementation, if strictly maintained, is capable of preventing further renal impairment in pyridoxine resistant patients. Urine magnesium levels must be checked regularly to ensure that sufficient concentrations are being achieved since long-term compliance is again a problem.

Transplantation. Unfortunately, many patients with primary hyperoxaluria still present in end-stage renal failure or progress rapidly toward it. The role of renal replacement therapy in this group of patients, thus needs to be considered. Conventional peritoneal or hemodialysis regimes are not capable of removing oxalate with the efficiency required to prevent continued oxalosis and the attendant dangers of crystal deposition in cardiac muscle, blood vessels, and bone;[143] thus they do not represent a satisfactory form of long-term therapy.

Transplantation has traditionally been considered unsuitable in patients with primary hyperoxaluria because of fears that oxalate deposition would rapidly reduce function in the allograft kidney, and this was certainly the impression from early reports.[35,152] However, our greater understanding of the disease and its treatment means that this view is no longer tenable in many patients.

In the subject who is fully responsive to pyridoxine, the body fluid oxalate levels can be reduced to the point at which there is little increased risk to the transplanted kidney, provided pyridoxine therapy is maintained.[107] Failure to sustain their pyridoxine dosage will probably lead to loss of graft function in these patients, and a history of good compliance is essential. It is important that pyridoxine responsiveness is not missed prior to comtemplating transplantation, and the procedure should not be attempted until 6 months of high-dose therapy has been tried.

In the non-pyridoxine-responsive group, transplantation should still be considered, although the potential problems are obviously much greater. Experience is still accumulating, but it appears that success in this group requires a combination of many approaches to reduce oxalate deposition in the newly transplanted kidney. In the patient with end-stage renal failure, a period of intensive hemodialysis immediately prior to transplantation is necessary to reduce the plasma oxalate to the minimum possible level. In the postoperative period, calcium oxalate precipitation in urine must be prevented by use of magnesium or phosphate coupled with a very brisk diuresis.

If renal function is slow to improve or deteriorates during this period, vigorous hemodialysis must be reintroduced to keep plasma oxalate levels down. Renal biopsy can be used if necessary to differentiate oxalate deposition from other causes of renal impairment in the post-transplantation period. Long-term graft survival has been reported with the use of a regime incorporating the above-mentioned approaches.[125]

The chances of successful transplantation would logically increase if an opportunity is provided to perform the procedure early in the course of the disease before plasma oxalate levels have climbed to the point at which oxalosis is inevitable. This probably occurs with plasma oxalate levels above 50 μmol/liter, but recent isotopic studies may help to clarify the point at which this complication develops.[142,143] One could speculate that it may be even more logical to perform early hepatic transplantation, thus correcting the underlying defect and abolishing oxalate overproduction before oxalosis becomes a problem. This has been attempted,[140] although not yet with successful outcome.

Type II

Although experience with this disease is limited because of its extreme rarity, it appears to be universally nonresponsive to pyridoxine. The approaches to treatment, including transplantation, are thus the same as those used for the pyridoxine-resistant type I patient, notably by use of magnesium plus high fluid intake. A 15-year followup of three siblings with this defect described in 1968[149] indicates that while one is now in end-stage renal failure, the other two have good preservation of renal function.[68]

Secondary Hyperoxaluria

Dietary Excess of Oxalate

The treatment of this problem seems obvious; however, there is a need to remind patients constantly about the range of oxalate rich foods and their derivatives (see previous section) and to check that dietary advice is being taken by regular monitoring of oxalate excretion. Responding to the need to increase fluid intake by consuming large amounts of tea can be a common mistake. The problem of patients being meticulous only with respect to oxalate and other dietary restrictions during those periods when urine collections are being made is well known. In this context it can be helpful to collect occasional spot urines during clinic visits for crystal studies and the measurements of urine oxalate:creatinine ratio. The dangers of calcium restriction without simultaneous oxalate restriction have already been referred to but must not be forgotten as many patients referred to metabolic stone clinics are found to be on low-calcium diets as a result of previous advice. The need to maintain high urine volumes applies as always.

Gastrointestinal Disorders

It must be realized that the hyperoxaluria in these patients can sometimes be very difficult to control for reasons that are not always clear. As the underlying problem is oxalate overabsorption, the logical first step is to restrict dietary oxalate as in the above group. Combining this with a low-fat diet if steatorrhea is present is usually necessary,[6] and these two approaches often produce a satisfactory fall in urinary oxalate. Some patients do fail to respond, however, and other measures have been tried when control is difficult. These include the use of anionic binding agents such as aluminium,[38,89] calcium,[76,77] and cholestyramine.[19,131] Since these bind not only oxalate but also bile acids and fatty acids, they may also minimize the effects of these latter substances on colonic permeability to oxalate.

Magnesium therapy seldom is practical, as it may aggravate existing diarrhea, and this is unfortunate because its use can lead to beneficial elevations in both urinary magnesium and citrate.[123] Calcium carbonate, either alone or in combination with other binding agents, is possibly the therapy of choice in difficult patients although a long-term compliance problem can be anticipated. The consequent alkalinization of the urine can also lead to a useful rise in urinary citrate. The difficulty in controlling hyperoxaluria in some of these patients raises the question as to whether other unsuspected mechanisms are contributing to the problem. Vitamin B_6 deficiency is conceivable in those patients with malabsorption, but against this is the finding, at least in our experience, that glycollate excretion is always normal, thus ruling out oxalate overproduction. In addition, we have been unable to produce a fall in urinary oxalate by giving 1 month of high-dose pyridoxine therapy (200 mg/day) to six such patients. Intestinal generation of oxalate by gastrointestinal flora has also been suggested, but there is little evidence to support this, although some reductions in oxalate excretion have been reported following a course of oral neomycin.[74] It has recently been shown that fecal samples from patients who have undergone jejunoileal bypass exhibit reduced baterial degradation of oxalate,[3] and this may be important.

In those patients with jejunoileal bypass whose hyperoxaluria remains refractory despite all the approaches mentioned above, surgical revision of the procedure may be the only permanent solution and should be seriously considered. The final point again concerns high fluid intake, but it is doubly important in these patients whose gastrointestinal disease may lead to chronic dehydration.

Mild Metabolic Hyperoxaluria

As this is a recently recognized syndrome, experience in its management is still limited, but a number of interesting aspects have emerged that have yet to be fully understood. The first line of treatment, as in primary hyperoxaluria, is with pyridoxine since virtually all patients show some response to this therapy. The dosage regime differs, however, because response in this group is often achieved with relatively low doses of pyridoxine, and 10–50 mg/day is the usual starting dose. Some patients can be controlled completely on this small dose, and although the hyperoxaluria usually returns within a few months if therapy has ceased, it can be rapidly recontrolled by restoring the same dose. These patients thus seem to have an increased requirement for vitamin B_6 with respect to its role in oxalate metabolism, as there is no other clinical or biochemical evidence of deficiency.

Other patients in this group have shown a more complex pattern of response to pyridoxine that is difficult to categorize. At least one patient, reported in detail elsewhere,[63] having responded to 10 mg/day of pyridoxine (but later given 100 mg/day for some months), then failed to relapse when therapy was stopped and has now remained normooxaluric for over 7 years. Subclinical vitamin B_6 deficiency could not be excluded here particularly as the requirement may have been increased by oral contraceptives, but this seems unlikely. Whatever the mechanism, a permanent "cure" seems to have been effected. In contrast to this, we have observed patients whose initial successful response to a low-dose regimen has been followed by relapse with rising requirements for pyridoxine in order to control their hyperoxaluria. They respond to each dose increment, therefore, but then relapse again such that one is sometimes forced to use a pyridoxine dose usually reserved for the primary hyperoxaluric. Even then control may not be achieved, and other therapy such as magnesium becomes necessary. A complete lack of response to pyridoxine, although seen by the authors, seems rare in this syndrome. Compliance with pyridoxine therapy must be monitored as outlined before.

It was stated earlier that a proportion of these patients were taking sodium cellulose phosphate, and in these patients it does seem necessary to discontinue the drug before a worthwhile pyridoxine response can be obtained. Although cellulose phosphate can cause hyperoxaluria by leading to overabsorption of dietary oxalate, this is not the mechanism here as glycollate excretion is also raised. The significance of this finding is not obvious, although the possibility that cellulose phosphate might reduce zinc absorption has been considered since this metal is necessary for the further metabolism of pyridoxine. No clinical evidence of zinc deficiency has been seen in this group, however, and plasma zinc levels, although accepted as a poor index of zinc status, have always been normal.

It is obvious that mild metabolic hyperoxaluria, although a very real entity that must always be looked for, is a poorly understood phenomenon at present. It does resemble primary hyperoxaluria in being more common in males and in some aspects of its response to pyridoxine. The recent report of primary hyperoxaluria apparently responding to much lower pyridoxine doses than are normally necessary is interesting in this context.[154] It is the spontaneous appearance at any age that most clearly distinguishes the mild metabolic syndrome from the genetic hyperoxalurias. We have seen the condition suddenly manifest, and responding to vitamin B_6, in a patient on long-term follow-up for idiopathic hypercalciuria whose urine oxalate had previously always been normal. It may be that some environmental factor is inducing a metabolic derangement that is similar to the defect present in primary hyperoxaluria, possibly via an effect on vitamin B_6 metabolism. Clearly, however, this is an area where further research is needed.

Summary

There is no question that hyperoxaluria always requires active treatment. From the preceding discussion it is clear that a logical approach to this requires a knowledge of the underlying cause. While pyridoxine is the key therapy in those groups indicated, the need for high fluid intakes, low-oxalate diets, and the liberal use of crystal inhibitors when necessary must always be appreciated. The need to preserve renal function is paramount, and this extends to all aspects of management; thus urinary tract infections must be detected early and treated vigorously. Surgical aspects of treatment are dealt with elsewhere in this volume, but it is important to remember the need for prompt diagnosis and relief of any obstructive episode.

CURRENT THOUGHTS AND PROBLEMS

It is hoped that this section has made readers aware of the role of urinary oxalate in the etiology of calcium oxalate urolithiasis. The importance of a thorough search for underlying hyperoxaluria in all patients, irrespective of any other diagnosis, cannot be overstated. The frequency with which mild metabolic hyperoxaluria is being found in the calcium stone formers attending the St. Peter's Hospitals supports this approach.

A rigid demarcation between normo- and hyperoxaluria must not be drawn on the basis of some of the currently quoted reference ranges. It is important for each laboratory to establish its own reference range; moreover, small elevations in urine oxalate, even within the "normal" range, can still represent a significant increase in the risk of stone formation, and attention has been drawn to the higher mean oxalate excretion seen in idiopathic calcium stone formers.[9,117] Similarly, a normal oxalate excretion in a stone-forming patient should not preclude attempts to reduce the level still further. The lower the urinary oxalate level the better must be the working rule. It may well be that our current practice of simply measuring daily oxalate excretion is not providing a sufficient index with respect to the risk from oxalate in some patients. Transient hyperoxaluria and crystalluria following high-oxalate meals does occur,[134] and it may be necessary to study oxalate excretion patterns throughout the day to uncover short-term changes not reflected in 24-hour collections. The search must continue for hitherto unrecognized sources of dietary oxalate and for factors that may alter its gastrointestinal absorption. In particular, the relationship between ascorbate and hyperoxaluria is again a completely open question badly needing answers.

The other area where research will hopefully contribute to future management and understanding is in unraveling the metabolic relationship between oxalate and vitamin B_6. Current improvements in analytical techniques with respect to both the B_6 vitamers and plasma oxalate should aid this process. It is important that any differences in vitamin B_6 metabolism that may exist between pyridoxine responders and nonresponders with metabolic hyperoxaluria are recognized in both the genetic and the mild metabolic groups. This would allow a more logical approach to treatment in these patients as well as directing much needed future developments in therapy.

EDITOR'S NOTE

An interesting, if uncommon, source for hyperoxaluria and resulting stone formation in the United States is the consumption of illegally produced apple brandy where it is produced by passing it through the radiator of an automobile where ethylene glycol (antifreeze) is present. The ethylene glycol is notorious for bringing about the precipitation of oxalate stones in experimental animals and in some individuals that consume the illegally prepared apple brandy.

REFERENCES

1. Akcay T, Rose GA: The real and apparent plasma oxalate. Clin Chim Acta 101:305–311, 1980
2. Albright F, Henneman P, Benedict PH, et al: Idiopathic hypercalciuria. Proc Roy Soc Med 46:1077–1081, 1953
3. Allison MJ, Cook HM, Milne DB, et al: Oxalate degradation by gastrointestinal bacteria from humans. J Nutr 116:455–460, 1986
4. Anderson DA: A survey of the incidence of urolithiasis in Norway from 1853–1960. J Oslo City Hosp 16:101, 1960
5. Andersson H, Gillberg R: Urinary oxalate on a high oxalate diet as a clinical test of malabsorption. Lancet 2:677–679, 1977
6. Andersson H, Jagenburg J: Fat-reduced diet in the treatment of hyperoxaluria with ileopathy. Gut 15:360–366, 1974
7. Archer HE, Dormer AE, Scowen EF, et al: Studies on the urinary excretion of oxalate by normal subjects. Clin Sci 16:405–411, 1957
8. Atkins GL, Dean BM, Griffin WJ, et al: Quantitative aspects of ascorbic acid metabolism in patients with primary hyperoxaluria. Clin Sci 29:305–314, 1965
9. Baggio B, Gambaro G, Favaro S, et al: Prevalence of hyperoxaluria in idiopathic calcium oxalate kidney stone disease. Nephron 35:11–14, 1983

10. Bais R, Nairn JM, Potezny N, et al: Urinary glycollate measured by use of (*S*)-2-hydroxy-acid oxidase. Clin Chem 31:710–713, 1985
11. Bais R, Potezny N, Edwards JB, et al: Oxalate determination by immobilised oxalate oxidase in a continuous flow system. Anal Chem 52:511–514, 1980
12. Barhan D, Trinder P: An improved colour reagent for the determination of blood glucose by the oxidase system. Analyst 97:142–145, 1972
13. Barker BM, Bender DA: Vitamin B_6 in Vitamins and Minerals, Vol. 1. London, Heinemann, 1980, pp 348–380
14. Barrett JFB: The oxalate content of blood. Biochem J 37:254–256, 1943
15. Biehl JB, Vimitz HJ: Studies on the use of a high dose of isoniazid. Am Rev Tuberc 70:430–441, 1954
16. Briggs MH, Garcia-Webb P, Davies P: Urinary oxalate and vitamin C supplements. Lancet 2:201, 1973
17. Buttery JE, Ludvigsen N, Braiotta EA, et al: Determination of urinary oxalate with commercially available oxalate oxidase. Clin Chem 29:700–702, 1983
18. Butz M, Hoffman H, Kohlbecker G: Dietary influence on serum and urinary oxalate in healthy subjects and oxalate stone formers. Urol Internatl 35:309–315, 1980
19. Caspary WF, Tonissen J, Lankisch PC: Enteral hyperoxaluria. Effect of cholestyramine, calcium, neomycin and bile acids on intestinal oxalate absorption in man. Acta Hepato Gastroenterol 24:193–200, 1977
20. Chalmers AH, Cowley DM: Urinary oxalate by rate analysis compared with gas-chromatographic and centrifugal analyser methods. Clin Chem 30:1891–1892, 1984
21. Chalmers AH, Cowley DM, Brown JM: A possible etiological role for ascorbate in calculi formation. Clin Chem 32:333–336, 1986
22. Chalmers RA, Lawson AM: Organic acids in man. London, Chapman and Hall, 1982, pp 409–414
23. Chalmers RA, Watts RWE: The quantitative extraction and gas liquid chromatographic determination of organic acids in urine. Analyst 97:958–967, 1972
24. Chambers MM, Russell JC: A specific assay for plasma oxalate. Clin Biochem 6:22–28, 1973
25. Coburn SP, Mahuren JD: A versatile cation-exchange procedure for measuring the seven major forms of vitamin B_6 in biological samples. Anal Biochem 129:310–317, 1983
26. Cole FE, Gladden KM, Bennet DJ, et al: Human plasma oxalate concentration re-examined. Clin Chim Acta 139:137–143, 1984
27. Constable AR, Joekes AM, Kasidas GP, et al: Plasma level and renal clearance of oxalate in normal subjects and in patients with primary hyperoxaluria or chronic renal failure or both. Clin Sci 56:299–304, 1979
28. Costello J, Hatch M, Bourke E: An enzymic method for the spectrophotometric determination of oxalic acid. J Lab Clin Med 87:903–908, 1976
29. Danpure CJ, Purkiss P, Jennings PR, et al: Mitochondrial damage and the subcellular distribution of 2-oxoglutarate: glyoxylate carboligase in normal human and rat liver and in the liver of a patient with primary hyperoxaluria type I. Clin Sci 70:417–425, 1986
30. Dean BM, Watts RWE, Westwick WJ: Metabolism of [1-^{14}C] glyoxylate, [1-^{14}C] glycollate, [1-^{14}C] glycine, and [2-^{14}C] glycine by homogenates of kidney and liver tissue from hyperoxaluric and control subjects. Biochem J 105:701–707, 1967
31. Dent CE, Stamp TCB: Treatment of primary hyperoxaluria. Arch Dis Child 45:735–745, 1970
32. DeZegher F, Przyrembel H, Chalmers RA, et al: Successful treatment of infantile type I primary hyperoxaluria complicated by pyridoxine toxicity. Lancet 2:392–393, 1985
33. Dobbins JW: Nephrolithiasis associated with intestinal disease, in Schwille PO, Smith LH, Robertson WG, et al: Urolithiasis and Related Clinical Research. New York, Plenum Press, 1985, pp 119–126
34. Dobbins JM, Binder HJ: Importance of the colon in enteric hyperoxaluria. New Engl J Med 296:298–301, 1977

35. Donckerwolcke RA, Chantler C, Broyer M: Combined report on regular dialysis and transplantation in children in Europe 1979. Proceedings of the European Dialysis and Transplantation Association 17:87–115, 1980
36. Dowling RH, Rose GA, Sutor DJ: Hyperoxaluria and renal calculi in ileal disease. Lancet 1:1103–1105, 1971
37. Driskell JA, Geders JM, Urban MC: Vitamin B_6 status of young men, women and women using oral contraceptives. J Lab Clin Med 87:813–821, 1976
38. Earnest DL: Perspectives on incidence, etiology, and treatment of enteric hyperoxaluria. Am J Clin Nutr 30:72–76, 1977
39. Earnest DL, Williams G, Williams HE, et al: Hyperoxaluria in patients with ileal resection: an abnormality in dietary oxalate absorption. Gastroenterology 66:1114–1122, 1974
40. Faber SR, Feitler WW, Bleiler RE, et al: The effects of an induced pyridoxine and pantothenic acid deficiency on excretion of oxalic and xanthurenic acids in the urine. Am J Clin Nutr 12:406–412, 1963
41. Fairclough PD, Feest TG, Chadwick VS, et al: Effect of sodium chenodeoxycholate on oxalate absorption from excluded human colon—a mechanism for enteric hyperoxaluria. Gut 18:240–244, 1977
42. Finch AM, Kasidas GP, Rose GA: Urine composition in normal subjects after oral ingestion of oxalate-rich foods. Clin Sci 60:411–418, 1981
43. Fitzhugh OG, Nelson AA: Comparison of the chronic toxicity of triethylene glycol with that of diethylene glycol. J Indust Hyg Toxicol 28:40–43, 1946
44. Fitzpatrick JM, Kasidas GP, Rose GA: A complication of transurethral resection of the prostate. Hyperoxaluria due to intra-operative glycine absorption. Br J Urol 53:250–252, 1981
45. Flocks RH: Calcium urolithiasis; role of calcium metabolism in pathogenesis and treatment of calcium urolithiasis. J Urol 43:214–233, 1940
46. Foster PN, Will EJ, Kelleher J, et al: Oxalate loading tests to screen for steatorrhoea: an appraisal. Clin Chim Acta 144:155–161, 1984
47. France NC, Windleborn EA, Wallace MR: In vitro oxalogenesis and measurement of oxalate in serum. Clin Chem 31:335–336, 1985
48. Freidman AL, Chesney RW, Gilbert EF, et al: Secondary oxalosis as a complication of parenteral alimentation in acute renal failure. Am J Nephrol 3:248–252, 1983
49. Frommer JP, Ayus JC: Acute ethylene glycol intoxication. Am J Nephrol 5:40–44, 1985
50. Gershoff SN: Vitamin B_6 and oxalate metabolism. Vitamins & Hormones 22:581–589, 1964
51. Gershoff SN, Faragalla SK, Nelson DA, et al: Vitamin B_6 deficiency and nephrocalcinosis in the cat. Am J Med 27:72–80, 1959
52. Gibbs DA, Watts RWE: Biochemical studies on the treatment of primary hyperoxaluria. Arch Dis Child 42:505, 1967
53. Gibbs DA, Watts RWE: The variation of urinary oxalate excretion with age. J Lab Clin Med 73:901–908, 1969
54. Gibbs DA, Watts RWE: The action of pyridoxine in primary hyperoxaluria. Clin Sci 38:277–286, 1970
55. Gochman N, Schmitz JM: Automated determination of uric acid, with the use of a uricase-peroxidase system. Clin Chem 17:1154–1159, 1971
56. Hagler L, Herman RH: Oxalate metabolism I. Am J Clin Nutr 26:758–765, 1973
57. Hagler L, Herman RH: Oxalate metabolism V. Am J Clin Nutr 26:1242–1250, 1973
58. Hallson PC, Kasidas GP, Rose GA: Urinary oxalate in summer and winter in normal subjects and in stone forming patients with idiopathic hypercalciuria. Urol Res 4:169–173, 1976
59. Hallson PC, Rose GA: A simplified and rapid enzymatic method for the determination of urinary oxalate. Clin Chim Acta 55:29–39, 1974
60. Hallson PC, Rose GA: Seasonal variations in urinary excretion of calcium and oxalate in normal subjects and in patients with idiopathic hypercalciuria. Br J Urol 49:1–10, 1977
61. Hallson PC, Rose GA: A new urinary test for stone "activity." Br J Urol 50:442–445, 1978

62. Hallson PC, Rose GA, Sulaiman S: Magnesium reduces calcium oxalate crystal formation in human whole urine. Clin Sci 62:17–19, 1982
63. Harrison AR, Kasidas GP, Rose GA: Hyperoxaluria and recurrent stone formation apparently cured by short courses of pyridoxine. Br Med J 282:2097–2098, 1981
64. Hatch M, Brouke E, Costello J: New enzymic method for serum oxalate concentration. Clin Chem 23:76–78, 1977
65. Helin I: Primary hyperoxaluria—an analysis of 17 Scandinavian patients. Scand J Urol Nephrol 14:61–64, 1980
66. Herbert RW, Hirst EL, Percival EGV, et al: The constitution of ascorbic acid. J Chem Soc 1270–1290, 1933
67. Herring LC: Observations on the analysis of ten thousand urinary calculi. J Urol 88:545–562, 1962
68. Hicks NR, Cranston DW, Charlton CAC: Fifteen year follow up of hyperoxaluria type II. New Engl J Med 309:796, 1983
69. Hocking MP, Duerson MC, O'Leary P, et al: Jejuno-ileal bypass for morbid obesity. New Engl J Med 308:995–999, 1983
70. Hodgkinson A: Oxalic Acid in Biology and Medicine. New York, Academic Press, 1977
71. Hodgkinson A, Peacock M, Nicholson M: Quantitative analysis of calcium containing urinary calculi. Invest Urol 6:549–561, 1969
72. Hodgkinson A, Pyrah LN: The urinary excretion of calcium and inorganic phosphate in 344 patients with calcium stone of renal origin. Br J Surg 46:10–18, 1958
73. Hodgkinson A, Wilkinson R: Plasma oxalate concentrations and renal excretion of oxalate in man. Clin Sci Molec Med 46:61–73, 1974
74. Hoffman AF, Laker MF, Dharmsathaphorn K, et al: Complex pathogenesis of hyperoxaluria after jejuno-ileal bypass surgery. Gastroenterology 84:293–300, 1983
75. Hollister LE, Moore FF, Forrest F, et al: Antipyridoxine effect of D-penicillamine in schizophrenic men. Am J Clin Nutr 19:307–312, 1966
76. Holst-Pedersen J, Steen J: The effect of calcium on hyperoxaluria following jejuno-ileal bypass in morbid obesity. Scand J Gastroenterol 14:97–99, 1979
77. Hylander E, Janum S, Nielsen K: Calcium treatment of enteric hyperoxaluria after jejuno-ileal bypass for morbid obesity. Scand J Gastroenterol 15:49–52, 1980
78. Jaeger P, Portmann L, Jacquet A, et al: Influence of the calcium content of the diet on the incidence of mild metabolic hyperoxaluria in idiopathic renal stone formers. Am J Nephrol 5:40–44, 1985
79. Kasidas GP: Factors affecting the levels of oxalate and glycollate in the urine and plasma of normal subjects and calcium stone formers. PhD thesis, University of London, 1980
80. Kasidas GP, Rose GA: A new enzymatic method for the determination of glycolate in urine and plasma. Clin Chim Acta 96:25–36, 1979
81. Kasidas GP, Rose GA: Oxalate content of some common foods: determination by an enzymatic method. J Hum Nutr 34:255–266, 1980
82. Kasidas GP, Rose GA: Metabolic hyperoxaluria and its response to pyridoxine, in Ryall, R, Brockis JG, Marshall V, et al (eds): Urinary Stone: New York, Churchill Livingstone, 1984, pp 138–147
83. Kasidas GP, Rose GA: Spontaneous in vitro generation of oxalate from L-ascorbate in some assays for urinary oxalate and its prevention, in Schwille PO, Smith LH, Robertson WG (eds): Urolithiasis and Related Clinical Research. New York, Plenum Press, 1985, pp 653–656
84. Kasidas GP, Rose GA: Continuous flow assay for urinary oxalate using immobilised oxalate oxidase. Ann Clin Biochem 22:412–419, 1985
85. Kasidas GP, Rose GA: Measurement of plasma oxalate in healthy subjects and in patients with chronic renal failure using immobilised oxalate oxidase. Clin Chim Acta 154:49–52, 1986

86. Kasidas GP, Rose GA, Samuell CT: Mild but clinically significant metabolic hyperoxaluria and its response to pyridoxine, in Gasser G, Vahlensieck W (eds): Pathogenese und Klinik der Harnsteine XI. Darmstadt, Steinkopf, 1985, pp 394–399
87. Koch J, Stokstad ELR, Williams HE, et al: Deficiency of 2-oxoglutarate: glyoxylate carboligase activity in primary hyperoxaluria. Proc Natl Acad Sci (USA) 57:1123–1129, 1967
88. Kohlbecker G: Direct spectrophotometric determination of serum and urinary oxalate with oxalate oxidase. J Clin Chem Clin Biochem 19:1103–1106, 1981
89. Laker MF, Hoffman AF: Effective therapy of enteric hyperoxaluria: In vitro binding of oxalate by anion-exchange resins and aluminium hydroxide. J Pharm Sci 70:1065–1068, 1981
90. Lamden MP, Chrystowski GA: Urinary oxalate excretion by man following ascorbic acid ingestion. Proc Soc Exp Biol Med 85:190–192, 1954
91. Larson JF, Philip J: Studies on the incidence of urolithiasis. Urol Internatl 13:53, 1962
92. Liao LL, Richardson KE: The synthesis of oxalate from hydroxypyruvate by isolated perfused rat liver. Biochem Biophys Acta 538:76–86, 1978
93. Ljunghall S, Bachmann U, Danielson BG: Epidemiology of renal stones in Sweden, in Brockis G, Finlayson B (eds): Urinary Calculus. Proceedings of the International Urinary Stone Conference, Perth, Australia, PSG, 1981, pp 13–24
94. Ljunghall S, Hedstrand H: Epidemiology of renal stones in a middle aged male population. Acta Med Scand 197:439–445, 1975
95. Lui A, Lumeng L, Li TK: The measurement of plasma vitamin B_6 compounds: Comparison of a cation exchange HPLC method with the open column chromatographic method and the L-tyrosine apodecarboxylase assay. Am J Clin Nutr 41:1236–1243, 1985
96. Mason DY, Emerson PM: Primary acquired sideroblastic anaemia: Response to treatment with pyridoxal-5-phosphate. Br Med J 1:389–390, 1973
97. Mayer GG, Chase T, Farvar B, et al: Metabolic studies on the formation of calcium oxalate stones with special emphasis on vitamin B_6 and uric acid metabolism. Bull NY Acad Med 44:28–44, 1968
98. Morris MC, Chambers TL, Evans PWG, et al: Oxalosis in infancy. Arch Dis Child 57:224–228, 1982
99. Mudd SH: Pyridoxine responsive genetic disease. Proc Am Soc Exp Biol 30:970–976, 1971
100. McDonald GB, Earnest DL, Admirand WH: Hyperoxaluria correlates with fat malabsorption in patients with sprue. Gut 18:561–566, 1977
101. Nath R, Thind SK, Murthy MSR, et al: Sources of oxalic acid, intermediary metabolism and physiology of oxalate, in Baum H, Gergely J, Fanburg BL (eds): Molecular Aspects of Medicine, Vol 7. Medical Aspects of Idiopathic Urolithiasis. New York, Pergamon Press, 1984, pp 55–88
102. Nime FA, Hutchins GA: Oxalosis caused by Aspergillus infection. John Hopkins Medical J 133:183–194, 1973
103. Nordin BEC, Peacock M, Wilkinson R: Hypercalciuria and calcium stone disease. Clin Endocrinol Metab 1:169–183, 1972
104. Nuret P, Offner M: A new method for determination of oxalate in blood serum by gas chromatography. Clin Chim Acta 82:9–12, 1978
105. Obzansky DM, Richardson KE: Quantification of urinary oxalate with oxalate from beet stems. Clin Chem 29:1815–1819, 1983
106. O'Regan PFB, Constable AR, Joekes AM, et al: The management of the primary hyperoxaluric patient, in Rose GA, Robertson WG, Watts RWE (eds): Oxalate in Human Biochemistry and Clinical Pathology. London, Wellcome Foundation, 1979, pp 209–219
107. O'Regan P, Constable AR, Joekes AM, et al: Successful renal transplantation in primary hyperoxaluria. Postgrad Med J 56:288–293, 1980
108. Pak CYC, Chata M, Lawrence EC, et al: The hypercalciurias: Causes, parathyroid functions and diagnostic criteria. J Clin Invest 54:387–400, 1974

109. Pak CYC, Galosy RA: Fasting urinary calcium and adenosine 3′5′-monophosphate: A discriminant analysis for the identification of renal and absorptive hypercalciurias. J. Clin Endocrinol Metab 48:260–265, 1979
110. Pak CYC, Kaplan R, Bone H, et al: A simple test for the diagnosis of absorptive, reabsorptive and renal hypercalciuria. New Engl J Med 292:497–500, 1975
111. Prenen JAC, Boer P, Darhout Mees et al: Renal clearance of ^{14}C oxalate: Comparison of constant infusion with single injection techniques. Clin Sci 63:47–51, 1982
112. Rampton DS, Kasidas GP, Rose GA, et al: Oxalate loading test; a screening test for steatorrhoea. Gut 20:1089–1094, 1979
113. Roberts JA, Siebold HR: Ethylene glycol toxicity in the monkey. Toxicol Appl Pharmacol 15:624–631, 1969
114. Robertson WG, Nordin BEC: Activity products in urine, in Hodgkinson A, Nordin BEC (eds): Renal Stone Research Symposium. London, Churchill, 1969, pp 221–232
115. Robertson WG, Peacock M: The cause of idiopathic calcium stone disease: Hypercalciuria or hyperoxaluria. Nephron 26:105–110, 1980
116. Robertson WG, Peacock M, Heyburn PJ, et al: Risk factors in calcium stone disease of the urinary tract. Br J Urol 50:449–454, 1978
117. Robertson WG, Peacock M, Heyburn PJ, et al: The significance of mild hyperoxaluria in calcium stone formation, in Rose GA, Robertson WG, Watts RWE (eds): Oxalate in Human Biochemistry and Clinical Pathology. London, Wellcome Foundation, 1979, pp 173–180
118. Robertson WG, Rutherford A: Aspects of the analysis of oxalate in urine—a review. Scand J Urol Nephrol (Suppl) 53:85–95, 1980
119. Rose GA: Urinary stones: Clinical and laboratory aspects. Lancaster, MTP Press, 1982
120. Rose GA: The role of pyridoxine in stone prevention in hyperoxaluric patients, in Rous, SM (ed): Urology Annual, 1987, New York, Appleton Century Crofts, in press
121. Rose GA, Arthur LJH, Chambers TL, et al: Successful treatment of primary hyperoxaluria in a neonate. Lancet 1:1298–1299, 1982
122. Rose GA, Harrison AR: The incidence, investigation and treatment of idiopathic hypercalciuria. Br J Urol 46:261–274, 1974
123. Rudman D, Dedonis JL, Fountain MT, et al: Hypocitraturia in patients with gastrointestinal malabsorption. New Engl J Med 303:657–661, 1980
124. Schaumburg H, Kaplan J, Windebank A, et al: Sensory neuropathy from pyridoxine abuse. New Engl J Med 309:445–448, 1983
125. Scheinman JI, Najarian JS, Mauer SM: Successful strategies for renal transplantation in primary oxalosis. Kidney Internatl 25:804–811, 1984
126. Scott R, Frealand R, Mowat W, et al: The prevalence of calcified upper urinary tract stone disease in a random population—Cumbernauld Health Survey. Br J Urol 49:589–595, 1977
127. Scriver CR, Hutchison JH: The vitamin B_6 deficiency syndrome in human infancy: Biochemical and clinical observations. Paediatrics 31:240–250, 1963
128. Silver L, Brendler H: Use of magnesium oxide in management of familial hyperoxaluria. J Urol 106:274–279, 1971
129. Silverberg DS, McIntyre JWR, Ulan RA, et al: Oxalic acid excretion after methoxyflurane and halothane anaesthesia. Can Anaesth Soc 18:496–504, 1971
130. Simmonds HA, Van Acker KJ, Potter CF, et al: Influence of purine content of diet and allopurinol on uric acid and oxalate excretion levels, in Smith LH, Robertson WG, Finlayson B (eds): Urolithiasis: Clinical and Basic Research. New York, Plenum Press, 1981, pp 363–367
131. Smith LH, Fromm H, Hoffman AF: Acquired hyperoxaluria, nephrocalcinosis and intestinal disease. New Engl J Med 286:1371–1375, 1972
132. Standal BR, Kao-Chen SM, Yang GY, et al: Early changes in pyridoxine status of patient receiving isoniazid therapy. Am J Clin Nutr 27:479–484, 1974

133. Stauffer JQ: Hyperoxaluria and intestinal disease. The role of steatorrhoea and dietary calcium in regulating intestinal oxalate absorption. Am J Digest Dis 22:921–928, 1977
134. Strenge A, Hesse A, Bach D, et al: Excretion of oxalic acid following the ingestion of various amounts of oxalic acid-rich foods, in Smith LH, Robertson WG, Finlayson B (eds): Urolithiasis: Clinical and Basic Research. New York, Plenum Press, 1981, pp 789–794
135. Takenouchi K, Aso K, Kawase K, et al: On the metabolites of ascorbic acid, especially oxalic acid, eliminated in urine following the administration of large amounts of ascorbic acid. J Vitaminol 12:49–58, 1966
136. Tiselius H, Ahlstrand C, Lundstrom B, et al: ^{14}C-oxalate absorption by normal persons, calcium oxalate stone formers, and patients with surgically disturbed intestinal function. Clin Chem 27:1682–1685, 1981
137. Tomlinson B, Cohen SL, Al-Khader A, et al: Further reduction of oxalate excretion by allopurinol in stone formers on a low purine diet, in Smith LH, Robertson WG, Finlayson B (eds): Urolithiasis: Clinical and Basic Research. New York, Plenum Press, 1981, pp 513–516
138. Vahlensieck EW, Bach D, Hesse A: Incidence, prevalence, and mortality of urolithiasis in the German Federal Republic. Urol Res 10:161–164, 1982
139. Watts RWE: Oxaluria. J Roy Coll Physicians London 7:161–174, 1973
140. Watts RWE, Calne RY, Williams R, et al: Primary hyperoxaluria (type I): Attempted treatment by combined hepatic and renal transplantation. Quart J Med 57:697–707, 1985
141. Watts RWE, Chalmers RA, Gibbs DA, et al: Studies on some possible biochemical treatment of primary hyperoxaluria. Quart J Med 190:259–272, 1979
142. Watts RWE, Veall N, Purkiss P: Sequential studies of oxalate dynamics in primary hyperoxaluria. Clin Sci 65:627–633, 1983
143. Watts RWE, Veall N, Purkiss P: Oxalate dynamics and removal rates during haemodialysis and peritoneal dialysis in patients with primary hyperoxaluria and severe renal failure. Clin Sci 66:591–597, 1984
144. Watts RWE, Veall N, Purkiss P, et al: The effect of pyridoxine on oxalate dynamics in three cases of primary hyperoxaluria (with glycollic aciduria). Clin Sci 69:87–90, 1985
145. White-Stevens RH: Interference by ascorbic acid in test systems involving peroxidase. I. Reversible indicators and the effects of copper, iron and mercury. Clin Chem 28:578–588, 1982
146. White-Stevens RH, Stover LR: Interference by ascorbic acid in test systems involving peroxidase II. Redox coupled indicator systems. Clin Chem 28:589–595, 1982
147. Will EJ, Bijvoet OLM: Primary oxalosis: clinical and biochemical response to high-dose pyridoxine therapy. Metabolism 28:542–548, 1979
148. Williams HE, Johnson GA, Smith LH: The renal clearance of oxalate in normal subjects and in patients with primary hyperoxaluria. Clin Sci 41:213–218, 1971
149. Williams HE, Smith LH: L-Glyceric aciduria. A new genetic variant of primary hyperoxaluria. New Engl J Med 278:233–239, 1968
150. Williams HE, Smith LH: Primary hyperoxaluria, in Stanbury JB, Wyngaarden JB, Fredrickson DS (eds): The Metabolic Basis of Inherited Disease, 5th ed. New York, McGraw-Hill, 1983, pp 204–228
151. Wilson JJ, Marshall RW, Hodgkinson A: Excretion of methoxyflurane metabolites. Br Med J 2:594, 1972
152. Wilson RE: A report from American College of Surgeons/National Institute of Health Renal Transplant Registry. Renal Transplantation in congenital and metabolic disease. JAMA 232:148–153, 1975
153. Woodring MJ, Fisher DH, Storvick CA: A microprocedure for the determination of 4-pyridoxic acid in urine. Clin Chem 10:479–489, 1964
154. Yendt ER, Cohanim M: Response to a physiological dose of pyridoxine in type I primary hyperoxaluria. New Engl J Med 312:953–957, 1985

155. Zarembski PM, Hodgkinson A: The fluorimetric determination of oxalic acid in blood and other biological materials. Biochem J 96:717–721, 1965
156. Zarembski PM, Hodgkinson A: Some factors influencing the urinary excretion of oxalic acid in man. Clin Chim Acta 25:1–10, 1969
157. Zerwekh JE, Drake E, Gregory J, et al: Assay of urinary oxalate: Six methodologies compared. Clin Chem 29:1977–1980, 1983

Stephen N. Rous

17

Determining the Success of Medical Therapy

Once the patient with recurrent urolithiasis has been evaluated and a therapeutic regime has been started, the clinician should have a means by which to follow the patient in order to determine the efficacy of the chosen therapy. Unsuccessful therapy (continued stone formation) can be attributed to the wrong treatment or can be due to noncompliance on the part of the patient.

Some physicians will use as the determinant for successful therapy the simple fact of whether the patient passes additional stones after therapy has started. This is less than ideal, however, because there will undoubtedly be some patients with stones already present in the kidney at the time that therapy begins, and the passage of such stones does not in any way suggest inadequate or unsuccessful therapy. Certainly, when careful tomograms of the kidneys do disclose calculi at the time that the therapy is started, it is most important to advise the patient that one or more of these calculi may pass but that this in no way should be considered as a reflection on the adequacy or inadequacy of the therapy.

Much more important, though, is if a newly formed and unexpected stone does pass, the patient will often tend to lose confidence in the physician's therapeutic excellence, and the physician also may have second thoughts about the drug treatment for this patient.

A better way to follow and evaluate the success of therapy is by observing the size and number of crystals in the urine of patients prior to and while undergoing therapy. Crystalluria rarely is found in normal patients, and its presence in stone formers, particularly when aggregates of crystals are found, portends the probability of future stone formation. When crystals are found in the urine, it suggests that one of the conditions for lithiasis is present, specifically, supersaturation. The more numerous the crystals, and particularly if present in clumps, the greater is the likelihood of stone formation. An examination of the urine of stone-forming patients on each visit to the physician's office

STONE DISEASE: DIAGNOSIS AND MANAGEMENT
ISBN 0-8089-1873-7

following the onset of therapy can give a good reading as to the success of therapy since the ideal goal of therapy (not always achieved) is to have the urine totally free of crystals. The fewer the crystals found in the urine, the more successful the therapy, and repetitive examination of the urine sediment for crystals should hopefully show these in decreasing numbers.[1–6]

The question remains, however, as to how best to determine the presence and the extent of the crystalluria. Simply counting crystals in the urine sediment would be misleading because on each and every visit the patient is likely to be in a different state of hydration, having been admonished to "drink a lot of water." Stated in other terms, the physician cannot logically make any statement about the therapeutic efficacy of the treatment rendered by comparing the numbers and sizes of crystals in a dilute urine on one visit with the crystal pattern found in a more concentrated urine that might occur on a subsequent visit. As a means of making meaningful comparisons between the crystalluria noted on a given patient visit and that noted on any other patient visit, the author has found it extremely helpful to use the urine evaporation technique developed by Hallson and Rose in 1978.[7] With this method, the urine passed at the time of each and every visit is evaporated to the same osmolarity (about 1250 mOsm/kg), thereby making it possible to compare the crystalluria found in the urine sediment on one day with that found on another day a month earlier or a month later.

On each physician visit, then, prior to therapy and once the patient is on therapy, a urine specimen is obtained, which will vary enormously from visit to visit in its osmolarity depending on how much fluid the patient has been drinking. This urine is collected in a thermos flask so that it remains at body temperature (37°C) and is then evaporated in a rotary evaporator to an approximate osmolarity of 1250 mOsm/kg (Fig. 17-1). It is then placed into a centrifuge tube and spun for 3 minutes. The supernatent fluid is then

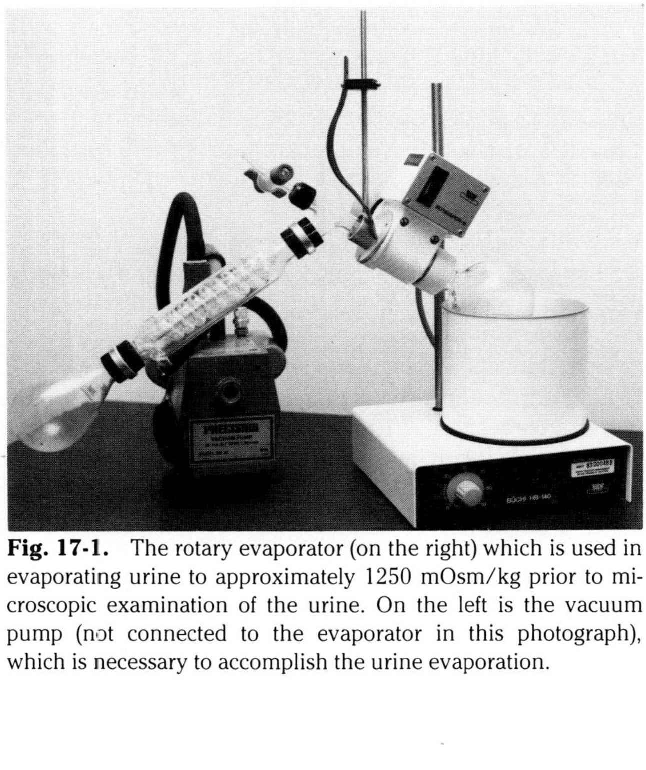

Fig. 17-1. The rotary evaporator (on the right) which is used in evaporating urine to approximately 1250 mOsm/kg prior to microscopic examination of the urine. On the left is the vacuum pump (not connected to the evaporator in this photograph), which is necessary to accomplish the urine evaporation.

poured off and the urine sediment examined by a binocular microscope under high dry power (400×). A grid manufactured by Zeiss and sold through the Georgia Instruments Company of Atlanta is placed in one of the oculars, and each box in the grid is approximately 12 μm in size, which is about the size of the largest calcium oxalate dihydrate crystals that will commonly be seen (not including clumping or aggregation of crystals) (Fig. 17-2). Ten different high-power fields are then observed, and in each field the number and the size (small, medium, and large) of crystals seen in the grid are counted and recorded. The average counts for the 10 high-power fields are then obtained and recorded, and this represents the study of a patient's crystalluria on a given day. By observing the crystalluria in this very specific and semiquantitative manner, a definite comparison can be made in the crystalluria that is noted each time the patient is seen, and the success of the therapy can be determined from this. As already noted, therapy should ideally eliminate the crystalluria entirely; in practice, it often does not, but it should certainly produce a downward trend in the number and size of the crystals from visit to visit as the therapy becomes effective, and the patient should then be maintained with minimal (or no) crystalluria. If occasional visits disclose a great upswing in the degree of crystalluria, the patient may safely be asked whether there has been adherence

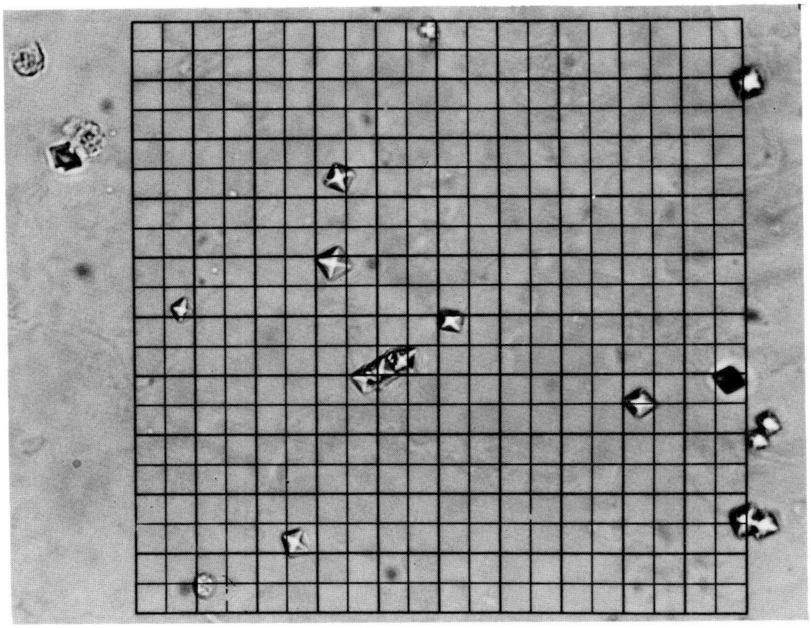

Fig. 17-2. Examination of the crystalluria under high dry magnification (400×). Each of the small boxes within the large grid is approximately 12 μm in size, and it can be seen that the largest crystals are approximately this size. A count of the number of crystals of each size (large, medium, and small) within the grid gives a semiquantitative value for the crystalluria of a specific high-power field. The average of such high-power fields is obtained at the time of each patient visit, and that average value represents the semiquantitative status of the patient's crystalluria on that day.

to the therapeutic regimen. Although the illustration of calcium oxalate dihydrate crystalluria has been used, the methodology is the same for any kind of crystalluria.

There are many different kinds and models of rotary evaporator that can accomplish the necessary urine evaporation. The author uses an instrument made by Buchi that is obtained from Fischer Scientific Instruments and a vacuum pump that is made and sold by the Precision Scientific Group of Chicago.

REFERENCES

1. Robertson WG: A method for measuring calcium crystalluria. Clin Chim Acta 26:105–110, 1969
2. Robertson WG, Peacock M: Calcium oxalate crystalluria and inhibitors of crystallization in recurrent renal stone formers. Clin Sci 43:499–506, 1972
3. Werness PG, Bergert JH, Smith LH: Crystalluria. J Crystal Growth 53:166–181, 1981
4. Rose GA: Crystalluria as an aid to the study of urinary stones. Lab-Lore (Wellcome Diagnostics) 9:738–740, 1982
5. Robertson WG, Peacock M, Nordin BEC: Calcium crystalluria in recurrent renal stone formers. Lancet 2:21–24, 1969
6. Hallson PC, Rose GA: Crystalluria in normal subjects and in stone formers with and without thiazide and cellulose phosphate treatment. Br J Urol 48:515–524, 1976
7. Hallson PC, Rose GA: A new urinary test for stone "activity." Br J Urol 50:442, 1978

PART III

Surgical Treatment and Management of the Urolithiasis Patient

Joseph W. Segura

18

Ureteroscopy, Including Lithotripsy and the Stone Basket

URETEROSCOPY

The last few years have witnessed a revolution in the surgical management of stone disease, and the treatment of ureteral calculi has shared in these changes. In 1981 Lyon and his colleagues started to use pediatric cystoscopes to examine the lower ureters in women and were able to remove ureteral calculi under direct vision utilizing forceps and baskets.[1,2] In that same year, Perez-Castro began to employ the first ureteroscope with which the entire ureter (and often the renal pelvis) could be examined.[3] Today, ureteroscopy is a routine procedure throughout the United States and Europe.[6]

Equipment

Both rigid and flexible ureteroscopes are available, although at the present time, the rigid units are the most technically developed and most commonly available. These units typically are 45 cm long (not including the lens) and vary in size from 8.5 to 13.5 French. The exact French sizes of different manufacturers' ureteroscopes has been the subject of some controversy, because for some of the older units, the actual size was larger than that stated by the manufacturer. The issue is further complicated because no ureteroscopes are circular, and hence, the French system of measurement is only approximately useful.

Rod-lens optics are used in all rigid units, and the quality of vision is outstanding, equal to that obtainable with the best cystoscopes. Equipment is available from three manufacturers: R. Wolf, K. Storz, and ACMI. Although there are more similarities than differences among these instruments, one may distinguish three groups of ureteroscopes. In the older, original equipment, the telescopes were placed directly down the ureteroscope sheath and the instrument was then passed up the ureter under direct vision, much like one passes a cystoscope into the bladder under vision. The smaller sheaths

STONE DISEASE: DIAGNOSIS AND MANAGEMENT

ISBN 0-8089-1873-7

accommodated only the telescope and could be used just for diagnostic purposes, although with removal of the telescope, an ultrasonic probe could be inserted up the sheath under fluoroscopic control until it made contact with a target stone. With the larger sheaths, space was also available for a basket or forceps in addition to the telescope.

In the next generation of equipment, the eyepiece was made an integral part of the instrument in order to accommodate both a working channel for a basket as well as space for an ultrasonic probe. The eyepiece was offset at a 30° angle. Although many people found this instrument difficult to use properly, it did enable the operator to employ an ultrasonic probe under direct vision. In currently available units, the eyepiece is offset at right angles so that the surgeon is looking in the direction in which the instrument is passed (Fig. 18-1). This yields a more natural "feel," and there is also adequate space for an ultrasonic probe as well as a basket.

The advantages of rigid ureteroscopes are in the unsurpassed and unequaled quality of the image obtained with rod-lens optics and also in one's ability to work through the instrument as well as look through it. The instruments' rigidity and size are relative disadvantages. Although all "rigid" ureteroscopes are somewhat flexible, some patients have enough curvature in their ureters to prohibit negotiation of the instrument through the areas of prominent curvature in the bony pelvis and over the femoral vessels. Also, the most useful instruments are the largest, and many ureters are simply not large enough for a 12.5–13.5-French device to pass.

The ureter may also be examined with a flexible ureteroscope. Devices are currently available from Olympus and ACMI. Image quality is excellent, but because fiberoptics are used, the image is not of the same standard as rod-lens optics. Flexible instruments may be difficult to pass up the ureter even though they are the same size as the rigid instruments (14 French). It is usually necessary to use an introducer. Flexible forceps and baskets may be used through the working channel, but if bleeding is present, their usefulness can be compromised by irrigating fluid pressure insufficient to clear the visual field of blood.

Disposable flexible ureteroscopes have recently been made by Van-Tec (Fig. 18-2) and Reichert. At the present time, these instruments seem suited more for a diagnostic

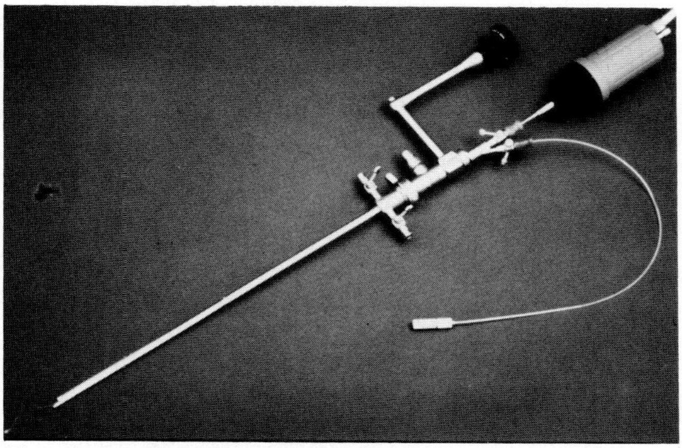

Fig. 18-1. The Wolf 12.5-French rigid ureteroscope. Both ultrasound and basket manipulation can be accomplished at the same time and under vision with also continuous irrigation.

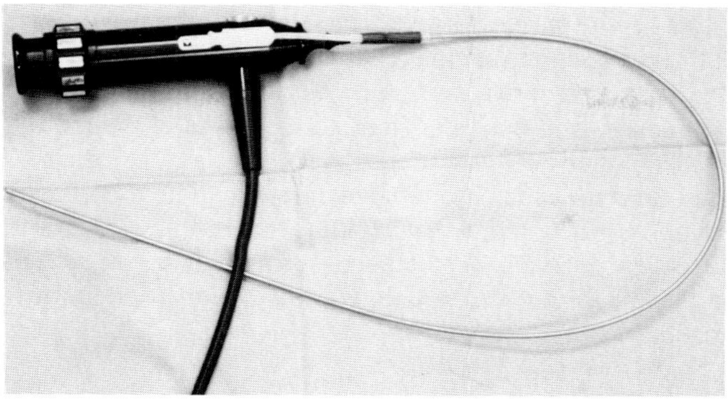

Fig. 18-2. The flexible Van-Tec ureteroscope. The flexible ureteroscopic portion is disposable and replaced after several uses. The handle is permanent.

rather than a therapeutic role. Nevertheless, their small size (6–9.5 French) is a feature of great appeal, and as baskets and other methods of stone removal, such as the laser (see below), become smaller and more widely available, these smaller ureteroscopes will become more important.

Indications for Ureteroscopic Stone Removal

Several factors enter into the judgment as to which stones should be removed, how they should be removed, and when this should be done.

Stone Size

Stones 4.0 mm or smaller will usually pass spontaneously, although often with colic or other symptoms. The present author usually allows patients to attempt to pass such stones, reserving intervention for those in whom pain has become intolerable, or in whom progress of the stone down the ureter has become too desultory. Fever or chills is usually a signal for early intervention, as is nonfunction on excretory urography.

As the size of the stone increases, the chances of spontaneous passage decrease markedly and spontaneous passage of a stone greater than 6.0 mm cannot reasonably be expected except in occasional individuals. Smooth stones are more likely to pass than are spiculated or irregular calculi.

The size of the stone per se does not affect the decision as to whether the ureteroscope should be used in a given case. Small stones are removed more easily and quickly than large stones, and while large stones may require more operating time and will usually require some form of power lithotripsy to reduce the calculus to manageable fragments, this all can effectively be done through the ureteroscope. Further, almost all ureteral stones are 1.5 cm or less in diameter, and stones of this size are manageable by ureteroscopic means.

Stone Location

In our opinion, stones in the lower ureter should be managed ureteroscopically. This is because in most patients it is possible to insert the ureteroscope as far as the femoral vessels. If the stone can be seen with the instrument, it should be possible either to remove it or to break it up into small pieces with the ultrasonic probe or the laser. When this is achievable, it seem senseless to push the stone all the way up to the kidney for shock-wave lithotripsy, much less operate on the patient.

The mid and upper ureter are accessed less easily with the ureteroscope, and for this reason our usual practice is to push the stone to the pelvis of the kidney and then use ESWL. In patients who have adequate ureters such that the ureteroscope can be readily passed to the stone, it seems simpler to remove the stone ureteroscopically. If the stone is associated with distal obstruction or a large-volume renal pelvic stone, or is otherwise not suitable for ureteroscopy or ESWL, percutaneous techniques are used. These latter procedures may be particularly useful for large stones that are impacted in the upper ureter or ureteropelvic junction.

Stone Type

Stone composition is usually not a consideration in deciding whether to use ureteroscopy. Calcium oxalate monohydrate, cystine, and uric acid stones that are too large to remove by manipulation will require some form of power lithotripsy.

Power Lithotripsy

Stones too large to manipulate through the dilated ureter will need to be reduced in size by using one of three techniques of power lithotripsy: (1) ultrasonic lithotripsy, (2) electrohydraulic lithotripsy, and (3) pulsed dye laser lithotripsy.

Ultrasonic Lithotripsy

The same equipment designed for percutaneous lithotripsy can be used through the ureteroscope with minor modifications. In general, the same ultrasonic generators and transducers are used, and the only difference is that the probe must be long and thin so that it will fit through the ureteroscope sheath. In the most recently developed models, the sheaths will accommodate the probe and a telescope and will also leave room for a basket. The probes are 41 cm long and 11.5 French in circumference. Most probes are hollow to allow for aspiration of fragments, but with the smaller probes, these lumina are too small to be particularly useful. The lumen on the older, 9-French Wolf probe is adequate to aspirate significant amounts of stony debris.

Pulsed Dye Laser

This new instrument has great promise for a future important role in ureteroscopic stone removal. Because the laser is fired in short, nanosecond bursts, very high energies can be transmitted without overheating and risking thermal damage to adjacent structures. The laser light is transmitted through a thin flexible quartz fiber that can be aimed at the stone under direct vision. Each time the laser hits the stone, energy is transmitted and bits of stone are gradually chipped away. As with other methods of lithotripsy, it is most effective with soft stones and less effective with hard, dense calculi. Its greatest disadvantage is that the pieces must be removed by some other technique, and with large stones, the recently created fragments may interfere with the destruction of the rest of the stone.

Because the fiber is flexible, it can easily be used with the flexible ureteroscopes described above or with standard flexible nephroscopes. It is in this area that pulsed dye lasers have an advantage over ultrasonic lithotripsy, and in the author's opinion, this is where their future lies.

Electrohydraulic Lithotripsy

Electrohydraulic lithotripsy (EHL) is particularly helpful in percutaneous stone removal when dealing with large, hard stones. In the ureter, its role is limited to the rare patient who has a large stone that has been refractory to the ultrasonic probe. It is absolutely essential that the EHL probe be used only under clear direct vision and that the operator be certain that there is clearance between the end of the probe and the ureteral walls. Further, the generator should be used on the single-pulse rather than the continuous-pulse setting.

If the probe is fired in close proximity to the ureteral wall, damage to the ureteral wall is likely. Bleeding from such injuries may complicate further efforts to remove the stone, and stricture may be a long-term result.

Technique

Most often, the ureteral orifices and intramural ureter must be dilated before the ureteroscope can be inserted. To accomplish this, we proceed as follows. As the first step, a 0.038 L-R torque wire is inserted up the ureter under fluoroscopic control. Once in place, the Gruenzig balloon is backloaded over the wire and positioned such that it will dilate the orifice as well as the intramural ureter. The author prefers a 6.0-cm balloon that expands to 16 French (Figs. 18-3 and 18-4).

Unless difficulty was encountered in inserting the wire, the author prefers to remove it and insert the ureteroscope only under visual control, using the 0° or 5° lens. The ureteroscope is carefully passed up to the stone, using the least amount of irrigating fluid consistent with good vision. If the force of the irrigating fluid is too great, or if the stone is not firmly positioned in the ureter, the stone may float up beyond the reach of the instrument.

Small Calculi

Once the stone is in the field of view, the operator must decide how best to remove it. When the calculus is smaller, usually 4.0 mm or less in size, a stone basket should be used under direct vision to engage and then extract the stone.

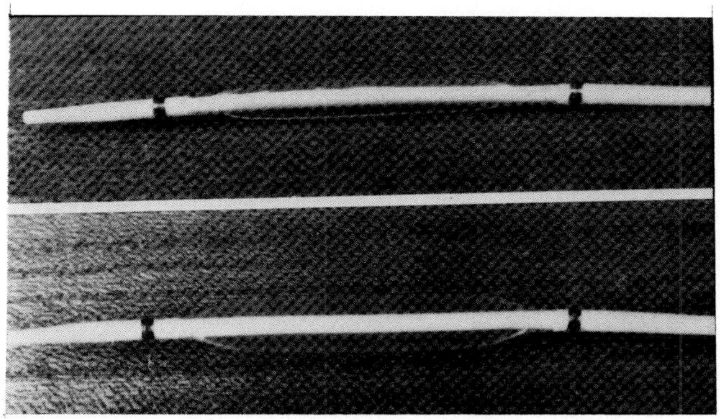

Fig. 18-3. The Gruenzig balloon. This is our preferred method for dilatation of the intramural ureter. We use a 6-cm balloon with the intramural ureter dilated to 16–18 French. The balloon will occasionally rupture with extravasation and mucosal tearing. There have been no complications from this.

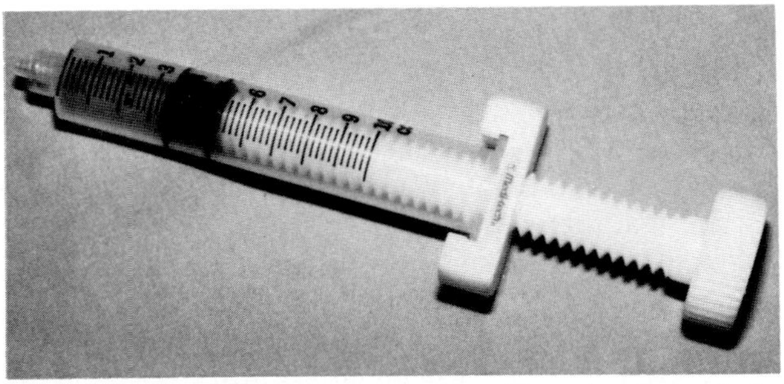

Fig. 18-4. There are various ways to dilate the Gruenzig balloon. This LeVeen syringe enables the operator to develop considerable pressure in inflating the balloon. It is both effective and easy to operate.

Stone Baskets

The urologic armamentarium contains an innumerable variety of urologic stone baskets and other devices designed to engage and remove stones. Many of these were designed in the days before manipulation under fluoroscopy and under direct vision was the rule. Also, the many baskets made by different manufacturers vary only slightly.

The most useful stone basket in my hands has been the flat-wire basket (Fig. 18-5). This device differs in several important respects from others and especially spiral retrievers. The flat wires tend to spring out more and distend the ureteral walls. Because the wires are vertical, and in the four-wire version, 90° apart, it is much simpler to engage a stone than with the spiral, helical basket. Owing to this feature, it is only necessary to place the basket adjacent to the stone and to rotate it in order to engage it. Also, it is easier to disengage a stone, in case a stone too large for removal has inadvertently been placed in the basket.

There are several varieties of flat-wire baskets all of which have been useful under various circumstances. One version of particular utility will pass over a guidewire. The most useful helical basket in our hands has been the Pfister-Schwarz. This is most

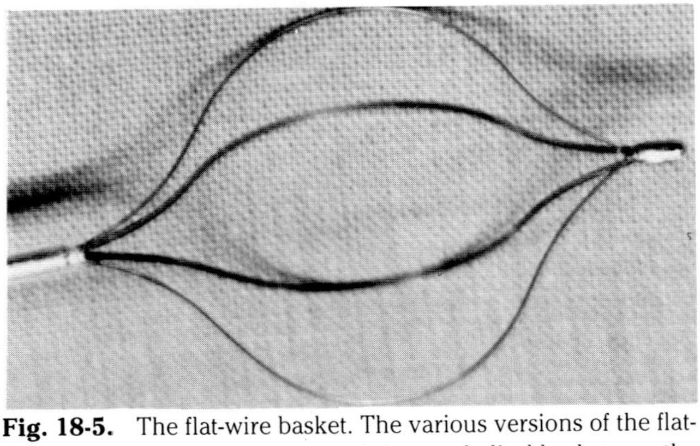

Fig. 18-5. The flat-wire basket. The various versions of the flat-wire basket, as well as the Pfister-Schwartz helical basket, are the author's preferred baskets.

practical in engaging very small stones and in removing small fragments generated by the ultrasonic probe. It is certainly true, however, that there is no perfect basket and no basket suitable for all circumstances. A variety of basket retrievers should be available to meet the challenge of a given situation.

With the stone under direct vision, the basket is positioned next to or beyond the stone. Unless the stone has been wedged in the ureter, virtually completely obstructing it, the surgeon will usually be able to insinuate the basket in such a position that the stone can be manipulated into the basket. Occasionally, only a wire can be passed beyond the stone. In this circumstance, the flat-wire basket that will pass over a guide wire will be helpful.

After the wire or the basket is passed beyond the stone, it is important to confirm the position of the device by fluoroscopy. It is surprisingly easy to perforate the ureter with a basket or wire and to open a basket outside the ureter and to pull it through the hole in the wall while it is still open.

Once the stone is in the basket, gentle traction should be exerted so that the calculus begins to move down the ureter (Fig. 18-6). It is at this point that the art of stone removal replaces the science. One must make several judgments important to the continuity of the procedure. The stone should have come free from any mucosal strands tending to fix it to the ureteral wall. It should be passing freely down the ureter without telescoping of the ureter in front of it. A judgment may be necessary that the stone can or cannot be safely pulled through an area of ureteral narrowing. When the stone reaches the intramural ureter, difficulty may be encountered in further progress, particularly if the stone is at or near the size to which the ureter was dilated. Passage may be optimized if the stone is irregular by rotating the stone-containing basket or by opening the basket and letting the stone move before closing it again.

At this point in the ureter, it is usually safe to place the basket under some traction to get it through the marginal intramural ureter. Exactly how much traction is safe in a given circumstance is impossible to describe and can be learned only from experience. After the stone has been removed, two No. 5 ureteral catheters are placed up the dilated orifice and tied around an 18-French Foley. These are left indwelling for 48 hours and then removed. The patient goes home that day.

Larger Calculi

The stone may be too large to allow removal from the ureter by manipulation, so some form of power lithotripsy will be necessary. Transureteral ultrasound is most commonly employed for this purpose.

Exactly how a given stone is approached depends on the instruments available. In all newer units, it is possible to use the ultrasonic probe under direct vision. This capability results in a precision of action not possible in the older units that had to be used under fluoroscopic control.

The first step is to engage the stone with a basket passed through the working channel that will not be used for the ultrasonic probe. This greatly facilitates the procedure by enabling the stone to be held in position so that the ultrasonic probe can be firmly placed on it. Further, it will keep the stone from moving up the ureter under pressure of the irrigating fluid after it becomes loose from the ureteral walls. As the stone begins to break up, the basket will tend to keep the pieces in one location so that they are easier to aspirate out the probe.

If the stone cannot be engaged with the basket, the ultrasonic probe can be directly

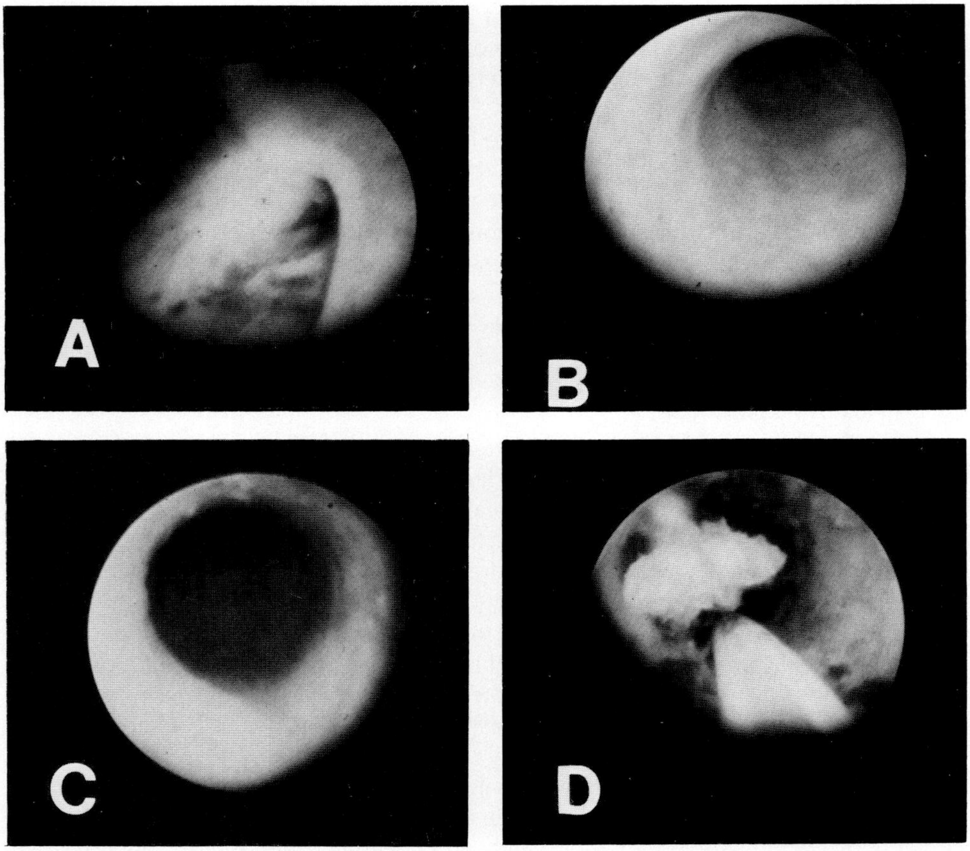

Fig. 18-6. (A) The left ureteral orifice has just been dilated and a 10.5-French ureteroscope will be introduced. (B) The pelvic ureter just as the ureter curves to go over the femoral vessels. The irrigating fluid is running and the ureter is slightly distended. (C) The ureter above the pelvic brim, below the stone. Passage cf the ureteroscope is straight up to the ureteropelvic junction (UPJ). (D) The stone is visible and a basket has been passed above the stone and the stone is being extracted inferiorly.

applied to the stone. The stone in this situation is usually fixed in the ureter, and it is generally possible to exert enough pressure to achieve destruction of the stone. Once the stone is freed from the ureter, the pieces are very likely to start floating upward, and the surgeon should be prepared to pass a basket to engage these fragments.

Ideally, the ultrasonic probe should reduce the stone to powder, which would then be aspirated down the lumen of the probe. In practice, this frequently does not happen, both because the lumena of the newer probes are too small to aspirate much debris and because the stone is often broken up only into large pieces. These fragments should be removed with the basket, a process that may require multiple passages of the ureteroscope up the ureter. Finally, one may be left with only a small amount of fine debris, which can be expected to pass in the postoperative period.

The ureter should be carefully inspected at the end of the procedure. The present author passes the ureteroscope as far cephalad as possible in an attempt to ensure that no residual stones are present.

As noted above, ureteral catheters are left indwelling for 48 hours and then removed. Patients should be warned that they may pass small fragments of stone or clots in the next few days. There is otherwise no particular disability associated with ureteroscopy.

Results

Success rates depend more on location of the stone than on size, composition, or other factors. When the stone is in the lower ureter, the success rate is about 98 percent, with failures only in the occasional case when the ureteroscope cannot be inserted through the ureteral orifice. Because of such results, blind manipulation in the traditional manner is no longer attempted in our institution.

In the mid and upper ureter, success rates are lower and related to the more frequent problem of getting the ureteroscope beyond the vessels. As a general rule, if the stone can be visualized with the rigid instrument, successful removal is likely.

Complications

Operative Complications

Occasionally, the intramural ureter cannot be dilated, despite efforts with balloons, rigid and flexible dilators, and so forth. While the situation can sometimes be salvaged by using the ureteroscope itself to dilate the recalcitrant segment, more often, safe dilatation is not possible. It is best to recognize this fact and terminate the procedure.

Even if the lower ureter can be entered, the size of the ureter may be marginal and such that the ureteroscope cannot be moved superiorly. This is suggested by a "telescoping" effect of the ureteral wall that one notices as the instrument is moved up. If a smaller sheath is not available, it may be wise to terminate the procedure as continued efforts could avulse the ureter.

It is amazing how easy it is to perforate the ureter with such instruments as guide wires, catheters, or the ureteroscope itself (Fig. 18-7). The operator is able to see these holes and thus is able to assess the situation and determine whether the procedure should be terminated. Ordinarily, the hole created by guidewire or ureteral catheter is not significant. Sometimes, however, manipulation of the instrument may exacerbate the

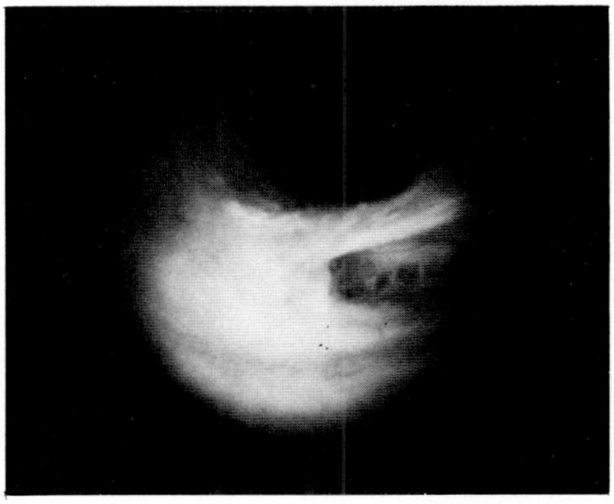

Fig. 18-7. A ureteral false passage. The true passage is superior in the film. This is in the pelvic ureter. This false passage was generated by trying to force a guidewire up the ureter. The tip caught the edge and the hole was started. Further efforts only enlarged the hole.

damage. If the ureteroscope itself is inadvertently pushed through the ureteral wall, the hole thus created is usually such that the case should be terminated.

There will be no short- or long-term sequelae from these perforations as long as a ureteral stent can be placed by the perforation, preferably as far as the renal pelvis. If a stent cannot be passed a percutaneous nephrostomy tube should be inserted as a temporary diversion.

Bleeding is sometimes so profuse that the operator can no longer see well and may be a reason for stopping the procedure. There is almost never enough bleeding for a significant drop in the patient's hemoglobin; it just does not take much blood in the confines of the ureter to cloud the field.

Long-Term Complications

No one knows whether ureteroscopy will generate any significant number of long-term problems. Intuitively, one would suspect that there would be a significant risk of ureteral stricture, but to date there has been no evidence of this.[4] Lyon has ureteroscoped a group of patients with upper urinary tract tumors on multiple occasions and noted no strictures.[1] We know of only one patient with a stricture in our series, but followup has certainly not been complete.[5] Forty-eight hours of stent placement postprocedure will likely prevent stricture formation.

Children

Ureteroscopy in children should be reserved for the occasional individual who has a large ureter for whatever reason. Currently available instruments are simply too large for the normal ureter, and attempts at dilatation of the child's orifice would most likely destroy the antireflux mechanism.

REFERENCES

1. Lyon ES, Bagley DH, Huffman JL: Eight year experience with rigid ureteroscopy: Indications, techniques, and results. J Urol 131:219A, 1984
2. Huffman JL, Bagley DH, Lyon ES, et al: Endoscopic diagnosis and treatment of upper tract urothelial tumors—a preliminary report. J Urol 131:204A, 1984
3. Perez-Castro-Ellendt E, Martinez-Pineiro JA: Transurethral ureteroscopy—a current urological procedure. Arch Esp Urol 33:445, 1980
4. Greene LF: The renal and ureteral changes induced by dilating the ureter. J Urol 52:505, 1944
5. Blute ML, Segura JW, Patterson DE: Ureteroscopy at the Mayo Clinic, manuscript in preparation

Stephen P. Dretler

19

Laser Fragmentation of Ureteral Calculi

Continuous-wave lasers (argon, CO_2, neodymium:YAG) vaporize urinary calculi. The temperatures necessary to cause vaporization are very high, ranging from 300°C for uric acid, 700°C for calcium oxalate, and 1200°C for magnesium ammonium phosphate. It is apparent that with the energy necessary to cause vaporization, surrounding tissue is injured: therefore, continuous-wave lasers have proven to be a poor method of treatment for urinary calculi.[1]

Pulsed lasers tend to fragment, rather than vaporize, urinary calculi. If laser energy is produced at a wavelength that is absorbed by the calculus and not by surrounding tissue, and this energy is pulsed at sufficiently short intervals, the stone will absorb the energy and the surrounding tissue will be spared. This is the principle on which tunable pulsed-dye laser photofragmentation of urinary calculi is based.[2]

At a wavelength of 504 nm, laser energy is absorbed by the calculi and not by the surrounding hemoglobin and ureteral tissue. With rapid frequency of laser energy production at a rate of 5–20 Hz, the stone absorbs energy and fragmentation occurs. The mechanism of fragmentation is similar to that created by a shock wave. The tensile strength of the stone is overcome by the repeated absorption of the light energy, and crumbling and fragmentation occur.

The problems that were required to be solved to allow laser fragmentation of urinary calculi in patients were multiple. A wavelength had to be found that could be absorbed by the stone and not by surrounding tissue, that could fragment the stone into 1- and 2-mm fragments so that stone destruction could occur efficiently, and that could be carried safely down a fiber so that energy could be delivered by a catheter or endoscope to the stone without destroying the fiber.

The parameters that were discovered to be the most efficient for fragmenting calculi were: a wavelength of 504 nm, which is in the green light range. This is achieved by exciting a dissolved dye, coumarin green, as the source of laser light energy. This energy

STONE DISEASE: DIAGNOSIS AND MANAGEMENT

ISBN 0-8089-1873-7

is then passed down a 250-μm silica-coated quartz fiber, and the light is pulsed at 5–20 Hz. This results in fragmentation of calculi into pieces of 1–2 mm. If a larger fiber is used for fragmentation, the pieces are too large. Different stones vary in their ability to be fragmented. Calcium oxalate dihydrate, uric acid, and struvite are the most fragile, while calcium oxalate monohydrate and cystine are less easily fragmented calculi. The latter require more energy, longer bursts of pulsations, and more total overall time for fragmentation. The softer stones may be fragmented within a few seconds; the larger require a few minutes.

The technique developed for the use of laser fragmentation of ureteral calculi currently involves the use of the endoscope. The laser-generating equipment may be kept in a room in a remote location. It does not need to be in proximity to the patient. The energy may be passed hundreds of yards along the 250-μm fiber that may run through the walls or the ceilings of the hospital. The laser fiber comes into the ceiling of the Cysto Room in a rubber tube; it is then coiled, soaked, and sterilized in a basin. The fiber is very flexible and may be coiled; however, it is brittle if "snapped." The current method includes the use of the 9.5-French ureteroscope and passing the fiber under direct vision through the working channel of the ureteroscope. The advantage of using the laser is that the 9.5-French ureteroscope may be used and there is no need to use the larger bore ureteroscopes.

The ureteroscope is introduced in the usual fashion, and when the ureteral stone is in view, the laser fiber is passed within a 4-French ureteral catheter and passed through the working element of the 9.5-French ureteroscope. Under direct vision, the stone may be fragmented. A small yellow filter should be worn over the operator's eye for protection from the action of the laser light. This is placed over the end of the viewing element of a ureteroscope. personnel in the room do not require protection. Depending on the fragility of the calculus and the ability to touch the tip of the fiber to the surface of the calculus, fragmentation may take a few seconds to a few minutes.

It is necessary to continuously infuse water through the irrigating channel because the mechanism of laser fragmentation requires water to facilitate the fragmentation process. It is hypothesized that the laser energy is absorbed by the stone and creates small fissures in the stone. In order to keep this energy confined, surrounding water causes confinement of the energy process and promotes fragmentation. The fragmentation process is thought to be the result of the absorption of the light energy with electrons bouncing off one another in a chain reaction with rapid expansion and contraction phases, creating what is known as a *plasma*. This repeated occurence results in weakening of the bonds between the aggregated crystals and fragmentation of the calculus.

If the calculus is hard and not fragile, the process of stone fragmentation, of course, is more difficult. The method that appears to work best for the harder black calcium oxalate monohydrate calculi and the dense brushite calculi is to use the 9.5-French ureteroscope and under direct vision, engage the stone in a stone basket. This specially designed "laser basket" has been previously drilled with a central channel to allow the laser fiber to pass through the middle of the wire and emerge in the basket (Fig. 19-1). With the stone held in position in the basket, the laser energy is then used to "chip" the stone until it is small enough to withdraw with the basket.

My initial experience with 60 patients has produced 58 of 60 successful treatments.[3] A successful treatment is that in which a stone has either been fragmented so that all the pieces or fragments can pass spontaneously, fragmented so that the remaining stone core may be extracted or an impacted stone, previously nonamenable to extracorporeal

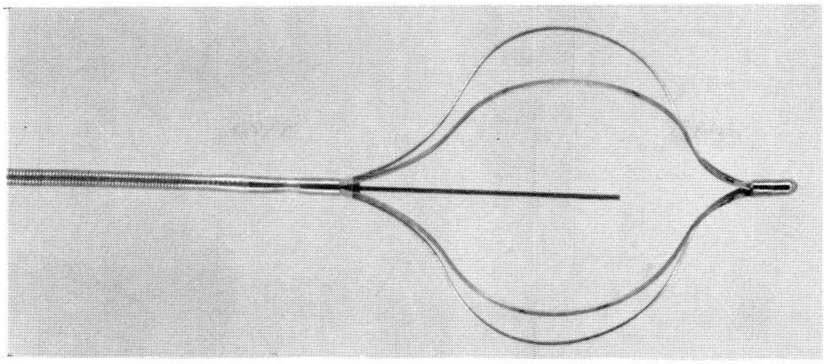

Fig. 19-1. Newly designed laser basket.

shock-wave lithotripsy (ESWL), has been disimpacted with resultant successful ESWL. Two very hard stones have been unable to be broken by the laser. They were both brushite [$CaPO_4(H_2O)_2$] stones, and both stones failed to fragment with ESWL even though a catheter was passed by the stones.

The laser is especially useful for fragmentation of calculi impacted in the ureteral tunnel as it is not necessary to bypass and basket these stones prior to fragmentation and removal. Also, the laser is extremely useful for large calcium oxalate dihydrate, struvite, and uric acid stones in the ureter, which are easily fragmented by laser energy. In addition, the laser is useful to disimpact ureteral pelvic junction stones. Furthermore, it is the use of the small instrumentation that has been very helpful in patients whose ureters are unable to be dilated to accept the larger bore instruments necessary for ultrasonic lithotripsy. The present author has used the laser with the flexible ureteroscope in ureters that could not otherwise be approached with rigid instrumentation and in double ureters. The difficulty at the present time is that, because of the limitations of the flexible endoscopes, one may not both guide and laser at the same time; thus the mechanics of using these flexible scopes are not yet sufficiently developed for reliable stone fragmentation.

The use of the tunable pulsed-dye laser for stone fragmentation is the first use of laser for biologic photofragmentation; however, it will not be the last. Work is currently being done to use the laser for fragmenting common duct stones. Furthermore, the selective absorption of tunable dye laser by arteriosclerotic plaque and the sparing of normal artery walls, hold promise for future utilization of pulsed-dye lasers utilizing the principles of photofragmentation for intra-arterial treatment of arteriosclerotic plaque.

With the development of smaller and more flexible instrumentation that will accommodate the 250-μm laser fiber, the pulse tunable dye laser should be an effective tool for stone fragmentation in the ureter and the upper urinary tract, the common duct and possibly the gallbladder, and the small blood vessels, including the coronary arteries and even more remote previously inaccessible parts of the human anatomy.

REFERENCES

1. Mulvaney WP, Beck CW: The laser beam in urology. J Urol 99:112–115, 1968
2. Watson GM, Murray S, Dretler SP, et al: The pulsed dye laser fragmentation of urinary calculi. Invest Urol, in press
3. Dretler SP, Watson GM, et al: Pulsed dye laser fragmentation of ureteral calculi: Initial clinical experience. J Urol, in press

Joseph W. Segura

20

Percutaneous Nephrolithotomy and Ureterolithotomy

In 1976 Fernstrom and Johannson established a percutaneous tract with the specific intention of removing a renal pelvic stone.[1] A year later, Smith and his colleagues began to remove selected renal and ureteral stones through matured tracts,[2] and by 1981 Alken and colleagues reported a series of patients with kidney stones removed by means of an ultrasonic probe.[3] It soon became apparent that it was possible to perform percutaneous procedures through an acutely dilated tract,[4] and since then percutaneous methods of stone removal have become widely available throughout the world.[5–8] Before the advent of shock-wave lithotripsy, such percutaneous methods were the only alternatives to an open surgical procedure for kidney stone removal, and today, in an era when shock-wave lithotripsy is widely available, the role of percutaneous stone surgery has contracted but still remains an important method of stone removal with a distinct role in the treatment of stone disease.

INDICATIONS FOR PERCUTANEOUS STONE REMOVAL

The patient with a "surgical" stone should have a stone that is symptomatic, or a stone that is obstructive or threatening to become so, or the stone should be a source of infection. Despite the fact that less invasive forms of stone removal are available, one should restrict one's efforts to patients whose calculi fit into the categories mentioned above. Nevertheless, the newer methods of stone removal available today have permitted the physician to consider elective nephrolithotomy in patients who would never have been candidates for open surgical procedures.

STONE DISEASE: DIAGNOSIS AND MANAGEMENT
ISBN 0-8089-1873-7

Very few patients at the Mayo Clinic today undergo an open surgical stone procedure. Those who do are either patients with unusual clinical problems or patients with certain staghorn calculi, where in the surgeon's judgment, complete stone removal cannot be achieved by percutaneous lithotripsy, shock wave, or a combined procedure.

Most of the time, a decision as to what procedure to employ in a given patient boils down to a decision as to whether the patient's interests are best served by extracorporeal shock-wave lithotripsy (ESWL). In general, stones under 2.0 cm are preferentially treated with shock-wave lithotripsy. This is based on our experience and the experience of others who have found that such stones will usually break up into pieces small enough that spontaneous passage can be reasonably expected, without the necessity for a second procedure, and with a total stone fragment burden that is readily manageable by a normal ureter. Residual stone rates in these patients are acceptable at the 9 percent level, and clinically such patients have done well.

As the stone becomes larger, the noninvasive advantage of ESWL becomes less pronounced and the chances that a secondary procedure may be required to complete a patient's treatment, or the chance that multiple shock-wave treatments will be necessary, or that the residual stone rates will be high become much greater. In the author's opinion, stones that are over 3.0 cm in size, whether metabolic or infected, should be treated by percutaneous lithotripsy (Fig. 20-1*A–G*).

In patients who have stones of intermediate size, treatment should be individualized depending on a variety of circumstances. Because the success of shock-wave lithotripsy depends on the patient's ability to pass the fragments, there must be no obstruction at the level of the infundibulum, ureteropelvic junction (UPJ), or elsewhere in the ureter. If the patient has had previous surgery at the ureterovesical junction or elsewhere, one should consider whether such surgery represents a contraindication to ESWL and whether there may be limitations on the patient's ability to pass the stoney fragments.

Table 20-1 lists the indications for percutaneous stone removal in the first year of operation of the shock-wave machine at the Mayo Clinic.[10] Of interest is the large number of patients undergoing a percutaneous procedure for a large-bulk stone or staghorn calculus, or those undergoing percutaneous lithotripsy as part of a combined procedure. There are a variety of other miscellaneous indications for such surgery. As a percentage, 86 percent of the group underwent shock-wave lithotripsy and 14 percent underwent percutaneous procedures. In the same time period another 180 patients underwent ureteroscopic stone removal only. It is probably true that many of the patients who underwent shock-wave lithotripsy in this first year of our experience with this machine should, in fact, have undergone a percutaneous procedure and the percentage distribution of stones should have been more like 80 percent shock wave and 20 percent percutaneous.

Before the advent of ESWL we routinely removed mid and upper ureteral stones by percutaneous routes. Today, such stones are removed percutaneously only when they are associated with a renal stone that is being approached percutaneously or in the event of failure of shock-wave lithotripsy to destroy a ureteral stone, or for an occasional patient with a very large ureteral stone in which successful shock-wave lithotripsy seems unlikely.

The "typical" upper ureteral stone is treated first by an attempt to push the stone into the renal pelvis for subsequent shock-wave lithotripsy, or failing that, by an attempt to shock it in situ, or perhaps to manage it ureteroscopically, as noted in Chapter 18.

Table 20-1
Indications for Percutaneous Techniques in 143 Patients

	Total	Percent
Obstruction	23	16
Ureteral	4	
UPJ	14	
Infundibular	5	
Stone volume	66	46
Large pelvic stone volume	17	
Staghorn	18	
Combined ESWL and percutaneous	31	
Body habitus	10	7
Patient too large	7	
Patient too small	1	
Scoliosis	2	
Other modality failures	21	15
Ureteroscopic failures, ureteral stones	4	
ESWL failures		
Stone did not break	3	
Retained significant fragments	12	
Hemorrhage after ESWL	1	
Hypotension in bath	1	
Miscellaneous	23	16
Cystine	11	
Cardiac pacemaker	4	
Calcified renal artery aneurysm	1	
Indwelling nephrostomy tube	3	
Patient request percutaneous removal	4	

TECHNIQUE

Percutaneous stone removal may be divided into two parts: (1) percutaneous access or nephrostomy tube insertion and (2) percutaneous stone removal. The exact relationship of these two events to each other, whether they are done on different days or the same day, and where in the hospital they are done and by whom, are not terribly relevant considerations and vary widely from place to place. The technique summarized below has worked well at Mayo in a large number of percutaneous procedures.[9]

Access

Percutaneous nephrostomy tube insertion is performed by the interventional radiologist in the Department of Diagnostic Radiology under IV sedation and local anesthesia either the afternoon before or the morning of the attempt at lithotripsy (Fig. 20-2*A–D*). The details of nephrostomy tube insertion have been well described elsewhere.[9–11] Nephrostomy tube insertion may also be done in a retrograde fashion as described by Hunter and Hawkins[12] and independently by Lawson.[13]

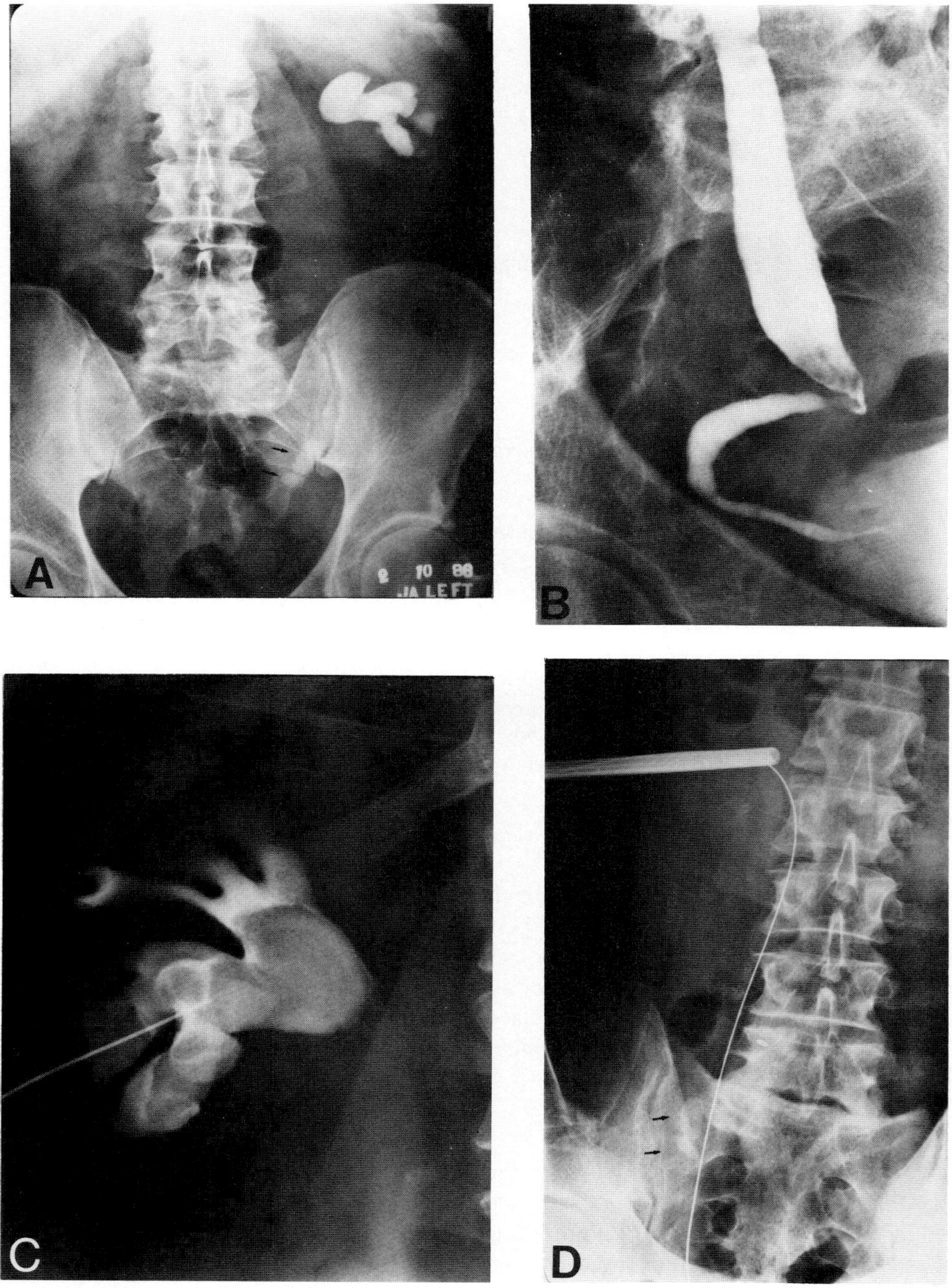
A
8 10 88
JA LEFT
B
C
D

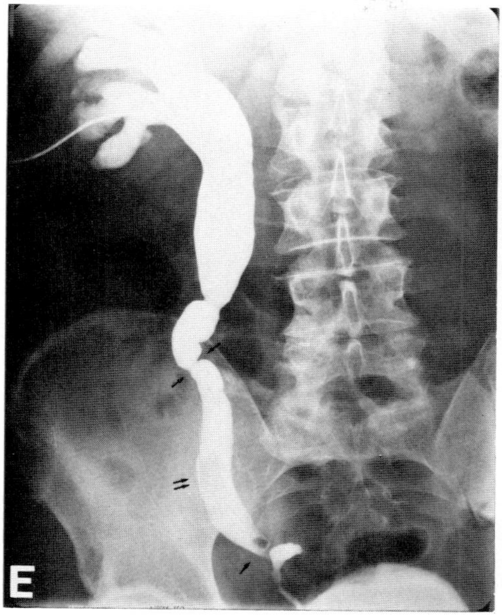

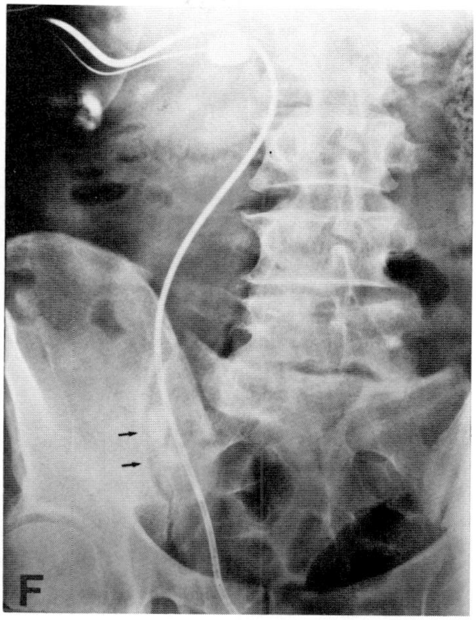

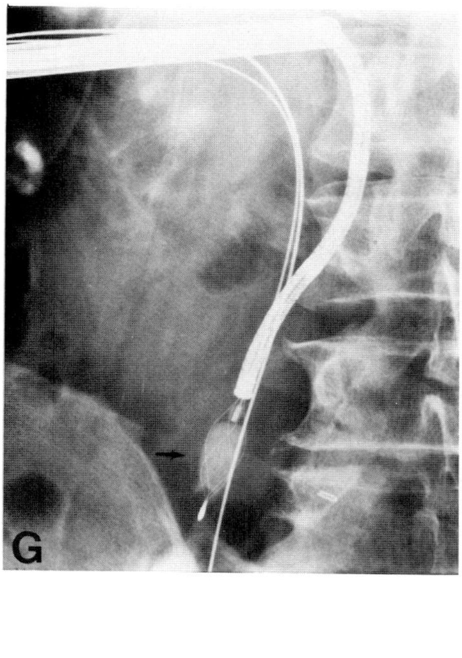

Fig. 20-1. Films *A–G* are of the same patient. (*A*) KUB showing large stones filling most of the left collecting system, plus very large ureteral calculi over the femoral vessels. (*B*) Postoperative stricture at the area of the pelvic ureter with fixation of the distal ureter preventing ureteroscopy. (*C*) Percutaneous access to the stone was achieved. (*D*) The renal pelvic stone was cleaned out and attention directed toward the ureter. (*E*) Midureteral strictures are present, although much of the ureter is dilated. (*F*) The stone is engaged in a stone basket but cannot be pulled up past the stricture and cannot be disengaged. (*G*) Flexible nephroscope is passed down the ureter and the electrohydraulic probe used to break the stone up.

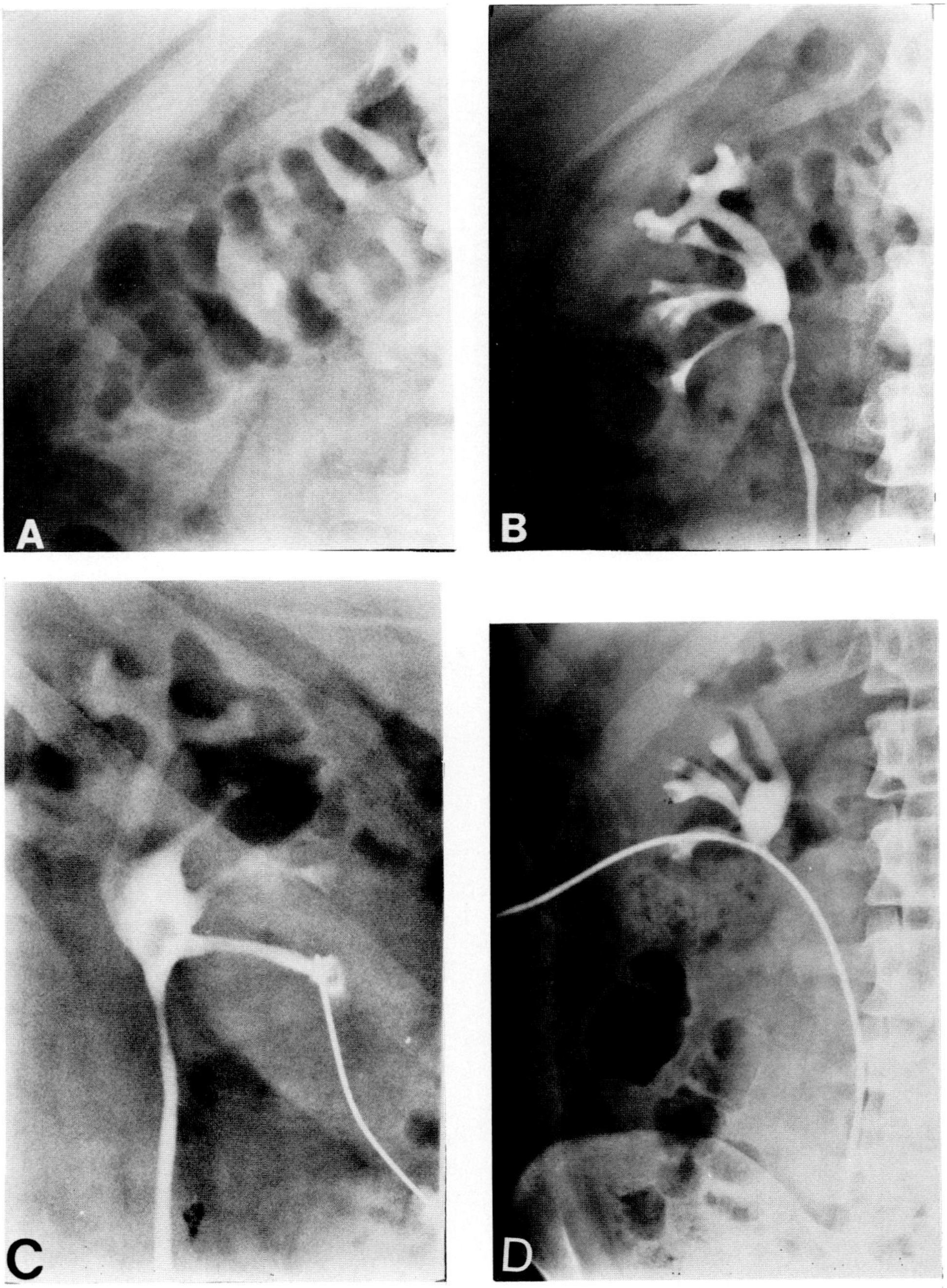

Fig. 20-2. The key to successul percutaneous stone removal is accurate guidewire placement (*A*, *B*). This small renal pelvic stone was removed by PUL before use of the shock-wave machine (*C*, *D*). Success depended on accurate placement of the guidewire through the lower pole calyx and narrowed infundibulum. All films are of the same patient.

Recently, Hosking in the *Journal of Urology* summarized experience with this technique in a large number of patients with successful access in 95+ percent.[14]

The patient is then brought to the operating suite, and under general anesthesia the nephrostomy tube is replaced with a guidewire and the tract dilated with flexible fascial dilators to 24 French. Although other dilating systems are available, we prefer the flexible fascial dilators because of ease of use, safety, and low cost. We proceed to 24 French because the instrument through which we perform all our percutaneous procedures is the Wolf nephroscope, which is 24 French in outside circumference. The nephroscope itself is placed over the guidewire as a final event in the dilatation and the nephroscope sheath itself provides insulation between the tract and the patient's flank. It is possible to use this instrument through an Amplatz sheath, but we have found it more convenient to do it through the nephroscope sheath alone.

Once the stone is visualized with the nephroscope, a decision must be made as to which method of stone removal is most efficacious under the circumstances. In general, smaller stones should be removed en block, without using power lithotripsy to reduce them in size. The largest stone that can be removed intact through the Wolf nephroscope is approximately 7 mm in diameter, although in the other dimension the stone can be longer. This is because the inside circumference of the Wolf sheath is approximately 21 French. Larger, more symmetrical stones up to a centimeter in size can be removed intact by securely engaging the stone in a basket and pulling it through the tract intact along with the sheath. If an Amplatz sheath is used, larger tracts can be created and larger stones removed intact.

Our preferred instrument for reduction in size of large stones is the ultrasonic probe (Fig. 20-3*A–C*). Its advantages include ease of use, but also the fact that the ultrasonic probe removes all stony particles as they are created. Particularly with softer stones, destruction of a stone may be, in fact, quite rapid and the stone may be quickly removed while it is being destroyed. Stones that are very hard, very large, or both will place the ultrasonic system at a disadvantage as the time required for stone breakup increases considerably. Ultrasound is effective with large, hard stones—it simply takes a long time to break the stone up or remove it bit by bit (Figs. 20-4*A–D*, 20-5*A–E*). We have, in these circumstances, used the electrohydraulic probe to break up pieces of the larger stone and then use the ultrasonic probe on these smaller, newly created pieces, as ultrasound is usually effective as the stone becomes smaller.

As long as the stone can be seen with the nephroscope, removal is virtually assured. Indeed, in some 1400 percutaneous lithotripsies at the Mayo Clinic there have been only two stones, both of them quite large, which could not be broken up by any method available to us. If the stone cannot be seen with the rigid instrument, another method of removal is indicated. In these circumstances we have preferred the flexible nephroscope because of its ability to access sequestered areas of the renal pelvis. If the stone can be seen with the flexible instrument, it may be engaged with forceps, engaged with a basket, or failing that, destroyed with the 5-French electrohydraulic probe. Lately, we have begun to use the pulsed-dye laser to destroy such stones visualized with the flexible instrument.

When the stone has been completely removed as determined by direct inspection and x-ray control, or when the surgeon has decided that no further manipulations are indicated, a nephrostomy tube is left indwelling and an angiographic catheter placed down the ureter. We have preferred a 22-French nephrostomy with a hole cut in the end that may be passed over one of the guidewires. A 6–7-French stent is placed in the ureter to ensure that the upper ureter does not close off as a result of edema or become plugged

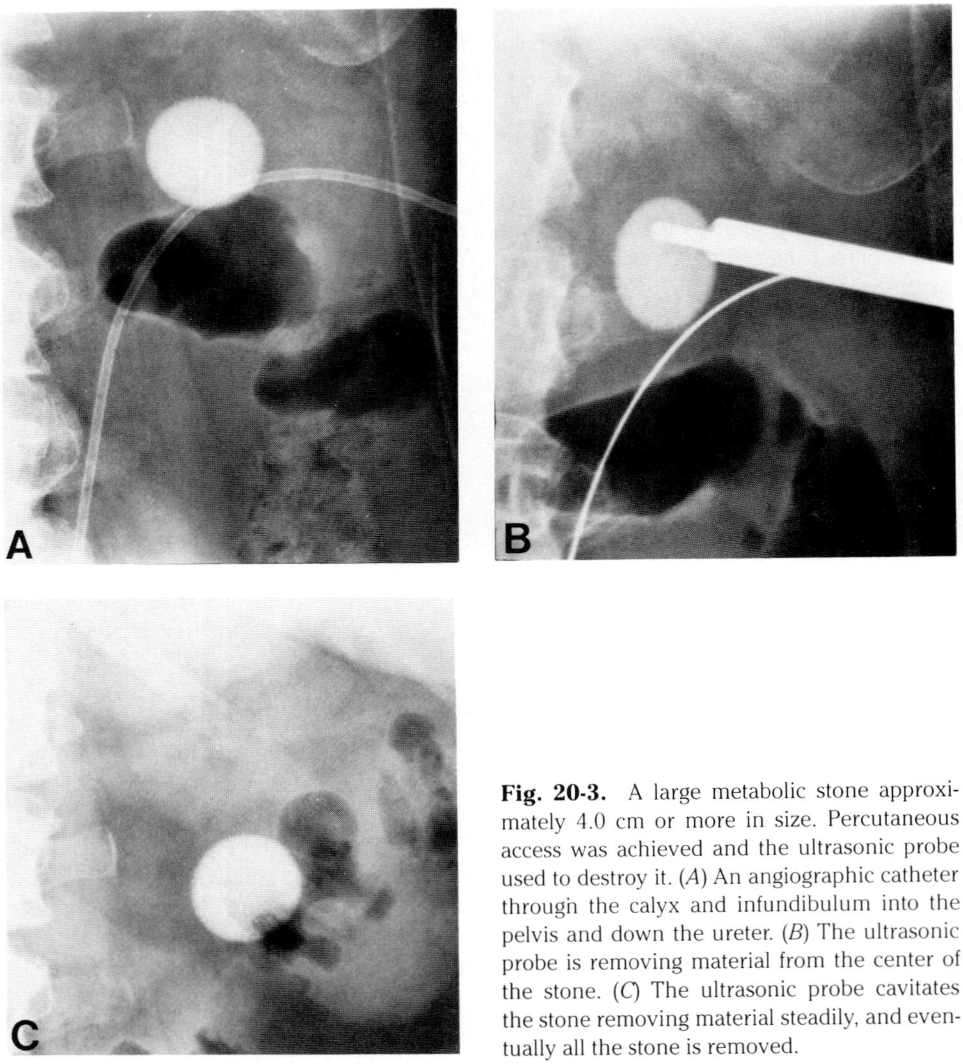

Fig. 20-3. A large metabolic stone approximately 4.0 cm or more in size. Percutaneous access was achieved and the ultrasonic probe used to destroy it. (*A*) An angiographic catheter through the calyx and infundibulum into the pelvis and down the ureter. (*B*) The ultrasonic probe is removing material from the center of the stone. (*C*) The ultrasonic probe cavitates the stone removing material steadily, and eventually all the stone is removed.

with clots or other debris. At 48 hours an x-ray film of kidneys, ureters, and bladder (KUB) is obtained, a nephrostogram performed, and the stent removed. If all looks good, the nephrostomy tube is clamped, and if the patient tolerates it, the nephrostomy tube is removed 8–10 hours later. The patient goes home the next morning.

URETERAL STONES

Some modifications of this technique are necessary to manage ureteral stones. If the ureteral stone is in the upper ureter, it is preferable to deal with it directly with ultrasound if possible. To optimize this and indeed to optimize treating the ureteral stone with any technique, a more lateral approach to the kidney is indicated. By orienting the nephroscope down the ureter, hopefully, one can directly visualize the stone and employ the ultrasonic probe to remove it. This is preferable to basket manipulation, as many of these stones are fixed in the ureter and attempts to remove them with the basket may result in perforations of the ureter and delays in the final resolution of the problem. When the ultrasonic probe is used in the ureter, the technique is the same as with renal pelvic stones, except that when the stone is finally removed, one must be sure to pass the basket down the ureter at the end of the procedure in order to retrieve small fragments. If the stone cannot be seen directly, it may respond to basket manipulation under fluoroscopic control. Failing such basket manipulation, it may be possible to wiggle the flexible nephroscope down the ureter and manipulate the stone under vision with the flexible instrument or perhaps use a small electrohydraulic probe on the stone as it sits in situ to break it up for subsequent basket manipulation.

RESULTS

In the era when percutaneous procedures were used on essentially all stones that were not treated ureteroscopically, our success rates were 98.3 percent for successful removal of renal pelvic and UPJ stones and 88 percent for removal of ureteral stones. This included all cases from the first to the thousandth case.[9] Success was defined as removal of the targeted renal or ureteral stone. The residual stone rates have varied with the complexity of the clinical situations in our patients. In our original best selected cases the residual stone rates were 3 percent but averaged out at about 9 or 10 percent when we dealt with stones at all levels of complexity. These residual calculi are all small and of a size that one could reasonably expect to pass without difficulty. Currently, residual stone rates tend to be higher because of the large number of difficult large stones which form the major part of our percutaneous stone practice. The typical patient leaves the hospital on the fourth postprocedure day (the day of surgery is day 1), mean 5.2 days, range 2–17 days). This figure has not changed despite the change in complexion of our more recent cases.

COMPLICATIONS

Complications may take a variety of forms and occur at any point in the process of stone extraction. Review of Table 20-2 reveals the number and type of complications occurring in the first 1000 patients done at the Mayo Clinic. Complications may, in general, be divided into two groups, those associated with the process of percutaneous access and those associated with the process of lithotripsy, although the distinction between the two is not always apparent.

Complications Related to Access

This subject is covered in detail elsewhere.[9] Inaccurate placement of the percutaneous nephrostomy tube may result in adjacent organ injury, particularly to the spleen and colon and possibly the duodenum. Two injuries to the colon occurred in our series, both of which were managed conservatively without difficulty. Pleural injuries, which are more common with supra-twelfth-rib approaches (8 percent in our experience) were

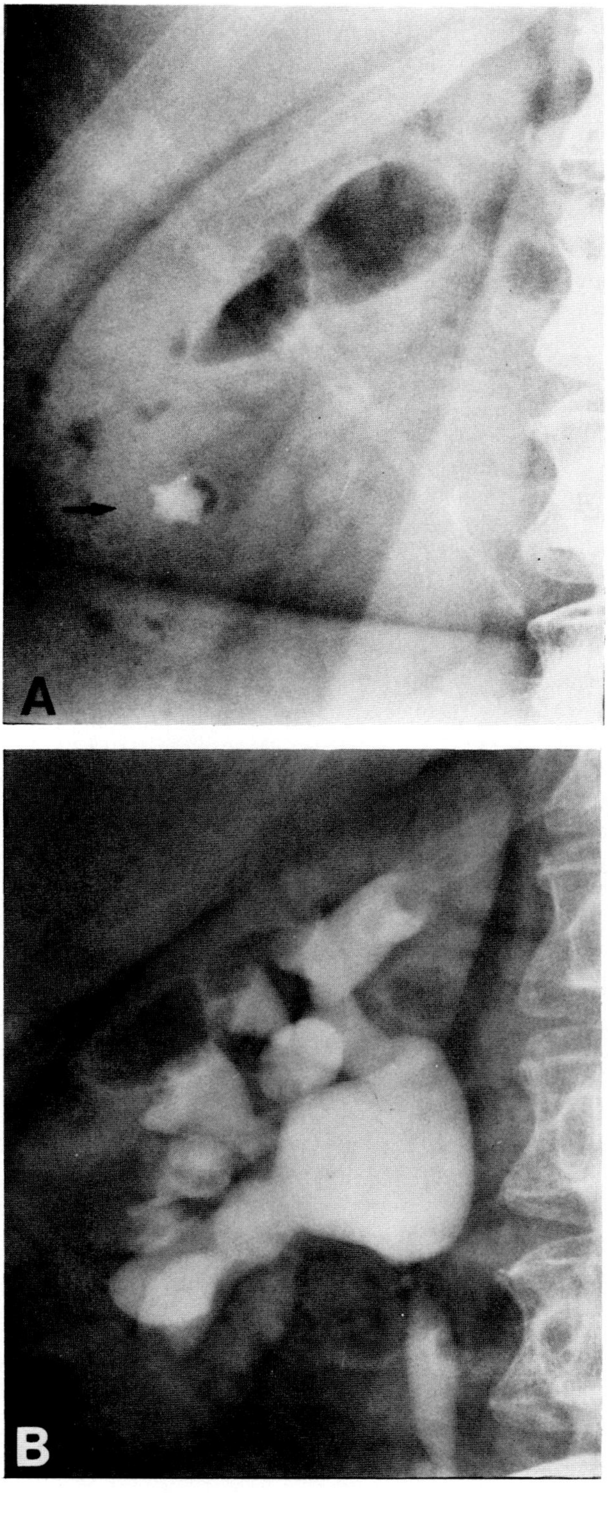
A
B

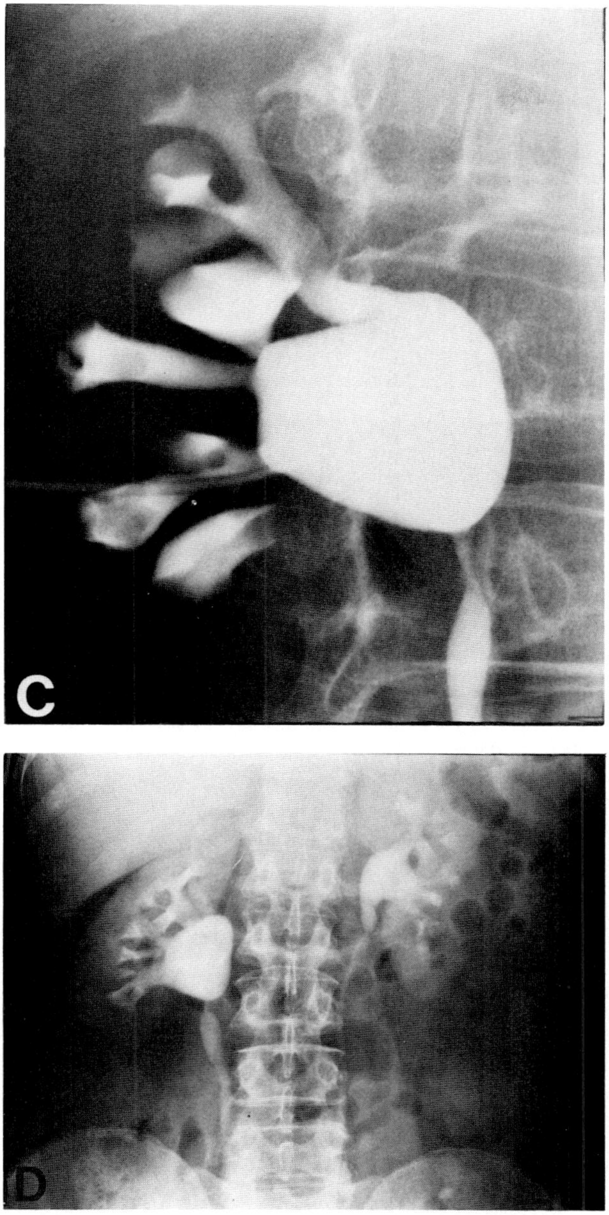

Fig. 20-4. (*A*) A Jackstone calculus in the lower pole of the right kidney. (*B*) There also is associated UPJ obstruction of uncertain provenance. (*C, D*) Percutaneous access is achieved through the calyx wherein lies the stone. The UPJ was dilated, and films taken 4 months later (*D*), show a persistent full renal pelvis, but the caliectasis has disappeared.

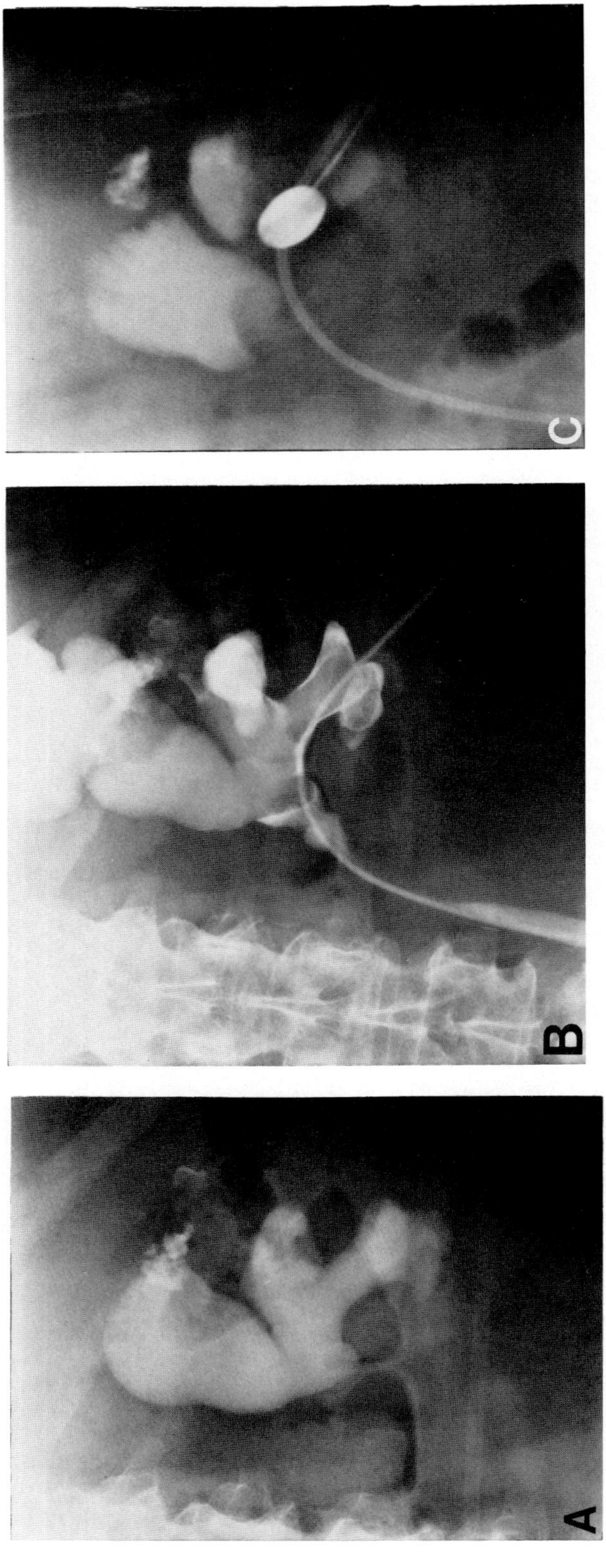
C
B
A

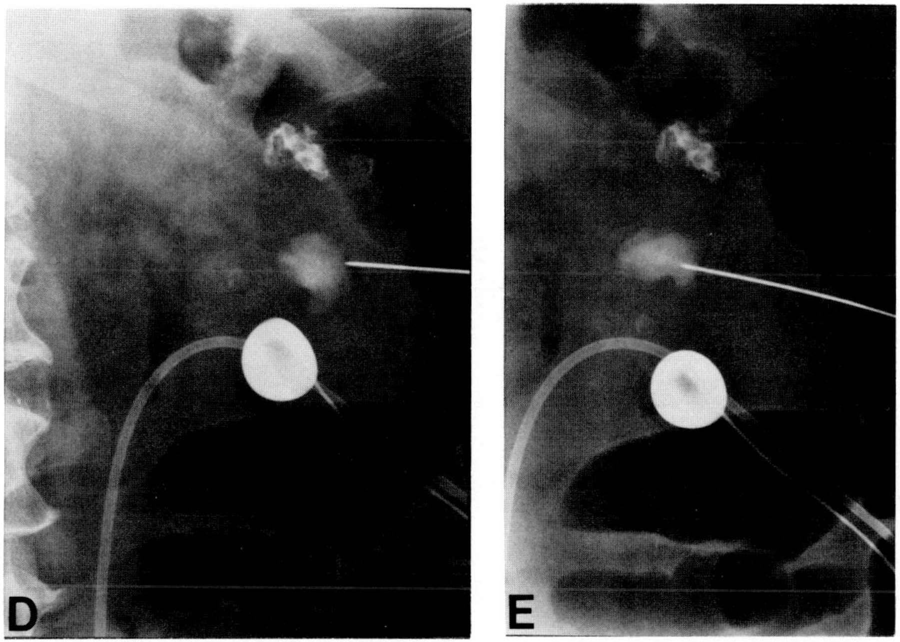

Fig. 20-5. (*A*) A cystine staghorn calculus. (*B*) Percutaneous access is achieved. (*C*) Much of the stone is removed. (*D*) After a second procedure, all the remaining stone is removed, except for two calyceal fragments that are pushed into the collecting system with a needle and destroyed with the ultrasonic probe. (*E*) A residual piece just above the balloon is removed with the ultrasonic probe.

Table 20-2
Significant Complications and Their Treatment in 1000 Cases of Percutaneous Removal of Surgical Stones

Complication	Treatment	Number of Patients
Arteriovenous fistula	Embolization	6
Significant postoperative bleeding	Nephrectomy (elsewhere)	1
Excessive intraoperative bleeding	Procedure stopped	6
Improper scope insertion	Procedure stopped	1
Mild postoperative UPJ stricture	No treatment (yet)	1
Dilators lacerated parenchyma	Surgery	2
Colocutaneous fistula	Conservative treatment	2
Postoperative pneumothorax	Conservative treatment	1
Ureteral separation	Surgery	1
Ureteral perforation, stone in retroperitoneum	No treatment	1
Ureteral basket impaction, could not remove	Surgery	1
Immediate postoperative septic shock	Medical treatment	2
Postoperative candidemia	Medical treatment	4
Too many ureteral stones in basket, could not remove stones or basket	Patience, removed basket and stones easily through tract 2 days later	1
Pelvic tear and extravasation	Conservative	2

identified in only 0.001 percent but may actually occur more often as an asymptomatic event. Bleeding associated with the process of access is uncommon, and although—at least in theory—the process of nephrostomy tube placement might inadvertently result in arterial injury, in fact, in some 1400 percutaneous nephrostomy tube placements for renal stone extraction, no instance of bleeding could be ascribed to arterial injury (see Tables 20-3 and 20-4).

Table 20-3
Causes of Failure in 15 of 805 Patients with Renal Stones Who Underwent Percutaneous Removal

	Number of Patients
Problems of access	
Inadequate tract placement	3
Could not access	2
Instrument not in kidney	2
Laceration from dilatation	1
Could not dilate (obesity)	1
Could not dilate (obesity and scar)	1
Problems of lithotripsy	
Stone too hard	1
1-cm pelvic tear	1
Could not move scope (retroperitoneal fibrosis)	1
Could not visualize stone (extravasation)	1
Extravasation	1

Table 20-4
Causes and Treatment of Failure in 23 of 195 Ureteral Stone Patients Managed by Percutaneous Methods

	Number of Patients
Causes of failure	
Could not engage stone	17
Could not disengage stone	1
Bleeding	1
Trauma to lower pole and pelvis	1
Could not dilate (obesity)	2
Ureteral perforation	1
Treatment of failure	
Ureterolithotomy	16
Ureteroscopic stone manipulation	3
Transurethral stone manipulation	1
No treatment	3

Complications Related to Lithotripsy

All patients undergoing percutaneous lithotripsy bleed to a greater or lesser extent, much as is the case in those patients undergoing transurethral resection of the prostate. Usually the amount of bleeding is not great, although the mean hemoglobin loss in our patients is 1.2 g. Large amounts of bleeding from the procedure may simply be due to intravenous extravasation. This possibility is suggested by large amounts of dark venous blood visible while little or no irrigating fluid is running but a visual field entirely free of blood when the irrigating fluid is flowing. Treatment is straightforward: simply plugging the nephrostomy tube for 30–40 minutes and then administering mannitol is effective. We have performed this maneuver many times without any problem.

Certainly the most significant problem associated with lithotripsy is arterial bleeding associated with arteriovenous (AV) fistula formation. Patterson has reviewed our cases in detail.[15] The incidence is approximately 0.5 percent. The patient may present with sudden serious arterial bleeding that requires immediate treatment with transfusion and supportive measures. Definitive treatment is by arteriography with embolization of the injured peripheral vessel. The author has had the impression that most of these cases are associated with trauma at some point in the procedure, but two of our cases had seemingly uncomplicated percutaneous access or lithotripsy. Surgery should be avoided if possible because of the distinct possibility that the operation may result in nephrectomy.

Long-Term Complications

There are no known long-term complications associated with percutaneous stone removal. Studies by Marberger et al.[16] and Segura et al.[17] reveal no increased incidence of new stone formation in followups up to 1–4 years. The review by Marberger involved a detailed evaluation on a group of patients whose followup was up to 4 years in length. We have one instance of an acquired UPJ stricture secondary to percutaneous stone removal. Although certainly not every patient who had a percutaneous ultrasonic lithotripsy (PUL) has had a follow-up excretory urogram, the vast majority of these patients who have had such an evaluation have had normal urinary tracts.

REFERENCES

1. Fernström I, Johannson B: Percutaneous pyelolithotomy. A new extraction technique. Scand J Urol Nephrol 10-257, 1976
2. Smith AD, Reinke DB, Miller RP, et al: Percutaneous nephrostomy in the management of ureteral and renal calculi. Radiology 133:49–54, 1979
3. Alken P, Hutschenreiter G, Günther R, et al: Percutaneous stone manipulation. J Urol 125:463, 1981
4. Segura JW, Patterson DE, LeRoy AJ, et al: Percutaneous removal of kidney stones: Preliminary report. Mayo Clin Proc 57:615–619, 1982
5. White EC, Smith AD: Percutaneous stone extraction from 200 patients. J Urol 132:437, 1984
6. Clayman RV, Surya V, Miller RP, et al: Percutaneous nephrolithotomy: Extraction of renal and ureteral calculi from 100 patients. J Urol 131:868, 1984
7. Brannen GE, Bush WH, Correa RJ, et al: Kidney stone removal: Percutaneous versus surgical lithotomy. J Urol 133:6, 1985
8. Wickham JEA, Kellett MJ, Miller RA: Elective percutaneous nephrolithotomy in 50 patients: An analysis of the technique, results and complications. J Urol 129:904, 1983
9. Segura JW, Patterson DE, LeRoy AJ, et al: Percutaneous removal of kidney stones: Review of 1,000 cases. J Urol 134:1077, 1985
10. LeRoy AJ, Segura JW, Williams JH Jr, et al: Percutaneous renal calculus removal in an ESWL practice. J Urol, in preparation
11. Segura JW, Patterson DE, LeRoy AJ, et al: Percutaneous lithotripsy. J Urol 130:1051, 1983
12. Hunter PT, Hawkins IF, Finlayson B, et al: Hawkins-Hunter retrograde transcutaneous nephrostomy: A new technique. Urology 22:583, 1983
13. Lawson RK, Murphy JB, Taylor AJ, et al: Retrograde method for percutaneous access to kidney. Urology 22:580–582, 1983
14. Hosking DH: Retrograde nephrostomy: Experience with two techniques. J Urol 135:1146, 1986
15. Patterson DE, Segura JW, LeRoy, et al: The etiology and treatment of delayed bleeding following percutaneous lithotripsy. J Urol 133:447, 1985
16. Marberger M, Stackl W, Hruby W, et al: Late sequelae of ultrasonic lithotripsy of renal calculi. J Urol 133:170, 1985
17. Segura JW, Patterson DE, LeRoy AJ, et al: Long-term follow-up of patients undergoing percutaneous ultrasonic lithotripsy. J Urol (abstract for North Central Section of AUA, November 3–9. 1985, Palm Beach, FL)

David A. Diamond
Mani Menon

21

Pyelolithotomy and Ureterolithotomy, Including the Dorsal Lumbotomy

The surgical management of renal and ureteral calculi is in the process of rapid evolution. With success rates of percutaneous ultrasonic lithotripsy (PUL), ureterorenoscopy, and extracorporeal shock-wave lithotripsy (ESWL) approaching those of open stone surgery and entailing less morbidity, the indications for open pyelolithotomy and ureterolithotomy have become far more restricted. Nonetheless, there remain specific clinical situations, which we will discuss, that warrant an open surgical approach. Furthermore, in our era of cost containment, it behooves us more than ever to use the most direct surgical approaches that result in minimal postoperative morbidity and rapid patient convalescence. In this chapter, we will discuss the use of the dorsal lumbotomy for exposure of the renal pelvis and proximal ureter, the clinical situations in which pyelolithotomy and ureterolithotomy seem indicated, and surgical approaches to stones in the distal ureter.

DORSAL LUMBOTOMY

We prefer the dorsal lumbotomy approach for most open renal stone surgery. With proper technique, it can afford excellent exposure while making for "very comfortable and grateful patients."[22] We have used an extended dorsal lumbotomy for anatrophic nephrolithotomy, renal vascular surgery, and adrenal surgery. It is also an ideal approach to the proximal third of the ureter.[14]

ANATOMY

The lumbar region, which is traversed during pyelolithotomy and proximal third ureterolithotomy, is located between the lowermost ribs above and the iliac crest below (Fig. 21-1). It is bounded posteriorly by the vertebral column and anteriorly by a vertical

STONE DISEASE: DIAGNOSIS AND MANAGEMENT
ISBN 0-8089-1873-7

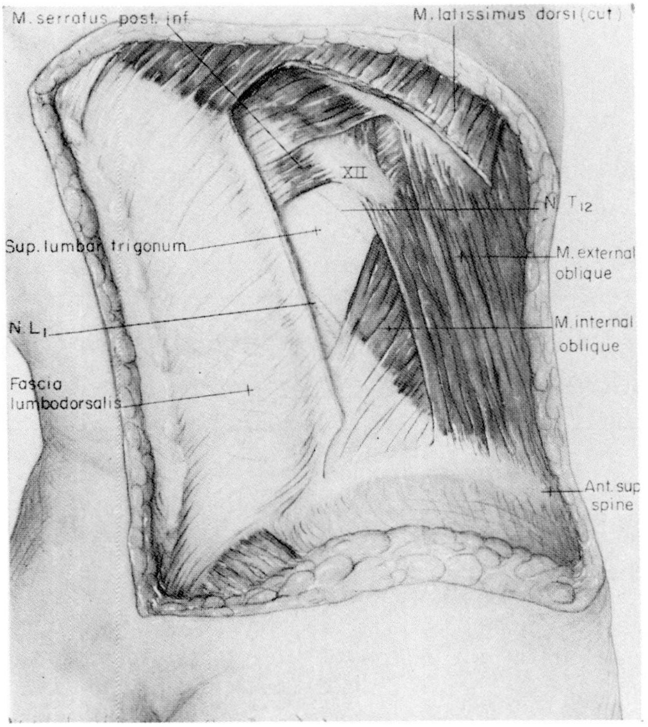

Fig. 21-1. Anatomy of the lumbar region. (Reprinted from Dodson AI: Anatomy and surgical approach to the urogenital tract of the male, in Campbell M [ed]: Urology. Philadelphia, Saunders, 1954, pp 1–35. With permission.)

line connecting the costal margin to the anterior superior iliac spine. In the course of a lumbar incision, the major superficial muscles encountered are the sacrospinalis, the latissimus dorsi, and the external oblique. The latissimus traverses the posterior aspect of the lumbar region, and the external oblique crosses the anterior, inferior aspect of the iliocostal region, creating two of the boundaries of Petit's triangle. The internal oblique muscle is deep to the external oblique and crosses anteriorly and superiorly. In the same plane as the internal oblique are the sacrospinalis and serratus posterior inferior. The sacrospinalis is adjacent to the spinous processes of the vertebral column and is encased in a fascial sheath created by the posterior and middle layers of lumbodorsal fascia (Fig. 21-2). A dorsal lumbotomy incision allows an approach just lateral to the sacrospinalis muscle. The serratus posterior inferior overlies the inferior lumbocostal ligament, which may be divided to displace the lowermost rib upward for enhanced exposure during dorsal lumbotomy. One must remember that the pleura is in the proximity of this ligament when dividing it.[15]

The deepest muscle in the posterior wall is the quadratus lumborum, which lies beneath the sacrospinalis. It, too, is contained within a fascial sheath created by the middle and ventral layers of lumbodorsal fascia. The ilioinguinal and iliohypogastric nerves course along the inner surface of the muscle and should be avoided during a lumbodorsal approach.

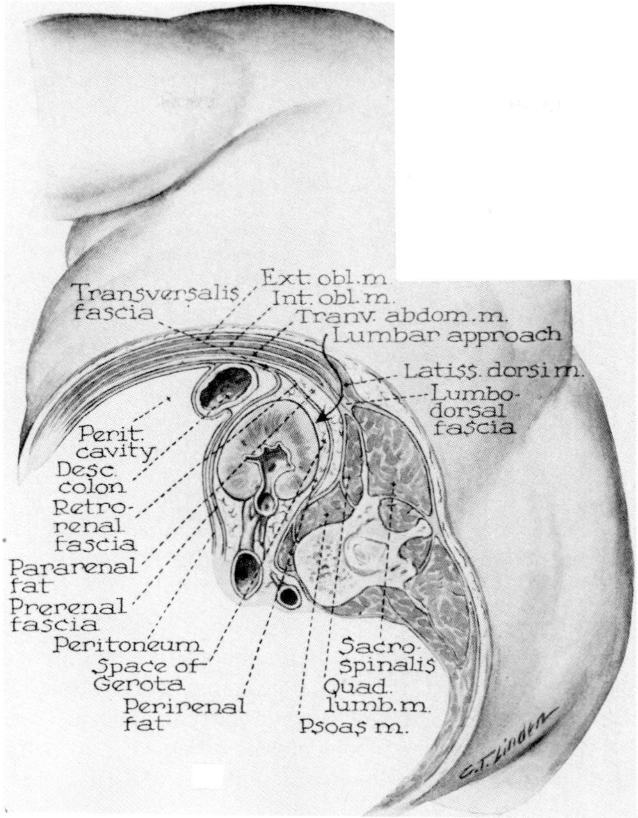

Fig. 21-2. Cross-sectional anatomy of the lumbar region. (Reprinted from Thorek P: Anatomy. Philadelphia, Lippincott, 1962. With permission.)

SURGICAL TECHNIQUE FOR DORSAL LUMBOTOMY

The patient is placed in position for a conventional flank incision; however, the table is not flexed. The dorsal lumbotomy incision is vertical, and flexing the table puts the muscles on stretch impeding retraction. A small sandbag or a plastic intravenous bag supports the dependent shoulder. The up shoulder and the bony pelvis are allowed to drop forward so that the torso of the patient is at an angle of 45° away from the surgeon who stands on the same side of the patient as the kidney to be exposed (i.e., on the right side of the patient for a right renal operation).

A vertical incision is made about two to three fingerbreadths lateral to the spine extending from the eleventh rib to the sacroiliac joint (Fig. 21-3). The incision may be curved gently at its lower end. The incision thus runs over the middle of the prominence formed by the sacrospinalis muscle. The subcutaneous tissue is divided, and the glistening fibers of the lumbodorsal fascia are identified in the middle and lower part of the incision (Fig. 21-4). This fascia encloses the sacrospinalis muscle and is the strongest fascia in the body. The fascia must be incised sharply so that it can be formally closed at the completion of the operation. Superiorly, the fascia thins out over the twelfth and

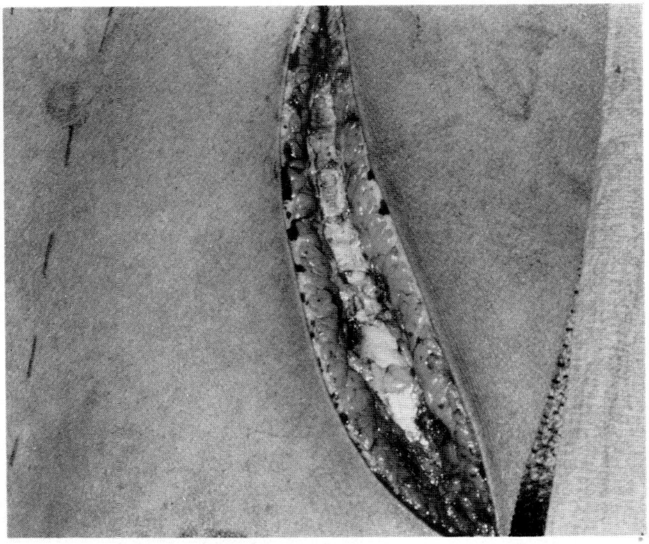

Fig. 21-3. Dorsal lumbotomy incision extending from the eleventh rib to the sacroiliac joint.

eleventh ribs, where a few fibers of the latissimus dorsi, the serratus posterior inferior, and the trapezius are incorporated into it. The incision extends through these fibers onto the eleventh rib. The lateral leaf of the incised lumbodorsal fascia is lifted up with Kocher or Allis clamps, and the fleshy sacrospinalis muscle is dissected away from its undersurface. The muscle does not adhere to the overlying fascia and can be easily swept away with a Kuttner dissector or a sponge holding forceps. The muscle is inserted through fleshy tendons to the inferior borders of the angles of the last six or seven ribs. The

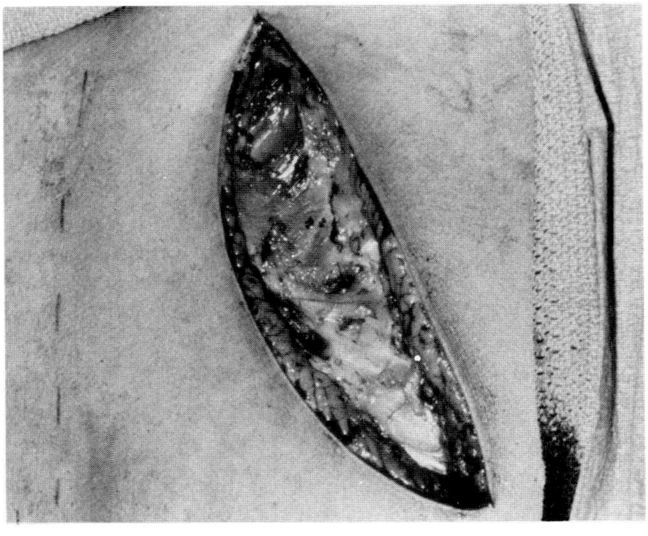

Fig. 21-4. Exposure of the lumbodorsal fascia through dorsal lumbotomy incision.

tendinous insertion to the twelfth and the eleventh ribs are incised sharply about 5 mm away from the inferior margin of the ribs so that the subcostal and intercostal bundles are not injured. This enables the muscle to be retracted medially (Fig. 21-5).

A self-retraining retractor such as a Buchwaldter or a Finochietto retractor is now inserted. The quadratus lumborum muscle can now be seen at the lower part of the incision, under the middle layer of the dorsal lumbar fascia. Lateral to the quadratus lumborum, the middle and anterior layers of the dorsal lumbar fascia fuse. The fused layer is incised with the scalpel at this point. Retracting the quadratus lumborum medially enables one to identify the fused layers of transversalis fascia and Gerota's fascia. This layer, which most often is not distinctly seen through a flank incision, is almost invariably clearly identifiable with the dorsal approach. Identification of this layer is necessary before proceeding further.

At this stage the exposure is limited superiorly by the twelfth rib and inferiorly by the iliac crest. Better exposure is needed in order to perform major renal surgery. The initial step in obtaining added exposure is subperiosteal resection of the twelfth rib. A 1-inch segment of rib is removed posterior to the angle. The ribs run obliquely upward posterior to their angle, and hence much more incisional length can be obtained by resecting the rib posteriorly than anteriorly. Care should be taken to avoid injury to the subcostal vessels during this maneuver. Once this segment of rib has been removed, the origin of the diaphragm from the rib can be identified. The pleura extends close to the rib this far posteriorly. The diaphragm is now incised sharply up to the level of the eleventh rib. The pleura can be dissected away or opened in the line of the incision. This maneuver effectively doubles the exposure obtained. Two nerves can be identified traversing the incision from its superomedial to inferolateral aspect: the iliohypogastric and the subcos-

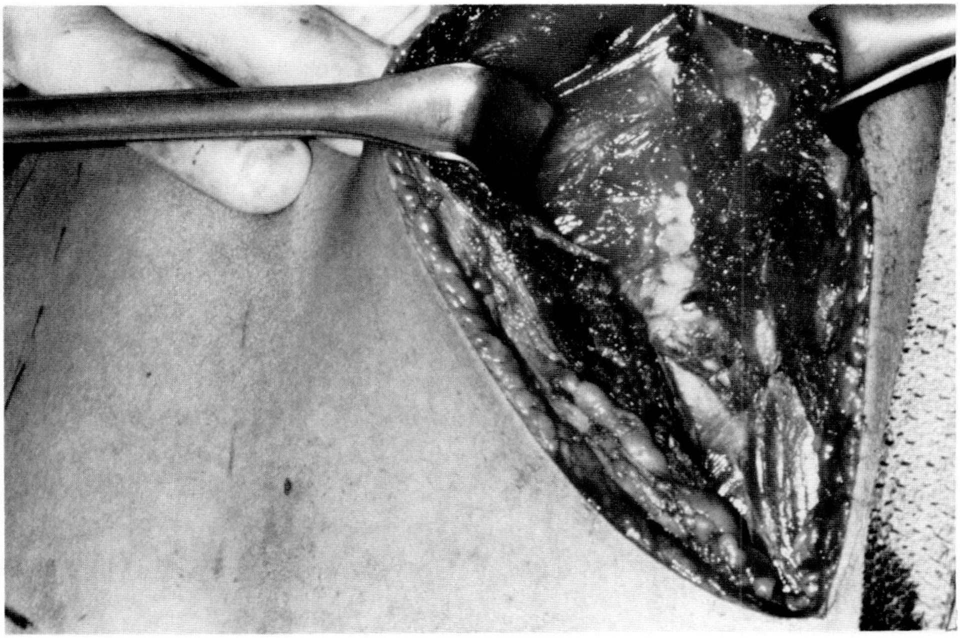

Fig. 21-5. Medial retraction of sacrospinalis muscle, exposing quadratus lumborum.

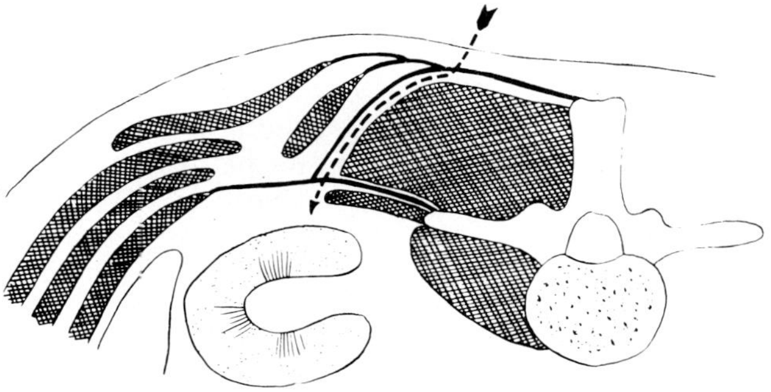

Fig. 21-6. Direct approach to Gerota's fascia lateral to paraspinous muscles. (Reprinted from Gil-Vernet JM: Pyelolithotomy, in Roth RA, Finlayson B (eds): Clinical Management of Urolithiasis, International Perspectives in Urology, Vol 6. Baltimore, Williams & Wilkins, 1983, pp 297–332. With permission.)

tal nerves. The nerves must be skeletonized and preserved. Sacrificing the subcostal nerve is sometimes unavoidable, with varying degrees of analgesia and muscle weakness resulting; however, the iliohypogastric nerve can and should be preserved in all instances.

Gerota's fascia can now be opened in the line of the incision (Fig. 21-6) and the kidney identified under the perinephric fat. The kidney can now be mobilized completely and the planned surgical procedure completed. The exposure obtained usually is sufficient for the performance of intraoperative roentgenography and sonography if necessary. Indeed, roentgenography often is easier through this approach than through the standard flank incision. The x-ray plate can be placed directly anterior to the kidney. This enables the x-ray tube to be placed vertically above the table and usually results in a better radiograph than one obtained through a conventional flank incision.

The closure of the incision is relatively simple. If the pleural cavity has been entered, a 14-French red rubber catheter is placed in the cavity and one end brought out through the incision. No attempt is made to close the filmy pleural layer, but the diaphragm is apposed to the more superficial intercostal muscles with a running layer of 2-0 chromic catgut, obliterating the dead space. The retractor is removed and perinephric fat is placed around the kidney. The incision in the dorsal layer of the dorsolumbar fascia is closed with a single layer of interrupted sutures. Once this layer is closed, the anesthesiologist is requested to hyperinflate the lung. The end of the catheter is dipped in a basin of water. As the lung is inflated, air will bubble through the water. Once no more bubbles are seen, the tube is clamped and removed. The skin is then closed in the usual manner.

REMARKS ABOUT EXTENDED DORSAL LUMBOTOMY

In the extended dorsal lumbotomy, the exposure obtained with a conventional dorsal lumbotomy is increased by the resection of the twelfth rib and diaphragm. This minor modification doubles the exposure and enables the performance of almost any renal operation through this incision. Although the concept is straightforward, several minor details need to be stressed. It is definitely more difficult and time consuming to expose the kidney with this incision than with the traditional flank incision; however, closure is considerably quicker. Although recuperation is much easier than with a standard flank incision, with most patients requiring oral analgesics alone within 24 hours, they do have more pain than patients who have a simple dorsal lumbotomy without rib resection.

Certain details of the operative technique deserve particular attention:

1. One should make the skin and fascial incisions on the belly of the sacrospinalis muscle rather than lateral to it.
2. One should reflect the fibers of the sacrospinalis muscle off of the twelfth and eleventh ribs.
3. The middle layer of the dorsal lumbar fascia should be incised lateral to the quadratus lumborum muscle.
4. The twelfth rib should be resected posterior to its angle.
5. One should incise the diaphragm up to the eleventh rib. While this may require making a pleurotomy, the additional exposure obtained is well worth this maneuver.
6. One should identify the posterior layer of Gerota's fascia, which leads one directly to the kidney.

RESULTS WITH DORSAL LUMBOTOMY APPROACH

The purpose of using the dorsal lumbotomy incision for pyelolithotomy is to take the most direct route to the renal stone while causing the least morbidity by avoiding the cutting of muscle. This was appreciated by Simon in 1870 and has been emphasized by Lurz[37] and Gil-Vernet.[24,59] Therefore, the results of the dorsal lumbotomy approach have been expressed in terms of decreased operative time, decreased postoperative analgesic requirements, and shortened recuperative periods, as well as the frequency of successful stone removal relative to the standard flank approach, percutaneous approach, or ESWL.

Comparing the dorsal lumbotomy to the standard subcostal incision in two groups of 20 patients, Gardiner et al. noted significantly quicker patient mobilization and a significant reduction in the number of major analgesic injections postoperatively.[22] Freiha and Zeineh evaluated 100 patients, half of whom underwent dorsal lumbotomy and half of whom had a standard flank incision.[20] The dorsal lumbotomy group required one-third the postoperative analgesia, experienced one-third the period of postoperative ileus, and had one-third the postoperative hospital stay of those patients treated with a flank incision. In general, the flank approach required 50 percent more operative time than did the dorsal lumbotomy approach. Das and associates compared 11 patients undergoing pyelolithotomy by dorsal lumbotomy to 11 patients undergoing pyelolithotomy through a standard flank incision.[10] In this small group of patients, dorsal lumbotomy required significantly less operative time and less postoperative analgesia.

Gittes and Belldegrun compared the duration of postoperative hospitalization among patients having pyelolithotomy or ureterolithotomy through a dorsal lumbotomy incision to patients undergoing similar stone removal by percutaneous nephrolithotomy or ESWL (Table 21-1).[28] Since this favorable comparison between dorsal lumbotomy and the alternative approaches, increased experience has allowed for the performance of percutaneous nephrolithotomies as well as ESWL on an outpatient basis.[52] Nevertheless, Gittes made certain important comparative points. With pyelolithotomy through a dorsal lumbotomy incision, there is no failure to retrieve a calculus and thus no need for a repeat procedure. (Gittes successfully removed the calculus in all 22 patients studied.) In addi-

Table 21-1
Comparison of Postoperative Hospitalization Following Dorsal Lumbotomy Pyelolithotomy Compared to Percutaneous or Extracorporeal Stone Management—Duration of Hospitalization in Published Reviews

Technique	Author	No. of Days
Percutaneous	Wickham†	8.3
Percutaneous	Alken‡	7
Percutaneous	Clayman§	4*
Extracorporeal	Chaussy‖	4*
Postlumbotomy	Freiha¶	2.96
Postlumbotomy	Gittes and Belldegrun	4.1

Reprinted from Gittes RF, Belldegrun A: Posterior lumbotomy: Surgery for upper tract calculi. Urol Clin N Am 10:625–628, 1983. With the permission of W.B. Saunders.
*Current practice; likely to be lower.
†Wickham JEA, Kellett MJ, Miller RA: Elective percutaneous nephrolithotomy in 50 patients: Analysis of technique, results and complications. J Urol 129:904, 1983
‡Alken P: Percutaneous ultrasonic destruction of renal calculi. Urol Clin North Am 9:145, 1982
§Clayman R: Personal communication to Gittes and Belldegrun, 1983
‖Chaussy C: Personal communication to Gittes and Belldegrun via Dr. Dretler, 1983
¶Freiha F, Zeinehs: Dorsal approach to upper urinary tract. Urology 11:15, 1983

tion, there is no radiation (or shock wave) exposure to the patient or physician. There is no fragmentation of calculi, resulting in small residual postoperative fragments that may cause delayed problems.

In summary, therefore, the dorsal lumbotomy approach allows for pyelolithotomy as well as other renal and upper ureteral surgery to be successfully performed more rapidly, with excellent exposure and with diminished morbidity, relative to the standard flank approaches.

PYELOLITHOTOMY

Classically, pyelolithotomy has been utilized for single renal pelvic stones (simple pyelolithotomy), branched staghorn calculi (extended pyelolithotomy), and single renal pelvic stones with associated caliceal stones, using a coagulum (coagulum pyelolithotomy).

Simple Pyelolithotomy

Surgical Technique for Simple Pyelolithotomy

Simple pyelolithotomy for the single renal pelvic stone has traditionally been one of the most satisfying procedures in urologic surgery. It is with a twinge of sadness that we describe a procedure that is performed relatively rarely today.

The normal renal pelvis is readily accessible through a dorsal lumbotomy incision. Alternative traditional approaches include a subcostal or twelfth rib incision, both of which provide excellent retroperitoneal exposure but entail more postoperative pain than does the dorsal lumbotomy approach.[31,46]

After exposing the retroperitoneal space, Gerota's fascia is incised vertically, on its lateral aspect, well away from the peritoneum. The lower pole of the kidney is palpated and the proximal ureter identified. The ureter is then traced upward to the renal pelvis. Dissection of perihilar fat surrounding the renal pelvis should be carried out on the posterior aspect of the renal pelvis, thereby avoiding injury to the renal artery and vein anteriorly.[55] After exposing the renal pelvis and the margin of the renal sinus, the stone should be palpable. Traction sutures of 5-0 absorbable suture are placed, and a transverse pyelotomy is made with a No. 15 blade. The pyelotomy should be extended laterally with Potts scissors and should be made in the configuration of a transverse smile, thereby following the direction of the muscle fibers of the renal pelvis.[24] The pyelotomy should be well away from the ureteropelvic junction (UPJ) in order to avoid inadvertent injury to the UPJ and the proximal ureter (Fig. 21-7).

Following the pyelotomy, the stone is grasped with forceps and removed. It is prudent to obtain a culture of the renal pelvic urine when there has been obstruction.[3]

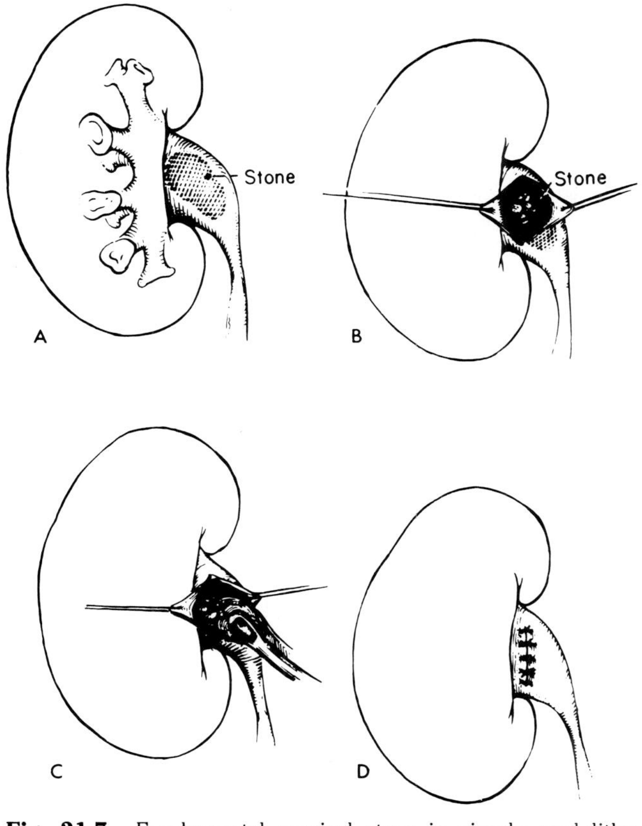

Fig. 21-7. Fundamental surgical steps in simple pyelolithotomy. (Reprinted from Juengst KN, Kursh ED: Pyelolithotomy. Urol Clin N Am 10:649–658, 1983. With permission.)

The renal pelvis is copiously irrigated with saline to flush out residual fragments. An 8-French red rubber catheter should then be passed down the ureter to ensure its patency. If doubt exists as to the presence of residual fragments, intraoperative x-rays are mandatory.

After determining the patency of the ureter and the clearance of all stone, the pyelotomy is reapproximated using interrupted 4-0 or 5-0 absorbable suture. A Penrose drain should be left in the retroperitoneum in the vicinity of the renal pelvis but not in direct contact with it.

SUCCESS RATES IN MANAGING SINGLE RENAL PELVIC CALCULI

While management of the single renal pelvic stone is eminently successful regardless of whether one chooses open surgery, percutaneous nephrolithotomy, or ESWL, the residual stone rate is probably the lowest with open surgery.[56] This is because a surgical pyelolithotomy is the only technique available for removal of a large stone without fragmentation.

Two recent studies have compared the results of percutaneous and open surgical lithotomy. Brannen et al. studied 250 patients treated percutaneously and 100 patients treated with open surgical lithotomy.[6] Half of each group of patients had renal pelvic stones. These investigators found that overall success rates for ultimate stone clearance by either technique were similar (97 percent for percutaneous, 96 percent for surgical lithotomy). This success rate for percutaneous techniques was comparable to that reported by White and Smith,[65] and represented significant improvement on Wickham's early report of a 71 percent success rate for simple renal pelvic or caliceal calculi treated percutaneously.[67] Only 79 percent of patients in Brannen's series had complete percutaneous stone removal in one session, however, as compared to 100 percent of patients in the open surgical group. The patients selected for dorsal lumbotomy in this series had recovery rates comparable to patients treated percutaneously.

Preminger et al. found that the benefits of percutaneous nephrolithotomy as opposed to open surgery applied primarily to renal calculi less than or equal to 2.5 cm in diameter.[53] Above a stone diameter of 2.5 cm, there was no difference in hospital stay, complication rate, or patient satisfaction between the percutaneous and open approach. In addition, with an original stone diameter of greater than 2.5 cm, the incidence of stone remnants was 17 percent, whereas it was only 7 percent in stones originally less than or equal to 2.5 cm. The main advantage of the percutaneous technique was that it decreased the period of convalescence after hospital discharge.[61]

In the initial report of the ESWL cooperative study, 48 percent of 2501 patients had their largest calculus in the renal pelvis, and 73 percent of patients had a single stone.[17] Patients with a solitary calculus had a 77 percent chance of having no residual fragments at 3-month followup. However, the larger the stone the greater was the likelihood of fragments remaining.[57]

Notwithstanding the potential problem of residual stone fragments with either ESWL or percutaneous nephrolithotomy, ESWL is the treatment of choice for simple renal pelvic stones. The high percentage of residual stones has not been clinically significant over short periods of followup. For the vast majority of patients, ESWL is an innocuous procedure associated with minimal morbidity.

In the absence of ESWL, we recommend a percutaneous approach to the small ($\leq$2.5 cm) renal pelvic calculus and pyelolithotomy through a dorsal lumbotomy approach for the large solitary renal pelvic stone.

The one absolute indication in our center for open surgical lithotomy for a single renal pelvic stone would be its coexistence with an anatomic lesion—most commonly a ureteropelvic junction (UPJ) obstruction. While a UPJ obstruction is an unusual cause for a renal pelvic stone in an adult, it is not uncommon in children. A review of 270 pediatric stone cases with J. H. Johnston in Liverpool demonstrated 25 to be associated with primary ureteropelvic junction obstruction, all of which were managed successfully with an open pyelolithotomy and pyeloplasty.

Certain investigators have advocated the combination of percutaneous stone removal and endopyelotomy in the setting of a solitary renal pelvic stone and UPJ obstruction.[9,60] To date, there are no long-term results of this approach, and there have been complications; therefore, this is not our preferred form of management.

EXTENDED PYELOLITHOTOMY

In 1965 Gil-Vernet described the technique of extended pyelolithotomy through a dorsal lumbotomy approach.[24] This new surgical approach to the renal sinus allowed visualization of the intrasinusal portion of the pelvis and calyces without damaging renal parenchyma. It allowed for removal of branched staghorn calculi that otherwise would have required an extensive nephrolithotomy to be removed.

Anatomy

The renal sinus is an anatomic space that is lined by an internal extension of the renal capsule. Its dimensions are approximately 5 cm vertically, 2 cm from back to front, and 3 cm deep. The dense fibers of the renal capsule adhere to the extrarenal portion of the renal pelvis, forming a capsule or diaphragm. This serves to close the entrance of the renal sinus and isolate it from the retroperitoneal space.

The elasticity of normal renal parenchyma allows the edge of the renal hilus to be lifted, thereby uncovering a significant portion of the renal pelvis for dissection. There is a well-defined plane between the adventitia of the renal pelvis and the capsular diaphragm that encloses it. After opening the diaphragm with blunt dissection, the peripelvic space can be entered easily, without damage to vessels and parenchyma.

In the course of hilar dissection, the artery in closest proximity to the renal pelvis is the retropelvic artery, which branches acutely off of the renal artery and then courses along the superior edge of the renal pelvis, finally crossing behind it in its extrahilar or intrasinusal portion. If it is extrahilar, the branch may be vulnerable during dissection of an inflamed or scarred extrarenal pelvis. The branch should be palpable and avoidable in such situations in which intrasinusal dissection is not usually necessary. In all other cases, in which the vessel takes an intrasinusal course, there is little risk of damage to the retropelvic artery, which runs through the interior of the sinus at a safe distance from the posterior edge of the hilus. In 600 cases of extracapsular surgical approaches to the renal sinus, Gil-Vernet has inadvertently sectioned the retropelvic artery on only one occasion.[26]

Surgical Technique for Extended Pyelolithotomy

The extended pyelolithotomy is readily performed through a dorsal lumbotomy approach, as originally described by Gil-Vernet in 1965.[24]

The kidney is completely mobilized so that it can be delivered into the wound. The main renal artery is isolated and held with an umbilical tape, in the event that vascular control becomes desirable. The ureteropelvic junction should then be identified. Proper exposure of the renal pelvis entails separation of peripelvic fat bluntly and then dissection between the capsular diaphragm and pelvic adventitia, using blunt scissors to split the diaphragm. This exposes the renal sinus, and allows for a Gil-Vernet retractor to be placed under the peripelvic fat and posterior edge of the kidney (Fig. 21-8). Blunt dissection of the renal sinus with a moist gauze helps to develop the proper plane and allow for effective retractor placement, after gauze removal (Fig. 21-9). After adequate exposure of the renal pelvis, a transverse pyelotomy, in the direction of the renal pelvic muscle fibers,

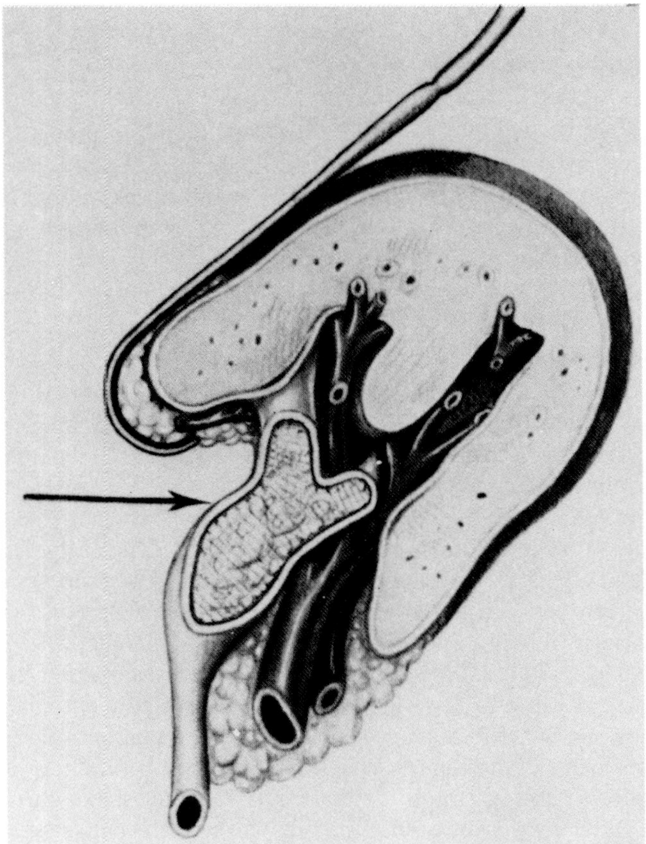

Fig. 21-8. Placement of Gil-Vernet retractor within renal sinus to expose pelvis. (Reprinted from Gil-Vernet JM: Pyelolithotomy, in Roth RA, Finlayson B (eds): Clinical Management of Urolithiasis, International Perspectives in Urology, Vol 6. Baltimore, Williams & Wilkins, 1983, pp 297–332. With permission.)

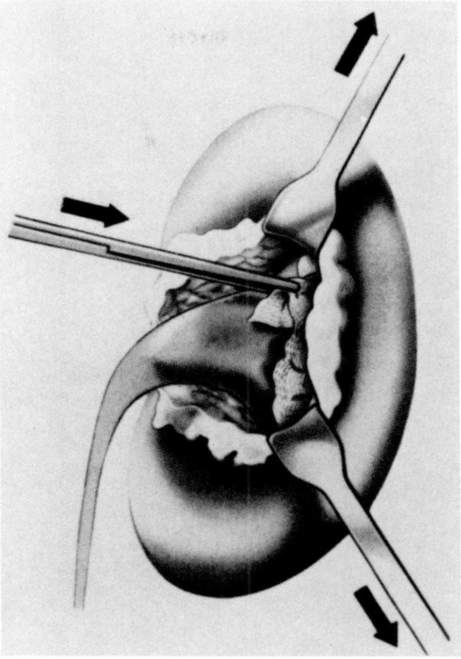

Fig. 21-9. Blunt gauze dissection of renal sinus, exposing renal pelvis. (Reprinted from Gil-Vernet JM: Pyelolithotomy, in Roth RA, Finlayson B (eds): Clinical Management of Urolithiasis, International Perspectives in Urology, Vol 6. Baltimore, Williams & Wilkins, 1983, pp 297–332. With permission.)

is performed. In order to avoid inadvertent tearing into the UPJ, the incision should be made as far as possible from the UPJ, while allowing sufficient exposure to remove the offending calculus.

When one is removing a large staghorn calculus, gentle mobilization often is required in order to extract the stone without injuring the kidney. Careful manipulation with a pituitary dissector or malleable probe is often effective. One should attempt to extract the shortest branch of the staghorn calculus first, following which the stone is more readily manipulated (Fig. 21-10). When removing difficult staghorn calculi, clamping of the renal artery with regional hypothermia may be helpful.[70] This results in some softening of the renal parenchyma and easier retraction and exposure of the pelvis and calyces. The operator is better able to palpate calyceal stones and make accurate radial nephrotomies if necessary. Intraoperative use of the nephroscope, pediatric cystoscope, and illuminated nasal speculum have all been useful in helping to identify elusive calyceal fragments.[27,40,43,66] In Gil-Vernet's large series, 25 percent of patients undergoing an extended pyelolithotomy required complementary radial nephrotomies.

Prior to completion of the procedure, the renal pelvis and calyces are copiously irrigated with saline.[68] The ability to produce a more powerful jet of saline by use of a Water-Pik may be helpful in some circumstances.[23,29] Intraoperative x-rays are essential to confirm complete stone removal. In the event of residual calcific fragments on x-ray, which cannot be localized intraoperatively, it is advisable to leave a nephrostomy tube indwelling for postoperative Renacidin irrigation.[45]

The renal pelvis should be closed with interrupted 4-0 or 5-0 absorbable suture, but no attempt is made to close incisions extending into the infundibula. A Penrose drain is left in the retroperitoneum for postoperative drainage.

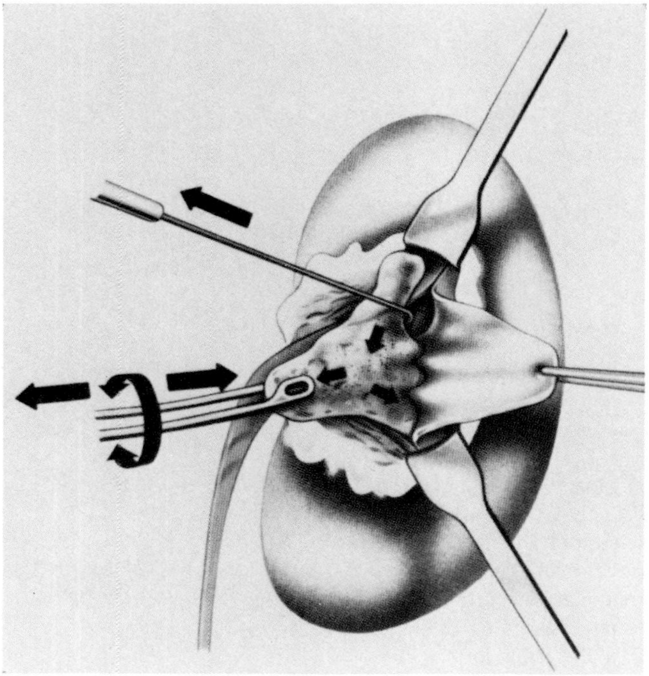

Fig. 21-10. Extraction of staghorn calculus through extended pyelolithotomy. (Reprinted from Gil-Vernet JM: Pyelolithotomy, in Roth RA, Finlayson B (eds): Clinical Management of Urolithiasis, International Perspectives in Urology, Vol 6. Baltimore, Williams & Wilkins, 1983, pp 297–332. With permission.)

Results with Extended Pyelolithotomy

The merits of extended pyelolithotomy must be assessed relative to the alternative techniques of managing branched staghorn calculi—anatrophic nephrolithotomy and combinations of percutaneous nephrolithotomy and ESWL.

The investigators represented in Table 21-2 evaluated their success rates at clearing branch staghorn calculi by means of extended pyelolithotomy, and the residual stone rate varied from 8 to 20 percent.

Certainly the advantage of the extended pyelolithotomy is preservation of maximal renal function as well as decreased operative time. Mean serum creatinine was measured

Table 21-2
Incidence of Residual Stones Following Extended Pyelolithotomy

Study	No. of Patients	Residual Stones (%)
Sleight and Wickham[60]	72	11
Blandy and Singh[4]	152	20
Gil-Vernet[24]	328	8
Woodhouse et al.[69]	189	11

Table 21-3
Incidence of Residual Stones Following Anatrophic Nephrolithotomy

Study	No. of Patients	Residual Stones (%)
Boyce and Elkins[5]	100	5
Wickham[66]	100	9
Redman[54]	56	21
James[30]	40	8

pre- and postoperatively by Sleight and Wickham and was found to be unchanged.[60] Woodhouse et al. noted improvement in renal function in those patients in whom renal function had not deteriorated beyond a critical point.[69]

By comparison, the success rates at clearing all stones by means of an anatrophic nephrolithotomy are demonstrated in Table 21-3 and are comparable to those with the extended pyelolithotomy.

Because one of the concerns of the anatrophic technique of nephrolithotomy is preservation of renal function, a comparison of pre- and postoperative renal function was carried out in three of the four series (Table 21-4).

Wickham found that mean postoperative renal function based on creatinine clearance was improved significantly over mean preoperative renal function in the 100 patients studied.[66]

From these data, it may appear that the results in terms of stone clearance using extended pyelolithotomy are comparable to those of anatrophic nephrolithotomy. It is not clear, however, whether the stone burdens were comparable in all the series studied. It is our belief that when an approach is decided on, that extended pyelolithotomy is most applicable to the staghorn calculus in an extrarenal pelvis with relatively few branches and in the absence of infundibular stenosis. If there are multiple caliceal extensions or infundibular stenosis, however, an anatrophic nephrolithotomy is the preferred form of treatment. In other words, while an extended pyelolithotomy without multiple nephrotomies is preferable to an anatrophic nephrolithotomy, anatrophic nephrolithotomy is better than an extended pyelolithotomy with multiple nephrotomies.

Recently, staghorn calculi that have been previously managed with extended pyelolithotomy, have been treated percutaneously or with ESWL. Staghorn calculi have been managed successfully by means of percutaneous nephrolithotomy alone or with ESWL in small series of patients.[8] Notwithstanding, the general consensus of opinion at the moment is that such stones are best treated with initial percutaneous stone debulking fo' owed by ESWL. A recent report describes the management of 87 patients with staghorn calculi who underwent such combined treatment. At 3 months, 80 percent of

Table 21-4
Relative Renal Function Pre- and Postanatrophic Nephrolithotomy

	Renal Function (%)		
Study	Improved	Stable	Deteriorated
Boyce and Elkins[5]	2	81	2
James[30]	8	66	25

patients had been cleared of their stones. The majority of patients required multiple procedures and the mean hospital stay was 19 days.[58] For this reason, we believe that the procedure of choice for patients with extensive staghorn calculi still remains the anatrophic nephrolithotomy.

COAGULUM PYELOLITHOTOMY

The technique of coagulum pyelolithotomy was described by Dees in 1943.[12,13] It is applicable to cases in which there are free lying stones within the renal collecting system, usually in association with a larger renal pelvic stone that has necessitated surgical exploration. The coagulum is injected into the renal pelvis intraoperatively in order to entrap calculi located inaccessibly in the depths of the collecting system, in order to facilitate their removal with minimal trauma to the kidney.

While the surgical principles of coagulum pyelolithotomy have remained unchanged since Dees' original description, the optimal formula for the coagulum has undergone considerable modification. The original formula utilized pooled human fibrinogen and bovine thrombin. Subsequently, cryoprecipitate was recognized as a superior source of fibrinogen to pooled human fibrinogen.[41] Cryoprecipitate, which results from the rapid freezing of plasma, is readily available in most blood banks and contains 10 times the fibrinogen concentration of that of untreated plasma. This high fibrinogen concentration enables cryoprecipitate to produce a coagulum with far greater tensile strength than that produced previously from pooled fibrinogen. Marshall has noted that the greater the concentration of fibrinogen, the stronger the tensile strength of the coagulum.[42] In addition to cryoprecipitate, the coagulum requires thromboplastin and calcium. Kalash has recommended that thrombin not be part of the formula for the coagulum.[34] Following massive pulmonary embolism in a patient after the injection of coagulum during pyelolithotomy,[49] dog experiments by Pence et al. demonstrated the association of thromboembolism with a high intrapelvic concentration of thrombin and overdistension of the pelvis.[50] In addition, Marshall found that tensile strength of the clot decreased with increasing thrombin concentration.[41] Because thromboplastin is present in all body tissues, including kidney, a clot of adequate tensile strength can be obtained by instillation of coagulum without thrombin into the renal pelvis. Calcium chloride is required to act as a cofactor to convert prothrombin to thrombin, to chelate citrate, the anticoagulant in cryoprecipitate, and to increase the tensile strength of the coagulum.[49] Marshall demonstrated that tensile strength of the coagulum is directly proportional to the concentration of the added calcium.[41] Kalash found that a ratio of 20 parts fibrinogen to 1 part 10 percent calcium chloride produced maximal tensile strength and the shortest clot generation time.[32]

The current recommendations for coagulum formula, therefore, are to use cryoprecipitate and 10 percent calcium chloride in a ratio of 20:1 by volume. Thrombin need not be added.

Surgical Technique for Coagulum Pyelolithotomy

The renal pelvis is exposed as if one were performing a single pyelolithotomy. The proximal ureter is identified and occluded with a vessel loop or Penrose drain. An 18-gauge angiocath needle is inserted into the renal pelvis and the obturator is removed.

The angiocath should provide a watertight fit into the renal pelvis, preventing leakage of coagulum without requiring purse string suturing.[42] One can assess the volume of the renal pelvis and calyces by measuring the urine which is drained by the angiocath. This volume of coagulum should then be mixed and usually is approximately 25 ml. Each unit of thawed cryoprecipitate is approximately 15 ml. The cryoprecipitate is mixed with calcium chloride in a ratio of 20 ml of cryoprecipitate to 1 ml of 10 percent calcium chloride and is drawn up in a single syringe (Fig. 21-11).[42] The addition of methylene blue dye to the formula aids in subsequent identification of the clot, particularly if there are retained clot fragments. The coagulum requires a minimum of 3 minutes to form, and therefore one can inject slowly, directing the angiocath into the upper and lower calyces. After 7 minutes the coagulum is firm, and the renal pelvis is incised between two fine absorbable holding sutures. The coagulum should then be extracted, with circumferential freeing of the pelvic and infundibular arms of the coagulum. Gentle tension with stone forceps or a right angle clamp should deliver the coagulum through narrow infundibula. Following coagulum extraction, an intraoperative x-ray should be performed to confirm complete stone removal. For difficult reoperative cases, Tanagho et al. have recommended the injection of coagulum by means of a ureteral catheter passed retrograde prior

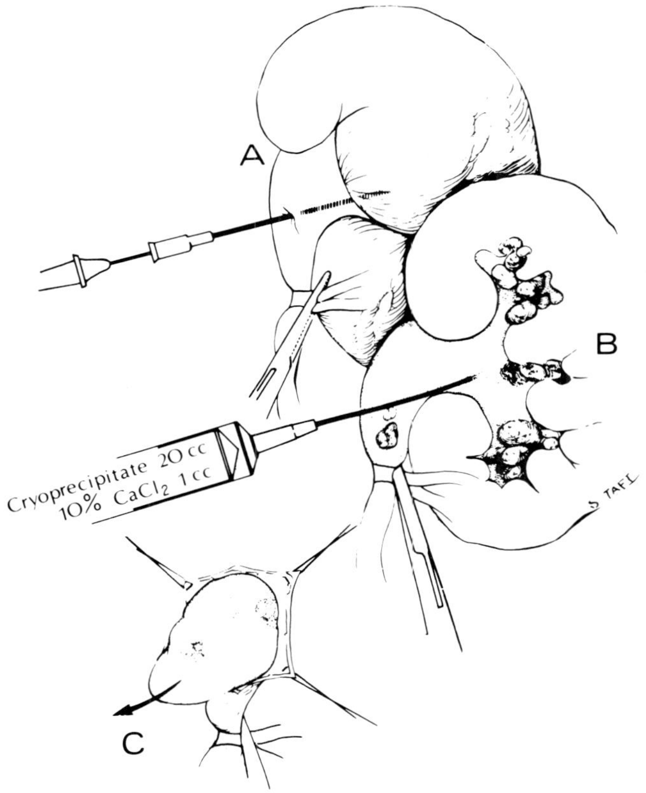

Fig. 21-11. Fundamental surgical steps for coagulum pyelolithotomy. (Reprinted from Marshall S: Coagulum pyelolithotomy. Urol Clin N Am 10:659–664, 1983. With permission.)

to the exploration.[63] The catheter is left in place to localize the UPJ and to occlude the ureter. The distension of the renal pelvis by the coagulum aids in the dissection.

Following radiographic confirmation of stone clearance, an 8-French red rubber catheter should be passed down the ureter, and the pyelotomy should be closed with interrupted 4-0 or 5-0 absorbable sutures. A Penrose drain should be left indwelling in the retroperitoneum.

Because coagulum will dissolve within 24 hours, retained fragments of clot do not represent a problem.

Results with Coagulum Pyelolithotomy

Fischer's series of 61 patients undergoing coagulum pyelolithotomy is the largest described. The technique was successful in 90 percent of cases.[18] A more recently published series of coagulum pyelolithotomies by Kalash and Young described 46 patients with 313 stones.[33] In this series, the authors extracted 99 percent of stones visualized preoperatively. They emphasized that the coagulum enabled them to extract additional stones that were not visualized preoperatively. The mean hospital stay for these patients was 4.8 days, which compares well with that of patients treated with percutaneous techniques.

URETEROLITHOTOMY

Upper Third Ureterolithotomy

Surgical exposure of the upper third of the ureter, from the renal pelvis to the third lumbar vertebra, is best achieved through a dorsal lumbotomy approach. The anatomy of this approach has already been discussed in detail.

Middle Third Ureterolithotomy

The middle third of the ureter may be approached through a lateral abdominal or Gibson incision, which is similar to the McBurney incision.[1] The incision is made at the junction of the middle and the outer thirds and at right angles to an imaginary line joining the anterior superior iliac spine with the umbilicus.

After the skin is incised, the muscles of the abdominal wall are encountered (Fig. 21-12). The fibers of the most superficial muscle layer, the external oblique, arise from the ribs, forming the costal arch, and pass downward and inward. The deep fibers form Poupart's ligament, and the anterior fibers insert into the xiphoid, linea alba, and pubic symphysis. The internal oblique muscle lies immediately beneath the external oblique. It arises from the lumbodorsal fascia, the anterior two thirds of the iliac crest, and the lateral half of the inguinal ligament. The posterior fibers of the internal oblique insert into the lower ribs and their cartilages. The fibers that contribute to the anterior abdominal wall form an aponeurosis before reaching the semilunar line. Above the semicircular line (located midway between the umbilicus and the pubis) the aponeurosis divides into two lamellae. The anterior lamella joins the aponeurosis of the external oblique to form the anterior rectus sheath and the posterior lamella fuses with the transversus abdominus to form the posterior rectus sheath. Inferior to the semicircular line, the aponeurosis of the

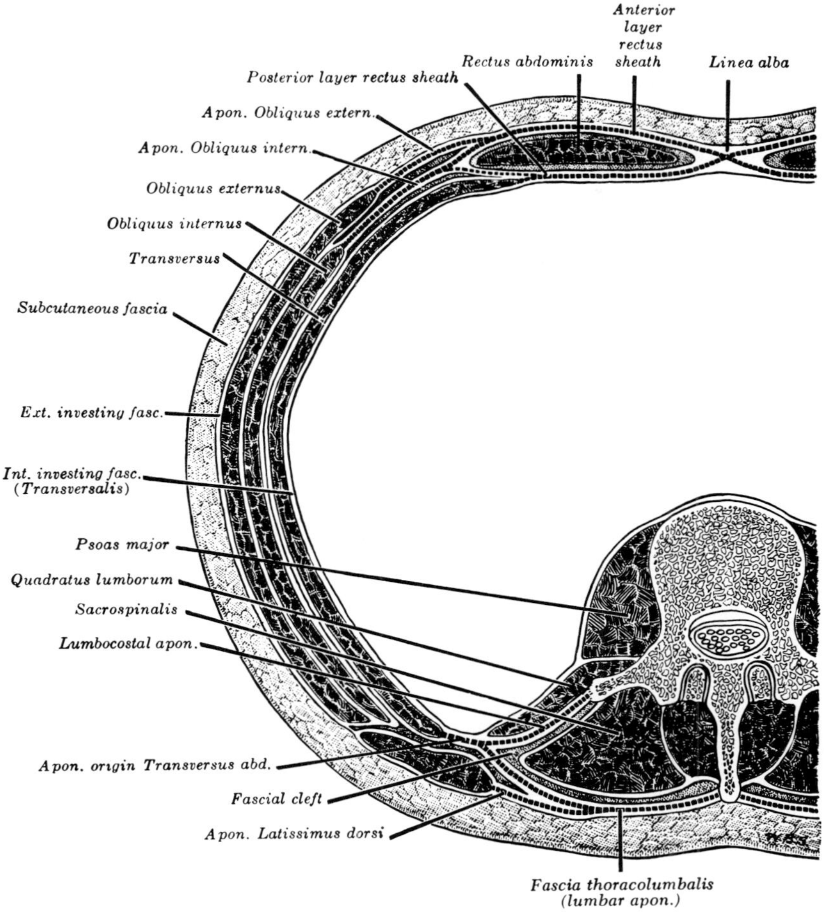

Fig. 21-12. Muscle layers of the abdominal wall. (Reprinted from Gray H: Gray's Anatomy. Philadelphia, Lea and Febiger, 1973. With permission.)

external oblique, internal oblique and transversus abdominus pass in front of the rectus muscle. These fibers of the internal oblique pass directly across the abdomen. The lowermost fibers blend with corresponding fibers of the transversus abdominus to form the conjoined tendon, which attaches to the pubic crest. The transversus abdominus muscle lies beneath the internal oblique. It arises from the lumbodorsal fascia (as the transversalis fascia), the iliac crest, the lateral third of the inguinal ligament, and the lower six costal cartilages. Its fibers pass directly across the abdomen. Its aponeurosis passes behind the rectus abdominus above the semicircular line and anterior to the rectus below the semicircular line. The transversalis fascia lies beneath the muscle and lines the abdominal cavity, with peritoneum just deep to it. Below the semicircular line, it is the only fascial covering of the posterior surface of the rectus abdominus muscle.[15]

It rarely should be necessary to cut the muscles. The external oblique, internal oblique, and transversus abdominus may be split in the direction of their fibers. When greater exposure is required, the combined aponeurosis of the lateral abdominal muscles may be cut downward along the lateral margin of the rectus muscle. The transversalis fascia is then divided and the parietal peritoneum is retracted medially. The ureter will be found attached to the peritoneum over the transverse process of the vertebrae (Fig. 21-13).

The blood supply to the ureter is relatively unusual in that it is segmental with overlap of the blood supply from nutrient vessels at essentially three levels (Fig. 21-14). The primary nutrient vessels arise from the renal vasculature via the ureteral branches, and from the vesical and middle rectal arteries distally via Waldeyer's sheath. Midway along the course of the ureter, nutrient branches arise from the gonadal and iliac vessels. Because of the segmental nature of the blood supply, overly aggressive mobilization of the ureter may result in devascularization and impaired ureteral healing.

Once the ureter is identified, careful palpation of the ureter should demonstrate the stone. If the ureter is dilated, a stone can be readily dislodged proximally. At this point, therefore, it is most critical to obtain proximal ureteral control with a vessel loop or umbilical tape. This is achieved following careful periureteral dissection with Metzenbaum scissors and a right-angle clamp. Distal ureteral control should then be achieved with similar technique. The ureter itself, should be mobilized as little as possible. After achieving proximal and distal ureteral control, holding sutures of 5-0 absorbable suture should be placed through the ureter on either lateral aspect of the stone. A longitudinal incision between the holding sutures and directly onto the stone is made with a hook knife. The incision should be extended if necessary with Potts scissors and the stone

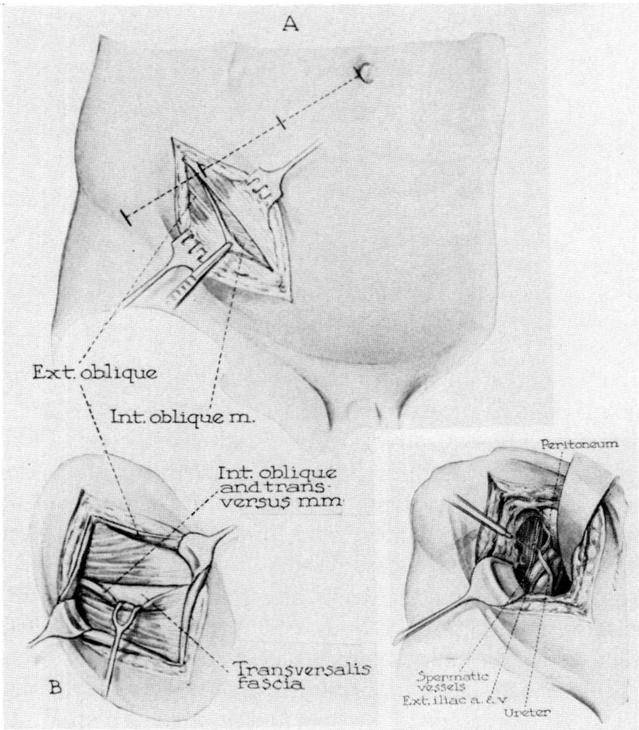

Fig. 21-13. Surgical exposure of distal ureter. (Reprinted from Thorek P: Anatomy. Philadelphia, Lippincott, 1962. With permission.)

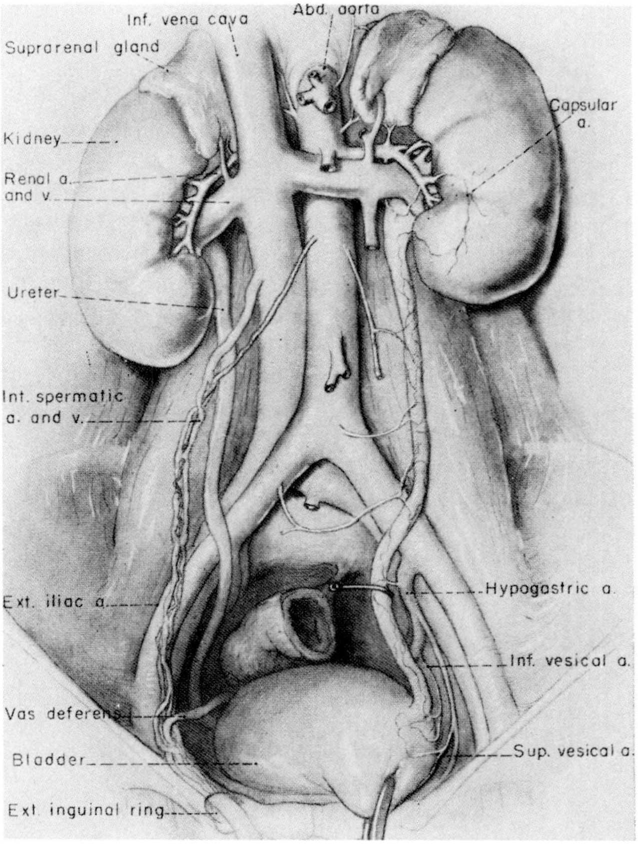

Fig. 21-14. Vascular supply to the ureter. (Reprinted from Dodson AI: Anatomy in the surgical approach to the urogenital tract of the male, in Campbell M [ed]: Urology. Philadelphia, Saunders, 1954, pp 1–35. With permission.)

gently removed with forceps or a pituitary dissector. A urine specimen should be sent for culture. Following stone extraction the distal ureter is calibrated with an 8-French red rubber catheter to rule out distal obstruction. The ureterotomy is gently reapproximated, and pliable tissue should be placed around the ureter to avoid fibrous adhesions to bone or fascia which may result in ureteral kinking.[62] A Penrose or Jackson-Pratt drain should be left in the retroperitoneum and be brought out through a separate stab wound. The muscle layers and skin are then reapproximated.

Gil-Vernet has advocated the use of a transverse ureterotomy, which he believes is less likely to result in ureteral narrowing and may better preserve ureteral peristalsis.[25] The transverse ureterotomy should be no greater than two-thirds the circumference of the ureter and should not be used in the distal 2 cm of ureter where the vascular supply is more tenuous. Gil-Vernet reported 72 of 73 transverse ureterotomies to be complication-free, with one patient having prolonged urinary drainage.

Orkin demonstrated that ureteral mucosa spans the defect of a clean longitudinal ureterotomy within 8–10 days.[48] A period of 6 weeks is required for smooth-muscle bridging of a longitudinal ureteral defect, when an intact segment of ureter remains.[11] Given the longitudinal, segmental nature of the ureteral blood supply, a clean longitudinal ureterotomy seems preferable to a transverse ureterotomy, following which reduced vascular supply may impair healing.

Some authors recommend that the ureterotomy should not be closed,[5] while others suggest that a few fine absorbable interrupted sutures be placed to approximate the seromuscular layer.[51,62] All authors agree that the mucosa should be left undisturbed and that a tight anastomosis, which may predispose to ureteral stricture, should be avoided. In a series of 100 patients who underwent ureterolithotomy with either no closure of the ureterotomy, a loosely approximated ureterotomy with interrupted absorbable suture, or a running closure of the ureterotomy, there was no significant difference in postoperative urinary drainage, morbidity, or subsequent narrowing of the ureter on IVP.[39]

If in the process of performing a ureterolithotomy the calculus is dislodged proximally, two techniques that allow stone retrieval without making an additional incision seem worth mentioning. Zaontz et al. have described the use of a coagulum ureterolithotomy, whereby one uses the same principles as in coagulum pyelolithotomy to entrap the loose calculus within the upper urinary tract and remove it through the ureterotomy incision.[71] Murchinson has described the intraoperative use of the ureterorenoscope to retrieve a proximally dislodged calculus.[44] The ureterorenoscope can be introduced through the ureterotomy in order to retrieve the dislodged stone.

Distal Third Ureterolithotomy

Of all portions of the ureter, the distal third is the most difficult to expose. Perhaps for this reason, various approaches have been recommended for distal third ureterolithotomy.

Standard Approach

The standard approach to distal third ureterolithotomy entails exposure of the ureter extraperitoneally through a Gibson, midline, paramedian, or Pfannenstiel incision. The bladder should be decompressed with a Foley catheter in order to retract it medially. The ureter is readily identified as it crosses the bifurcation of the iliac vessels. In order to obtain distal ureteral exposure, the superior vesical artery must be divided.[5] The calculus should be managed as described previously, but because of the difficult exposure it is often best to avoid suturing a distal ureterotomy.

Transperitoneal Approach

The transperitoneal approach to the distal ureter is particularly applicable to reoperative situations, in which the patient was previously explored retroperitoneally. The ureter is readily accessible through a peritoneal approach. A modification of the transperitoneal ureterolithotomy entails raising a flap of peritoneum with its base extending from the pelvic brim to the bladder.[7] With the flap raised, the iliac vessels and ureter are exposed (Fig. 21-15). Following ureterolithotomy, a drain is laid in the retroperitoneal space and brought to the skin in a plane between peritoneum and muscle. The peritoneal flap is reapproximated to the pelvic wall, returning ureter and drain to a retroperitoneal position. On the left side, it is occasionally easier to expose the ureter by reflecting the entire mesocolon from the pelvic side wall, with the mesocolon serving as the peritoneal flap.

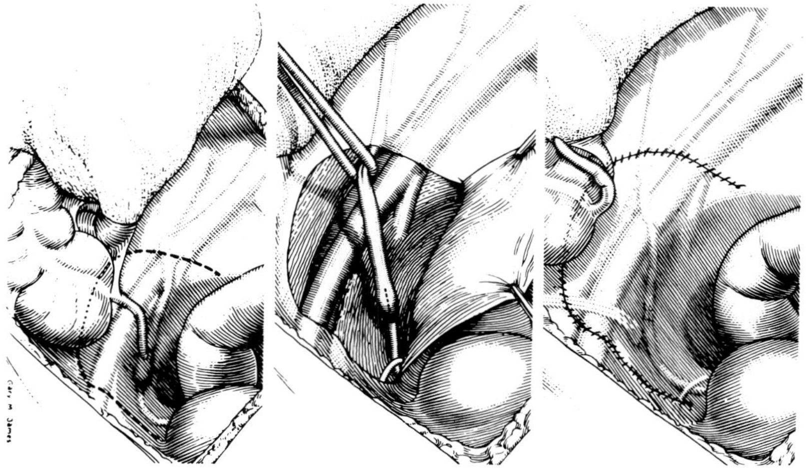

Fig. 21-15. Transperitoneal approach to distal ureter by raising peritoneal flap. (Reprinted from Bristol JB, Smith PJB: Transperitoneal ureterolithotomy for stones in the lower third of the ureter. Br J Urol 54:220–222, 1982. With permission.)

VAGINAL URETEROLITHOTOMY

A distal ureteral calculus, which is palpable vaginally, may be removed by a vaginal incision directly onto the calculus.[47,62] A weighted vaginal speculum and lateral tenaculum traction on the cervix provide adequate exposure. The ureters should be controlled proximally with a vessel loop, and ureteral dissection should avoid the uterine artery. Following stone extraction, the ureter and vagina should be closed separately to avoid fistula formation.

Approaches to the Intramural Stone

The two open approaches to the intramural stone entail either intravesical or extravesical ureteral exposure.

Intravesical Approach

Kropp has described a technique wherein the ureter is exposed and dissected as if one were performing a ureteral reimplantation.[35] The ureter is dissected from its hiatus and mobilized into the bladder, facilitating distal ureterolithotomy. The ureter can then be reimplanted following closure of the ureterotomy. A ureteral stent should be left indwelling for a few days postoperatively.

Many distal ureteral stones requiring ureterolithotomy will be impacted and produce ureteral erosion. The beauty of Kropp's approach is that it routinely allows for ureteral freshening and reimplantation under these circumstances.

An alternative intravesical approach to the intramural calculus is to incise down onto Waldeyer's sheath more proximally, without dissecting the ureteric orifice.[2] Following the ureterotomy, the ureter slips back into its normal position, and mucosa and bladder muscle are reapproximated. This approach avoids the need for ureteral reimplantation but entails more intraoperative bleeding.

If the periureteral inflammation is extensive, making distal ureteral dissection difficult, Straffon suggests that one consider bypassing the calculus by ligating the ureter proximal to the stone and doing a Psoas hitch reimplantation. As long as the ureter distal to the calculus is patent, no complications should result.[62]

Extravesical Approach

A juxtavesical ureterolithotomy has been described in which a right angle clamp is introduced between the ureter and bladder hiatus for a length of 1–2 cm at the 12 o'clock position. The detrusor muscle above the clamp is divided between chromic ligatures, placed in order to avoid bleeding. The intramural ureter is exposed, and an appropriate ureterotomy made. Following the ureterotomy, the detrusor muscle is reapproximated over the distal ureter as in a Lich-Gregoir extravesical ureteral reimplantation.[56]

While this procedure seems readily performed by its proponents, the intravesical approach seems more straightforward in achieving adequate exposure of the difficult intramural stone.

CURRENT INDICATIONS FOR URETEROLITHOTOMY

Ureterolithotomy should be performed only in circumstances where ESWL or ureteroscopic techniques are not indicated or have failed. Extracorporeal shock-wave lithotripsy is technically applicable to stones above the pelvic brim, and the recent cooperative report on ESWL noted that in 13 percent of patients the primary stones were in the upper or mid ureter.[17] As previously noted, however, 23 percent of patients with a solitary calculus had residual stone fragments at 3-month followup, the long-term significance of which is unknown.

Distal ureteral calculi within the bony pelvis are not technically treatable by ESWL. Ureteroscopic extraction or lithotripsy has been most valuable in managing this group of patients. While success rates with ureteroscopic techniques will vary depending on the aggressiveness of the center in recommending stone manipulation, the majority of reports describe a 56–77 percent success rate.[19,29,38] One recent report describes a success rate of 94 percent with ureteroscopic extraction or lithotripsy of 159 ureteral stones located below the pelvic brim.[36]

In all series, those distal ureteral stones that were most troublesome to manage ureteroscopically had been impacted. The complications associated with ureteroscopic stone extraction are considerable, with Lingeman et al. reporting a 14 percent complication rate in 206 procedures.[36] The most common complication is ureteral perforation, requiring stent placement, but false ureteral passages and ureteral avulsion have occurred as well. In comparison, Furlow reported a complication rate associated with 1061 open ureterolithotomies to be 17.5 percent. When one subtracts the cardiovascular complications from Furlow's series, the rate of complications from ureterolithotomy is identical to that of ureteroscopic stone extraction (14 percent).[21]

Stones that are inaccessible to ESWL because of their location in the distal ureter and stones that cannot be retrieved by means of ureteroscopy because they are impacted, or as a result of ureteral or urethral anatomy, may require open ureterolithotomy. The same situations which mitigate against transuretheral instrumentation of the distal ureter would be indications for open ureterolithotomy. As noted by Drach, these include:

> abnormal ureteral anatomy such as bifid ureter, ectopic or transplanted ureteral orifice; ureteral orifice in a diverticulum; significant prostatic hypertophy; impassable urethral stricture; or stones in children whose urethra (and ureter) is too small for adequate instrument passage.[16]

COMPLICATIONS OF OPEN STONE REMOVAL

The complications experienced with open stone removal include persistent urinary drainage, urinoma formation, wound infection, and urinary fistula formation.

Persistent Urinary Drainage

In the vast majority of pyelo and ureterolithotomies, Penrose urinary drainage lasts for less than 4–5 days.[47] If copious urinary drainage persists for significantly longer periods, one must suspect distal obstruction. This can be assessed initially with an x-ray film of kidneys, ureters, and bladder (KUB) looking for distal stone fragments and subsequently by performing an intravenous pyelogram (IVP) and retrograde ureteropyelogram. If no obstructing distal fragment is found but significant extravasation is documented, a ureteral stent should be left indwelling for a number of days until the leakage subsides. If obstruction is noted it must be promptly relieved.

Urinoma Formation

A urinoma may form as a result of premature drain removal or a poorly functioning drain.[62] Significant amounts of urine can collect in the retroperitoneum before symptoms such as nausea or vomiting arise. The management of the urinoma entails broad-spectrum antibiotic coverage, stenting of the ureter to reduce extravasation, and percutaneous drainage of the urinoma. If massive extravasation is documented, open drainage and Penrose drain placement may be necessary.

Wound Infection

Wound infection is second only to persistent drainage of urine as the most common surgical complication of ureterolithotomy.[21] Management entails systemic antibiotics, if the infection is diagnosed early. If a positive urine culture has been obtained, it is reasonable to presume that the same organism is responsible for the infection until wound cultures return. Management of the more advanced wound infection entails drainage and local care.

Urinary Fistula

Prolonged urinary extravasation can result in the formation of a urinary tract fistula. A fistula is usually the result of ureteral obstruction, due to either a retained stone fragment or stricture or kinking of the ureter at the site of the ureterotomy.[47] The evaluation of a fistula is identical to that for persistent urinary drainage. An IVP with delayed and oblique films should delineate the site of the fistula and the presence of obstruction. Retrograde ureteropyelography confirms these findings.

The optimal management of a fistula entails the relief of distal obstruction and the placement of a soft, double-J stent around which the ureter may heal. If healing does not occur despite ureteral stenting for 4 weeks, one must consider performing an open surgical repair. At the time of fistula closure it is important to cover the repair with pliable tissue. Omentum is ideal for wrapping such a ureter to promote healing,[64] but retroperitoneal fat usually is satisfactory and avoids the need to enter the peritoneal cavity. In addition, a soft internal ureteral stent and retroperitoneal drain should be left at the time of open repair.

REFERENCES

1. Anderson EE: The management of ureteral calculi. Urol Clin N Am 1:357–363, 1974
2. Barnhouse DH, Marshall M Jr, Price SE Jr: Ureterolithotomy for juxtavesicular stone. J Urol 129:944–945, 1983
3. Blandy JP: The ureter, in Blandy JP (ed): Urology. Philadelphia, Lippincott, 1976, p 83
4. Blandy JP, Singh M: The case for a more aggressive approach to staghorn stones. J Urol 115:505–506, 1976
5. Boyce WH, Elkins IB: Reconstructive renal surgery following anatrophic nephrolithotomy: follow up of 100 consecutive cases. J Urol 111:307–312, 1974
6. Brannen GE, Bush WH, Correa RJ, et al: Kidney stone removal: percutaneous versus surgical lithotomy. J Urol 133:6–12, 1985
7. Bristol JB, Smith PJB: Transperitoneal ureterolithotomy for stones in the lower third of the ureter. Br J Urol 54:220–222, 1982
8. Clayman RV, Surya V, Miller RP, et al: Percutaneous nephrolithotomy—an approach to branched and staghorn renal calculi. JAMA 250:73–75, 1983
9. Clayman RV, Surya V, Miller RP, et al: Percutaneous nephrolithotomy—extraction of renal and ureteral calculi from 100 patients. J Urol 131:868–871, 1984
10. Das S, Harris CJ, Amar AD, et al: Dorsovertical lumbotomy approach for surgery of upper urinary tract calculi. J Urol 129:266–270, 1983
11. Davis DM: Intubated ureterotomy: A new operation for ureteral and ureteropelvic stricture. Surg Gynecol Obstet 76:513, 1943
12. Dees JE: The use of an intrapelvic coagulum in pyelolithotomy: Preliminary report. South Med J 36:167–175, 1943
13. Dees JE, Fox H: The properties of human fibrinogen coagulum: Preliminary report. J Urol 49:503–511, 1943
14. Diamond D, Johnston, JH: Unpublished data.
15. Dodson AI: Anatomy and surgical approach to the urogenital tract in the male, in Campbell M (ed): Urology. Philadelphia, Saunders, 1954, pp 1–35
16. Drach GW: Stone manipulation. Urology 12:286–289, 1978
17. Drach GW, Dretler S, Fair W, et al: Report of United States Cooperative Study of Extracorporeal Shock Wave Lithotripsy. J Urol 135:1127–1133, 1986
18. Fischer CP, Sonda LP, Diokno AC: Further experience with cryoprecipitate coagulum in renal calculus surgery: A review of 60 cases. J Urol 126:432–436, 1981
19. Ford TF, Watson GM, Wickham JEA: Transurethral ureteroscopic retrieval of ureteric stones. Br J Urol 55:626–628, 1983
20. Freiha F, Zeineh S: Dorsal approach to upper urinary tract. Urology 21:15–16, 1983

21. Furlow WL, Bucchiere JJ: The surgical fate of ureteral calculi: review of Mayo Clinic experience. J Urol 116:559–561, 1976
22. Gardiner RA, Naunton-Morgan TC, Whitfield HN, et al: The modified lumbotomy versus the oblique loin incision for renal surgery. Br J Urol 51:256–259, 1979
23. Gibbons RP, Correa RJ, Cummings KB, et al: Use of Water-Pik and nephroscope. Urology 4:605, 1974
24. Gil-Vernet JM: New surgical concepts in removing renal calculi. Urol Internatl 20:255–288, 1965
25. Gil-Vernet JM: Transverse ureterotomy. J Urol 111:755–756, 1974
26. Gil-Vernet JM: Pyelolithotomy, in Roth RA, Finlayson B (eds): Clinical Management of Urolithiasis, International Perspectives in Urology, Vol 6. Baltimore, Williams & Wilkins, 1983, pp 297–332
27. Gittes RF: Operative nephroscopy. J Urol 116:148–152, 1976
28. Gittes RF, Belldegrun A: Posterior lumbotomy: Surgery for upper tract calculi. Urol Clin N Am 10:625–628, 1983
29. Huffman JL, Bagley DH, Lyon ES: Treatment of distal ureteral calculi using rigid ureteroscope. Urology 20:574–577, 1982
30. James R, Novick AC, Straffon RA, et al: Anatropic nephrolithotomy for removal of staghorn or branched renal calculi. Urology 15:108–111, 1980
31. Juengst KN, Kursh ED: Pyelolithotomy. Urol Clin N Am 10:649–658, 1983
32. Kalash SS, Campbell EW, Young JD: Sources of fibrinogen for coagulum pyelolithotomy, without thrombin. Urology 22:486–492, 1983
33. Kalash SS, Young JD: Coagulum pyelolithotomy: Impact on unrecognized stones. J Urol 134:1082–1085, 1985
34. Kalash SS, Young JD, Harne G: Modification of cryoprecipitate coagulum pyelolithotomy technique. Urology 19:467–471, 1982
35. Kropp KA: Surgical approaches to renal and ureteral calculi. Urol Clin N Am 10:617–623, 1983
36. Lingeman JE, Sonda LP, Kahnoski RJ, et al: Ureteral stone management: emerging concepts. J Urol 135:1172–1174, 1986
37. Lurz H: Ein muskelschonender lumbalschnitt zur freilegung der niere. Chirurg 27:125, 1956
38. Lyon ES, Huffman JL, Bagley DH: Ureteroscopy and ureteropyeloscopy. Urology 23:29–36, 1984
39. Maddocks R, Jewell E, Decenzo JM, et al: Management of the ureterotomy incision in 100 consecutive ureterolithotomies. J Urol 116:422–423, 1976
40. Marshall FF: Intraoperative localization of renal calculi. Urol Clin N Am 10:629–635, 1983
41. Marshall S: Commercial fibrinogen, autogenous plasma, whole blood and cryoprecipitate for coagulum pyelolithotomy: A comparative study. J Urol 119:310–311, 1978
42. Marshall S: Coagulum pyelolithotomy. Urol Clin N Am 10:659–664, 1983
43. Miki M, Inaba Y, Machida T: Operative nephroscopy with fiberoptic scope: preliminary report. J Urol 119:166–168, 1978
44. Murchison RJ: Intraoperative use of ureterorenoscope. J Urol 134:728, 1985
45. Nemoy NJ, Stamey TA: Use of Hemiacidrin in management of infection stones. J Urol 116:693–695, 1976
46. Novick AC: Posterior approach to the kidney and ureter. J Urol 124:192–195, 1980
47. O'Flynn JD: Clinical management of ureteral calculi, in Roth RA, Finlayson B (eds): Clinical Management of Urolithiasis, International Perspectives in Urology, Vol 6. Baltimore, Williams & Williams, 1983, pp 441–452
48. Orkin LA: Experimental studies on the repair of ureteral injuries, in Trauma to the Ureter: Pathogenesis in Management. Philadelphia, FA Davis, 1964, Chapter 3
49. Pence JR II, Airhart RA, Novicki DE: Coagulum pyelolithotomy (letter). J Urol 125:134, 1981

50. Pence JR II, Airhart RA, Novicki DE, et al: Pulmonary emboli associated with coagulum pyelolithotomy. J Urol 127:527–573, 1982
51. Persky L, Hoch WH, Kursh ED: Surgical management of the ureter, in Harrison JH, Gittes RF, Perlmutter AD, et al (eds): Urology, 4th ed. Philadelphia, Saunders, 1979, pp 2188–2210
52. Preminger GM, Clayman RV, Curry T, et al: Outpatient percutaneous nephrostolithotomy. J Urol 136:355–357, 1986
53. Preminger GM, Clayman RV, Hardeman SW, et al: Percutaneous nephrostomy versus open surgery for renal calculi. JAMA 254:1054–1058, 1985
54. Redman JF, Bissada NK, Harper DL: Anatrophic nephrolithotomy: Experience with complications of the Smith and Boyce technique. J Urol 122:595–597, 1979
55. Resnick MI, Grayhack JT: Simple and extended pyelolithotomy. Urol Clin N Am 1:319–332, 1974
56. Rosemberg SK: Extravesical transmural ureterolithotomy. Urology 23:336–339, 1984
57. Roth RA: Residual stones, in Roth RA, Finlayson B (eds): Clinical Management of Urolithiasis, International Perspectives in Urology, Vol 6. Baltimore, Williams & Wilkins, 1983, pp 422–440
58. Schulze H, Hertle L, Graft J: Combined treatment of branched calculi by percutaneous nephrolithotomy and extracorporeal shock wave lithotripsy. J Urol 135:1138–1141, 1986
59. Simon G: Extripation einer niere am menschen. Deutsche Klin 22:137, 1870
60. Sleight MW, Wickham JEA: Long term follow-up of 100 cases of renal calculi. Br J Urology 601–604, 1977
61. Smith AD: Percutaneous ureteral surgery and stenting. Urology 23:37–42, 1984
62. Straffon RA: Surgery for calculus disease of the urinary tract, in Walsh PC, Gittes RF, Perlmutter AD, et al (eds): Urology, 5th ed. Philadelphia, Saunders, 1986, pp 2478–2504
63. Tanagho EA, Diamantopoulois A, Marshall S: Simplified approach to cryoprecipitate coagulum pyelolithotomy. Urology 27:532–533, 1981
64. Turner-Warwick R: The use of the omental pedicle graft in urinary tract reconstruction. J Urol 116:341–347, 1976
65. White EC, Smith AD: Percutaneous stone extraction from 200 patients. J Urol 132:437–438, 1984
66. Wickham JEA, Coe N, Ward JP: One hundred cases of nephrolithotomy under hypothermia. J Urol 112:702–705, 1974
67. Wickham JEA, Kellet MJ, Miller RA: Elective percutaneous nephrolithotomy in 50 patients: An analysis of the technique, results and complications. J Urol 129:904–906, 1983
68. Wickham JEA, Mathur VK: Hypothermia in the conservative surgery of renal disease. Br J Urol 43:648–657, 1971
69. Woodhouse CRJ, Farrell CR, Davis AMI, et al: The place of extended pyelolithotomy (Gil-Vernet Operation) in the management of renal staghorn calculi. Br J Urol 53:520–523, 1981
70. Wulfsohn MA: Extended pyelolithotomy: The uses of renal artery clamping and regional hypothermia. J Urol 125:467–470, 1981
71. Zaontz MR, Banfield WL, Pahira JJ: Uses of coagulum for displaced ureteral calculi. J Urol 130:548–549, 1983

M. J. Vernon Smith

22

Anatrophic Nephrolithotomy and Extended Pyelolithotomy

Surgery on the normal kidney for stones has enjoyed exactly 100 years of life. On February 11, 1880, Sir Henry Morris removed the first kidney stone through normal kidney tissue, and in February 1980, Chaussy and his colleagues began their experimental work in humans using shock-wave techniques. Today, the interrelationships of each new technique and those other evolving energy forms remain in their infancy. While consideration of the comparisons of cost, length of stay, or time out of work are involved in optimal care, these are factors that bear no relationship to the overall goal, which is the prevention of any further stone formation, and preservation and improvement of renal function, so that, in effect, the patient is cured of the disease by lifelong management.

The exact role of open surgical lithotomy is no longer entirely clear; nevertheless, urologists will explore kidneys for stone disease, and the management and prophylaxis of stones will involve surgical intervention, but perhaps not as frequently as in earlier times.[8] The meticulous techniques involved in the operations known as *anatrophic nephrolithotomy* and *extended pyelonephrolithotomy* will be a required part of our armamentarium. This chapter will not espouse a particular approach but will discuss the various techniques in detail and pay particular attention to the various ancillary modalities such as intraoperative nephroscopy, ultrasonography, radiography, and cooling that are essential for successful surgery of stone disease.

RENAL ANATOMY

The surgeon must have a clear understanding of intrarenal anatomy and distribution of the lobules, renal artery and vein, and their relationships to each other before undertaking intrarenal surgery.[2,10,12,25,26]

Some find difficulty in understanding that there exists constant anatomic arrange-

STONE DISEASE: DIAGNOSIS AND MANAGEMENT
ISBN 0-8089-1873-7

ment within any kidney. The apparent deviation from the normal thus is, in fact, a manifestation of the bimodal embryological origin of the kidney. The metanephric duct induces a change in the surrounding mesoderm to form the metanephric tissue, and this metanephron is not influenced by the divisions of the collecting system, but rather drains into it. Kidney parenchyma is divided into 14 lobulations; 7 anterior and 7 posterior. Fundamentally, three anterior and three posterior calyceal groups exist in the midkidney. There are two anterior apical and two posterior apical groups with two anterior and posterior basilar lobulations. Some of these may compound, but the same basic underlying anatomic arrangement exists. Although the infundibula or pelvic arrangement can show tremendous variation, this basic 7/7 arrangement can be seen (Fig. 22-1).

The kidney has a segmental arterial blood supply that conforms to this basic lobular configuration. It does not interconnect. One needs to think in this manner so that the concept of so-called aberrant or accessory blood vessel is no longer a part of the anatomic language. The kidney can be divided into four segments: apical, basilar, anterior, and posterior, each with its individual primary arterial supply. Each kidney has a peculiar anatomic arrangement that is unique but predictable (Fig. 22-2). Seventy percent of kidneys have a single artery. Studies show that branching occurs in the proximal third of the renal artery in 7 percent; in the middle third, in 12 percent; in the distal third, in 48 percent; and, finally, within the sinus, in 32 percent. In at least one-third of kidneys,

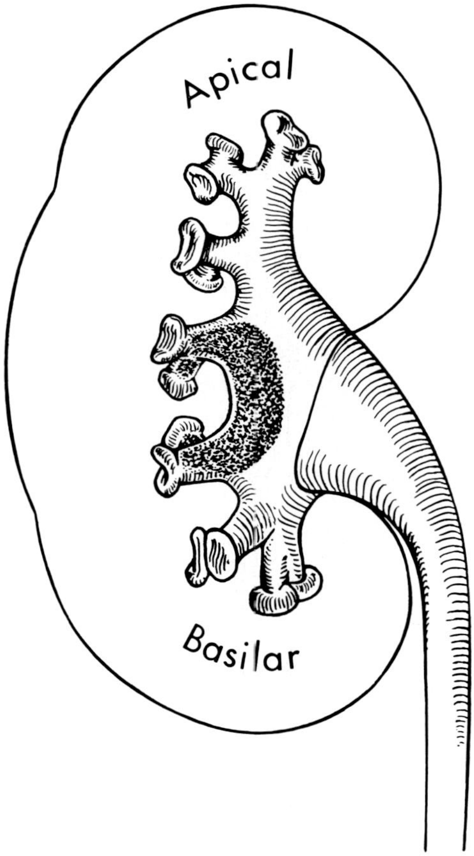

Fig. 22-1. The basic arrangement of calyces with apical and basilar segments with two anterior and posterior calyceal groups. The midportion of the kidney has three posterior calyces and three anterior calyces. this basic 7/7 arrangement persists even though infundibula or pelvic variation is not unusual.

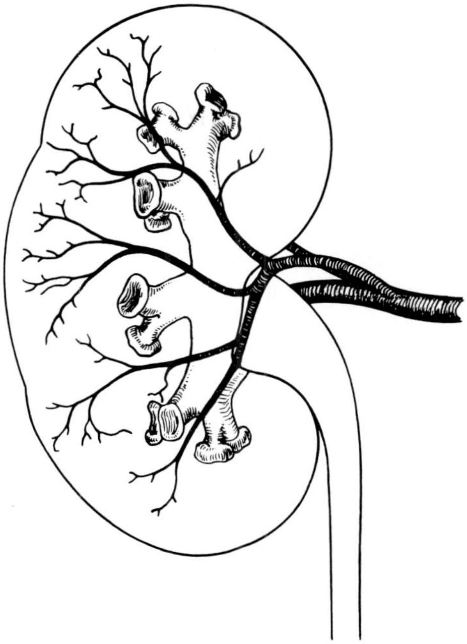

Fig. 22-2. The posterior segmental renal artery usually is the first division and turns down parallel to and under the hilar lip, giving branches off its lateral border.

therefore, the renal artery shows no extrarenal branch. If two branches are extrahilar, the cephalic one is the posterior division. Any dissection of a main or renal artery should be done as far from the renal hilus as possible, since in at least 80 percent of cases no risk of damage of important renal arteries exists. A common problem when viewing arteriograms lies in trying to make the decision as to which is the anterior and which is the posterior division. The posterior segmental artery usually is the first branch and curves away from the main artery. Also, this has a smaller caliber than all the other first-order branches and usually crosses in the renal sinus just above the pelvis and then descends parallel to the axis of the hilar lip. This branch characteristically appears to cross the ventral or anterior branches, and the divisions always come off the lateral border. The anterior divisions divide equally each time and fan out across the kidney (Fig. 22-2).

The segmental arteries and their first-order branches all lie within the renal sinus, not within the renal parenchyma; that is, they are protected in the fatty tissue surrounding the infundibula of the collecting system. The presence of a staghorn does not alter this arrangement. The posterior segmental arterial branches lie on the cephalic and caudal aspect of the infundibulum, while the anterior segmental vessels have a different relationship. When they acquire their interlobar configuration, they can lie on the anterior and posterior aspects of the anterior group of infundibula. Great care thus must be taken to avoid the point of crossing, which usually is located at the base of the infundibulum as it joins the pelvis. If an incision is contemplated at the posterior aspect of the anterior infundibula group, particular care must be exercised not to divide or damage an arterial vessel that lies in the renal sinus tissue at this point. All incisions in the pelvis near the infundibulum should be kept posterior.

An arteriogram is mandatory when there has been previous surgery on the kidney, or trauma to that kidney or when the intravenous pyelogram (IVP) suggests that there is a peculiar calyceal arrangement; that is, a pelvic bifurcation or similar variations may warn of underlying anatomic abnormalities. Early work suggests both percutaneous lithotriopsy and extracorporeal shock-wave lithotripsy (ESWL) qualify as previous surgical events. Therefore, an arteriogram should be obtained before an open surgical lithotomy in these patients.

The arrangement of the venous arcades should also be kept in mind by all surgeons; these interconnect, yet appear to be concentrated in three anatomic areas. An intrarenal layer of venous channels probably at the corticomedullary junction, another at the level of calyceal fornices, and, finally, one at the level of the pelvis run along the axis of the kidney. The veins must be sutured in a fashion that parallels the axis of the kidney. Vessels that run at right angles to this axis are arterial bleeders. These relationships of vessels to the collecting system should be clearly remembered when closing the calyceal system. It is very easy to inadvertently obstruct a major vessel during this surgical exercise; therefore, use of surgical magnification loupes and a head lamp is suggested.

PREOPERATIVE EVALUATION AND PREPARATION

Surgery for a renal calculus rarely is an emergency. Surgery should always follow a careful preoperative evaluation. This must include a medical evaluation as to whether the patient is an operative candidate. An appropriate metabolic and bacteriological evaluation should be carried out so that the surgical procedure is not turned into a surgical exercise. The patient with uric acid or cystine stones should have shown no decrease in size in spite of appropriate intensive medical regimen over an 8-week period. The metabolic stone should also have been controlled (i.e., no increase in size) over a similar time period.

Precise localization of renal calculi is carried out prior to surgery. This requires a careful, plain film with tomographic cuts and an IVP in the anteroposterior (AP), posteroanterior (PA), and oblique positions. It is helpful to have at least one lateral view of the kidney. This will show the calyceal anatomy and its relationship to the contained stones. If a clear appreciation of the intra- and extrarenal anatomy is not obtained by these studies, retrograde studies must be done. Most patients will benefit from a voiding cystourethrogram since occasionally reflux occurs in the presence of staghorns. This requires appropriate management during the postoperative period. Catheter drainage needs to be prolonged until suture lines have healed. Recently CAT scans have been helpful in assessing intrarenal anatomy. Future work could show that they may be used routinely.

Renal surgery may result in the loss of functioning renal tissue; thus renal clearance studies become a mandatory preoperative evaluation. It is simple to measure creatinine clearance, and this will provide a baseline if the patient encounters problems in the postoperative period. These initial studies are done in a basal state while those obtained after the surgery are affected by increased fluid intake and tissue damage, which may give rise to misleading values. In some cases the surgeon needs to alert the renal service that dialysis may be necessary during the postoperative period and, certainly, if clearances are low or if there is bilateral disease then differential studies are warranted. This is particularly true in a patient who is over the age of 60, because if radioisotope studies show that one kidney is contributing less than 10 percent of overall renal function, nephrectomy may be the operation of choice even though the aim of all calculous surgery is conservation of renal tissue.

All patients should undergo bacteriologic studies. The patient should discontinue all antibiotics for 1 week prior to these studies, so that the appropriate antibiotic can be given. This should be started 48 hours prior to surgery. If the preoperative evaluation of the urine shows no growth of bacteria, these patients are treated in the normal fashion with a prophylactic antibiotic, usually an IV cephalosporin given 2 hours before surgery and continued for 48 hours. The infected patient is then switched to suppressive oral medications that are continued for at least 3 months.

The author prefers to give 2000 ml of intravenous fluids in the 8 hours prior to surgery. This gives maximal renal perfusion.

OPERATIVE ADJUNCTS

Hypothermia

There are many methods of instituting hypothermia of the kidney, and these have been reviewed recently. All staghorn surgery should be done under hypothermia.[15,16] This way the team understands that this will happen every time a staghorn is approached. Surgical exercises always proceed much more smoothly when the surgical team has a routine that they follow.

Slush is made in the following manner: 8 liters of normal saline or lactated ringers are placed in individual one liter bottles at 4 degrees centigrade and left overnight. When the nursing staff comes on in the morning, the bottles are placed in the freezer section and agitated every 20–30 minutes so as to keep their contents liquid. It is wise to handle these bottles wrapped in a towel; otherwise, ice will crystallize. These supercooled solutions can then be taken to the operating room and poured into an appropriate sterile basin and slush will form immediately.

We have had the opportunity to use the sterile surgical slush machine by the Taylor Freeze Company, Rockton, Illinois and, like Boyce,[3–7] have been pleased. This consistently produces excellent sterile slush and facilitates precise temperature control in 30–40 minutes.

Intraoperative Radiology

Each individual surgeon and radiologic technician should work out an appropriate technique for his or her circumstance. These techniques should be clearly displayed in the radiologic area. Unless the radiologic technique is excellent, achieving the aim of surgery—a kidney free of calculus—cannot be expected. The technique developed by Roth[19] and Griffith[11] is useful. A liter of IV fluid is placed so that half of the film surface is covered. A few stones are taped on this container (see Fig. 22-3). The x-ray machine that is to be used in the operative suite is then placed a standard distance from the film (usually 30 inches) and multiple exposures obtained until the appropriate technique is achieved. The technician and the clinician should remember when testing Polaroid positive film, that light means overexposure.

The following techniques provide excellent roentgenographic evaluation of stones in situ. The Kodak X-O MAT KS film is the standard against which all other studies should be measured. This film can be sterilized and it is wise to have at least 10 available. It is not unusual for sterilization to have been forgotten. In these circumstances a sterile,

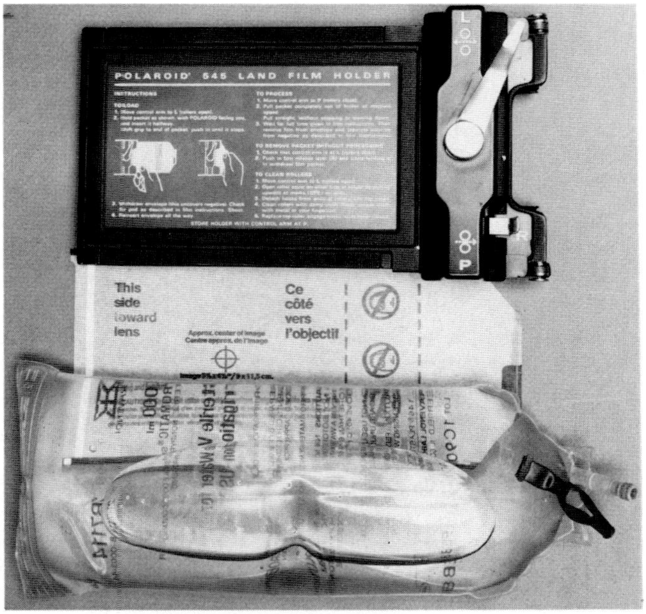

Fig. 22.3. The 545 Polaroid film (below) and developer (above) that are used for intraoperative x-rays. The bag of fluid is the same density as a kidney and is used in the standardization of film-taking technique (see text).

small intestinal bag is obtained, and an assistant nurse drops the unsterile film into this, which is now a sterile package. It is important that the kidney x-ray be supported in the hernia tapes or whatever sling the surgeon elects to use. The author believes that the notch in this film should not be placed around the renal hilum, because there is a real danger of missing a stone in the pelvis. Usual exposure using this film is 50 kV and 150 milliampere seconds (mAS), with a distance of 30 inches from the x-ray source. This film is then developed and is very useful because it gives both the high- and low-contrast film.

It is easier to manipulate the head of the x-ray machine than the kidney, so the kidney should be appropriately suspended and then *not* moved until the developed film is brought to the suite. This is done by clamping the supporting lap pads in place.

Recently, various workers have been using Polaroid film that can be readily processed in a 545 Polaroid 4 × 5-inch holder. Type 52 Polaroid Pan is a panchromatic fine-grain positive-print film. Polaroid Type 57 is a panchromatic medium-grain positive print film with an ASA of 3000. There is also an experimental type TPN, produced by the Polaroid Company, which gives transparent radiographic film (Fig. 22-3). Each film has its various advantages; certainly the most important is that the control of the image returns to the surgeon and the frustrating wait for the return of films is cut to 60 seconds. All of these films and developing cassettes are available from photographic stores. Type 52 Polaroid film is a standard for intraoperative organ studies because there is rapid development with very clear definition. The surgeon must be trained to look at a photograph rather than a radiographic transparency; for example, stones appear black rather than white.

Other Aids

The Water-Pik has been recommended as a useful method to free the kidney of residual fragments. It should never be used when there is "bare" renal tissue present since the jet will cut through parenchyma like a knife. Thus it is inadvisable to use the powerful Water Pik during anatrophic nephrolithotomy, but it is used when the collecting system remains intact. This pulsatile jet is used on occasion to work through the cortex and medulla instead of a blunt instrument, but it is so uncontrollable that one should probably use a Cavitron instead; however, neither technique has a great deal to recommend it.

Every calyx should be inspected and flushed with cold saline. There are a host of methods for this; the important activity is to endeavor to cleanse every papilla and calyceal neck of debris. If a stone is difficult to locate, it is clear that there is forniceal stenosis, and this should be corrected.

The new real-time ultrasonic probes are very exciting;[17] however, air in the collecting system can be misleading. It requires some experience to localize a stone, and it is important to relate stone position to the collecting system and to the vascular segments of the parenchyma; otherwise, stone removal may become traumatic. Sometimes it is helpful to use the ultrasonic probe in the placement of Randall's forceps. The stones and forceps can be visualized and directed toward each other under ultrasonic control.

Some would suggest that the nephroscope has a place in anatrophic nephrolithotomy. The author disagrees, since exposure of the stone by wide incisions is the basis of this operation. It does, however, have a place in extended pyelolithotomy when finding a stone may be difficult.

Recently, there has been a great deal of interest in Doppler flow meters with pencil probes to map out the renal blood flow and to locate the avascular plane. When these open operations are undertaken occasionally, this adjunctive technique will be used commonly. Limited experience with kidneys previously submitted to percutaneous or extracorporeal lithotripsy suggests that there is remarkable fibrotic reaction in the area of the renal hilum. Finding the major vessels thus may become a hazardous undertaking, and Doppler probes might be useful.

Coagulum lithotomy is useful. Since 1978 cryoprecipitate (type-specific) in a mixture of 25:1 with 10 percent calcium chloride has been used. This is usually colored with a few drops of methylene blue so it can be easily seen. The mixture is injected cold into the pelvis prior to any incision. It takes approximately 5–10 minutes to form a good coagulum of sufficient tensile strength to remove any small calculi and provides a readily visible roadsign to the site of unsuspected infundibulum or calyx. One should remember that the coagulum is slightly radioopaque but has a typical homogenous appearance and should not be confused with matrix, which is more speckled.

Anatrophic Nephrolithotomy*

This operative approach is indicated when there is:

1. A complex branched calculus in a kidney with an intrarenal pelvis
2. The presence of a large or dominant posterior segmental artery, which might be damaged in an extended pyelotomy

*References 13, 14, 18, 20–24

3. The demonstrated need for intrarenal repair of scarring or stricture of an infundibulum causing obstruction
4. Need for papillary excision
5. Malignant stone disease secondary to extensive matrix formation
6. Previous open surgery on that kidney (a relative indication)

The classic flank approach to the kidney is most often utilized, although some prefer to use the anterior approach. A small urethral catheter is placed under aseptic conditions and connected to straight drainage before the operation is started. The patient is then placed on the table in the lateral position and the table flexed. The kidney rest should not be used. After this the patient should be taped in place. Unfortunately, some people tape the patient on the table and then break the table. This can result in a fractured rib and interference with lung function on the down side. There are certain surgeons who would insist that the break of the table be placed at or near the level of the iliac crest. The possibility of damage to the laterofemoral cutaneous nerve exists; therefore, the break should always be placed squarely in the flank. Any sandbags that are used for support of the abdomen should be 1- or 3-liter, plastic-covered, fluid containers wrapped in an appropriate towel. These give better support and are less damaging to tissue. It must be remembered that the patient may spend some 3–6 hours in this extraordinarily unphysiologic position, so careful padding of all potential pressure points must be done.

After the patient is satisfactorily placed on the table, the kidney is most easily approached through a twelfth rib incision. If there has been previous surgery in the area, then a supracostal or an incision over the tenth or eleventh rib is the most appropriate approach. The anterior aspect of the wound should be extended nearly to the border of the rectus sheath. Many surgeons leave themselves inadequate exposure, because it is forgotten that the kidney must be lifted out and forward in the wound in order to give adequate exposure of the posterior aspect of the kidney. It is here, after all, that most of the important dissection will take place. The kidney should be mobilized out of Gerota's fascia by sharp dissection. The fat should not be torn or shredded because it remains the bed and support of the kidney after surgery. It is essential that the upper and lower poles be completely freed of surrounding fat but at the same time entrance of the renal capsule should be avoided because it maintains the tamponade at the completion of the operation. If the capsule is entered, it should be closed immediately; this will obviate troublesome oozing during the procedure.

The kidney is then best suspended in a sling made of 0.5-inch hernia tape. The radiopaque tags attached to the conventional lap pad are an extremely useful way to suspend the kidney. These have a gauze portion that provides sufficient weight to hold the kidney out of the wound without any undue traction. The assistant can hold the kidney up, thus exposing the hilar area so that the artery may be exposed proximally. The aim is to avoid injuring the arterial supply to the posterior segment of the renal pelvis. No effort is made to expose the renal vein. The ureter should be obstructed with silastic tape, or possibly a rubber shod clamp. Complete mobility of the kidney on its pedicle is the keystone to successful surgery (Fig. 22-4).

Once the artery has been identified and the kidney is fully mobilized, a rubber or watertight dam is prepared. A large intestinal bag is the most convenient way to do this. The bag is passed over the suspended kidney and the tapes tightened to obtain a watertight closure around the hilum. The body is shielded with dry lap pads. The closed end of the bag is then opened and draped over the previously placed self-retaining

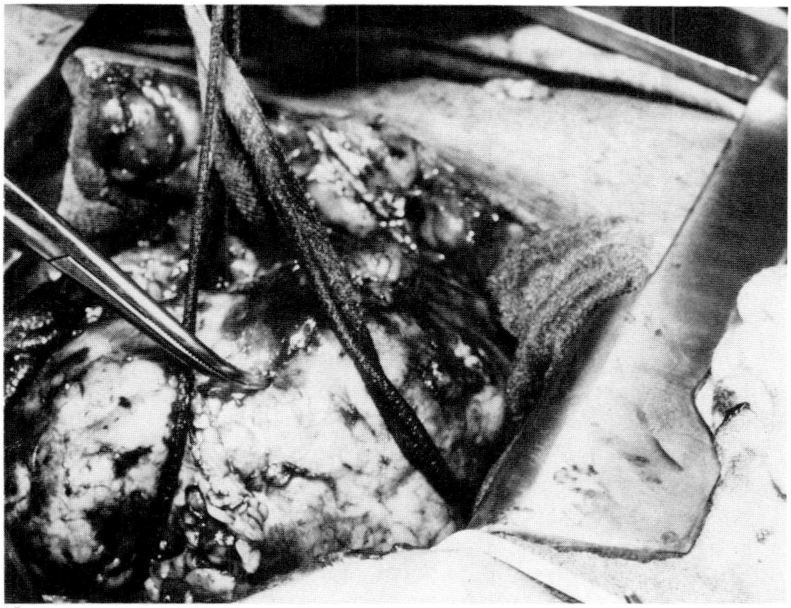

Fig. 22-4. The kidney is completely mobilized and suspended by tapes. the hemostat indicates the site of the intersegmental incision.

retractors. This well is then filled with slush. Just prior to this maneuver, the patient receives 12.5 g of mannitol intravenously and the artery is clamped. The arterial clamping should be continuous (not intermittent) and should not exceed a period of 3 hours.

Before an incision is made, the first x-ray should be obtained. This will act as a scout film and also ensure that the technique has been correctly developed for this particular kidney, rather than waiting for a more stressful moment in the surgical procedure. Boyce has developed a technique in which the anterior or posterior division of the renal artery is occluded, and then a bolus of methylene blue is given intravenously in order to outline the line of the incision more accurately. This is an intriguing addition to the technique of preventing atrophy in any kidney substance; however, it presents the anesthesia team with severe problems because it is difficult to determine the oxygenation of their patient. The site of the incision in the renal capsule is determined in several ways. First, the shrunken renal parenchyma after arterial occlusion will often allow easy palpation of the middle group of posterior calyces. Second, Brodel's white line can be located by the attachment of the perirenal fat to the capsule. This represents the fusion of the anterior and posterior embryological anlage. Frequently, a perforating vessel will leave the kidney in this area. The incision is located one fingerbreadth (1–2 cm) posterior to this line. The incision is always confined to the junction between the anterior and posterior segments and must not stray into the apical or basilar areas. Individual determination is aided by the preoperative arteriograms and calyceal anatomic arrangement that will determine the site of incision in the posterior segment (Fig. 22-2). The capsule is incised with the scalpel blade. The handle of the knife is then used to bluntly dissect away the renal parenchyma and deepen the wound until the most prominent anterior portion of the posterior calyceal group is reached. the collecting system of this particular calyx is then opened down into the pelvis, and then the pelvis is outlined. It is probably a matter of good surgical technique that the collecting systems should be opened both anterior and posterior before any attempt is made to remove any staghorn or calculus material (Fig. 22-5). The surgeon should explore all anterior and posterior calyces and make absolutely certain that all have been accounted for. If a vein is entered, at any time, it should be closed with a running suture of 6-0 absorbable material.

When the major portions of the stones have been removed, the inside of the pelvis should be carefully checked, making sure that no stone is present. At this stage, it is wise to pass a silastic catheter down into the bladder, thus proving no ureteral obstruction.

Attention should be directed in a formal and logical manner to inspecting the interior of *every* calyx that was seen on the preoperative x-ray to ensure that no stones or debris are present. Usually it is easy to inspect the lower pole calyces directly through the wound. It is important to resist the tendency to extend the nephrotomy wound. If there are stones that cannot be extracted through this nephrotomy wound, a new nephrotomy in the apical or basilar segment should be made in the lines of the arteries, and *not* by extending the anatrophic incision. It is important to stay away from the junction of the middle and the upper pole calyces, for it is here that the confluence of the vessels takes place and damage to the main arteries and veins can occur with catastrophic results. Whenever an obvious open vessel is seen, this should be suture ligated with 6-0 plain catgut. When these ligatures are inserted, the suture will hold only on the vessel while cutting through renal parenchyma.

The kidney may then be flushed free of all stone particles with cold saline. It is wise to add some antibiotic solution to the final flush in hope that this will sterilize the interior of the collecting system. An x-ray should be taken at this juncture preferably in two planes. While these are being developed, the kidney should again be flushed and all identifiable vessels suture ligated.

If the preoperative x-rays had shown that there was obstruction of any calyceal neck, this should be repaired by plastic calyrhaphy. This is usually done carefully with magnify-

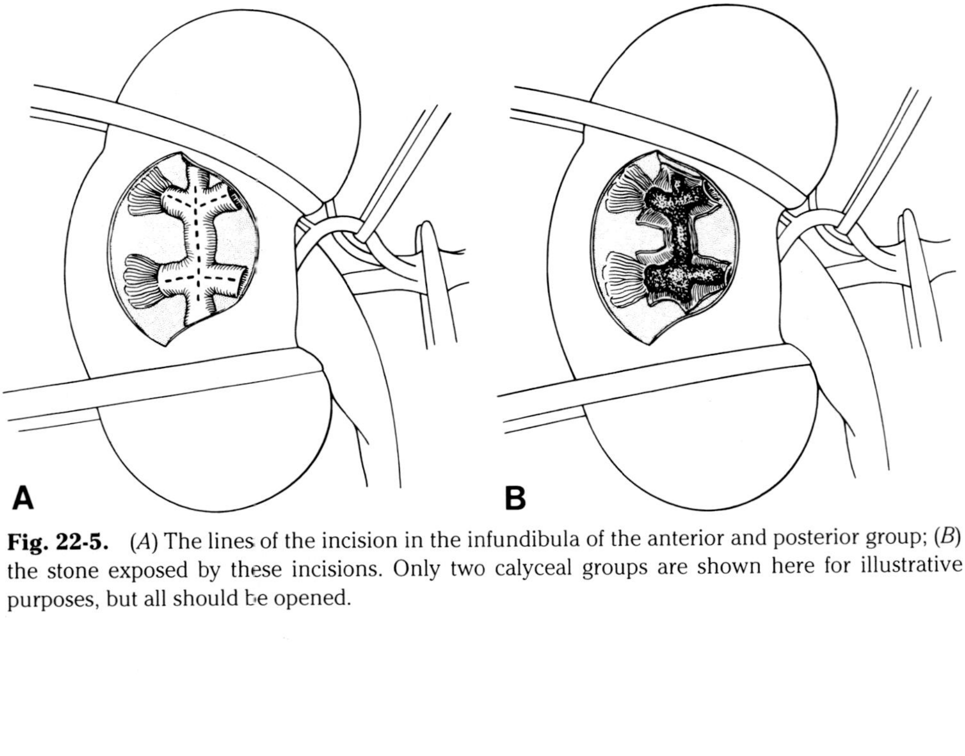

Fig. 22-5. (*A*) The lines of the incision in the infundibula of the anterior and posterior group; (*B*) the stone exposed by these incisions. Only two calyceal groups are shown here for illustrative purposes, but all should be opened.

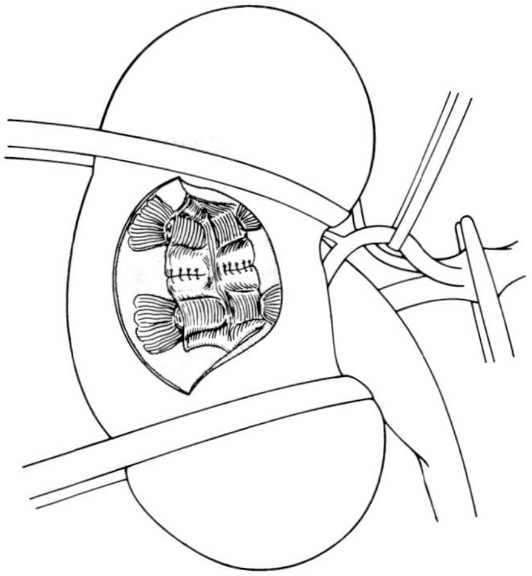

Fig. 22-6. This figure shows the plastic repair of calyrhaphy where the incised portions of the infundibula are sewed to adjacent infundibulum. This procedure has been carried out in both the anterior and posterior segments.

ing loupes and very fine sutures. It is important to remember that all knots must be *outside* the collecting system and the sutures should not obstruct the lobar arteries as they run in the paracalyceal sinus. It is sometimes difficult to remember that if a plastic repair is necessary on a calyx, it is also necessary to carry out a like procedure on the corresponding calyx that lies anteriorly, so that the anterior and posterior calyces will eventually be joined into one compound calyx with a common wide open drainage into the pelvis (Figs. 22-6 and 22-7). If no formal repair of the calyces is necessary, the next step is to close the pelviocalyceal incision in a watertight fashion. There are some who would not try to do this because of the danger of arterial occlusion. In this case approximation of the collecting system is adequate.

The x-rays should demonstrate that there are no stones before the collecting system is closed. If there is any question as to the complete integrity of the closure, a silastic or double-J stent should be placed. No nephrostomy tubes are left as these have no place in anatrophic nephrolithotomy. The capsule is then closed with a running 4-0 chromic catgut and the arterial clamp released. If there is no undue bleeding from the renal incision, the wound may be closed. It is very important to make sure that Gerota's fascia is closed around the kidney so that it may be comfortably placed in its bed. One of the problems with surgery on structures in the retroperitoneum is that the incision site is

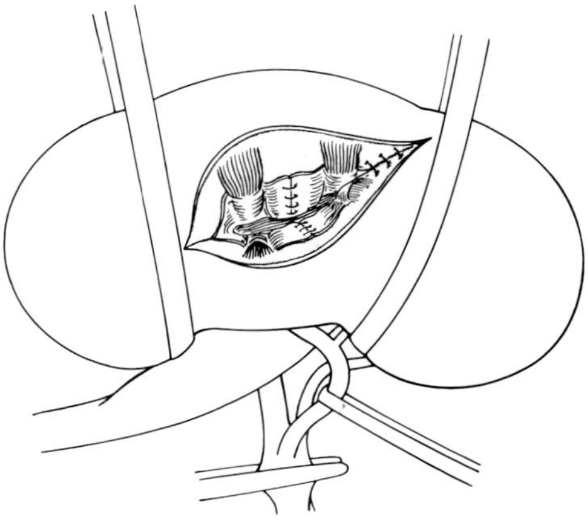

Fig. 22-7. Closure of the collecting system has been started at the apical portion of the intersegmental incision. This will create a large pelvis with compound calyces and excellent drainage.

allowed to come in close contact with the muscle and a physiologic obstructed area will develop.

The area should be drained with a Penrose drain that can be advanced at an appropriate time. After the release of the arterial clamp, 12.5 g of mannitol are given intravenously. This ensures a continuing diuresis, which is probably helpful in preventing obstruction of any of the tubules in the papilla by blood or matrix collections. A continuing flushing diuresis is a very important part of this operative procedure.

MODIFICATION OF THE EXTENDED PYELOLITHOTOMY

In 1965 Gil-Vernet advocated (1) the use of a posterior lumbotomy, (2) performance of the operation through this incision without undue mobilization of the kidneys, (3) use of intrasinus approach to the renal calyces, and (4) a transverse pyelotomy.[9]

The posterior lumbotomy is an excellent approach with a short postoperative recovery; however, it is useful only in less complex situations where the stone involves the pelvis and one calyx only. Any stone larger than this will require more mobilization and vascular control, which is difficult through a posterior lumbotomy incision; thus, most of these procedures are done through the flank. It is helpful to add to the Gil-Vernet procedure clamping of the renal artery because this allows the kidney parenchyma to shrink away from the stone and gives better dissection up the infundibular areas and within the renal sinus.

The pyelotomy incision is placed underneath the hilar lip whenever possible; in this way the major arteries of Margarucci are avoided. Damage to these arteries gives rise to prolonged ureteral atony and may contribute to recurrent stone formation and infection. There is a tendency when doing this operation to try to go straight to the hilum of the kidney. This is a hazardous approach. It is far more efficient to mobilize the upper portion of the ureter, occlude this structure with silastic tape, and then work along the surface of the ureter over the pelvis and then into the sinus. The dissection should be gentle, and the effort is to separate the adventitia from the underlying ureteropelvic and infundibular muscles, so that the vessels that run in the renal sinus will be retracted out of the way. The so-called Gil-Vernet retractors must be used during this procedure, and not the Cushing-type retractors sometimes found in laparotomy sets. This differentiation is very important since the design of these instruments is such that they ensure that the retractor pulls the hilar lip and the intrasinusal fat off the pelvis, thus avoiding any damage to vascular structures. When ordering these retractors, it is useful to get an extra two or three and have the machine shop place a smooth, 60° angle in the middle of the shaft. This makes retraction more efficient and also keeps the assistant's hands out of the operator's field of view. The best exposure is obtained by using two or three of the smaller retractors rather than a single large one (Fig. 22-8).

The incision into the pelvis should be located under the hilar lip if at all possible. The placement of this incision is predicated on obtaining the best exposure. A hooked blade knife or the angled Potts scissors are very useful for this incision. The incision can be carried down the infundibula to the fornices if necessary (Fig. 22-8). Exposure is again improved by gentle traction on the staghorn, which usually is best applied at the inferior pelvioinfundibular junction with a right angle clamp, rather than on the main bulk of the stone. Sometimes it is difficult to visualize and/or deliver the anterior extension of the stone, in which case it should be broken rather than ruptured. During incisions in the

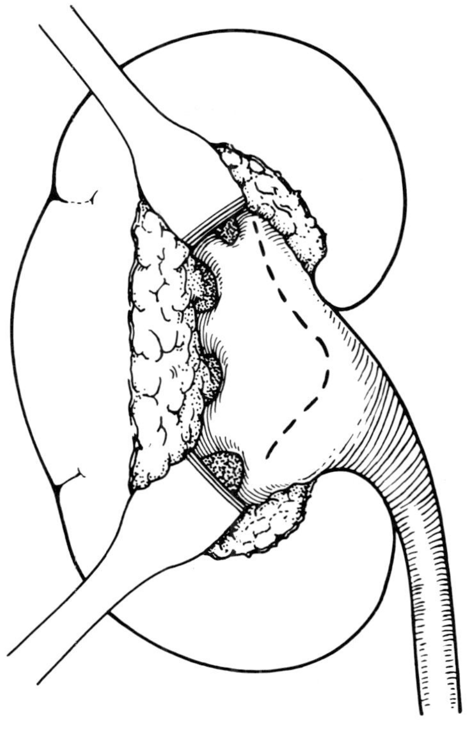

Fig. 22-8. The two smaller Gil-Vernet retractors give excellent visualization of the collecting system. Notice that incisions can be carried down the infundibulum to the fornices if necessary.

infundibulum it is important for the operator to understand that the junction between the upper pole collecting system and the middle portion of the kidney is, in fact, at the major site for the confluence of the venous return from the kidney, and any overzealous dissection toward the veins can result in catastrophic bleeding. Following extraction of the stone, every calyx should be explored. This can be helped by the nasal speculum, vein retractors, and nerve hooks. A nephroscope may be required. Radiographic evaluation is carried out in a similar manner in all nephrolithotomies. (This procedure is no exception.) Sometimes nephrotomy in a radial fashion has to be combined with this procedure so as to ensure complete removal of stones. The pyelotomy and infundibulotomy site should be closed with continuous running sutures of 5-0 absorbable material and the fat closed over the pelvis. It is interesting that if one can manage to keep the suture line so that it lies under the hilar lip, watertight closure is much easier to obtain. In contrast to anatrophic nephrolithotomy, where the placement of a nephrostomy tube potentially removes a tamponade, it is possible to place a nephrostomy tube in these patients. On occasion, a small feeding tube can be placed through the lower calix. This access can be used later to allow passage of a guidewire and dilation of the tract for postoperative chemolysis if necessary.

Infundibular strictures must be incised. They are probably best left open. On occasion they can be closed in a transverse manner. The pelvis should be closed watertight with 5-0 or 6-0 sutures. A stent is probably advisable and can be removed after 5–7 days.

Two logical extensions of these techniques are sometimes useful. First, it is possible to make a nephrotomy between the inferior border of the posterior segmental artery and the basilar portion of the kidney. The incision can be extended all the way to the posterior inferior calyx. This, incidentally, is the correct anatomic site for the placement of a nephrostomy that will do the least damage. (Fig. 22-9). This incision should be closed in layers. The second variation is an incision that is made through the parenchyma of the medial inferior border of the kidney as an extension of an incision that begins on the lateral (inferior) border of the renal pelvis. This approach should not be undertaken unless the arteriogram has clearly shown that this is a relatively avascular approach. As before, the incision in the capsule should be by sharp dissection while the renal parenchyma is separated by handle of the scalpel (blunt dissection). This incision should be closed by anastomosis of the cut infundibula edges to the edges of the divided pelvis.

POSTOPERATIVE CARE

The single most important aspect of the postoperative management of patients with large calculus is elimination of urinary infection. This must be treated vigorously and continuously; otherwise, the surgery is doomed to failure. This means repeated urinary cultures and careful attention to the use of appropriate antibiotics.

In the immediate postoperative period, the diuresis must be encouraged. It is probably wrong to utilize Lasix to encourage this since this causes hypercalciuria. It is preferable to use hydrochlorothiazide 50 mg bid.

The use of 0.5 percent buvicaine placed around the intercostal nerve bundles along the skin edges has significantly reduced narcotic use postoperatively. Recently, it has become apparent that patients who are managed with epidural analgesia have a considerably easier postoperative course.

No patient should leave the hospital until a flat plate has been reviewed. If persistent calculi are present they represent retained or residual calculi and are sometimes referred to as a "false recurrence." The surgeon must decide what is the most appropriate course of action, because a residual stone means that the operation has failed and the second

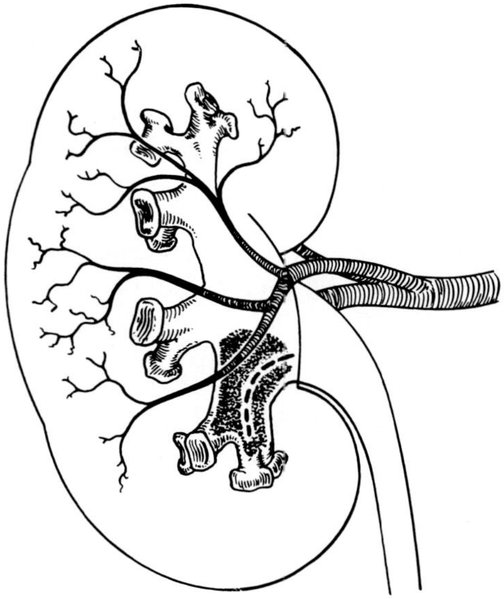

Fig. 22-9. Extension of a parenchymal incision into the inferior collecting system is possible if one remembers that there is an intersegmental line between the posterior segmental artery and the posterior branch of the basilar segmental artery.

aim of maintaining the patient infection free is doomed to failure. All patients should be studied with renal clearance studies and a pyelogram at 6 weeks. The patients require continuous close followup with repeated urine cultures and x-ray study for the rest of their lives.

COMPLICATIONS

Complications are listed in Table 22-1, and some are discussed so that the reader may be forewarned and hopefully avoid these problems. It is impossible to predict when these will occur nor can percentages or probabilities be assigned. Even those with extensive experience with these operations have not necessarily had similar problems; thus Boyce[1] has not reported major arterial problems (cf. Medical College of Virginia (MCV) experience, Table 22-2), while we have fortunately not been aware of nephrocutaneous fistula or the need to explore for postoperative bleeding.

The urinary tract in all nephrolithotomies should be closed watertight, and the stent should provide unobstructed drainage down the ureter. A properly positioned Penrose drain will take care of the minimal leakage that will occur. If it is not appropriately placed, however, a retroperitoneal collection of urine can occur and prolonged ileus is a warning that this is happening. The Penrose drain should be evaluated. If the urinary fistula occurs, the surgeon should pay particular attention to the position of the stent; on occasion, the proximal end of a double-J may have moved so that it is holding the calyceal or pelvic wall open and thus drainage is occurring. Alternatively, severe edema or migratory calculus at the ureteral pelvic junction may be causing obstruction. This should be handled appropriately. If the fistulous drainage persists beyond 8 days, it is appropriate that the internal stent be replaced. Fortunately, this complication has not persisted beyond 14 days in our hands. If this should occur, however, a percutaneous nephrostomy can be placed in the patient approximately 21 days postoperatively. If this does not heal the fistula, a complete reevaluation might be necessary since one of the conceivable causes might be complete occlusion of an infundibulum and thus urinary drainage into the retroperitoneum has occurred.

Bleeding during the first 48 hours after surgery is not unusual. If it persists longer than 5 days and transfusions are necessary, however, reevaluation of bleeding and clotting times should certainly be carried out. Significant hematuria that appears for the first time at 10–14 days will sometimes be associated with intrarenal vascular problems and selective renal angiography is useful, and indeed may be therapeutic. Rarely, surgical exploration may be required.

Retained calculi or so-called "false recurrence" should not occur, but as Table 22-3 demonstrates, this still happens on occasion. These calculi are usually in minor calyces

Table 22-1
Complications

Pulmonary	Down lung, pneumothorax, embolus
Infection	Persistent urinary septicemia
Wound, prolonged pain	Delayed healing
Postoperative bleeding, urinary fistula, retained calculi	

Table 22-2
Nephrolithotomy, Medical College of Virginia, 1968–1982

		Anatrophic	Gil-Vernet
Total		173	114
Deaths		1	0
Nephrectomy		4	0
Recurrence	True	27	13
	False	14	9
Infections	Preop	168	101
	Postop	35	12

with very stenotic infundibula so they were missed at surgery. Leaving a nephrostomy tube postoperatively in the renal pelvis in such a case would be a waste of effort because irrigating fluid would never reach the stones.

True recurrence is usually associated with urinary tract infections that cannot be cleared out with aggressive antimicrobial therapy. The surgeon in this case will have to decide whether further therapy with antiurease drugs or repeat surgery is needed.

MEDICAL COLLEGE OF VIRGINIA SERIES

This experience represents the combined work of nine faculty members and their resident trainees; thus there are some deviations in management and differing philosophies over 20 years. Nevertheless, it is clear that a variety of small but significant scientific advances have been incorporated into our approaches and the improved results are evident. These are shown in Tables 22-2 and 22-3. It will be noted that the period from 1982 is not reported in detail because full analysis and appropriate followup (5 years) has not yet been completed. This group of people includes those who have been managed percutaneously or by ESWL. All of these patients were carefully informed of the availability of these procedures and the possible complications and with the help of their attending made a decision as to which was the appropriate management. During this period of time, we have only done six open procedures; the remainder have been managed with the newer modalities.

Table 22-3
Anatrophic Nephrolithotomy Followup

	Prior to 1970	1970–1973	1973–1976	1976–1979	1979–1982
Deaths	1	0	0	0	0
Nephrectomy	1	1	1	0	1
Recurrence					
True	20.0%	24%	8.1%	8.4%	6.4%
False	11.7%	8%	6.08%	5%	3%
Infection					
Preop	95%	92%	98.0%	97%	98%
Postop	31.6%	24%	16.3%	14%	16%
Total patients	60	25	48	8	21

The one death in our series occurred very early in the experience and was due to septicemia from a resistant pseudomonas.

As mentioned before, all cases of nephrectomy have been secondary to difficulties with the renal artery, not renal hemorrhage. In one patient, the renal artery was cut when clamped with a Satinsky clamp; revascularization was unsuccessful. In two patients, subintimal tears were caused presumably by the arterial clamp and stretching of the renal pedicle just prior to occluding it with the clamp. In one patient, there was no renal blood flow following the removal of the arterial clamp. The exact cause of this is not known. We were unable to flush the kidney out, and despite vigorous efforts to revascularize this kidney, we were unsuccessful. The only abnormality found at pathologic evaluation was an intimal tear and extensive thrombosis.

As Table 22-3 demonstrates, there has been a remarkable drop in recurrence. This is ascribed to the improvement in the surgical technique and the ability to visualize the intrarenal structures. There are those who would suggest these results represent a difference in followup. It is still apparent that recurrences usually happen within the first 4 years. We must, however, acknowledge 15 percent of the patients that are lost to followup.

REFERENCES

1. Assimos DG, Boyce WH, Harrison LH, et al: Post-operative anatrophic nephrolithotomy bleeding. J Urol 135:1153–1156, 1986
2. Boijsen E: Angiographic studies of the anatomy of single and multiple renal arteries. Acta Radiol Suppl 183:1–35, 1959
3. Boyce WH, Harrison LH: Complications of renal stone surgery, in Smith RB, Skinner DG (eds): Complications of Urologic Surgery. Philadelphia, Saunders, 1976, pp 87–105
4. Boyce WH: Nephrolithotomy, in Glenn JF (ed): Urologic Surgery, ed 3. Philadelphia, Lippincott, 1983, pp 181–193
5. Boyce WH, Elkins IB: Reconstructive renal surgery following anatrophic nephrolithotomy. J Urol 111:307–312, 1974
6. Boyce WH: Surgery of urinary calculi in perspective. Urol Clin N Am 10:585–594, 1983
7. Boyce WH, Russell JM, Webb R: The management of the papillae during intrarenal surgery. Trans Am Assoc Genitourin Surg 71:76–82, 1979
8. Deming CL: Renal circulation following various types of nephrotomies. Am J Surg 4:424–431, 1928
9. Gil-Vernet J: New surgical concepts in removing renal calculi. Urol Internatl 20:255–288, 1965
10. Graves FT: The Arterial Anatomy of the Kidney. Baltimore, Williams & Wilkins, 1971
11. Griffith DP: Struvite stones. Kidney Internatl 13:372–382, 1978
12. Hodson J: The lobar structure of the kidney. Br J Urol 44:246–261, 1972
13. James R, Novick AC, Straffon RA, et al: Anatrophic nephrolithotomy for the removal of staghorn or branched renal calculi. Urology 15:108–111, 1980
14. Kerr WS Jr: Surgical management of renal stones with emphasis on infundibulotomy. J Urol 103:130–133, 1970
15. Luttrop W, Nelson CE, Nilsson T, et al: Study of glomerular and tubular function after in-situ cooling of the kidney. J Urol 115:133–135, 1976
16. Metzner PJ, Boyce WH: Simplified renal hypothermia: An adjunct to conservative renal surgery. Br J Urol 44:76–85, 1972

17. Pahira TJ, Elyaderani MK: Intraoperative localization of renal calculi. Urol Clin N Am 12:787–798, 1985
18. Redman JF, Bissada NK, Harper DL: Anatrophic nephrolithotomy: Experience with simplification of Smith & Boyce Technique. J Urol 122:595–597, 1979
19. Roth RA: Current surgical management of branched renal calculi. Surg Clin N Am 56:753–766, 1976
20. Smith MJV: Anatrophic nephrolithotomy, in Roth RA, Finlayson B (eds): Stones: Clinical Management of Urolithiasis. Baltimore, Williams & Wilkins, 1983, pp 349–371
21. Smith MJV, Boyce WH: Anatrophic nephrotomy and plastic calyrhaphy. Trans Am Assoc Genitourin Surg 59:18–24, 1967
22. Spirnak JP, Resnick MI: Anatrophic nephrolithotomy. Urol Clin N Am 10:665–675, 1983
23. Stephenson TP, Bauer S, Hargreave TB, et al: The technique and results of pyelocalycotomy for staghorn calculi. Br J Urol 47:751–758, 1986
24. Straffon RA: The surgical management of staghorn calculi, in Novick AV, Straffon RA (eds): Vascular Problems in Urologic Surgery, Philadelphia, Saunders, 1982, pp 99–108
25. Sykes D: The correlation between renal vascularization and lobulation of the kidney. Br J Urol 36:549–555, 1964
26. Vordermark JS II: Segmental anatomy of the kidney. Urology 17:521–531, 1981

Stephen P. Dretler

23

Extracorporeal Shock-Wave Lithotripsy

Extracorporeally produced focused shock waves for the destruction of urinary calculi was first reported by Chaussy and associates in 1980.[1] Since that time, approximately 300 lithotriptors have been installed around the world, and perhaps 200,000 to 300,000 patients have had extracorporeal shock-wave lithotripsy (ESWL) for treatment of urinary calculi (Fig. 23-1).

HISTORY OF SHOCK-WAVE RESEARCH

The advent of ESWL was not the result of a brief innovative investigation but rather the result of many years of intense laboratory and clinical research by Dornier Systems GMBH, a West German aerospace and engineering company, and the urology group at Munich's Grosshadern Clinic. The Dornier research team was led by Drs. Wolfgang Hepp and Bernt Forssman, and the urology group was led by Dr. Christian Chaussy.

The effect of shock waves on metal spheres was being investigated at the Dornier Company as part of their aerospace program. It was realized during these studies that when the metal spheres passed through the sound barrier and a shock wave hit the sphere, small pits occurred under water droplets on the surface of the metal spheres; similarly, there were small pits on the inside of the sphere at the interface of air and metal. It was recognized by the Dornier scientists that shock waves had an action at the interface of two surfaces of differing accoustical impedance, in this instance, water and metal on the outside of the sphere and metal and air on the inside. How this concept became translated into the treatment of kidney stones has not been clearly enunciated, but it appears that speculative conversation by Dornier engineers was the genesis for the concept. They thought that if shock waves acted on surfaces of differing acoustical impedance, then perhaps shock waves could be focused in the body. If so, they could act at the junction of kidney stones and tissue—two surfaces of differing acoustical impedance. Initial tests on the biologic effects of shock waves were carried out in the Dornier laboratory by Dr. Wolfgang Hepp.[2] The Dornier engineers then studied the effect of shock

STONE DISEASE: DIAGNOSIS AND MANAGEMENT
ISBN 0-8089-1873-7

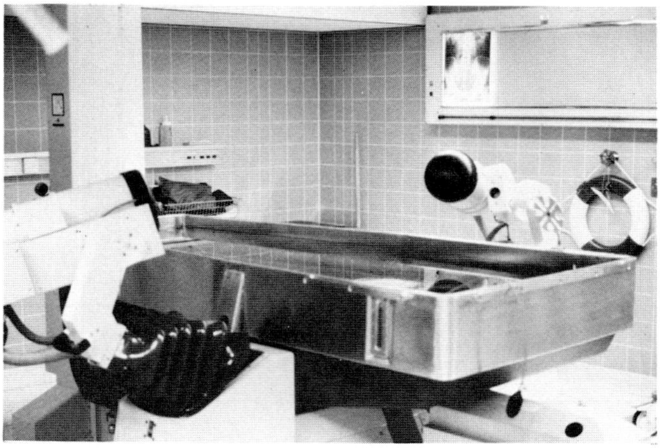

Fig. 23-1. Dornier lithotriptor in Grosshadern Clinic, Munich, West Germany.

waves on in vitro kidney stones and, encouraged by the initial results, presented their preliminary findings at a combined medical-industry conference in Munich.[3] Dr. Egebert Schmiedt, a professor of Urology at Ludwig Maximillian University in Munich and Chairman at the Grosshadern Clinic, recognized the clinical possibility of extracorporeal destruction of kidney stones, and he, Dr. F. Eisenberger, and Dr. C. Chaussy began to investigate the possibilities of ESWL as a clinical entity.

The initial laboratory investigations relative to the problems of producing a usable shock wave had been carried out by Drs. Forrsman and Hepp. They used a detonating wire to provide shock waves. At that time (1972), there was not yet a clinically acceptable method of generating shock waves. The invention of the underwater spark gap method of generating shock waves was the next advance in the development of a clinical prototype.[4]

SHOCK WAVES AND ULTRASOUND WAVES

Both shock waves and ultrasonic impulses behave according to the laws of acoustics; however, there are differences in the physical properties of ultrasound and shock waves. When examining the pressure/time diagram of ultrasound and shock waves, it is seen that the shock wave has a very high intensity pressure spike, a steep onset and a gradual relaxation, whereas the ultrasonic wave has a single, well-defined frequency and a sinusoided pressure variation with alternating tension and compression (Fig. 23-2).[5]

When shock waves and ultrasound waves are passed through biologic materials, the tissue dampens the effect of high-frequency impulses. The extensive low-frequency range of the shock wave and the lack of tissue dampening makes depth of tissue penetration greater with shock waves than with ultrasound. Because tissue has a dampening effect on ultrasonic waves, long exposure to high-frequency ultrasonic waves will result in cellular degradation. Tissue damage does not occur from exposure to the amount of low-frequency shock waves used for clinical stone destruction. The observations that low-frequency shock waves did not produce cellular degradation or alteration in tissue culture

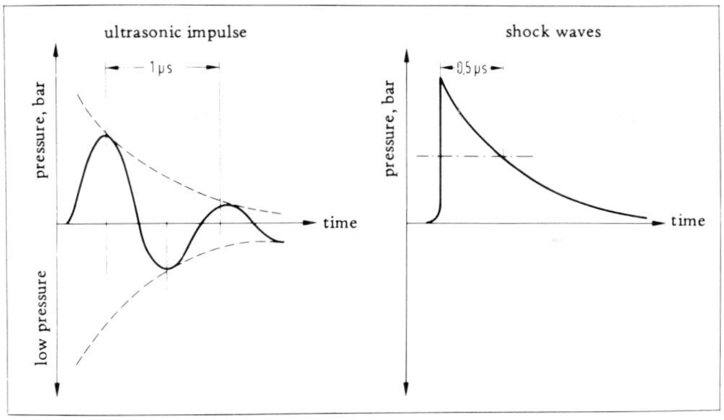

Fig. 23-2. Schematic representation of pressure/time diagram for shock waves and ultrasound waves.

growth made the application of shock waves to destroy kidney stones a clinical possibility.

The first aspect Chaussy studied of shock-wave kidney stone destruction was the fundamental physical changes that occurred when the shock wave met the stone. The externally generated shock wave passes through a tube of water and then tissue and then meets the stone. Since body tissue, including bone, is acoustically similar to water, the shock wave interprets body tissue as water and exerts no physical action until it meets a surface of differing acoustic impedance, in this case, a stone. All lithotriptors, both first- and second-generation, use some coupling apparatus so that the shock wave does not act at the surface of the body and cause injury or dissipate (Table 23-1).[6]

When the shock wave meets the stone, it interprets the junction of stone and tissue or the interface between stone and fluid as an alteration in acoustic impedance. The pressure wave of the shock is then reflected by the stone. When the shock hits the front side of the stone, it causes compression, and this pressure acts on the front surface of the stone. The wave is then transmitted through the stone, and a tensile wave is created on

Table 23-1
Basic Data for Lithotriptors Currently Developed and Under Development

Manufacturer	Generation	Focusing	Coupling	Localization	Positioning
Dornier	Spark Gap	Ellipsoid	Bath	Biplane fluoro	Move patient
EDAP	Piezoelectric	Spherical	Membrane	Ultrasound	Move generator
International biomedics	Exploding liquid conductor	Ellipsoid	Membrane	C-arm fluoroscope	Move patient; multipurpose table
Medstone	Spark gap	Ellipsoid	Membrane	Plane x-ray films	Move patient
Northgate	Spark gap	Ellipsoid	Membrane	Ultrasound	Move reflector
Siemens	2 electromagnetic generators	Acoustic lens	Membrane	2 fluoroscopes	Move generator of patient; multipurpose table
Technomed	Spark gap	Ellipsoid	Pool	Ultrasound	Move generator

the back surface of the stone. Both compression and tensile waves, when they exceed the strength of the stone, cause crumbling and fragmentation. This occurs almost simultaneously on both sides of the stone.

FOCUSING THE SHOCK WAVE

If a method had not been developed to focus the power of the shock wave and then direct the focused shock wave at a stone, clinical use of shock waves would have been impractical. Without focusing, the amount of power necessary to break a stone would have been greater than tissue tolerance. The focusing of the shock wave diminishes the amount of energy necessary to produce stone destruction and is accomplished by the use of a symmetrical semiellipsoid in the Dornier machine. An acoustic lens is used by the Siemans model. The shock wave is produced by underwater spark discharge in the Dornier model. When the spark occurs, water is vaporized at the site of the spark and a pressure wave is created that spreads until it hits the side walls of the semiellipsoid. The waves are then reflected by the walls of the semiellipsoid and converge at a second focal point, F_2 (Fig. 23-3). The power that occurs at the site of wave convergence (F_2) is equal to the sum of the reflected waves. The size of the focal point is 1.5 cm^3. Most of the effective energy is focused in the 1.5-cm^3 space with rapid falloff in pressure outside the focal point. The energy generated at the focal point is dependent not only on the curvature of the semiellipsoid but also on the distance of the gap between the sparking electrode tips. As the space between the electrode points widens, the pressure amplitude increases significantly. Also, as the distance between the tips widens, the geometry of the wave reflection is altered, and the site of the focal point (F_2) changes.

The shock waves may be dampened by body mass. For instance, 6 cm of muscle tissue will cause a decrease of 10–20 percent in pressure amplitude. Since lithotriptor voltage is adjustable, modifications in the amount of power per shock are able to be made and depend on the operator's assessment of patient mass between the energy source and the stone as well as the anticipated stone hardness.

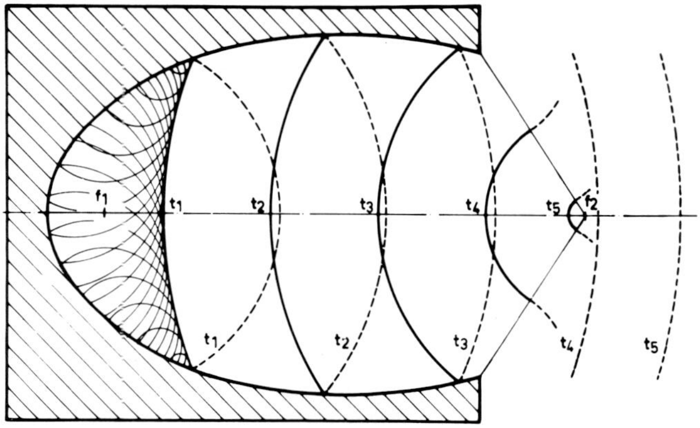

Fig. 23-3. Diagram of reflected pressure waves from the walls of the semiellipsoid indicating site of shock-wave generation (F_1) and site of convergence at F_2.

Experimental studies of the effects of shock waves on stones of various compositions showed that fragmentation occurred at energies that created kinetic energy in the stone fragments of only 2×10^{-3} joules, or the power of a raindrop hitting the pavement. There is no explosive effect on the stone, and fragments do not become lodged in mucosa. The power of the shock wave itself is 300–600 bar (a pressure measurement). This is similar to 300–600 atm of pressure. If patients are not anesthetized, the treatment is quite painful.

BIOLOGIC EFFECTS OF SHOCK WAVES

Although the shock wave causes hemolysis, the amount of blood present at the focal point of each shock wave is too small in relation to total circulating blood volume to cause any systemic effects. Furthermore, since the blood is flowing, only one shock wave hits each blood cell, minimizing hemolysis. However, the hemolyzing effect of shock waves can be seen clinically. Hematuria occurs during stone destruction, and the cherry-colored blood in the urine is obviously hemolyzed, presumably because of the time the cells spend in the renal pelvis or calyces at the focal point of the shock wave.

The shock wave has had no observable effect on cell growth in lymphocyte culture; however, the lungs of experimental animals have shown significant change as a result of shock-wave application. The multiple air-tissue alveolar interfaces in the lungs create surfaces at which the shock wave encounters a change in acoustic impedance; therefore, energy is released, resulting in tissue damage. With proper patient positioning the lung is rarely seen during stone treatment and, when seen, is easily recognizable. No report of lung damage has been reported in over 50,000 treatments. Similarly, no observable damage to the intestine has been reported, despite the air-tissue interfaces.

The record of the effect of shock waves on renal function in laboratory animals appears limited to micro- and macroscopic studies 48 hours after exposure and a few treated animals followed for 1 year. In these studies, there is no record of adverse effects on renal function following shock wave application; however, the quantitation of how much shock could be given before tissue damage occurs is not available.

CLINICAL APPLICATION OF SHOCK WAVES

Once the shock wave was found to be effective against renal calculi, was discovered not to be damaging to adjacent tissue, and could be focused, the problem of accurate clinical localization and aiming of the focused wave was addressed. Chaussy found ultrasound techniques to be ineffective for localizing stone fragments following the application of shock waves. Repeatedly, artifacts were seen by ultrasound, and it could not be determined when the stone was fragmented sufficiently to allow spontaneous passage of all pieces; therefore, biplanar fluoroscopy was chosen as the localization method. Stone fragments of 2–3 mm could be visualized, thus assuring that fragmentation could continue until it appeared that all stone fragments could be passed via the ureter. The x-ray units were mounted on swivel arms and the point at which they intersected was fixed to be the same at the F_2 focal point of the shock wave (Fig. 23-4). The objective then became to move the stone to the focal point of the shock wave with proper stone visualization. To accomplish this, the patient is placed in a chair controlled by hydraulic lifts. The patient is

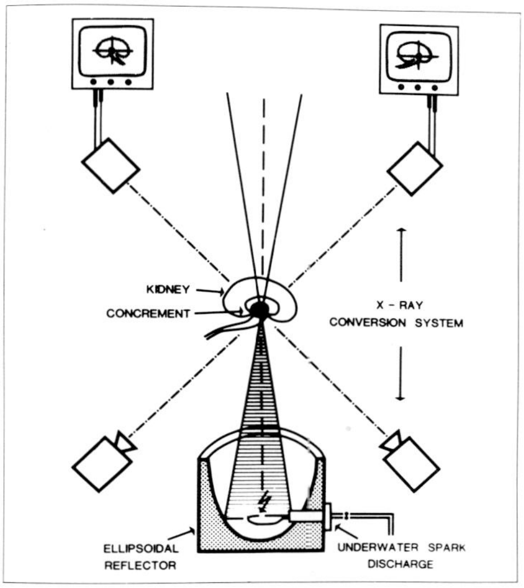

Fig. 23-4. Diagramatic representation of the coordination of shock-wave focusing and x-ray visualization.

able to be moved forward and backward, up and down, side to side, and diagonally along the axis of the x-ray tubes. This imaging system is sufficient for visualization of most calculi and to coordinate the placement of the stone at the focal point. There are limitations to the positioning of patients. A patient who is shorter than 4 ft will be difficult to secure in the chair, and in a patient taller than 6 ft 6 inches, the kidney may be difficult to place at the focal point F_2. Small children have been treated, but additional supports are needed to properly position the patient. If the patient weighs more than 280 pounds, the sensitive hydraulic lift will be stressed, and if the patient is too rotund, the x-ray tubes may be unable to be placed in proper position or the patient may be unable to be lowered deep enough in the tub for the kidney and the stone to be placed at F_2. Many hours of struggle have been waged to get large patients into proper position in the tub so that the kidney stone is at the focal point of the shock wave. The experienced machine operator may, by repositioning the patient or vectoring with the controls, win the battle. Despite these efforts, however, some patients cannot be positioned properly for stone treatment. The chair in which they are placed hits the bottom of the tub before the kidney with the stone can be lowered into the F_2 focal point. Some of these technical problems may be circumvented with the use of second generation technology.

The tub in which the treatment occurs is made of stainless steel and is coated with resins to decrease x-ray exposure to personnel in the area. Persons standing 5 feet away from the tub have no lead apron requirement. Similarly, although each discharge of a shock wave makes a loud noise, the water and the tub insulation dampen the sound so that it is not in the decibel range that produces auditory damage. Protective ear coverings are not required.

For effective treatment, the tub in the Dornier machine is filled with heated, degassed water. If regular tap water is used, the CO_2 bubbles in the tap water allow *pseudocavitation* to occur. The CO_2 bubbles create air–water interfaces, and the shock wave becomes partially absorbed by these interfaces. By the time the shock wave reaches the stone, it is thus of insufficient force to break the calculus. Therefore, it is necessary to use distilled, degassed water in the tub for effective shock wave treatment. If the water is "hard," a desalting process is also necessary to remove minerals from the water as they interfere with the power and propagation of the shock wave.

The water temperature in the tub is also of significance. The higher the water temperature, the higher the partial pressure of dissolved gases. When the water temperature in the tub is heated to the patients' body temperature, gas in the water expands and is more likely to allow pseudocavitation. Since the shock wave discharges energy at the interface of water and gas bubbles, bruises may occur on the patients' skin if air bubbles are on the skin surface. To prevent both the skin bruises and the dissipation of the shock wave, vaseline is put on the skin over the target area before the patient is submerged. If the patient has body hair that traps bubbles, it must be shaved prior to treatment. Care must be taken both at the entry point (posterior) of the shock wave and the exit point (anterior) to minimize bruising that may occur.

SUMMARY OF PRECLINICAL INVESTIGATION OF THE DORNIER LITHOTRIPTOR

Shock waves are produced by a spark gap in the F_1 focal region of a water-filled semiellipsoid and, by reflection on the inner wall of the semiellipsoid, are focused at a second focal point (F_2). It was found that the power of the shock wave is affected by tissue layers, the distance between electrode points, gas in the water, heat of the water, and kilovoltage of the electrical discharge, and that these variables needed to be controlled for safe treatment to be administered. It was noted that the only significant tissue damage was to alveolae, and that cells and blood were not clinically affected. Chaussy and investigators found that stone destruction could be achieved in vivo, and that in dogs the particles would pass down the ureter spontaneously. The x-ray visualization system was developed to detect fragments down to 2 mm in size so that fragmentation could be sufficiently complete to allow spontaneous passage of all concretions. Animal renal function studies showed no discernible renal impairment at shock-wave pressure levels necessary to destroy implanted calculi. Patient studies were then carried out.

CLINICAL STUDIES

The initial successful results of shock-wave therapy for cherry-sized renal pelvic calculi as reported by Chaussy et al.[7] allowed expansion of the clinical indications to include calculi in the pelvis and calyces and upper third of the ureter. A summary of the first 1012 shock-wave treatments by Chaussy and coinvestigators were reported just before clinical trials were begun in the United States.[8] Chaussy and Schmiedt reported that shock-wave treatment was carried out on 896 patients. The 896 patients included 39 cases of partial staghorn, 6 cases of total staghorn, 108 patients with multiple calculi, and 13 patients with bilateral calculi. They followed patients for 2–3 months after treatment and found that 9.3 percent had small retained stone fragments, mostly in dilated lower calyces. Subsequent surgery was necessary in only 5 percent of their patients. Glomerular filtration and clearance studies on 50 patients prior to ESWL, and then 3 months and 18 months after ESWL, showed overall improvement in function of the treated kidney. Approximately 3 percent of their patients required endoscopic procedures to treat obstructing ureteral stone debris (Fig. 23-5). The only other significant complications re-

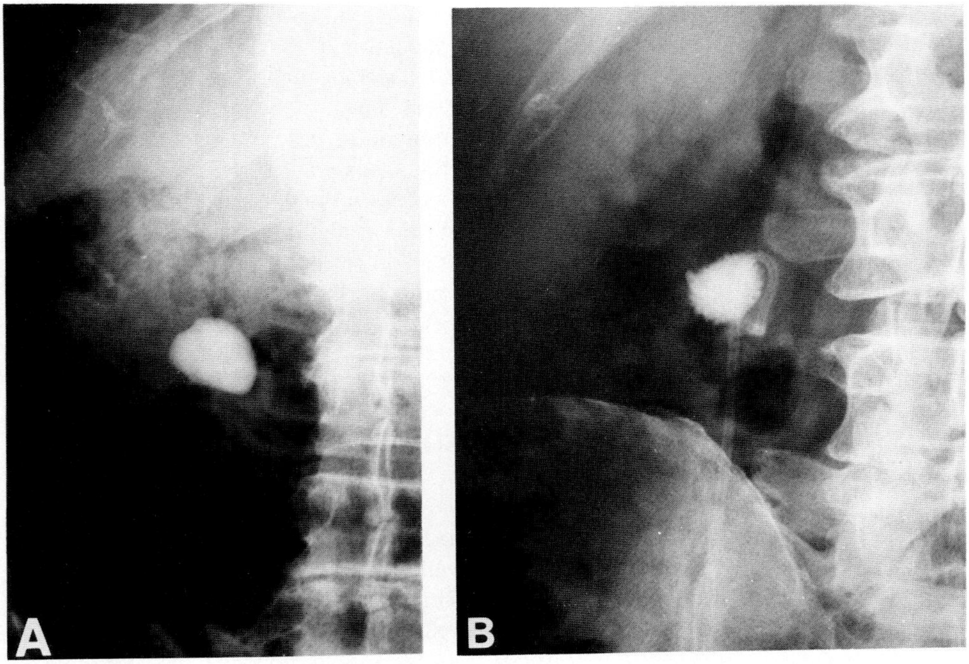

Fig. 23-5. (*A*) Smooth, dense monohydrate stone (not fragile). (*B*) Spiculated typical fragile calcium oxalate dyhydrate stone. Note delicate architecture.

ported were six instances of subcapsular renal bleeding, one of which required operative intervention. Chaussy initially did not include patients with infected calculi. Later, however, he found that antibiotics administered for 1–2 days prior to treatment allowed ESWL of infected calculi without precipitating an acute septic episode. Percutaneous nephrostomy, for treatment of sepsis, was only rarely required; therefore, the easily fragmentable struvite calculi were included in the treatment protocols.

Ureteral calculi lodged in position for less than 4–6 weeks that were above the iliac crest were treated successfully. Chaussy treated 83 patients with ureteral calculi and reported that only four failures occurred. He deduced that treatment failure occurred only in patients whose stones were lodged in the ureter for over 4–6 weeks.

United States Experience

In 1984 an investigation was started by six U.S. centers that collaborated in a cooperative study of ESWL.[9] Initially, all stones treated by each study center were solitary, located in the renal pelvis or calyces, and were less than 2 cm in diameter. After each investigator treated 50 patients, calculi larger than 2 cm, multiple calculi, and upper ureteral calculi were also included. A total of 2501 patients were treated in the combined U.S. group study, and 3-month followup was completed for 926 patients.

There were 885 calculi less than 1 cm in size; 1225 had stone volume totaling 1–2 cm, and 296 patients had a calculus burden of 2–3 cm. Of these patients, 65 had staghorn calculi and 30 were inadequately reported. The duration of treatment varied considerably, but most treatments required over 60–90 minutes of operating time. Anesthesia given was either epidural or general. Fluoroscopic exposure time varied from 15 to 600 seconds, but recordings did not account for the radiation from the spot films, only fluoroscopy. Recent studies by McCullough have shown that radiation exposure from ESWL, including fluoroscopy and spot films, may average 17 rads per treatment, considerably more than the 3 rads for an IVP. He noted that this compared favorably to the average of 33 rads for cardiac catherization and 25 rads for percutaneous ultrasonic treatment.[10]

The number of shocks necessary to fragment calculi averaged about 1200 but varied for different sizes and composition of calculi. Initially, there was a limit of 1500 shocks per kidney. This was eventually raised to 1800, then 2000. Undoubtedly, the average shocks per treatment would have been higher if there had been no limits set. The number of shocks increased as stone volume increased; however, it was apparent that some stones fragmented easily while others were more resistant. Increasing experience with ESWL allowed for increasingly accurate predictions relative to the number of shocks necessary to fragment a stone.

In the group study, it was found that a second treatment was necessary for approximately 8–10 percent of patients with a stone of less than 1 cm, 15–20 percent retreatment for calculi of 1–2 cm, and a higher percent required retreatment when calculus volume was greater than 2–3 cm. The retreatment rate reported from one center showed that for solitary pelvic stones of under 2 cm, 7 percent needed retreatment, but if stones were over 2 cm, then 32.7 percent needed retreatment.[11]

Small calculi lodged in the ureter or sequestered in a calyx may necessitate second treatments, not because of volume, but because the fragments can not separate. Multiple fragments around a central core of stone will prevent action of the shock wave on the central portion. Large stones often require more than 2000 shocks for complete fragmentation; therefore, more than one treatment is necessary. Some stones are harder and more difficult to fragment than others. Data generated at the Massachusetts General Hospital indicate that the calculi with over 60 percent of calcium oxalate monohydrate (COM) or predominantly calcium phosphate dihydrate (brushite) fragment with more difficulty than struvite, uric acid, apatite, or calculi that are composed predominantly of calcium oxalate dihydrate (COD). The COD calculi fragment into crumbs, while the monohydrate often breaks into small chunks. The harder calculi require more shocks and higher kilovoltage to complete fragmentation than do the more fragile calculi. After experience with a number of calculi, an observant operator can begin to accurately predict the number of shocks necessary to complete treatment, the size of fragments, and the clinical course of the patient by the radiographic appearance of the stone and the position of the stone in the collecting system. This is very helpful when selecting patients for treatment and for anticipating which patients may need a supplemental form of therapy including percutaneous debulking, percutaneous drainage, ureteral stone manipulation, or adjunctive chemolysis. Whether a patient with a stone over 2 cm is a candidate for percutaneous treatment or ESWL is determined by both the size and the anticipated chemical composition of the stone. Therefore, a new distinction has been introduced into the diagnostic area—the distinction of "stone fragility." Undoubtedly, the fragment retention rate is also affected by stone composition or "fragility" as well as size. Lingeman et al. reported a 37 percent fragment retention rate at 3 months for calculi over 2 cm.[11] It is clinically apparent that if stratified for composition, pure COD calculi would have fewer remnants than COM.

In the U.S. investigation, patients with calculi less than 1 cm in diameter had less pain following treatment than patients with larger calculi. Sixty percent of patients with calculi less than 1 cm had pain post ESWL treatment; 65 percent of patients with calculi 1–2 cm and 70 percent of patients with calculi 2–3 cm had pain following ESWL treatment. The pain was due to local trauma of the shock wave and colic from passage of fragments. Currently, there is a body of opinion that the use of double-J stents may alleviate pain and allow outpatient management of calculi. Of the U.S. study patients, 809 of the 2501 had partial (792) or complete (17) ureteral obstruction noted at the time of discharge. Most patients passed these fragments without the need for intervention; however, 96 (3.8 percent) of 2501 patients required cystoextraction attempts of obstructing fragments prior to discharge from the hospital, and undoubtedly, many patients underwent other unrecorded procedures to treat ureteral obstruction in the followup period. Data collected from the Massachusetts General Hospital demonstrated that experience and patient selection decreased the number of endoscopic manipulations necessary following ESWL treatment. The first 721 patients treated at that hospital had a 3.7 percent incidence of "Steinstrasse" that required endoscopic intervention. Of the next 300 patients, however, only 1 percent required ureteral fragment manipulation.[12] Including surgical intervention, endoscopic manipulation, and percutaneous procedures, only 7 percent of patients in the U.S. investigation required additional urologic treatment following treatment and prior to discharge.

In the immediate post-ESWL period, radiographs showed that 72 percent of calculi were pulverized, so that all fragments measured less than 2 mm in diameter. Five percent of the patients had some fragments greater than 5 mm, and 2 percent of stones failed to show any change at all. In all likelihood, the stones that failed to show change were either caught in an obstructed calyx or diverticulum, were impacted in the ureter, or were composed of the more difficult to fragment COM, brushite, or cystine. At the time of hospital discharge, fragments of calculi were still present in 85 percent of the patients and 34 percent of all patients had retained fragments at 3 months following ESWL. Of significance is that, at 3 months, residual fragments were noted in 18 percent of calculi less than 1 cm, 22 percent of calculi 1–2 cm, and 47.5 percent of calculi 2–3 cm in size. Although it is as yet unclear what this means relative to future stone recurrence, it is a foreboding statistic and is particularly noteworthy when considering therapy for infected calculi.

Complications other than urologic occurred in 7 percent of the patients treated. Four deaths occurred within 6 weeks of ESWL treatment. Two were related to cerebrovascular accidents and hypertension. One death was from liver carcinoma and one from suicidal depression. There were no deaths directly attributed to shock-wave treatment.

The shock-wave delivery is tripped by the *QRS* complexes of the ECG. As a result, the shock wave is delivered during the refractory period of the cardiac pulsation, decreasing the possibility of electronically induced cardiac electrical discharges. Pacemaker patients, although excluded from treatment by product labeling, have been treated without consequence by a number of centers in the United States and Europe.

Each patient entered in the U.S. study had a renogram performed pretreatment and 3 months posttherapy. Of the 494 studies completed and available, 241 patients showed some deterioration of renal function while 248 showed improved clearance post therapy. For 5 patients, function was unchanged. The analysis of this data is preliminary and requires much more evaluation prior to drawing conclusions. It is not known whether this decrease in function noted for 241 patients is only 1–2 percent and within the scope of variation in test results or is truly significant. Patients have been noted to have segmented decrease in renal function following multiple ESWL treatments; therefore, caution should be exercised when administering multiple ESWL treatments until all this information has been thoroughly evaluated. Furthermore, a recent data update from the American group circulated in August 1986 stated that followup data on 300 patients showed that 3 percent had developed hypertension. The significance of this observation is as yet unclear and uncorroborated.

Kaude et al. studied 33 patients pre- and post-ESWL by intravenous pyelogram (IVP), renogram, and magnetic resonance imaging within 48 hours of ESWL treatment. They found seven asymptomatic perirenal hematomas, and in all patients with hematomas renal plasma flow was significantly diminished. Furthermore, all seven hematoma patients showed intrarenal obstructive patterns not seen with other patients.[13] Again, the long-term significance of these observations has not yet been determined.

The maximum number of shock waves per treatment, the kilovoltage at which they are administered, the safe interval between first and subsequent treatments, and the total number of treatments that can be given without causing renal impairment or the common denominators that render one susceptible to renal damage have not been clearly established. At the present time, medical centers are giving 2000 shocks per treatment without any specified time interval between first and subsequent treatments. Usually, an ultrasound is done between treatments to rule out the presence of a subcapsular or perinephric hematoma. At present, there are no safety guidelines established for the total number of treatments or the time interval between individual treatments to the same kidney.

PATIENT SELECTION AND TREATMENT METHOD

The patients usually selected for treatment are those with calculi less than 3 cm in diameter, who have adequate outflow tract for fragment egress, and who have normal bleeding and clotting parameters. These patients must also fit the previously noted physical criterion that allows proper positioning for calculus treatment. Patients with calcified renal artery aneurysms have been excluded. Calcifications in the aorta have not been a contraindication, and no untoward effects have been noted. Patients with infected urine or a history of struvite calculi are treated with appropriate antibiotics before, during, and after ESWL therapy. Urosepsis has occurred on rare occasions and has usually been due to obstruction by infected fragments. Preoperative antibiotic therapy is usually adequate to prevent sepsis in patients who have had urinary infection. Percutaneous tube placement may avoid sepsis in those with struvite calculi and also provide an entry port for chemolysis following treatment.

Preoperative preparation for ESWL is not elaborate. Heavy hair-bearing areas over the entrance and exit site of the shock wave are shaved to prevent air bubble accumulation and subsequent skin damage from shock-wave action. Preoperative enemas are not given so as to prevent excess air from being introduced in the intestinal tract. Preoperative low-roughage diet to decrease intestinal air is recommended. If intestinal air is excessive, fluoroscopic visualization of the calculus may be impaired. No damage has been noted by action of the shock wave at the air–intestinal wall interface and does not appear to be a consideration.

The patients are given epidural or general anesthesia. A review of the patients treated in the U.S. study showed no difference in complications for these two types of anesthesia. Local anesthesia by extensive subcutaneous paraspinous block has been reported[11] and appears to be a possible successful method for anesthesia for some patients.

Once anesthetized, the patient is placed in the patient gantry in an oblique position so that the stones do not overlie the spine on the oblique radiographic projections that are taken during the procedure. Once the calculus is in the focal point on both fluoroscopes, 100 shocks at a time are administered, and between each 100 shocks, repeat fluoroscopic examination is carried out. Shock-wave treatment is carried out until fragmentation is considered to be complete. Lucent, poorly visualized, or small calculi require pretreatment ureteral stent placement to aid visualization. Unexpectedly poor visualization of the calculus may require removal of the patient from the tub and stent placement or an intravenous urogram during the procedure. Large calculi, which appear to require two treatments for total fragmentation, are best treated by indwelling or external stent placement prior to the first treatment so that fragments do not obstruct the ureter between the two treatments.

In the U.S. group study, 26 percent of patients stayed in the hospital for 1 day following ESWL, 42 percent stayed for 2 days, and 13 percent stayed for 3 days. Following treatment, 16 percent of patients required more than 4 days of hospitalization. Recently, there has been some impetus for outpatient treatments. The success of outpatient ESWL in some centers may be attributed to the use of double-J stents, which minimize the obstruction and pain in the early posttreatment period.

CLINICAL CIRCUMSTANCES

Extracorporeal shock-wave lithotripsy treatment strategies are evolving for a variety of clinical circumstances, including calculi less than 2 cm, calculi greater than 2 cm, staghorn calculi, ureteral calculi, cystine calculi, calculi in diverticula, lucent calculi, medullary sponge kidney, and nonstaghorn calculi larger than 2.5–3 cm in greatest diameter.

Calculi Under 2 cm

Almost all calculi less than 2 cm, except cystine calculi and those sequested in a diverticulum, are amenable to ESWL therapy. Approximately 7–10 percent of patients with stones under 2 cm need retreatment. Posttreatment pain and time in the hospital is less than for patients with larger calculi. Residual calculi at 3 months' followup were seen in 18 percent of patients with calculi under 1 cm in size and in 22 percent of patients with calculi of 1–2 cm. Posttreatment ureteral obstruction requiring cystoscopic extraction occurred in 1.6 percent of those with calculi under 1 cm and in 3.3 percent of those with calculi of 1–2 cm.[9]

Calculi Over 2 cm

Calculi over 2 cm that are less than the size considered to be staghorn are those that present somewhat of a therapeutic dilemma. The cystoscopic extraction rate posttreatment in this group is 12.5 percent and the fragment retention rate at 3 months is 47.5 percent. Many patients require more than one treatment. Increasingly, percutaneous ultrasonic techniques are being considered as an alternative in this group of patients. Certainly for those with cystine calculi, the percutaneous approach is more effective. The ability to determine by radiographic appearance which stones are more fragile will be the distinction that will allow assignment of patient to ESWL or percutaneous ultrasonic lithotripsy (PUL) therapy (Figs. 23-5*A* and 23-5*B*). The more fragile calculi, of course, will be able to be fragmented more completely by ESWL; therefore, fewer residual fragments, less ureteral obstruction, and a decreased incidence of retreatment will occur in this group of patients. Patients with large calculi who undergo planned retreatment should have a stent placed prior to treatment to prevent fragments from occluding the ureter between the first and subsequent treatments.

Staghorn Calculi

It was quickly determined by Chaussy and the other German and U.S. investigators that most staghorn calculi were inappropriate for ESWL treatment because the large bulk of stones prevented adequate or complete fragmentation and the large volume of stone debris caused upper and lower ureteral obstruction. ESWL as monotherapy for staghorn calculi usually required multiple treatments and unless combined with a debulking procedure, caused lengthy hospital stays and post-ESWL complications, including obstruction and sepsis.

Kahmoski et al. have reported experience with 36 patients (50 renal units) with staghorn calculi who underwent PUL for debulking and ESWL of portions of the calculus unable to be removed percutaneously.[14] They reported that 30 of 50 patients had a single percutaneous procedure, 14 of 50 required two percutaneous procedures, and 6 renal units required three percutaneous approaches. Following PUL for staghorn calculi, 25 renal units required only a single ESWL, 10 had two ESWL(s), and 3 had three ESWL(s). Seven renal units also required ureteroscopy. In total, there were 2.6 procedures performed per renal unit. They reported that 44 of 50 renal units were rendered stone-free. It should be noted that, in their series, debulking procedures averaged 202 minutes. This combination of procedures (ESWL + PUL) does offer an alternative to traditional surgical operations for staghorn calculi. Other investigators are reporting similar experience as that reported by Kahmoski. Data reported by Schultz et al.[15] showed that 50 percent of patients with staghorn required a total of two treatments (PUL + ESWL); 30 percent required three treatments; 13 percent required four treatments; 4 percent required five treatments, and 1 percent required six treatments. The average number of treatments per patient was 2.6, the same as reported by the Indianapolis group. The mean hospital stay was 19 days.

If staghorn calculi are present in previously operated kidneys that do not have stenotic infundibula or calculi sequestered in bulbous obstructed calyces, the patient is probably a good candidate for combined ESWL + PUL. The patient should be aware of the need to wait 3–5 days between treatments, the possibility for multiple procedures, and the lengthy hospitalization entailed in this choice.

Some patients have staghorn calculi that occupy obstructed calyces and are difficult to reach percutaneously. In those patients, combined therapy is a poor choice. Operative intervention may be more appropriate. For patients with struvite and uric acid calculi, a period of post–ESWL + PUL chemolysis is necessary, or rapid recurrence may be the result.

Ureteral Calculi

Calculi above the iliac crest can be treated successfully by ESWL. The success rate is 58 percent for unstented calculi and close to 100 percent for stented calculi or calculi pushed up into the renal pelvis.[16] The management of the upper two-thirds of ureteral calculi by ESWL now includes preliminary ureteral catheter placement. For some as yet unexplained reason, the presence of the ureteral catheter facilitates the effect of the shock wave. It may be that the presence of a stent allows space for separation of fragments or for fluid to suffuse around the stone. The presence of fluid around the stone improves fragmentation. For instances where the ureteral catheter cannot bypass the calculus, Chaussy has suggested that 2 percent xylocaine jelly may be injected as a lubricant to facilitate catheter passage. Angled wires and ureteral catheters have also been used to facilitate passing the catheters by the impacted calculi. For the 20–30 percent of calculi that cannot be bypassed by a stent, the ureteroscope must be used to dislodge the calculus or to pass a catheter in preparation for ESWL therapy. For impacted calculi, the percutaneous approach is favored by the afficionados of the percutaneous method, while ureteroscopic dislodgement and ESWL is the choice for others. Each method is likely to produce success in 90–95 percent of patients.

Extracorporeal shock-wave lithotripsy is difficult for lower-third ureteral calculi; the patient chair is difficult to position in such a way that the lower third of the ureter is over the focal point (F_2) of the shock wave. The bony pelvis and head of femur make the lower-third calculi difficult to visualize. Jenkins and Gillenwater stented and treated six lower-third calculi and reported that three subsequently required operative intervention.[17] Lower ureteral calculi, approached with ureteroscope and chased into the mid or upper ureter, may then be stented and treated by ESWL. Because ESWL of lower-third calculi requires passage of a stent and then the patient must still pass the fragments, removal of lower-third ureteral calculi by ureteroscopy appears to be a more effective treatment method and, currently, remains the treatment of choice of most endourologists.

Calculi in Diverticula

When is a calyceal infundibulum too small to allow passage of shock-wave-pulverized stone fragments from a diverticulum? If the infundibulum and calyx can be identified and outlined by retrograde urography, it is possible for fragments to work their way out. Also, the ability for fragments to pass also depends on the composition of the calculus. Since the harder calculi, like COM and calcium phosphate dihydrate, break into larger pieces than do COD or struvite calculi, they are more difficult to pass from a partially obstructed segment. Approximately 20 percent of patients with a 1-cm calculus lodged in outpouching of upper calyces can be expected to have fragments work their way out and become stone free. Fifty percent of patients will have residual calculi, but the pain that necessitated treatment will disappear.[18] If pain or infection persist, either operative intervention or skilled percutaneous extraction will be necessary. If there is any possibility for fragments to work their way out, ESWL treatment should be attempted and then a few months given for the fragments to be passed.

Medullary Sponge Kidney (MSK)

The patient with pain from calculi in a kidney afflicted with medullary sponge disease may benefit from ESWL if the calculi are not sequestered in cystic cavities. The patient with MSK who repeatedly passes ureteral calculi may benefit from ESWL treatment to decrease the load of stone disease. Those calculi that are open to the collecting system will fragment and pass; those that are not will not be affected by shock wave therapy. Success in relieving pain or decreasing stone load for MSK patients is anecdotal, but it has occurred.

Uric Acid Calculi

Ureteral catheters or percutaneous tubes and contrast infusion must be utilized to successfully treat lucent uric acid calculi; otherwise, the stone can not be seen and targeted on the ESWL fluoroscopic system. During attempted visualization, however, the infused contrast media can obliterate moderate sized fragments. Consequently, the end point for uric acid fragmentation is difficult to determine. Therefore, it is useful to supplement the treatment of uric acid calculi with intravenous, retrograde, or antegrade infusion of an alkaline solution until ultrasound studies demonstrate that all uric acid fragments are small enough to be able to be passed spontaneously. We have used chemolysis with bicarbonate or tromethamine-E (pH 10.4) as a useful adjunct to ESWL. Also, ESWL may be combined with PUL for removal of large uric acid calculi (Fig. 23-6). Ureteral stents passed at the time of treatment are left in place for 24–48 hours after ESWL, and infusion with alkaline solutions are given until documentation of adequate fragmentation of uric acid calculi is complete.

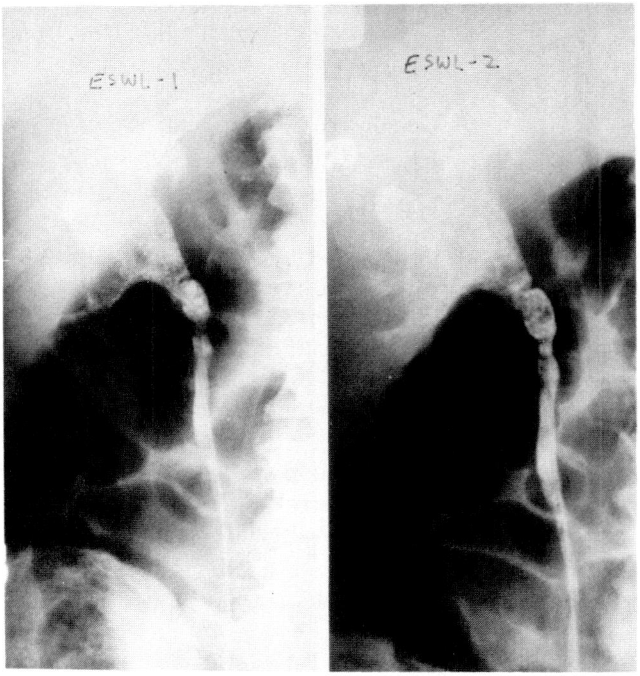

Fig. 23-6. Obstructing upper ureteral stone debris after first and then second ESWL treatment of large uric acid stone.

Struvite ($MgNH_4PO_4$) Calculi

Struvite calculi, unless composed mostly of lucent mucoid matrix, are successfully treated by ESWL. Although large struvite calculi may be easily fragmented, the problem remains as to how to manage the large fragment volume. For larger calculi, initial percutaneous tube placement should be done to relieve outlet obstruction caused by the sludge of struvite or as a port for post-ESWL hemiacidrin irrigation. Hemiacidrin irrigation can be a helpful supplement to ESWL therapy. It may reduce fragment burden or be used to dissolve otherwise poorly accessible ureteral fragments, especially in the ureters of patients with an ileal or sigmoid conduit, in partially obstructed calyces, or in small calyceal diverticula. As it has become apparent that large struvite calculi will fragment with ESWL, chemolysis of residual fragments has begun to play a bigger role in planned staged therapy, both with and without percutaneous debulking. It is likely that unless chemolysis is used to supplement the treatment of struvite calculi, the recurrence rate will be unacceptable, especially for the larger calculi.

The reasoning to support this approach is based on the fact that there is a 47.5 percent fragment retention rate for calculi over 2 cm in size after ESWL treatment and there is a 30 percent recurrence rate (after surgery), as reported by Griffith when he reviewed the results of staghorn surgery for struvite calculi.[19] If the recurrence rate is 30 percent under the best of circumstances, one can expect the recurrence rate of large struvite calculi following ESWL alone to be unacceptably high. Silverman and Stamey reported a 5 percent recurrence rate of struvite calculi for patients with struvite calculi who have undergone postsurgical hemiacidrin irrigation until no calculi were seen on 0.5-cm tomographic cuts.[20]

This appears to be the treatment that should be employed to supplement ESWL therapy for large struvite calculi. We have, therefore, started to administer routinely hemiacidrin following ESWL for large or recurrent struvite calculi.

Cystine Calculi

Cystine calculi are particularly resistant to ESWL therapy. It is likely that this resistance is due not only to the crystal structure of crystine but also to the fact that crystine is organic rather than inorganic and the change in acoustic impedance is not as marked as for other types of calculi. Initial experience showed that cystine calculi could be fractured by ESWL, but the resulting fragments were too large to pass spontaneously. Treating cystine stones of larger than 1 cm may result in a ureter full of unpassable calculi that then requires lengthy percutaneous dissolution to complete therapy. Initially, we treated 13 patients successfully by combining ESWL of cystine calculi with acetylcysteine or tromethamine-E post-ESWL chemolysis. If the calculi were greater than 1 cm, multiple ESWL treatments were required and dissolution resulted in lengthy hospitalizations. We now recommend percutaneous removal for accessible cystine calculi.

MAJOR COMPLICATIONS OF ESWL THERAPY

There are three major complications of ESWL treatment: pain, ureteral obstruction, and subcapsular or perinephric hematoma. In the U.S. study, 2415 patients were evaluated for pain following ESWL therapy. Following the procedure, 904 (37 percent) had no pain. On a scale of 1–10, where 10 represented excruciating pain, 774 (32 percent) had pain in the 1–3 level, 413 (17 percent) had pain on the 4–6 level, and 324 (13 percent) had pain at the 7–10 level. If patients had a sized calculus of under 1 cm, 17 percent had pain from the 5–10 level, but if the calculus was 1–3 cm in size, 24 percent had pain in the 5–10 level.

Ureteral obstruction occurs when fragments are too large to pass the ureter or the accumulation of a bulk of fragments obstruct the ureter. When multiple fragments line the ureter, the line or aggregate of calculi is known as "Steinstrasse" or, in translation, "stone street." The presence of fragments lining the ureter is not necessarily a problem. The stones may not be obstructing or symptomatic, and if not, no treatment is necessary. If left alone, most fragments will pass spontaneously. If sepsis occurs and ureteral obstruction is present, emergency treatment must be carried out. Placement of a percutaneous drainage tube is the therapy of choice. The sepsis is treated by percutaneous drainage and the obstructing fragments given 2–4 weeks to pass. If they do not pass, endoscopic treatment is necessary. Significant obstruction or pain secondary to ureteral fragments are also an indication for treatment. In the absence of sepsis, primary ureteroscopic management or primary percutaneous tube placement are the initial treatments of choice for persistent pain. If percutaneous tube placement is chosen as primary therapy, 3–4 weeks are given to allow fragments to pass. If the fragments remain obstructing, they require endoscopic management.

The fragments of Steinstrasse are usually packed in the ureter like sand in a straw. It is usually futile to try to bypass the obstruction with a stent and successful placement of a guidewire to dilate the ureter prior to ureteroscopic insertion is rarely achieved. The fragments are simply packed too closely to allow stent placement. The distal ureter may be cleared by pulsating saline through a ureteral catheter until some of the distal fragments wash out of the ureter. The 9.5-French rigid ureteroscope can then be placed in the ureteral meatus and the fragments irrigated under direct vision. The distal ureter may then be dilated with a 12-French dilating balloon placed via the ureteroscope. Then, once the distal ureter is dilated, the ultrasonic ureteroscope can be used to clear the lower ureter of fragments. Blind ureteral basketing will result in false passages through the ureteral wall and is not recommended. To clear a ureter of Steinstrasse can take a few hours and must be performed with extreme caution. A large volume of fragments must be treated, and the ultrasonic ureteral probe often obstructs with stone fragments. Experience in predicting stone fragility and careful patient selection for ESWL can reduce the incidence of obstructing ureteral fragments and the need for intervention.

The incidence of significant perinephric or subcapsular hematoma following ESWL is approximately 1 in 500 patients. A significant hematoma is one that requires intervention or transfusion or is symptomatic. In an initial review of 1650 lithotriptor patients in the U.S. study, only 4 patients had a significant perinephric or subcapsular hematoma. Undoubtedly, the incidence of perinephric bruising and small asymptomatic hematomas is larger than 1 out of 500, but they do not require treatment.

There is no underlying etiology identified to be able to pick out the patients who will sustain perinephric or subcapsular bleeding following ESWL. In view of this possible complication, however, all patients should be carefully screened for intake of aspirin, Advil (ibuprofen; Whitehall Labs, New York, NY), Persantin (dipyridamole; Geigy), and other antiinflammatory drugs prior to ESWL treatment. Clotting parameters are measured on all patients pre-ESWL, and in those who may have been taking antiinflammatory drugs within 2 weeks of treatment, a bleeding time should be obtained. When bleeding is suspected, ultrasound evaluation of the perirenal area should be done prior to contemplated repeat ESWL treatments. Perirenal bleeding is usually noted within 24–48 hours of treatment. Most perinephric hematomas caused by ESWL may be treated by observation and transfusion. Rarely, if ever, is renal exploration required, and renal loss is extremely unlikely. Evaluation of the patients in the U.S. study who developed perirenal bleeding showed no specific predisposing factors. The only identifiable factor was that 80 percent of the calculi in patients with perinephric bleeding were in the left lower pole of the kidney. It is not clear that there is any significance in that observation.

MINOR COMPLICATIONS OF ESWL THERAPY

Brachial palsy has occurred as a result of the abduction of arms during therapy. In some centers this has been averted by floating the arms in inflatable plastic splints during the procedure. Anesthetic complications appeared to be related to patients' condition and anesthetic used, not to the use of the machine. Cardiac arrhythmias, although few, were occasionally due to the electrical activity of the electrode discharge. There is no absolute relationship between shock waves and cardiac arrhythmia because the electrical shock discharge is tripped by the *QRS* complex of the ECG, and therefore the shock wave occurs during the refractory period of the cardiac pulse. Consequently, irregularities and arrhythmias are few.

Pancreatitis was reported in 1 of 2500 patients and appeared to be due to faulty electrode placement and resultant shock-wave focal point malalignment. There have been no specific findings of pulmonary injuries or infarcts due to shock-wave injury; however, it is known that if lung is hit by shock waves, the multiple air–tissue interfaces will allow the shock wave to cause damage. This may be more likely to occur when small children are treated and the lungs are not protected by the metal back on the patient support. It has not been a problem in adults.

Slight hemolysis with small hemoglobin elevations may occur as a result of the shock-wave action on red blood cells. This is expected because of the known hemolytic effect of shock waves on red blood cells; however, so little blood volume is at the focal point of the shock wave that this is not clinically significant.

The data from the combined U.S. group study produced interesting and, as yet, unclear data related to kidney function following treatment. As noted previously, approximately half of the patients followed for 3 months had an improvement in renal function following treatment. The other half had a decrease in function following treatment. What is unclear is whether the patients with decreased function had decreases of just a few percent so that, in effect, function was actually unchanged. More detailed investigation of the renal function data is being performed to obtain accurate and reliable data on possible renal functional abnormalities related to single or multiple ESWL therapies.

INPATIENT-OUTPATIENT TREATMENT

There has been considerable discussion about the appropriateness of ESWL as an outpatient procedure. Outpatient treatment centers have been formed and have successfully treated patients, and in one series of 700 patients, only 1 percent required hospitalization following treatment.[21] Other experience suggests that even in the most carefully selected patients, approximately 20–30 percent will require admission to the hospital the night of the procedure for colic or abdominal symptoms. It may be that the use of indwelling stents to allow drainage and to prevent stone passage in the immediate post-ESWL period makes this period more tolerable and allows more successful outpatient treatment. Also, selection of healthy patients with decreased stone burden allows for successful outpatient treatment. Some centers use same-day admitting procedures and then decide at the end of the day whether it is appropriate for the patient to go home. The major contraindication for outpatient therapy is the rare patient who will develop blood loss and shock secondary to perinephric hematoma occurring within 24 hours of ESWL treatment. Thus far, no deaths have been reported. The occurrence of a serious complication may dull the enthusiasm for outpatient treatment.

Placement of indwelling double-J stents have found great usefulness: to prevent obstruction when treating a solitary kidney, to prevent sepsis, to prevent obstruction when giving bilateral treatments, for patients who come from afar, for patients with large stone burden, for those with ureteral calculi, and to dilate a ureter in preparation for large volume fragment passage.

MULTIPLE TREATMENTS

There is a limit of 2000 shock waves per kidney per treatment in the United States. This limit was agreed to by the U.S. investigators and supported by the FDA. It is relatively arbitrary as it does not include the kilovolt dosage. For example, 1200 shocks at 24 kV (upper kilovolt limit) is about the same amount of energy as 2000 shock waves at 18 kV. However, there is no renal function data relative to the safety of giving higher dosages. If multiple treatments are to be given, it is appropriate to check an ultrasound between the two treatments to ensure that a perinephric hematoma has not occurred. Second treatments may be done within 24–48 hours without apparent short-term problems. Whether a longer time interval between treatments would have an effect on renal function has not yet been determined.

OTHER USES FOR SHOCK WAVES

The extracorporeal shock wave used to fragment urinary calculi is the first use of shock waves in a biologic system. Work is currently in progress using ultrasound as the imaging modality to fragment biliary calculi, and it is likely that within the next 2–3 years, this will be a method for treating gallstones. McCullough reports fracturing a common duct stone with ESWL therapy.[22] Research is also being done by Fair[23] and Chaussy[24] on the effect of shock waves on in vitro tumor and cell cultures. It appears that the shock wave has a greater effect on rapidly dividing cells than on normal cells and in the future may possibly be used in conjunction with other therapies for some aspects of tumor treatment. Although there is considerable industrial secrecy about the possible uses for shock waves, it is rumored that more than 200 different uses for shock waves in medicine have been contemplated by the Dornier Company. It is likely that what we are seeing is the initial use of shock waves in medicine. It may be that there will evolve a specialty of shock-wave therapy similar to that seen with radiation therapy. The evolutionary cycle of this modality is not yet clear.

SECOND-GENERATION MACHINES

U.S., French, and German companies are using shock-wave technology, adding an alternative imaging system, and doing laboratory and clinical studies on their effect on urinary calculi to gain access to the American market. These machines promise to be in the $400,000–$1,000,000 price range and require less patients to be treated per machine to be economically feasible than the $1.7 million Dornier machine. Whether these machines will be as accurate and effective as the Dornier machine remains to be determined.

Utilization of the ESWL machines thus far has been limited to major medical centers. This will change. Newer, less expensive models and mobile units will spread the use of shock-wave technology to all geographic areas and most hospitals of 200 or more beds within 2–3 years. Most urologists will have access to one or another of these models and referral, and patient distribution patterns will doubtless revert to some semblance of those present before the introduction of the Dornier machines.

EDUCATION PROGRAMS

For the first time, the American Urologic Association (AUA) recommended a structured training program to certify urologists in the use of new technology. The criteria for training are involvement with 20 cases in a certified urologic training program supervised by a urologist with experience in at least 250 cases. This training program takes from 5 to 10 days and is designed not only to teach the use of the equipment but also to educate urologists to the shift in management of stone disease that has occurred as a result of the introduction of the extracorporeal shock-wave lithotriptor. Although the initial response by urologists was negative, most who have participated in the training program have reported that they agree with the necessity of this recommendation by the AUA.

COSTS AND ECONOMICS OF ESWL

At the time of this writing, approximately 100 Dornier lithotriptors are installed in the United States. It is expected that 150 machines will be in place by the end of 1986. Mobile machines will also be used. No second-generation machines have been approved by the FDA. The cost estimates for the technical component of lithotripsy compiled by the Blue Cross and Blue Shield Association and the American Hospital Association suggest a cost of $1240.00–$1730.00 per case. The estimates are based on yearly case levels of 800 and 1000 cases. These numbers will change as the caseload falls and the number of machines increases, especially with the advent of second generation machines.

The newer machines are all priced below one million dollars or approximately one-half the cost of the Dornier machine. Costs of operation for second-generation machines that do not require expensive electrodes promise to be less than that of the first-generation equipment.

As the competition for patients gets more intense and as health-maintenance organizations (HMOs) contract with individual providers, some expensive ESWL equipment may be in rare use. The final chapter on the economics of ESWL has not been written.

CONCLUSION

Although some centers initially contemplated the idea of separating "button pushers" from referring urologists, it is clear that ESWL is one of a number of therapies available for the treatment of a patient with stone disease and that the treatment cannot be separated from the urologists making the decisions about their patients. Extracorporeal shock-wave lithotripsy is an art, and the results will depend on patient selection, educated and thoughtful choice of combinations of therapy, meticulous technique, and attention to the details of patient care, just as it does in the operating room. It would be a serious error for urologists and a significant impediment to patient care if this fact was overlooked.

REFERENCES

1. Chaussy C: Extracorporeal shock wave lithotripsy. Presented at the American Urologic Association meeting, Boston, MA, May 1981
2. Hepp W: Vorversuche zur Zerkleinerung von Niesensteindurch Stobwellen Dornier System Versuch-sbericht 638, 1972
3. Hausler E, Kiefer W: Destruction of kidney stones by means of auto focused guided shock waves. Second European Congress on ultrasonics in Medicine, Munchen, 1975
4. Forssmann B, Hepp W, Chaussy C, et al: Zertrummerung von Nierensteinen mit Bokussierten Stobwellen Verhandl, DPG (VI) II:K4, 1976
5. Chaussy C (ed): Extracorporeal Shock Wave Lithotripsy—New Aspects in the Treatment of Kidney Stone Disease. Basil Karger, 1982, p 95
6. Report of the AUA Ad Hoc Committee to Study the Safety and Clinical Efficacy of Current Technology of Percutaneous Lithotripsy and Noninvasive Lithotripsy, May 22, 1986, p 1
7. Chaussy C, Brendel W, Schmiedt E: Extracorporeally induced destruction of kidney stones by shock waves. Lancet 2:1265–1268, 1980
8. Chaussy C, Schmiedt E: Extracorporeally shock wave lithotripsy for kidney stones: An alternative to surgery. Urol Rad 6:80–87, 1984
9. Drach GW, Dretler SP, Fair W, et al: Report of the United States Cooperative Study of Extracorporeal Shock Wave Lithotripsy. J Urol 135:1127, 1986
10. McCullough DM: Radiation Exposure During ESWL. Second Symposium on Extracorporeal Shock Wave Lithotripsy, Indianapolis, IN, March 1, 1986
11. Lingeman JE, Newman D, Mertg JH, et al: Extracorporeal shock wave lithotripsy: The Methodist Hospital of Indiana Experience. J Urol 135:1134, 1986
12. Dretler SP: Management of "Steinstrasse." Presented at the American Urological Association, Annual Meeting, New York, May 1986
13. Kaude JV, Williams CM, Millner MR, et al: Renal morphology and function following extracorporeal shock wave lithotripsy: Preliminary observations. Am J Roentgenol 145:305–313, 1985
14. Kahmoski RJ, Lingerman JE, Coury TA, et al: Combined percutaneous and extracorporeal shock wave lithotripsy for staghorn calculi. Second International Symposium on ESWL, Indianapolis, IN, March 1, 1986
15. Schultz H, Hertle L, Graff J, et al: Combined treatment of branched calculi by percutaneous nephrolithotomy and extracorporeal shock wave lithotripsy. J Urol 135:1138, 1986
16. Dretler SP, Keating MA, Riley J: An algorithm for the management of ureteral calculi. Presented at the Second Symposium on Extracorporeal Shock Wave Lithotripsy, Indianapolis, IN, March 1, 1986
17. Gillenwater J: Personal communication

18. Psihramis K, Dretler SP: ESWL and calyceal diverticula. Presented at the New England Section, American Urological Association, St Thomas, Virgin Islands, October 25, 1986
19. Griffith DP: Struvite stones. Kidney Internatl 13:371, 1978
20. Silverman DE, Stamey TA: Management of infection stones: The Stanford experience. Medicine 62:44–51, 1983
21. Reid CF: Outpatient ESWL. Second Symposium on Extracorporeal Shock Wave Lithotripsy, Indianapolis, IN, March 1, 1986
22. McCullough D: Personal communication
23. Fair WR: Effect of shock wave on tumor cells. Second Symposium on Extracorporeal Shock Wave Lithotripsy, Indianapolis, IN, March 1, 1986
24. Chaussy C, Fuchs GJ, Randazzo RF, et al: In vitro and in vivo results of ESWL treatment on cancer cells. Second Symposium on Extracorporeal Shock Wave Lithotripsy, Indianapolis, IN, March 1, 1986

Warren H. Chapman, Michael E. Mayo
Barton F. Norton, Robert E. Breidenthal
Robert D. Brooks, and David A. Russell

24

Alternative Forms of Extracorporeal Shock-Wave Lithotripsy (ESWL)

There can be no question about the effectiveness of the Dornier lithotriptor. As with all new technology, however, there is a rush to "improve" on the original, and indeed there have been numerous competitive suggestions as to how the technology might be made safer, more effective, and less expensive. In this chapter we will review some of the basic principles of shock-wave lithotripsy, discuss what might be some of the characteristics of an ideal lithotriptor, list what constitutes public knowledge about the various second-generation machines, and give a brief description of the historical development of the device that has been worked on by International Biomedics and the University of Washington.

The concept of using externally produced focused shock waves to noninvasively disrupt body tissues was described as long ago as the late 1940s by Rieber (Fig. 24-1), who used them to produce localized injuries in the brains of laboratory animals for brain function studies, but nothing further was heard until the Dornier machine appeared some 30 years later. Even with the lithotriptor in wide use, there has been remarkably little in the literature about the physics of lithotripsy, and a short review of what is known in this area seems appropriate.

FLUID-WAVE MECHANICS

Shock Waves Versus Ultrasound

It is important to distinguish between ultrasound and shock waves. Ultrasound is composed of relatively low-amplitude, high-frequency pressure waves, originally above the frequency that can be heard by the human ear (>20,000–30,000 Hz). In medicine, however, it has come to denote the frequency range used for diagnostic imaging (2–15

STONE DISEASE: DIAGNOSIS AND MANAGEMENT
ISBN 0-8089-1873-7

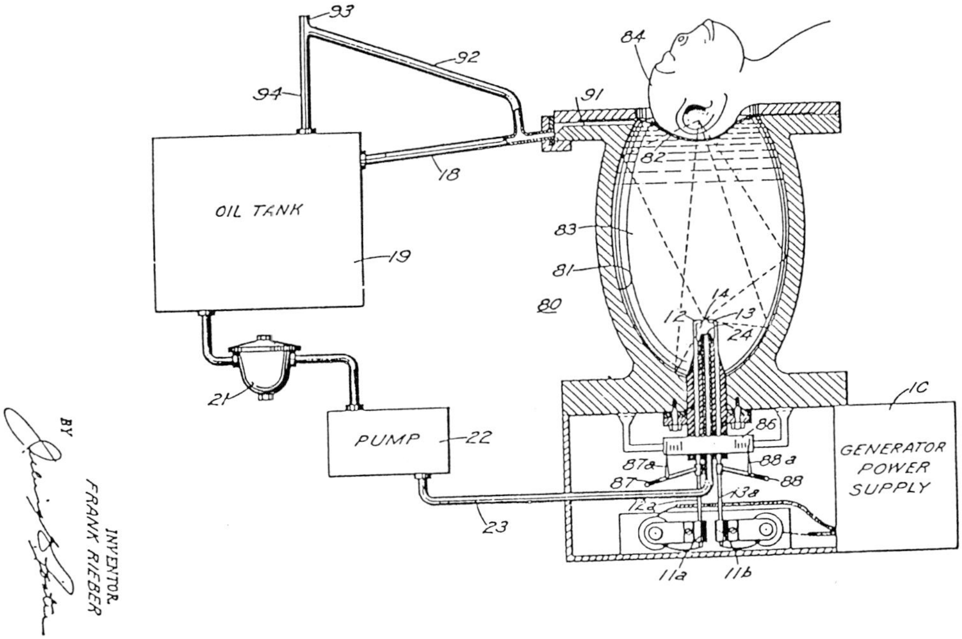

Fig. 24-1. Rieber's original illustration for the first use of focused shock waves. This illustration was in the original patent obtained by Rieber (patent number 2,559,227, filed on May 24, 1947; issued on July 3, 1951).

MHz). All parts of the small-amplitude acoustic waves travel at the same speed, the undisturbed speed of sound, so the wave shape is unchanging in time as the wave train propagates. Since the local speed of sound in a solid or liquid depends on the local pressure, however, for large-amplitude waves the local sound speed varies from high-pressure crests, where it is speeding up, to low-pressure troughs, where it is slowing down. Consider the analogy of an ocean wave. If it is of small amplitude, the local speed is the same throughout the wave and the wave travels without change. Now imagine a large-amplitude water wave in shallow water. The local wave speed is greater at the crest than the trough, so the crest overtakes the trough. The wave shape changes, steepens, and eventually breaks. The analogous process for a pressure wave within a solid or liquid is the formation of a very steep shock wave (Fig. 24-2). Not only do large-amplitude shock waves change shape as they move, but they do not propagate in the easily predictable manner of sound waves. Their behavior can be predicted to some extent, but it is much more complicated than the optical ray-tracing geometry and diffraction of sound waves. If a periodic, sinusoidal pressure wave is strong enough, the successive wave peaks will steepen and try to catch up with one another, compressing the wave in time and increasing the maximum pressure.

In contrast, an expansion wave (a sudden reduction in pressure) smears out in time, rather than becoming steeper as a shock wave does. This is a result of the forward component of the expansion wave being at normal pressure while the expansion component is at lower pressure and therefore going slower, so that they separate with time.

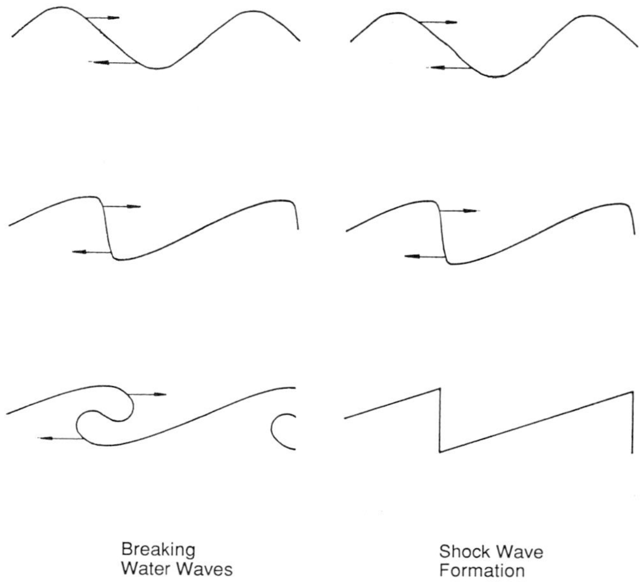

Fig. 24-2. Analogy between surface wave breaking and shock-wave formation.

Penetration of Sound Waves

Another property of sound waves is their absorption in liquid media or tissue, because the attenuation rate is inversely proportional to the square of the wavelength; or the higher the frequency, the less distance the wave will travel before it is absorbed. For penetration through the body to the stone, there should be as little attenuation (absorption) as possible before the wave reaches the stone, and this implies that the wave should have a relatively low frequency.

Sound Waves at Interfaces

The behavior of these waves at an interface of two materials of differing density or speed of sound must also be considered. As with optical behavior, at each such interface some of the wave is transmitted through the interface, but the greater the mismatch in acoustic impedance (the product of density and sound speed), the more of the wave will be reflected. This property can be used to advantage in focusing waves where the marked difference in acoustic impedance between a metal ellipse and water is used to focus waves at the second focal point of the ellipse. In this instance the mismatch between the metal and the water is so great that the interface acts like a mirror, reflecting essentially the whole wave. Alternatively, differences in sound speed rather than acoustic impedance may be used to advantage in an acoustic lens, focusing the wave in much the same fashion as an optical lens.

Although this is a useful effect, the phenomena at the interface are not always so benign. As a strong wave is passed through an interface with tissue, its reflection may damage the tissue. During lithotripsy the most obvious effect is at the skin surface. As the pressure wave enters the body, if there is not good contact between the water and the body, an air-skin interface results. Then there can be significant damage to the skin with hemorrhage and separation of the layers of the skin (blistering). The same effect can take place at the site of the exit of the wave from the body, and this area must be protected by the application of gel or a waterlike substance that takes the air–water interface out away from the body. Inside the body this phenomenon takes place in the lung, where there is an air-fluid interface in each alveolus, and if the lung is exposed to the shock, a hemorrhagic pneumonitis may be produced.

Stone Destruction

Although little is yet known about what breaks up the stone, several facts are clear. The stone itself must be brittle. The stresses produced by the passage of the wave through the stone must not be accommodated by an elastic stretching, which then returns to normal after the wave has passed through. This was illustrated clinically in the treatment of cystine stones, which are relatively soft and resist breaking apart. They are therefore, the most difficult type of stones to treat with extracorporeal shock-wave lithotripsy (ESWL). The exact mechanism of the breakdown is not well understood. It was originally thought that the shock wave reflected off both surfaces of the stone, causing multiple stress fractures. There has been debate about whether it is the sudden rise in pressure that is effective or the drop in pressure that occurs as the wave goes by. The actual pressures that are generated are also in dispute. The transducers used in most of the measurements have a response time in the microsecond range, and they may be missing many of the highest pressures. The newer, faster transducers are expensive and fragile enough that only a few high-pressure measurements may destroy them. Too little energy (usually considered equivalent to the square of the peak pressure times the duration of the impulse at a pressure of one-half of the maximum peak) will not break up the stone, while too much energy will produce unacceptable levels of tissue damage in the patient. A curve of stone breaking probability versus energy level is shown in Fig. 24-3. The maximum pressure should be in the range of 700–1000 bars.

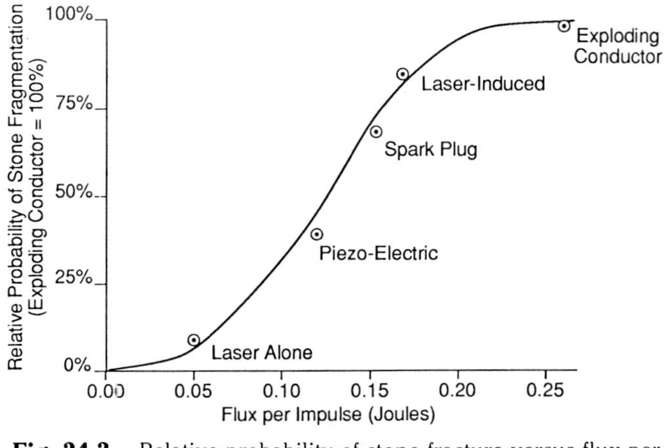

Fig. 24-3. Relative probability of stone fracture versus flux per impulse in joules for various ESWL shock-wave generators.

The group at the University of Florida under Dr. Finlayson has done some interesting experiments in which they placed ceramic platens at various positions along the z axis near the second focal point. When they placed the disks nearer to the origin of the wave than the focal point, there was cavitation on the near side of the disk with the production of small fragments from this side of the disk. When the platen was placed beyond focal point F^2, there was spallation or erosion of the far side of the disk. When the platen was placed right at the F^2, however, the disk was split transversely as though there had been an internal explosion pushing the two sides apart. There is obviously a lot still to be learned about the phenomenon, and it seems likely that with increased knowledge, many improvements can be made.

Cavitation

Cavitation is nothing more than boiling. It occurs at room temperature in water when the pressure is low enough for the necessary time interval. The time interval is necessary for nucleation sites of bubbles to form and grow. The waveform must have a large negative pressure component to cavitate.

Cavitation has been shown to occur not only with ultrasound generators but also with the single shock-wave generator. The phenomenon is a highly complex one and is not well understood despite the fact that it has been known for over 100 years. Multiple bubbles are produced that influence each other. After the negative wave passes and the pressure rises, the cavitation bubbles begin to collapse. The resulting implosion produces very large pressure and temperatures at the center. These temperatures are sufficiently high to produce free radicals in living tissue, and these may have profound chemical activity in spite of their very short life. The collapse of the bubble is not perfectly, spherically symmetric because of instabilities, so that a high-speed jet of liquid is formed. This jet is responsible for the rapid erosion of cavitating marine propellers and may have an effect on living tissue, including breaking down of cell walls.

The Ideal Shock Wave

The ideal shock wave as understood at the present time has a pressure between 700 and 1000 bars. Since this is a fairly narrow range, it must be consistent. The volume of the effective pressure zone at the focal point must be large enough to cover the average stone (1–2 cm) but not be so small that it is difficult to aim or will miss the stone completely during respiratory movements.

COMMERCIAL PROPOSALS

While each lithotriptor manufacturer involved has taken an approach designed to differentiate its approach to lithotripsy, all shock-wave generators proposed to date may be grouped into two classes. The first class relies on a spherically radiating shock wave driven by a bubble of expanding gas or plasma. An ellipsoid reflector focuses the spherical shock wave to a small zone inside the kidney. The second class creates plane waves by mechanically displacing a fluid medium very rapidly. This can be done with either piezoelectric or magnetostrictive devices. These plane waves are then focused into the body either with an acoustic lens or by coordinating the timing (as in a phased array) or by the placement of the various generators in a hemispherical fashion. The proposed machines differ mainly in the methods used for generation and focusing of the wave and to some extent in the methods used for coupling the wave to the patient. Lesser differences exist between the methods of localizing and positioning the stone within the patient.

Spherical Expanding Shock Wave with Ellipsoid Focusing

Spark Gap Generators

The Dornier spark gap generator is the most familiar of this type of device. The two electrodes are spaced 1 mm apart in treated water at the first focal point of the ellipse. A capacitor is charged to a voltage that can be varied from 16 to 30 kV with an energy of 10–30 joules. The potential difference between the two opposing electrodes is concentrated by the conically pointed electrode tips. When this voltage is discharged, the water in the gap is dissociated or ionized and a bubble of hot gas or plasma is formed that expands and accelerates out into the surrounding fluid, forming a spherical shock wave. A portion of this wave is directed toward the outlet of the ellipsoid and escapes as the *spherical wave.* The majority of the wave, however, is reflected from the ellipsoid and is focused at F^2, the second focus of the ellipsoid. This reflected wave reaches the F^2 focal point somewhat later than the spherical or unreflected wave and the two separate waves can be detected with appropriate transducers. As the bubble expands, it cools and then collapses. The collapse of the bubble produces a second shock wave that has its own spherical and reflected portion detectable at F^2. The principle is quite simple. In practice, however, there is a 50 percent variation in pressure from one shock wave to the next. This probably results from the arcing between the electrodes to produce a discharge in a position that is not confined to F^1 and thus not focused at F^2. In their present conformation the metal of the pointed electrode tips is eroded by the electrical discharge, and Dornier suggests that these electrodes be changed every 700 shocks.

Exploding-Liquid Conductor

An improvement in the electrohydraulic generator called the *exploding-liquid conductor* (ELC) has been developed to deal with the lack of repeatability and relatively short electrode life of the spark gap designs. The principle of operation of the ELC is to inject a conductive medium at high pressure across the gap normally found in the spark plug. One side of the plug injects the conductive fluid, while the other side uses a vacuum to withdraw the fluid and some of the surrounding water. This removal of a small amount of excess fluid creates a laminar flow along the stream of conductive fluid that prevents it from mixing with the deionized water and preserves a tight cylindrical shape of the injected fluid. Since the current will be channeled along the conductive fluid, the shape of the electrode is different. Instead of being sharply pointed, the ELC electrodes are hemispherical in shape. As the current flows, it stays in the pathway of the conductive fluid and does not arc out of this pathway into the water. The result is a more stable shock wave that is more accurately positioned at F^1 and thus better focused at F^2. Because of their shape, the larger electrodes are more uniformly eroded, and electrode use is estimated at 5000 impulses.

Focused Laser

The use of a focused laser has been investigated by the University of Washington and International Biomedics, Inc. This technology is well known from atomic fusion experiments. In the experimental apparatus a 3-joule ruby laser with a pulse 20 ns in length is focused at F^1 of an ellipsoid. The concentration of the light at F^1 breaks down the water in the same fashion as the spark gap discharge, stripping the electrons off the water and producing a similar expanding bubble of plasma. There are several attractive aspects to this technology. There is no high-voltage current near the patient, suggesting that the shock waves might not have to be gated to the EKG, the F^1 is unobstructed so that the focus of the pressure at F^2 can be tighter, and there are no electrodes to wear out. (The flash lamps do have a finite life, but if not pushed to capacity, this life can be in the 100,000-impulse range.) The limitations of this technique in practice, such as obtaining enough power and increasing the repetition rate, will be described in more detail later.

The difference between this focused laser and the dye laser that is used for disintegrating ureteral calculi should be mentioned. In the latter the laser guide is introduced in the ureter and placed directly on the calculus. The small target area is heated up to a plasma, and a miniature explosion is created that chips away small pieces of the stone. Because it is directly on the stone, the wave need not be nearly so strong as the shock that is used in ESWL.

Micro Explosions

Perhaps the simplest principle of shock-wave generation is the use of a conventional chemical explosion. Workers in Japan[1] have placed a 10-mg lead azide pellet at the F^1 focus of an ellipse and detonated it with a 12-V current. The shocks produced are very powerful, breaking renal stones in 100–200 explosions. Initial reports suggest that the damage to the lung and kidneys may be more than that produced by the spark gap device, but the Japanese have treated more than 50 patients without reporting any major problems.

Mechanically Created Plane Wave

Piezoelectric

The most commonly proposed device to mechanically produce a wavefront involves the use of the piezoelectric effect, in which an appropriate material is constricted by the passage of an electric current through it. The crystal face need not achieve sonic velocities but must accelerate rapidly to form wavefronts that steepen into shock waves. To achieve this, a single pulse rarely is used, but rather short bursts of very high frequency discharge are used to produce a series of waves. These generators (transducers) may be arranged in a hemispherical array so that they focus on a single point that is the center of the sphere. An alternative is to align the transducers on a flat plane and have them activate in succession (a phased array) so that they produce a focus where the waves meet. The advantages to this are that there are no electrodes to wear out and there is no high-voltage current near the patient. There are some concerns about the amount of cavitation and possible damage produced by the cavitation either mechanically or by the free radical release. Within these limits of damage the repetition rate is limited only by the presence of the bubbles of cavitation that would interfere with the next impulse.

Magnetostrictive

The Siemens Company has built a machine that uses the magnetostrictive principle. In this device a strong magnetic field is applied to a metal plate or diaphragm that accelerates to push a shock wave in front of it. In the Siemens device this wave is then focused by an acoustic lens on the desired target area, but this function could also be performed by an appropriate shape of the diaphragm. The concept has most of the same advantages as does the piezoelectric device, specifically, no expendable parts such as the electrodes and no high-voltage current near the patient.

Coupling

Water Bath

The Dornier water bath is probably the simplest in principle. It assures a good contact. If the patient is completely under water, it also takes care of the exit wave. Nevertheless, it is the most consistently revised part of the second generation machines. It requires large amounts of treated water, the weight of which often necessitates expensive reinforcing of the floor before installation. The gantry to move the patient in and out of the bath requires extra height in the room. The amount of water spilled during immersion and removal of the patient from the tank requires a floor drain, and the immersion of the patient in the large tub makes adequate access awkward for the anesthesiologists.

Telescopic Coupler

All except one of the known proposals for new devices have a coupler to connect the patient to the shock wave. The only exception to this is the Sonolith machine, which uses a shallow basin type of coupler. The others vary from simple water-filled bags to complex telescopic devices with internal balloons that can be deflated for treatment or inflated for taking x-rays. The telescopic devices may have several insulating diaphragms to protect the patient from exposure to electric currents. When such an enclosed coupler is used in conjunction with one of the spherical wave generators, there must be a means of getting rid of the bubbles formed by the explosion. This is most often done by means of a current of water washing across the applicator cavity.

Localization and Positioning

X-Ray

The Dornier unit uses two fixed fluoroscopic heads set to center on F^2. These are moved aside to move the patient in and out of the tank. The console can display both images simultaneously for easy localization. The Siemens machine uses a similar setup. Other devices have used a single tube, and some have installed a C arm. The latter has the ability to track the stone in real time as the tube is moved and to select the best angle for visualizing the stone.

Ultrasound

The use of ultrasound for localizing is very attractive since it is potentially both safer and cheaper, but to date a satisfactory system has not been forthcoming. Northgate had a

Table 24-1
Basic Data for Lithotriptors Currently Developed and Under Development

Group	Model	Generator	Focusing
Dornier	HM-3 HM-4	Spark gap	Ellipsoid
EDAP	LT-01	Piezoelectric	Hemispherical
International Biomedics	Lasertripter	Focused laser	Ellipsoid
	Ultracrusher	Piezoelectric	Acoustic lens
	Jetstream	Liquid conductor	Ellipsoid
Medstone	1000	Spark gap	Ellipsoid
Northgate		Spark gap	Ellipsoid
Siemens	Lithostar	Magnetostrictive	Acoustic lens
Technomed	Sonolith	Spark gap	Ellipsoid
Wolf		Piezoelectric	Hemispherical
Johns Hopkins?			
Vanderbilt?			

proposal for a two-headed ultrasound unit that utilized the crossing point of the shadows of the stone to fix its position.

Marketplace

A review of the preceding material suggests that the next generation of machines will dispense with the large water bath, thus improving anesthesia access and reducing both equipment and installation costs. They will lower the cost of each individual treatment by improving or eliminating the elctrodes and will develop equipment that can be used for both cystoscopy and percutaneous nephrostomy, allowing the cost of the devices to be spread over all of these procedures. Table 24-1 lists the groups involved in the development of such devices.

History of the Seattle Machine

The University of Washington Department of Aeronautics and Astronautics and the Department of Urology have been interested in developing a machine for lithotripsy since 1978. Simple bench experiments using a spark gap electrohydraulic generator and a focusing ellipse produced adequate pressure at F^2, but one of the hazards of the unprotected spark gap was convincingly demonstrated when an anesthetized laboratory rat was placed at F^2 and convulsed right out of the bath at the first shock. It was felt that stray currents or induced voltages incited this and it was decided to look at another technique.

The use of a focused laser beam to produce an expanding plasma had been used for some time in nuclear fusion experiments, where it was necessary to compress a pellet of fuel for very short periods but at very high temperatures and pressures. The power required for the fusion experiments was several orders of magnitude greater than that needed for the focused shock wave, but the use of the principle was appealing as there were at least four theoretical advantages over the use of the spark gap. The most obvious of these was that the laser did not have any electrodes to wear out. While the laser did require replacement of flash lamps, this should only be about every 100,000 impulses rather than every 700 used by the Dornier machine. The focus at F^1 could be small (about 0.006 ml) and unobstructed by the cagelike structure of the Dornier electrode. This meant that the focus at F^2 should be sharper. Virtually all of the output of the laser is absorbed at F^1 during the very short (20-ns) pulse so that there can be better control over the power and the reproducibility from shock to shock. Finally, there would be no direct exposure of the patient to high-voltage current and induced voltages. If the cardiac irregularities that had been noted are due to induced depolarizing currents, it might not be necessary to gate the impulses to the EKG, allowing a repetition rate higher than the pulse rate, which, in turn, might allow a more gentle, less tissue-damaging shock to be used.

A 3-joule, Q-switched ruby laser, which has only a small proportion of its energy absorbed in the water, was chosen and the physical characteristics studied (Charko).[2] The maximum pressure found at F^2 was greater than 100 atm, and the half-maximum pressure width was 1 cm radially and 3 cm axially. The maximum pressure F^2 measured was found to be 3–4 cm nearer to the F^1 than was calculated geometrically.

In cooperation with IBI, stones were broken up in vitro, and experiments on 14 dogs with stones implanted in the kidney showed that stones of up to about 1 cm in diameter could be broken up with an average of 3600 shocks. The safety of the machine was well demonstrated. Fourteen thousand shocks were given to rabbits without significant damage to renal function as measured by dimercaptosuccinic acid (DMSA) scans, and shocks were given directly to the heart without any evidence of cardiac irregularity. At that time it was planned to use more but gentler shocks with a higher repetition rate (without cardiac gating) so that the time would be no longer than with the Dornier machine. After consultation with the FDA, however, it was decided that the arbitrary limit of 2000 shocks established by the FDA had to be adhered to, which meant that the shocks had to be made stronger. Part of this decision was the difficulty of proving the safety of these shocks to the heart without a long period of development.

An enhanced pathway device was developed in which the laser was focused on a point between two electrodes, and just as the laser-produced ball of plasma was expanding, an electrical impulse was sent across the spark gap, which then used the plasma as an enhanced pathway. This was termed a *turbo-charged* laser by the laboratory but seemed to have all the complexities of both the electrohydraulically and laser-generated devices.

The ELC was then developed and is the present prototype machine. Pressures can easily be generated up to over a thousand bar with variations between pulses in the neighborhood of 5 percent rather than 50 percent. Initial studies in dogs have shown the device to be effective in breaking stones with less than 500 shocks and minimal damage to kidneys. Further studies on animals are again under way in order to be able to use this device on humans.

REFERENCES

1. Kambe K, Kuwahara M. Kuvosu S, et al: Underwater shock wave focusing and application to extra-corporeal lithotripsy, in Bershader D, Hanson R (eds): Proceedings of the 15th International Symposium on Shock Waves and Shock Tubes. (Berkeley, California, July 28 August 2, 1985). Stanford University Press, 1986
2. Charko RE: Laser shock wave lithotripsy. MS thesis in Aeronautics and Astronautics, University of Washington, 1984

PART IV

Combined Medical and Surgical Management of Urolithiasis

Glenn M. Preminger

25

Management of Residual Stones

All urologists performing surgery for stone disease occasionally are confronted with the dilemma of residual stones. These embarrassing and often frustrating calculi may be left behind following open surgical procedures, endourologic stone manipulation, and extracorporeal shock-wave lithotripsy (ESWL). It is the purpose of this chapter to discuss the significance of residual calculi, explain why stones are left behind, and offer a logical management plan to deal with this problem.

SIGNIFICANCE OF RESIDUAL STONES

Residual calculi present two major problems, one immediate and real and the other long-term and theoretical. The first is that any remaining stone fragments can acutely become dislodged and cause significant obstruction with resultant pain and sepsis. While this problem has been previously described following open stone surgery, it was fortunately a rare occurrence since most residual stones following nephrolithotomy are located in obscure calyces. With the large number of percutaneous nephrostolithotomy (PNL) and ESWL procedures being performed, however, this complication is, unfortunately, a common problem in those patients in whom ureteral catheters are not utilized. In addition to causing obstruction of the collecting system, residual stones may also act as a source of persistent infection. This is especially true with struvite stones.

The second and more theoretical problem deals with the question as to whether residual stones act as a nidus for stone growth and recurrent stone formation. Recent advances in the pathophysiologic elucidation and medical diagnosis of nephrolithiasis suggest that a physiologic or environmental cause of stone formation can be identified in greater than 95 percent of patients.[25] In most cases, stone formation is secondary to either the supersaturation of stone-forming substances or lack of stone-inhibitor substances; therefore, if residual stones are present and the underlying physiologic or metabolic defects persist, growth of these stones and possibly formation of new calculi may be inevitable. This problem should also be true in both single stone formers and patients

STONE DISEASE: DIAGNOSIS AND MANAGEMENT
ISBN 0-8089-1873-7

with infection stones since both of these groups of patients have the same incidence and severity of underlying metabolic derangements (e.g., hypercalciuria, hyperuricosuria) as do patients forming recurrent calcium oxalate stones.[23] In addition, if a patient has a persistent anatomic abnormality, such as a stenotic calyceal diverticulum or ureteropelvic junction (UPJ) obstruction, urinary stasis will surely increase the risk of stone growth or recurrent stone formation.

These potential problems emphasize the importance of adequate metabolic evaluation and proper medical and supportive management of patients with nephrolithiasis. Utilizing selective medical therapy in patients with existing calculi, we have been able to inhibit new stone formation in 77 percent and reduce the stone formation rate in 98 percent of our patients with recurrent nephrolithiasis.[27] In addition, adequate medical therapy with appropriate followup in this same group of patients with existing stones was able to diminish the need for stone surgery from 58 percent prior to beginning medical therapy to 2 percent while on medical treatment.[27]

INCIDENCE OF RESIDUAL STONES

As mentioned previously, even with the advent of endourologic stone manipulation and extracorporeal shock-wave therapy, residual stones are still a fairly common problem. Residual stones may be present in 5–21 percent of open surgical procedures (Table 25-1). After percutaneous nephrostolithotomy, the incidence of residual stones is somewhat lower but has been reported to be as high as 8.1 percent.[37] In addition, many of the early reports concerning ESWL therapy have reported an incidence of upwards of 34 percent at 3 months following treatment.[10] The significance of these residual fragments has yet to be determined. While many physicians feel post-ESWL fragments may be insignificant, no hard data have been presented as to the long-term incidence of residual stone growth or new stone formation following ESWL therapy. Following open surgical

Table 25-1
Incidence of Residual Stones

Procedure	No. of Patients	Residual Stones (%)
Open surgery		
Anatrophic nephrolithotomy		
Boyce and Elkins[4]	100	5
Redman et al.[29]	56	21
Pyelolithotomy		
Gil-Vernet[16]	328	8
Blandy and Singh[2]	152	20
Percutaneous nephrostolithotomy		
Segura et al.[37]	1000	8.1
Preminger et al.[26]	82	7.4
Reddy et al.[28]	400	1.0
ESWL (3 months' posttreatment)		
Drach et al.[10]	1524	34
Lingeman et al.[20]	569	28

procedures, investigators have described the incidence of residual stone growth to range from 30–50 percent in sterile stones[2] to as high as 70 percent in infection stones.[38] Nonetheless, with aggressive medical management, it is anticipated that residual stone growth can be significantly reduced and that a universally poor outcome is not inevitable in patients with residual stones.

It must be pointed out that the introduction of the new modalities of stone removal (PNL + ESWL) have allowed combination therapy for many types of stones and that this "dual therapy" technique has significantly reduced the incidence of residual stones.

CAUSES OF RESIDUAL STONES

Most residual stones stem from one or a combination of the following four problems (Table 25-2). The most common and perhaps the most preventable is the improper selection of a surgical technique for stone removal. The urologist must be able to select the technique that will provide the most optimum access and best chance for complete stone removal. While this may entail a solitary surgical procedure such as anatrophic nephrolithotomy,[4,29] it also encompasses the combined techniques of initial percutaneous debulking and followup ESWL therapy of large staghorn calculi.[39] No one technique is appropriate for all situations and, therefore, improper selection of a certain procedure dramatically increases the likelihood of leaving behind residual stone fragments.

For example, a "complete" branched staghorn calculus with multiple calyceal extensions may be approached by anatrophic nephrolithotomy, PNL, ESWL, or a combination of PNL and ESWL. The urologist must decide which option offers the patient and the surgeon the best chance of success and the least possibility of problems. Some feel that, if this kidney has not been operated on previously, the anatrophic nephrolithotomy offers the patient the best chance of being rendered stone-free. In addition, this procedure allows intraoperative reconstruction of the collecting system, which is especially important in those patients who may have a stenotic calyceal infundibulum or calyceal diverticulum associated with the staghorn calculus.[4] Percutaneous nephrostolithotomy[8,26] and ESWL[10,20] or a combination approach of these two techniques[36] is also a viable option for treating this type of stone. Both the urologist and patient must realize, however, that although these techniques are "less invasive," they often require multiple procedures over an extended period of time, often at significant expense. In addition, for staghorn calculi, there is a reported residual stone fragment rate of 16–42 percent following PNL therapy[26,37] and 30–60 percent following ESWL therapy.[10,20] Most investigators now agree that a combined approach of percutaneous stone debulking followed by ESWL therapy of remaining fragments offers the patient with large stones the best chance of complete removal.[36]

Anatomic abnormalities, such as a stenotic infundibulum, calyceal diverticulum, UPJ

Table 25-2
Causes of Residual Stones

Improper selection of surgical technique
Anatomical abnormalities
Stone composition
Impatience and/or technical constraints

obstruction, or ureteral obstruction, will increase the incidence of residual stones. Here again, selection of the appropriate surgical technique may avoid the occurrence of residual stones. For example, while stones located in a dilated calyx behind a stenotic infundibulum may be broken up by ESWL, the stone fragments may not readily pass from the calyx and may be a source of continued infection, pain, or recurrent stone formation. These stones may be best treated by a percutaneous approach that would allow direct access to the obstructed calyx for stone removal and offer the option of balloon dilatation of the infundibulum. Other options would include open surgical procedures such as radial nephrotomy or in some severe cases, partial nephrectomy.[32,41]

Stone composition also has an important impact on the incidence of residual calculi. While this factor is not so important when considering open surgical procedures, the crystalline makeup of the stone plays a significant role in both percutaneous nephrostolithotomy and ESWL therapy. Cystine and calcium oxalate monohydrate calculi are much more difficult to fragment by PNL and ESWL techniques. The incidence of residual cystine calculi has been reported as high as 42 percent following monotherapy with percutaneous nephrostolithotomy.[37] In a recent study, calcium oxalate monohydrate stones produced larger particles after ESWL than did the dihydrate form.[30] In addition, cystine and uric acid stones required more than the average number of shock waves for disintegration, suggesting that these stones are more difficult to break up and thus more prone to resultant residual calculi.

The final problem concerns the surgeon's impatience, frustration, and various technical constraints, which may contribute to residual stones. Successful stone surgery requires an unusual degree of patience. It is not infrequent after a masterful open surgical procedure or percutaneous nephrostolithotomy that small residual stone fragments are discovered during intraoperative radiographs. It is, therefore, imperative that the surgeon meticulously hunt for any residual stones that may be discovered during the surgical procedure. Although this may add a significant amount of time to an already lengthy procedure, careful investigation and inspection following open surgery and endourologic manipulation may prevent repeat procedures for these residual stones. If time is running out on a "cross-clamped" kidney or significant bleeding develops during a percutaneous nephrostolithotomy, however, it would be better to terminate the procedure, knowing that there are residual calculi, than to possibly lose the kidney from ischemia or significant hemorrhage.

While the technical advances of ESWL have revolutionized the treatment of renal calculi, this technology does have certain limitations. When utilizing ESWL therapy, it often is difficult to see small residual stones due to the technical constraints of the fluoroscopy units being used within the large waterbath. Even though a stone appears to be sufficiently fragmented after a limited number of shocks, careful fluoroscopy with judicious use of x-ray filming in the waterbath[6] may allow the location of residual fragments and prevent the necessity for repeat ESWL procedures.

MANAGEMENT OF RESIDUAL STONES

A number of different factors must be taken into account when formulating a treatment plan for dealing with residual calculi. Stone location and composition are probably the most important considerations. If the stone is located within a calyceal diverticulum and does not appear to be in communication with the collecting system, further therapy may not be indicated. If, however, multiple stone fragments are located in a lower pole calyx that have potential for obstructing the ureter, more aggressive management may be warranted. The crystalline composition of the stone is important since struvite, cystine, and uric acid stone fragments may be dissolved by using a combination of oral medications and direct chemolysis. This would obviate the need for a repeat surgical procedure. Successful dissolution by irrigation is associated with a recurrence rate similar to complete stone removal.[15]

In addition, one must consider the adjunctive use of selective medical therapy for the "treatment" of residual calculi. As mentioned previously, the incidence of stone growth and new stone formation may be virtually eliminated while on selective medical therapy.[27] One may, therefore, elect to "medically manage" small residual stones that are not infected or causing significant discomfort. If the patient does develop recurrent infections, intermittent pain, and/or obstruction, appropriate surgical management may be warranted.

Intraoperative Management

Many adjunctive procedures are available to help locate small stone fragments during open stone surgery and eliminate the possibility of residual stones (Table 25-3). The most reliable means of stone localization remains intraoperative radiography. This entails the use of small x-ray film that can be placed directly against the kidney, allowing small fragments to be localized with certainty.[3] Some helpful hints in utilizing intraoperative radiography include making a radiograph of the kidney *before* removing the stone. This helps with orientation and with the quality of the radiograph so that small peripheral fragments can be clearly seen. Small needles placed in the renal parenchyma during the x-ray exposure will help to localize fragments within the kidney. Finally, one may use a calibrated grid interposed between the kidney and the cassette to provide an additional means of locating stones within the kidney.[31] This may avoid repetitive radiographic exposures. A more recent advance in locating residual stones intraoperatively is the use of B-scan ultrasound.[21] A 7-MHz ultrasonic probe can be used to noninvasively locate stones as small as 1mm. After observing the stone with its acoustic shadow, the surgeon can make a limited nephrotomy incision to remove the stone. With more advanced real-time ultrasound scanners, only limited expertise in reading ultrasound films is necessary to locate small stones, making this technique available to all urologists.

Pulsatile irrigation of the renal pelvis and collecting system should be a routine part

Table 25-3
Intraoperative Management Options

Stone localization
X-ray cassettes
Calibrated grids
Sonography
Irrigation
Nephroscopy
Partial nephrectomy

of any open surgical procedure for large calculi. A Water Pik dental irrigator or a large catheter with a flexible tip can be used to flush saline throughout the kidney and gently irrigate all portions of the collecting system. Low-pressure flushing should avoid any problems of renal damage or sepsis.

Intraoperative nephroscopy is another useful adjunct in trying to locate small stone fragments during open surgery. Careful inspection of the renal pelvis and calyceal system with a flexible nephroscope will help to confirm total removal of all stones. The development of new fiberoptic nephroscopes has allowed access to the entire collecting system through a single nephrotomy or renal pelvis incision. Either grasping forceps or baskets can then be used to extract stones that may be located in a distant calyx. If a stone can be located, but not removed with the scope, one may use the transmitted light from the nephroscope as a guide for a nephrotomy incision.

Partial nephrectomy does still have a role in the treatment of residual stones that cannot be located intraoperatively.[32,41] In a patient with a normal contralateral kidney who may have a large calyceal diverticulum containing stones that cannot be adequately cleaned out, partial nephrectomy may obviate the need for repeat surgeries and further adjunctive therapy.

Finally, the development of endourologic procedures as well as ESWL therapy has somewhat diminished the significance of residual calculi following open surgical procedures. In many instances, it may be possible to percutaneously remove residual stones following anatrophic nephrostolithotomy[24] and/or treat small stone fragments utilizing ESWL. While these treatment options are available, one must remember that they are not without complications and do add additional expense and possible morbidity to the initial surgical procedure.

Endourologic Management

The manipulation of residual calculi can be performed through either a previously established surgical nephrostomy tract or a newly placed percutaneous tract. A combination of baskets, flexible nephroscopy, rigid nephroscopy, fragmentation techniques, and forceps will allow the urologist to remove most residual calculi.

The most important aspect of the management of residual stones utilizing endourologic techniques is the proper placement of the percutaneous tract. Access is best achieved through the calyx closest to the residual stone. If a stone is located at the UPJ or in the proximal ureter, access through the mid or upper pole of the kidney is most desirable to lessen the angle to reach these stones. Flexible nephroscopy allows direct visualization of residual calculi in distant calyces or fragments that have migrated down the ureter. The stone may either be basketed under direct vision or retrieved by using alligator grasping forceps. If a stone has migrated down the ureter and cannot be visualized by means of the flexible nephroscope, stone baskets may be passed down the ureter under fluoroscopic guidance. Access to the ureter can also be gained in a retrograde fashion by using either rigid or flexible ureteroscopes.[18] These instruments also utilize stone baskets or grasping forceps. An ultrasonic lithotripsy probe or electrohydraulic lithotripsy probe can be utilized to fragment large stones within the ureter. In addition, new laser technology has been utilized to fragment ureteral stones.[13] Since the laser fiber is only 250 μ in diameter, this allows the usage of much smaller instrumentation, such as a 9-French flexible ureteroscope, and thus avoids excessive trauma to the ureter.

Irrigation of Stone Fragments

Irrigation or oral chemolysis may be used as adjunctive therapy after open surgery, PNL, or ESWL.[1,11] Primarily, uric acid, cystine, and struvite calculi are most amenable to dissolution; however, we are currently exploring the use of potassium citrate therapy for the dissolution of calcium containing stones (Table 25-4).

General Precautions

Certain elements of the chemolysis technique are important for all stones regardless of their composition.[14] It is essential that any urinary tract infection be eradicated prior to beginning irrigation. In addition, the patient should be placed on prophylactic antibiotics to prevent the possibility of sepsis during irrigation. Successful chemolysis requires the irrigating solution to flow over the stone and allow complete drainage to prevent excessive pressure within the renal pelvis. Any combination of ureteral catheters and percutaneous nephrostomy tubes may be used to accomplish adequate irrigation and drainage. However, ureteral catheters are not recommended in patients who may require chemolysis for longer than 3–4 days. Finally, the pressure in the renal pelvis must be high enough to bathe the stone in the chemolysis solution but not so high as to cause absorption or tissue damage. The intrapelvic pressure must be monitored during irrigation and kept at 20–25 cm of water pressure. This can be accomplished by using an open-ended manometer that does not permit intrarenal pressures to exceed 25 cm of water. Finally, a computer-monitored irrigation system has been devised that delivers intermittent irrigation to the collecting system.[19] In vitro tests have shown this low-pressure (15-cm H_2O) system to be more efficient in dissolving calculi when compared to continuous irrigation.

Uric Acid Stones

A combination of allopurinol (300 mg/day) and potassium citrate (20 mEq tid) is effective in controlling uric acid stone formation and may dissolve uric acid calculi. It is important to maintain urine pH between 6.5 and 7.0. In addition, adequate urine output must be maintained between 2500 and 3000 ml/day. Occasionally, direct irrigation with an alkaline solution is indicated for dissolution of residual uric acid calculi. Irrigation with sodium bicarbonate solution can be performed by placing 2 ampules of sodium bicarbonate in 1 liter of 1/2 normal saline. More rapid dissolution can be accomplished by using

Table 25-4
Dissolution of Residual Stones

Stone Composition	Chemolytic Agents	Oral Agents
Uric acid	Sodium bicarbonate Tromethamine Tromethamine-E	Potassium citrate Allopurinol
Cystine	Sodium bicarbonate Tromethamine Tromethamine-E Acetylcysteine	Potassium citrate D-Penicillamine α-Mercaptopropionyglycine
Struvite	Hemiacidrin Suby's Solution G	Acetohydroxamic acid
Calcium		Potassium citrate?

either tromethamine (THAM) or tromethamine-E (THAM-E).[5,33] In addition, these patients should be supplemented with oral potassium citrate therapy and allopurinol if indicated.

Cystine Stones

Cystine calculi also respond to both systemic alkalinization and direct irrigation with alkaline solutions. We begin oral alkali therapy with potassium citrate and maintain urinary pH between 6.5 and 7.0. In addition, *D*-penicillamine or Thiola (α-mercaptopropionylglycine; Santen) may be used to reduce the total cystine excretion by complexing cysteine, the monomeric form of cystine. Both *D*-penicillamine and Thiola undergo a thiodisulfide exchange with cystine to form soluble complexes that are much more soluble than cystine alone. The dose of *D*-penicillamine ranges between 750 and 1200 mg/day. Thiola, an investigational drug, has been demonstrated to cause significantly less side effects than *D*-penicillamine. Direct dissolution of cystine calculi is often successful and may be used as adjunctive therapy following PNL[12] and ESWL[35] to eliminate residual calculi. Currently used solutions include $1/2$ normal saline mixed with 60 ml of acetylcysteine (Mucomyst).[39] In addition, THAM or THAM-E can be used for dissolution of cystine calculi.[9,34]

Struvite Stones

Struvite calculi are soluble in an acid pH ($pH < 5.5$). Two commonly used solutions for the direct dissolution of struvite calculi are Suby's Solution G (Abbot Labs, North Chicago, IL, Cutter Labs, Emeryville, CA, Travenol Labs, Deerfield, IL) and hemiacidrin (Renacidin; Guardian Chemical Corp, Smithtown, NY). Both solutions contain acid to increase the solubility of struvite and citrate, which forms soluble complexes with the phosphate and calcium components of the stone. Renacidin may safely be used for renal irrigation; however, it is imperative that intrarenal pressures be kept below 25 cm of water.[22] In addition, serum magnesium and phosphate levels must be checked daily to prevent serious metabolic side effects.[7,40] Finally, urine cultures should also be checked daily to prevent possible sepsis during the chemolysis of these infected stones. Oral dissolution of residual struvite calculi may be attempted with a combination of antibiotic therapy and acetohydroxamic acid (AHA).[17] When given at a dose of 250 mg tid, AHA has caused dissolution in a limited number of patients; however, it appears that the current role for this medication is in the prevention of growth of residual stones or recurrence of newly formed stones in patients with chronic urea-splitting infections.

Calcium Stones

Potassium citrate may cause dissolution of calcium-containing stones in certain patients. Approximately 40 percent of our patients with calcareous calculi showed reduced stone mass following long-term therapy with potassium citrate. Since this effect has seemed to be most prominent in smaller stones, it may prove to be an ideal adjunct in the treatment of residual stones. Currently, long-term, randomized clinical trials are being performed to study the efficacy of calcium stone dissolution with potassium citrate.

Considerations with ESWL

Several important factors must be considered to prevent residual stones after ESWL therapy. The first is adequate localization/visualization of all stones to be treated. Prior to beginning lithotripsy, preoperative radiographs, including plain tomograms and possibly retrograde pyelograms, should be obtained to pinpoint all stones located within the collecting system. For small stones that are not easily seen on preoperative radiographs, one should consider the placement of a ureteral catheter prior to placing the patient on the machine. This will allow the urologist the option of injecting contrast to opacify the collecting system and thoroughly treat various locations within the kidney. Of course, utilization of a ureteral catheter and contrast is mandatory when treating radiolucent stones with ESWL.

At the beginning of ESWL treatment, the voltage of the shock wave should be as low as possible to initiate fragmentation of the stone. This will prevent explosive shattering of the stone, which may scatter fragments in multiple directions. We routinely begin treatment at 18 kV and then increase the power to a maximum of 24 kV as treatment progresses. If, however, the stone appears to be adequately fragmenting at the lower kilovolt setting, then increasing the power is probably not necessary.

After the stone appears to be adequately fragmented on the fluoroscopic images, one may consider the use of in-bath radiographs.[6] Our own experience with in-bath filming has shown these x-rays to be of some use in localizing small fragments that may have not been pulverized. However, the overall quality of these films is still not as good as those that can be obtained on normal x-ray tables. It is anticipated that the second-generation, "waterless," lithotripsy machines will allow more adequate radiologic stone localization and thus prevent the occurrence of residual stones.

As noted previously, ESWL monotherapy of large and/or staghorn calculi has resulted in a significant number of stone fragments. Most investigators now agree that combined percutaneous debulking of large stones followed by ESWL treatment of residual stones will offer the patient the most expeditious and cost-effective option for treating these stones.[36] If one is considering ESWL monotherapy for large stones, irrigating catheters may be utilized to flush out fragments during the ESWL procedure.

Stone fragments produced during lithotripsy may continue to absorb much of the shock-wave energy. Evacuation of stone fragments during an ESWL procedure may allow more shock waves to reach the "untreated" portion of a large stone, allowing complete pulverization. To aid in the intraoperative evacuation of stone fragments, one may utilize a series of irrigating catheters. These catheters may be placed either up the ureter, percutaneously, or in a combination of both approaches. Since a large amount of stone debris will be generated during the ESWL treatment, it is probably advantageous to place as large a drainage catheter as possible to help in removing these fragments.

If a percutaneous tube has been placed either before or after ESWL, this tract can be used for either stone manipulation or irrigation of chemolytic solutions if residual fragments are found. Many investigators now feel that routine irrigation of the renal collecting system should be employed with hemiacidrin or Suby's Solution G after treating infection stones with ESWL. Even though no stone fragments may be located on postoperative films, irrigation may prevent the enlargement of small stone fragments that cannot be visualized radiographically. Theoretically, this may also prevent the recurrent growth of struvite stones.

Finally, cystine calculi are difficult to adequately fragment with ESWL therapy because of their extreme hardness. Attempted treatment of cystine stones with ESWL monotherapy has resulted in a significant amount of residual stones. Here again, the current approach appears to be a combination method by first fragmenting the cystine stone utilizing ESWL and then either percutaneously removing any residual stone fragments or utilizing the percutaneous approach to instill chemolytic solutions to dissolve any remaining stone fragments.[35]

REFERENCES

1. Blaivas JG, Pais VM, Spellman RM: Chemolysis of residual stone fragments after extensive surgery for staghorn calculi. Urology 6:680–686, 1975
2. Blandy JP, Singh M: The case for a more aggressive approach to staghorn stones. J Urol 115:505–506, 1976
3. Boyce WH: The localization of intrarenal calculi during surgery. J Urol 118:152–157, 1977
4. Boyce WH, Elkins IB: Reconstructive renal surgery following anatrophic nephrolithotomy: Follow-up of 100 consecutive cases. J Urol 111:307–312, 1974
5. Burns JR, Gauthier JF, Finlayson B: Dissolution kinetics of uric acid calculi. J Urol 131:708–711, 1984
6. Bush WH, Gibbons RP, Brannen GE, et al: Facilitating extracorporeal shock wave lithotripsy (ESWL) application of x-ray filming in the water bath. J Urol 135:180A, 1986
7. Cato AR, Tullock AGS: Hypermagnesemia in a uremic patient during renal pelvis irrigation with renacidin. J Urol 111:313–314, 1974
8. Clayman RV, Surya W, Miller RP, et al: Percutaneous nephrolithotomy: An approach to branched and staghorn renal calculi. JAMA 250:73–75, 1983
9. Crissey MM, Gittes RF: Dissolution of cystine ureteral calculus by irrigation with tromethamine. J Urol 121:811–812, 1979
10. Drach GW, Dretler S, Fair W, et al: Report of United States cooperative study of extracorporeal shock wave lithotripsy. J Urol 135:1134–1137, 1986
11. Dretler SP, Pfister RC, Newhouse JH: Renal-stone dissolution via percutaneous nephrostomy. New Engl J Med 300:341–343, 1979
12. Dretler SP, Pfister RC, Newhouse JH, et al: Percutaneous catheter dissolution of cystine calculi. J Urol 131:216–219, 1984
13. Dretler SP, Watson GM, Murray S, et al: Laser fragmentation of ureteral calculi. J Urol 135:210A, 1986
14. Fostveldt GA, Barnes RW: Complications during lavage therapy for renal calculi. J Urol 89:329–334, 1963
15. Gavin R, Smith J: Recurrence of infected calculi following postoperative renal irrigation with stone solvents. Br J Urol 48:531–537, 1976
16. Gil-Vernet JM: Pyelolithotomy, in Roth RA, Finlayson B (eds): Stones clinical management of urolithiasis. Baltimore, Williams & Wilkins, 1983, pp 297–331
17. Griffith DP, Moskowitz PA, Carlton CE Jr: Adjunctive chemotherapy of infection-induced staghorn calculi. J Urol 121:711–714, 1979
18. Huffman JL, Bagley DH, Lyon ES: Extending cystoscopic techniques into the ureter and renal pelvis. JAMA 250:2002–2005, 1983
19. Kuwahara M, Kambe K, Takahaski K, et al: Intermittent irrigation system for dissolution of renal calculi monitored by computer. J Urol 128:1379–1383, 1982
20. Lingeman JE, Newman D, Mertz JHO, et al: Extracorporeal shock wave lithotripsy: The Methodist Hospital of Indiana experience. J Urol 135:1134, 1986
21. Lytton B: Intraoperative ultrasound for nephrolithotomy. J Urol 130:213–217, 1983

22. Nemoy NJ, Stamey TA: Surgical, bacteriological, and biochemical management of "infected stones." JAMA 215:1470–1476, 1971
23. Pak CYC: Should patients with single renal stone occurrence undergo diagnostic evaluation? J Urol 127:854–857, 1982
24. Palestrant AM, Sacks BA, Klein LA: Postoperative percutaneous kidney stone extraction. Radiology 134:778–779, 1980
25. Preminger GM, Pak CYC: The practical evaluation and selective medical management of nephrolithiasis. Sem Urol 3:170–184, 1985
26. Preminger GM, Clayman RV, Hardeman SW, et al: Percutaneous nephrostolithotomy versus open surgery for renal calculi. JAMA 254:1054–1058, 1985
27. Preminger GM, Peterson R, Peters PC, et al: The current role of nephrolithiasis: The impact of improved techniques of stone removal. J Urol 134:6–10, 1985
28. Reddy PK, Hulbert JC, Lange PH, et al: Percutaneous removal of renal and ureteral calculi: Experience with 400 cases. J Urol 134:662–666, 1985
29, Redman JF, Bissada NK, Harper DL: Anatrophic nephrolithotomy: Experience with complications of the Smith and Boyce technique. J Urol 122:595–597, 1979
30. Riehle RA Jr, Vaughn ED Jr: Chemical and crystallographic analysis of voided stone fragments after ESWL. J Urol 135:152A, 1986
31. Roth RA: Two aids for removal of renal calculi. J Urol 120:666–667, 1978
32. Rose MB, Follows OJ: Partial nephrectomy for stone disease. Br J Urol 49:605–610, 1977
33. Sadi MV, Saltzman N, Feria G, et al: Experimental observations on dissolution of uric acid calculi. J Urol 124:575–579, 1985
34. Salzman N, Gittes RF: Chemolysis of cystine calculi. J Urol 131:258–260, 1984
35. Schmeller HT, Kerting H, Schuller J, et al: Combination of chemolysis and shock wave lithotripsy in the treatment of cystine calculi. J Urol 131:434–438, 1984
36. Schulze H, Hertle L, Graff J, et al: Combined treatment of branched calculi by percutaneous nephrolithotomy and extracorporeal shock wave lithotripsy. J Urol 135:1138–1141, 1986
37. Segura JW, Patterson DE, LeRoy AJ, et al: Percutaneous removal of kidney stones: Review of 1000 cases. J Urol 134:1077–1081, 1985
38. Sleigh MW, Wickham JE: Long-term follow-up of 100 cases of renal calculi. Br J Urol 49:601–604, 1977
39. Smith AD, Lange PH, Miller RP, et al: Dissolution of cystine calculi by irrigation with acetylcysteine through percutaneous nephrostomy. Urology 13:422–424, 1979
40. Thompson IM Jr, Mora RV: Hypermagnesemia associated with hemiacidrin irrigation. J Urol 132:741–743, 1984
41. Wein AJ, Carpiniello VL, Mulholland SG, et al: Partial nephrectomy: Review of 80 cases emphasizing its role in management of localized renal stone disease. Urology 10:193–196, 1977

Stevan B. Streem

26

Bladder Calculi

HISTORY

Bladder calculi have afflicted humans since prehistoric times as Shattock reported Smith's findings of a calculus in a 7000-year-old mummified boy of 16.[21] While such stones were uncommon at that time, their prevalence apparently increased over the next 5000 years[26] so that by the European medieval period, bladder calculi had become so common that lithotomy became a surgical subspecialty.[24] The practice of lithotripsy has been first credited to Ammonios, who performed crude transurenthral procedures in the third century b.c. In the first century a.d., Celcus documented the earliest known techniques of perineal lithotomy.[10] By the eighteenth century, the open surgical techniques of perineal and suprapubic cystolithotomy were widely practiced. During the next 100 years, transurethral procedures were to be improved with the development of better instrumentation including the Bigelow lithotrite.[4] That instrument, introduced in the late 1800s, is still in use today.

The next advance in litholapaxy came through the addition of a lens system to the lithotrite for direct visual control during stone fragmentation. Such instruments have continuously been modified and refined and they are still widely used today in general urologic practice.

More recently, bladder stone fragmentation has become a province of high technology. The electrohydraulic lithotriptor, developed in Russia,[11] and ultrasonic lithotripsy, refined in West Germany, are finding increasing clinical use throughout the world. While a continued clinical role for these procedures currently seems secure, the future management of most bladder calculi may ultimately be relegated to extracorporeal shockwave lithotripsy (ESWL)[7] or, for some extremely large or hard stones, to "microexplosion" cystolithotripsy.[27]

STONE DISEASE: DIAGNOSIS AND MANAGEMENT

ISBN 0-8089-1873-7

EPIDEMIOLOGY AND ETIOLOGY

The incidence of bladder stones has decreased with time and industrialization. While bladder calculi represented 80 percent of the cases of urolithiasis in nineteenth century Europe, that percentage essentially reversed over the next 150 years; thus vesical stones now account for only 10 percent of urinary calculi in industrialized Europe and the United States. However, nonindustrialized and developing nations maintain high proportions of bladder calculi.[1] In some areas of the world, particularly in parts of the Middle and Far East, bladder calculi remain common in infants and children, but only those of lower socioeconomic background. Van Reen has extensively reviewed these primary or "endemic" bladder calculi.[26] Generally, they affect children under 10 years of age, with a disproportionately high incidence found in boys compared to girls. These stones are most often composed of ammonium acid urate together with calcium oxalate or phosphate. In some parts of the world, pure urate calculi may predominate.[5] Interestingly, it has been felt that these bladder stones are only rarely associated with upper tract calculi, though that finding has now been challenged by others.[16] In contradistinction to upper (urinary) tract disease, these calculi rarely recur following surgical removal.

The etiology of endemic bladder calculi remains unclear but appears to be multifactorial. In these affected children, obstruction or infection generally are not identifiable; however, dietary factors appear important in their pathogenesis. Deficiencies of dietary phosphates, chronic dehydration, and excessive protein or oxalate consumption have, among others, all been implicated at times.[26]

"Secondary" bladder calculi occur primarily in adults and most often are associated with urinary stasis with or without associated infection. In some cases, these stones begin as upper tract calculi that migrate to the bladder. In those cases, the primary etiology of the calculus might be related to any of the metabolic factors associated with renal stone formation. However, calculi that are able to spontaneously traverse the ureterovesical junction should be easily passed through the bladder neck and urethra with micturition. As such, all patients with bladder calculi, regardless of whether they are known to have associated upper tract calculus disease, must be suspected of having anatomic or functional bladder outlet obstruction. As will be discussed, therapy must then be directed not only to removing the calculus but also at correcting the voiding dysfunction.

The chemical composition of these bladder calculi is similar to the spectrum seen in the upper tract. They may be composed of calcium oxalate, calcium phosphate, urate, struvite, cystine, or any combination thereof. Like upper-tract stones, the chemical composition is affected by local urinary factors such as pH or the presence or absence of associated infection. As such, an acid urine predisposes to uric acid calculi, while an alkaline pH, with or without infection, promotes calcium phosphate or struvite. The finding of cystine bladder calculi, like upper-tract cystine stones, implies the presence of homozygous cystinuria.

Finally, a foreign body in the urinary tract, even without associated infection, may act as a nidus for stone formation. In these cases, phosphatic encrustation often is the initial factor in the stone formation. In patients with bladder calculi associated with foreign bodies, the most usual inciting factor is an indwelling Foley catheter. Recently, however, we have encountered cases of bladder calculi resulting from longstanding indwelling self-retaining ureteral stents (Fig. 26-1). This problem may become more frequent with the increasing use of such stents. Nonabsorbable suture material that has penetrated the urothelium following previous bladder or other pelvic surgery may also act as a nidus for bladder stone formation. A myriad of other foreign bodies have also

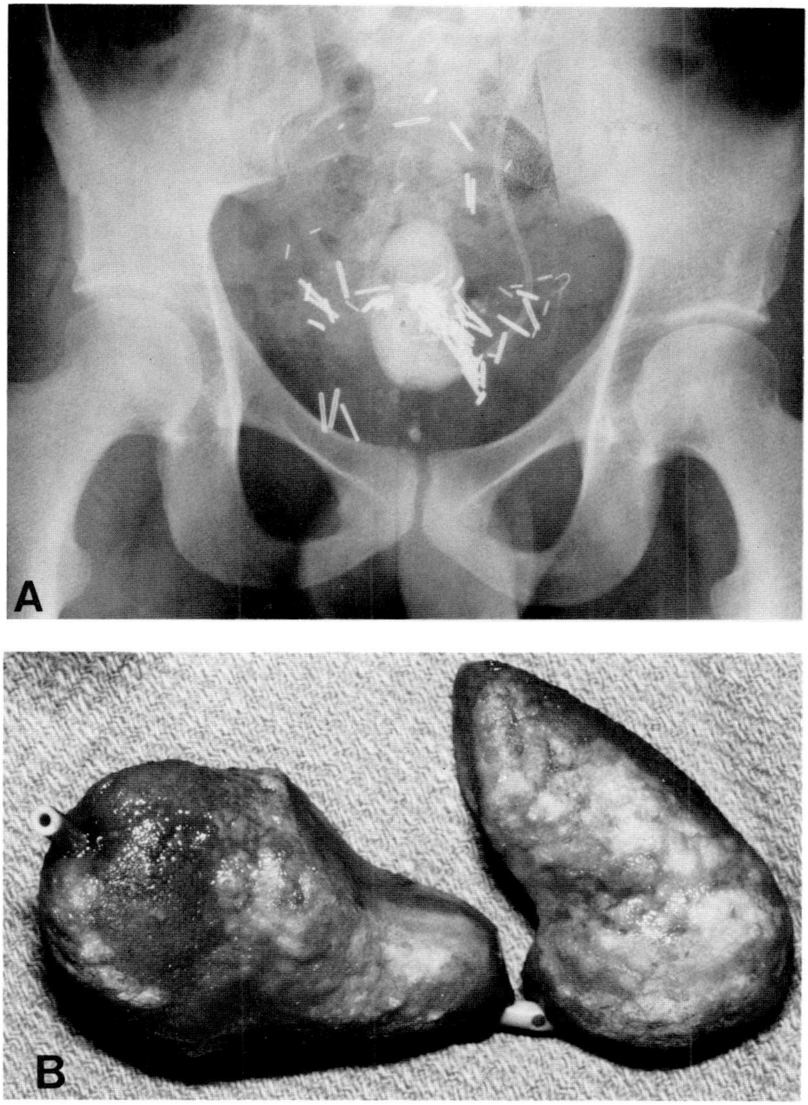

Fig. 26-1. (A) Plain film showing large bladder calculus intimately associated with self-retaining left ureteral stent. (B) Gross specimen revealing bladder calculus forming around the stent. (Courtesy of Anthony J. Thomas, Jr., M.D.)

been encountered in association with bladder calculi. Generally, these foreign bodies have been introduced transurethrally, either by the patient or iatrogenically such as in cases of retained Foley balloon fragments.[8]

DIAGNOSIS

The patient's history may provide a clue to the diagnosis. As mentioned earlier, however, with the exception of those calculi occurring in children in endemic areas, most of these stones are associated with urinary stasis with or without associated infection, or the presence of a foreign body. Patients with anatomic or functional outlet obstruction, therefore, such as males in the "prostatic" age group or patients with neurogenic bladder, are at increased risk of harboring bladder calculi. In most cases, then, the presenting symptoms are those of outlet obstruction or urinary infection. A history of hematuria, especially terminal stream, may be elicited. In these patients, the vesical calculi are found during the course of the routine urologic investigation. There are, however, some specific symptoms that are highly suggestive of vesical stones. In males, intermittent pain radiating toward the tip of the penis occasionally is noted. This results from the stone abutting on the bladder neck. This symptom generally is positional, occurring more often in the upright position or during activities such as descending a flight of stairs. The patient may note relief by assuming a reclining position. A patient might also complain of intermittent sudden interruption of the urinary stream, again the result of the stone rolling onto the bladder neck or into the prostatic urethra. Emperor Napoleon III, who died of complications of vesical calculus disease following litholapaxy,[9] has been depicted leaning at an acute angle against a tree in an attempt to void. Apparently, this position allowed the stone to roll away from the bladder neck, where it presumably was causing obstruction, pain, or both.

As mentioned, patients with neurogenic bladder are at high risk for vesical calculi. In these patients, the calculi may result from stasis of urine secondary to functional outlet obstruction or from the presence of indwelling catheter. The bladder calculi in these patients may even present as a need for more frequent catheter changes as the calculi or inspissations cause intermittent blockage of the catheter.

Finally, a history that suggests a potential foreign body in the bladder should be sought. This might have resulted from previous vesical or pelvic surgery with retention of a nonabsorbable suture. Another iatrogenic cause of a foreign body is a retained fragment of a Foley catheter balloon; thus even a remote history of catheterization for a short period of time is important. Foreign bodies may also be self-introduced in men or women, and such a history should again be sought. After a period of time, essentially all these foreign bodies become calculogenic and act as niduses for stones. Infection in those cases is almost inevitable.

Physical examination generally is unrewarding in a specific search for bladder calculi. Again, factors or conditions that predispose to urinary stasis such as benign prostatic hyperplasia, large cystoceles, or neurogenic bladder, should be sought. Occasionally, extremely large vesical calculi may be palpated suprapubically, transvaginally, or transrectally.

Laboratory studies are again nonspecific. An impairment of overall renal function would be unusual and more likely related to intrinsic renal disease or obstructive uropathy from the primary urologic condition that predisposed to the stones. Urinalysis generally will reveal at least microhematuria and pyuria, with or without infection. The cornerstone of noninvasive diagnosis lies in radiographic findings. The radiodensity of a bladder calculus is variable and depends mostly on the chemical composition. As the composition of bladder stones has the same spectrum as upper tract calculi, the radiodensity may vary between lucent and highly opaque. Those containing large amounts of uric acid will be relatively lucent and may only be noted as filling defects on the cystogram phase of an intravenous urogram or during formal cystography. Such filling defects may easily be differentiated from tumors, intravesical prostate, or blood clots by ultrasonography, which will demonstrate acoustic shadowing.[20] Computed tomography, performed without intravenous or intravesical contrast, can also differentiate vesical calculi, although this modality is only rarely required for diagnosis. As in the upper tract, struvite or calcium phosphate stones are relatively opaque and may appear laminated. Calcium oxalate stones are often spiculated and have been likened to a "jackstone" in their gross appearance[2] (Fig. 26-2).

At times, the radiographic diagnosis of a bladder calculus may be difficult or confusing because of a location within a vesical diverticulum. Oblique radiographs before and after administration of contrast generally will allow a definitive diagnosis in these cases.

Even with a high degree of suspicion, a significant proportion of bladder calculi will remain undiagnosed radiographically, and therefore the definitive diagnostic study is cystoscopic examination.

TREATMENT

Standard treatment options include chemodissolution; transurethral extraction with or without mechanical, electrohydraulic, or ultrasonic fragmentation; or open vesicolithotomy. In the future, microexplosion cystolithotripsy or, more likely, ESWL may find standard roles in management. With all the options available, the choice of therapy must be directed to a procedure that allows removal of the calculi in a manner that is both relatively noninvasive and expeditious. Furthermore, the choice of therapy should allow correction of the underlying disorder whenever possible so that stone recurrences can be minimized.

Chemodissolution is theoretically attractive because it is minimally invasive and

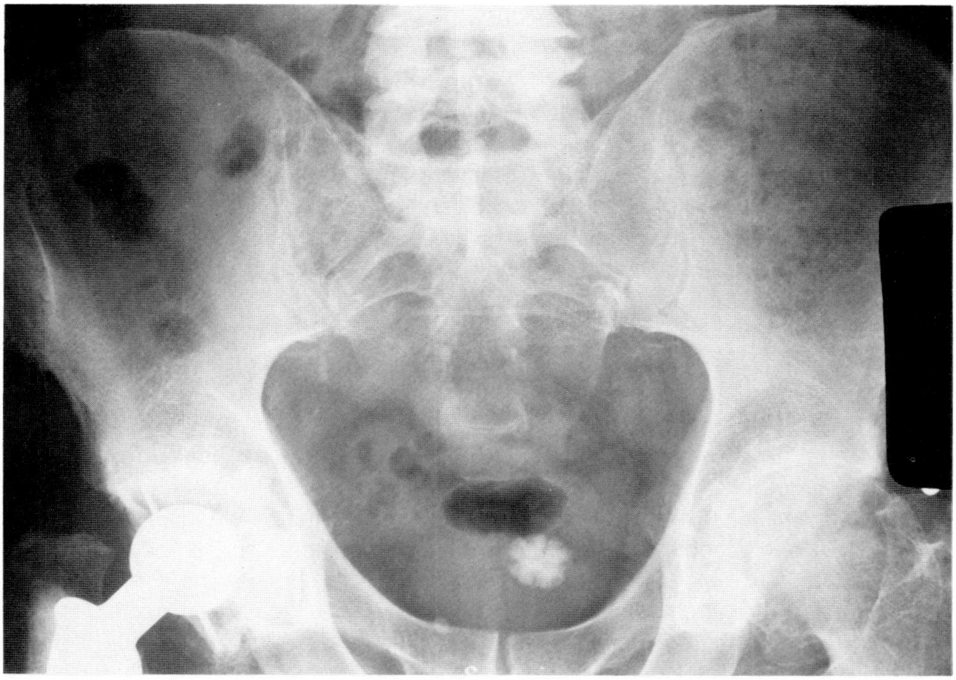

Fig. 26-2. Typical jackstone appearance of a calcium oxalate bladder calculus.

applicable to several varieties of calculi, including uric acid, struvite, and cystine stones. Unfortunately, the long periods of time generally required for this treatment modality often makes it impractical compared to other available options. Furthermore, chemodissolution may require the presence of an indwelling catheter placed either transurethrally or suprapubically. The long-term presence of such a catheter would be highly undesirable in a patient not already instrumented. In select situations, though, chemodissolution can play a role. In patients with uric acid or cystine bladder calculi, oral chemodissolution may be instituted, as it would be for such calculi in the upper tract, with alkalinizing agents. In cystinurics, d-penicillamine can be added to the regimen. It must be emphasized, again, however, that even in the presence of demonstrable underlying metabolic defects, the presence of these stones in the bladder implies urinary stasis and functional or anatomic outlet obstruction that should be searched for and corrected.

Bladder irrigations may be indicated in patients with struvite calculi, especially when the stones are associated with the preexisting presence of an indwelling catheter. In such cases, acidifying agents such as Suby's G Solution or hemiacidrin[17] may be administered. For dissolution of existing calculi, a continuous flow through a three-way catheter is preferable to intermittent irrigation, although the latter may be preferable or more practical in an outpatient setting or for simple prophylaxis.[28] Perhaps the most important part of therapy in patients who form these stones in the presence of an indwelling catheter is further evaluation and treatment to rid the patient of this nidus for infection and stones. When operative therapy is not indicated, consideration should be given to changing the patient to a regimen of intermittent catheterization wherever feasible. Such a program will vastly decrease the incidence and rate of bladder stone formation, although that complication has been reported even in this setting.[15,23]

In our practice, the majority of patients presenting with bladder calculi are treated with a transurethral procedure to extract the stones. In some patients, small calculi may simply be grasped under vision with a cystoscopic forceps or irrigated out with an Ellik-type evacuator. These small stones are often discovered incidentally during the course of cystoscopy performed at the outset of a planned transurethral procedure such as prostatic resection. In such cases, the stone extraction is performed during the same procedure, adding little, if any, potential morbidity. In females, urethral dilatation alone may allow extraction of larger calculi intact.[12] In males, however, calculi larger than 7 or 8 mm in smallest diameter require fragmentation before they can be evacuated. While fragmentation of bladder calculi were among the first surgical procedures recorded, current advances in this area continue to set a standard for surgical technology. Presently, urologists have at their disposal practical equipment for transurethral fragmentation of bladder calculi by mechanical, electrohydraulic, or ultrasonic means. The urologist's access to all these procedures and familiarity with their advantages and limitations in specific settings will help to ensure optimal treatment for the patient.

Lithotripsy became a part of contemporary urologic practice with the introduction of the Bigelow lithotrite.[4] This instrument (Fig. 26-3) is introduced blindly into the bladder and tactile means alone are used to grasp and crush the stone. Potential complications are numerous and generally relate to perforation of the bladder or even adjacent pelvic structures. The lack of visual control requires repeated insertions and removal of the instrument for intermittent visualization and evacuation of remaining fragments, and bleeding eventually obscuring vision is almost inevitable. The indication for tactile lithotripsy is the presence of a large, free-floating bladder calculus. To prevent bladder perforation, a normal bladder capacity must be present so that the bladder can be distended

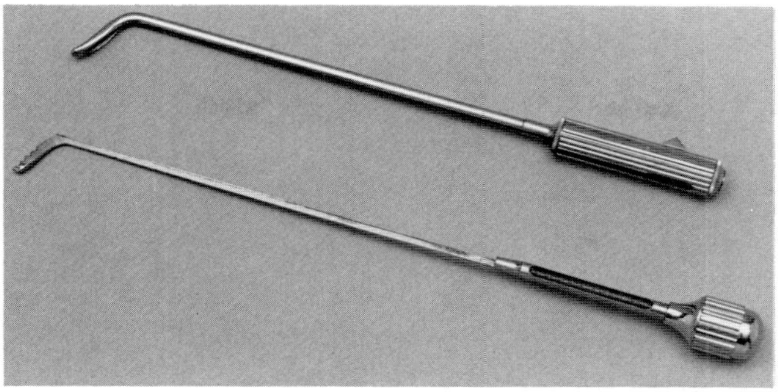

Fig. 26-3. Bigelow lithotrite allowing fragmentation of large calculi by tactile means alone.

prior to grasping and crushing of the stone. In current practice, fluroscopy can be added for better control of stone engagement, crushing, and determination of residual fragments; nevertheless, the potential complications are great compared to more recently introduced techniques. While some experienced urologists may still find tactile lithotripsy a useful part of their practice,[13,22] we thus no longer employ this technique and prefer instead current methodology that allows direct visual control.

The next advance in litholapaxy was the addition of a telescopic lens system to the lithotrite.[10] A variety of such instruments are currently available (Fig. 26-4), and all have in common the ability to allow engagement and crushing of the stone under direct vision. As with tactile lithotripsy, adequate bladder capacity is required to decrease the likelihood of vesical perforation. Lithotripsy under vision is applicable to most patients with bladder calculi and is preferable in almost all instances to tactile lithotripsy. The procedure does have its own limitations, in that some stones are simply too large or too hard to engage or crush with these instruments. Alternatives and adjunctive modalities are now available in those cases, however, and in our practice electrohydraulic and ultrasonic lithotripsy have rapidly become the preferred techniques for stone fragmentation in most patients.

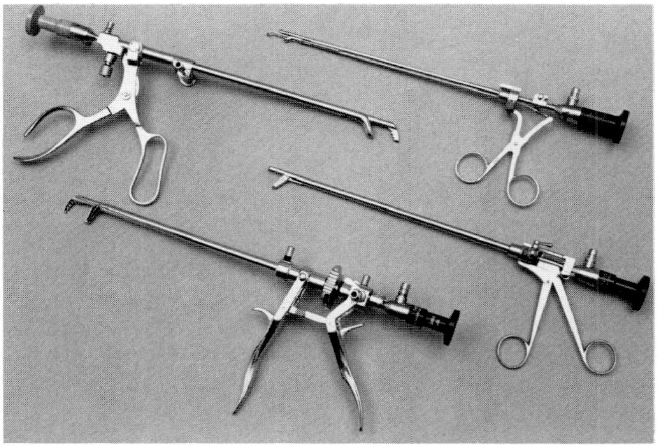

Fig. 26-4. A variety of modern lithotrites allow direct visual control during mechanical lithotripsy.

Since the early 1970s there has been increasing interest in the use of ultrasonic energy to fragment urinary calculi, and the excellent results that can be obtained with bladder calculi are well documented.[14] The procedure has several advantages over simple mechanical lithotripsy, but in our experience it has not been applicable to all patients. The ultrasonic energy is transmitted from a generator to a lithotrite (ultrasound wand). The lithotrite is placed directly on the calculus with direct visual control and ultrasonic energy is applied to fragment the stone. The rigid lithotrite must be passed through a cystoscope with an offset lens system. The instrument is easily introduced into the bladder transurethrally (Fig. 26-5) or, in patients with preexisting suprapubic tubes, through that tract. Continuous irrigation and suction are utilized throughout the procedure, thus allowing simultaneous evacuation of the stone particles during the procedure. The ultrasonic energy has no significant adverse effects on the vesical mucosa other than

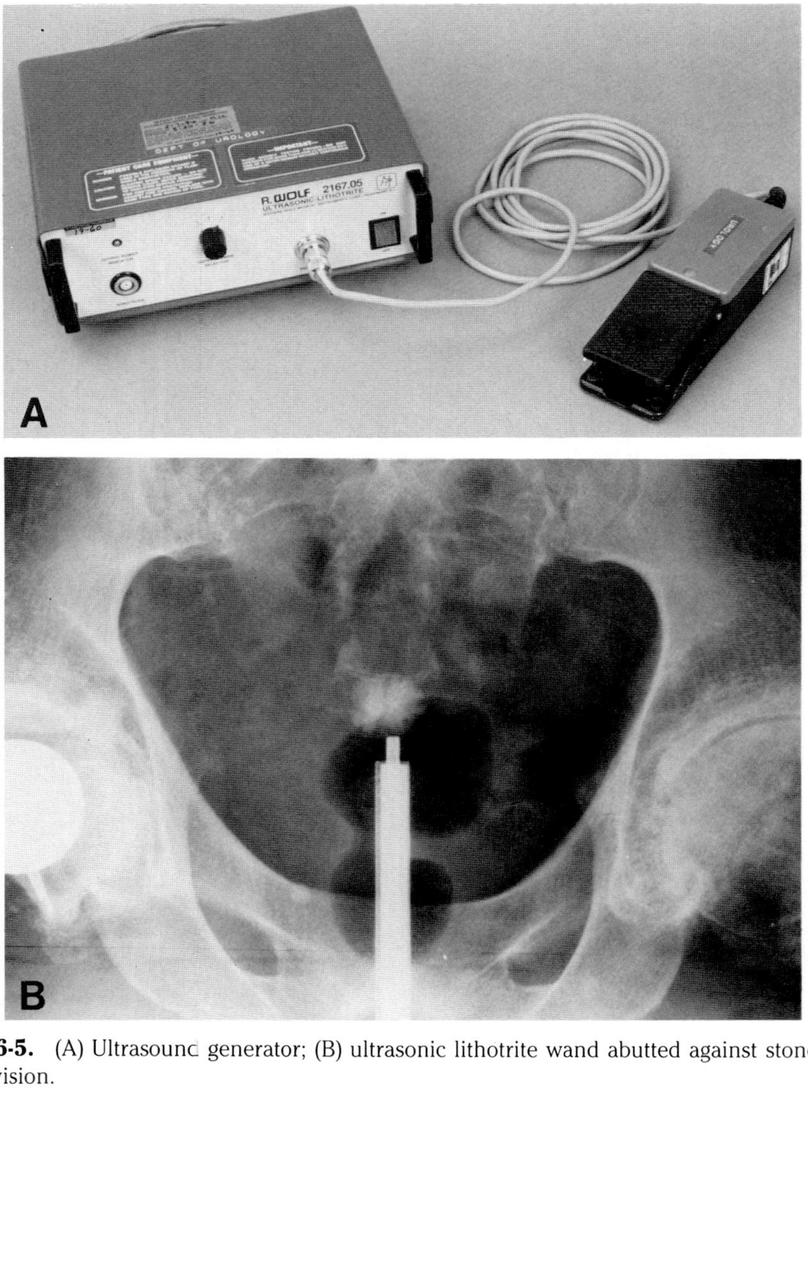

Fig. 26-5. (A) Ultrasound generator; (B) ultrasonic lithotrite wand abutted against stone under direct vision.

a local edematous reaction that resolves quickly. The bladder can be perforated by the wand itself, however, so direct visualization is required throughout the procedure.

We have found ultrasonic lithotripsy to be most valuable in patients with struvite calculi as they fragment readily. Calcium oxalate monohydrate and calcium phosphate stones are more difficult to fragment; however, those measuring up to 3 cm in diameter are managed well with this modality. Uric acid stones are even more resistant to ultrasonic fragmentation.

In some patients, the stones are too hard, because of either their size or chemical composition, for effective ultrasonic fragmentation. In most of those cases, we have found electrohydraulic lithotripsy to be the most efficacious procedure. This technique, developed in Russia in the 1960s[11] now has worldwide acceptance with few complications reported.[3,6,18,19,25] The procedure is again performed under direct vision. The electrohydraulic generator is used to transmit a series of high voltage sparks across the tip of a flexible probe (Fig. 26-6). Because the probe is flexible, standard cystoscopic equipment can be utilized, but distilled water or one-sixth normal saline must be used as an irrigant. The shock waves from the electrohydraulic lithotriptor are generated after the probe is placed cystoscopically 1–2 mm from the calculus. Repeated shocks result in fragmentation of the stone, during which time care must be taken to keep the probe from contact-

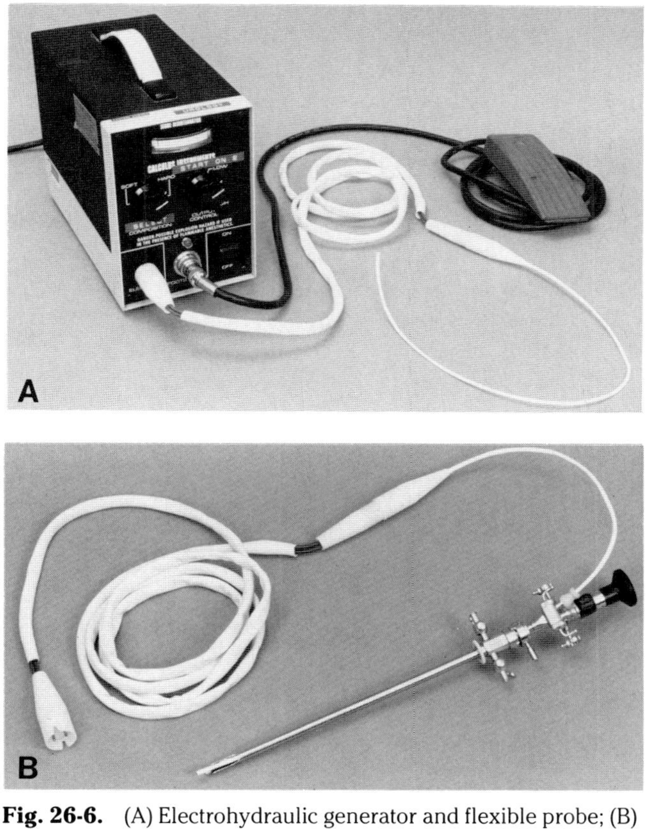

Fig. 26-6. (A) Electrohydraulic generator and flexible probe; (B) flexible probe is passed through standard cystoscopic instrumentation.

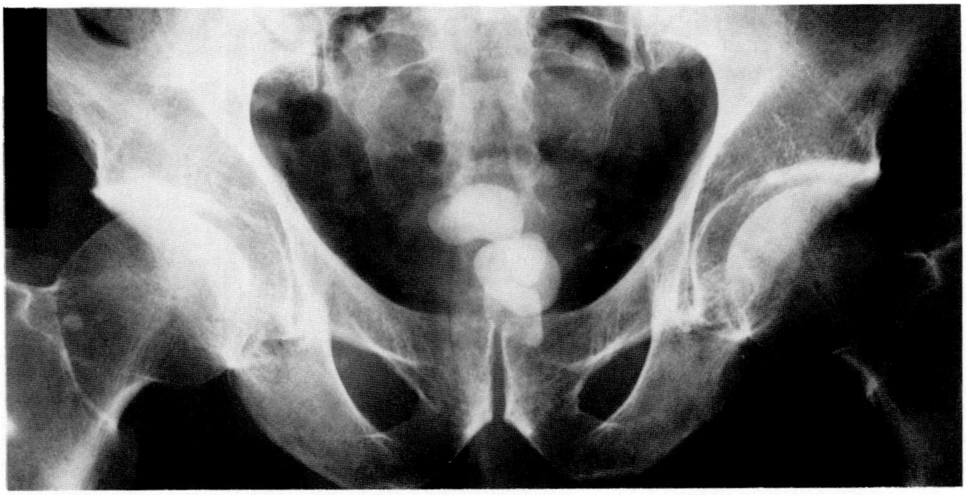

Fig. 26-7. Multiple large, hard stones such as these may at times still be managed most safely and efficiently with a simple open cystolithotomy.

ing the bladder mucosa directly. When the stone fragments are small enough, they are irrigated out with an Ellik evacuator.

In some cases, open cystolithotomy may still be the safest, most efficient treatment. This is especially true with extremely large or hard stones (Fig. 26-7) or in patients with relatively small bladder capacities that renders them prone to significant musocal injury with bleeding obscuring vision or even perforation. The other major consideration in choosing an open procedure is the associated pathophysiologic condition. Thus, for example, the surgeon might have to choose between staging a transurethral resection and cystolitholapaxy for even a moderate sized obstructing prostate and stones, or a simultaneous open prostatectomy and vesicolithotomy. Generally, the urologist's own experience and the preference of the patient will play the greatest role in such a decision.

THE FUTURE

Future advances in surgical technology will continue to be adapted to the management of patients with vesical calculi. While there are still some patients with stones too large or too hard to manage expeditiously by litholapaxy, modalities such as microexplosion cystolithotripsy might eventually gain a significant clinical role. Even more likely, noninvasive technology such as ESWL[7] will become the standard of treatment for most affected patients. Even in such cases, however, the urologist will have to continue to search for and correct the underlying metabolic, physiologic, and anatomic abnormalities that initially led to the formation of the bladder calculi.

REFERENCES

1. Asper R, Schmucki O: Socioeconomic aspects of urinary stone disease in Eurasia in the nineteenth and twentieth century in Ryall R, Brockis JG, Marshall V, et al (eds): Urinary Stone. New York, Churchill Livingstone, 1984

2. Banner MP, Pollack HM: Radiologic evaluation of urinary calculi, in Roth RA, Finlayson B (eds): Stones: Clinical Management of Urolithiasis. Baltimore, Williams & Wilkins, 1983
3. Bergman B, Nygaard E, Osterman G, et al: Vesical calculi: Experience of electrohydraulic lithotripsy with URAT I. Scand J Urol Nephrol 16:217, 1982
4. Bigelow HJ: Lithotrity—a single operation. Boston Med Surg J 98:259, 1879
5. Brockis JG, Bowyer RC, McCulloch TA, et al: Proceedings of the International Urinary Stone Conference. Littleton, MA, PSG Publishing Company, 1979
6. Bulow H, Frohmuller HGW: Electrohydraulic lithotripsy with aspiration of the fragments under vision—304 consecutive cases. J Urol 126:454, 1981
7. Chaussy C, Schmiedt E, Jocham E, et al: First clinical experience with extracorporeally induced destruction of kidney stones by shock waves. J Urol 127:417, 1982
8. Dalton DL, Hughes J, Glenn JF: Foreign bodies and urinary stones. Urology 6:1, 1975
9. Ellis H: The bladder stone of Emperor Napoleon III. Chirurgie 110:370, 1984
10. Glenn JF: Bladder stones: From lithotrity to ultrasound. Urol Clin N Am 1:375, 1974
11. Goldberg VV: On the history of the electrohydraulic lithotripsy method (E). Urol Nefrol (Moscow) 50:90, 1974
12. Gottesman JE, Flanagan MJ: Removal of bladder stones in females. Urology 11:636, 1978
13. Hadley HL, Barnes RW, Rosenquist RC: Tactile litholapaxy—safe and efficient. Urology 9:263, 1977
14. Hautmann R, Tehorst B, Rathert P, et al: Ultrasonic litholapaxy of bladder stones—10 year experience with more than 400 cases, in Ryall R, Brockis JG, Marshall V, et al (eds): Urinary Stone. New York, Churchill Livingstone, 1984
15. Kutscher HA, Vinson RK: Bladder calculi formation during clean intermittent catheterization. Urology 14:357, 1979
16. Malek RS: Urolithiasis, in Kelalis PP, King LR (eds): Clinical Pediatric Urology. Philadelphia, Saunders, 1976
17. Mulvaney WP: Prevention of calcification of indwelling catheters. Arch Phys Med Rehab 45:610, 1984
18. Raney AM: Electrohydraulic lithotripsy: Experimental study and case reports with stone disintegration. J Urol 113:345, 1975
19. Reuter HJ: Electronic lithotripsy: Transurethral treatment of bladder stone in 50 cases. J Urol 104:834, 1970
20. Rosenfield AT, Taylor KJW, Weiss RM: Ultrasound evaluation of bladder calculi. J Urol 121:119, 1979
21. Shattock SG: A prehistoric or predynastic Egyptian calculus. Trans the Pathol Soc London 56:275, 1905
22. Smith JM, O'Flynn JD: Transurethral removal of bladder stone: The place of litholapaxy. Br J Urol 49:401, 1977
23. Solomon HM, Koff SA, Diokno AC: Bladder calculi complicating intermittent catheterization. J Urol 124:140, 1980
24. Streitz JM, Aufderheide AC, El Najjar M, et al: A 1,500 year old bladder stone. J Urol 126:452, 1980
25. Trapeznikova MF, Borodulin GG: Electrohydraulic impulse lithotripsy of bladder stones with URAT I. Endoscopy 9:6, 1977
26. Van Reen R: Idiopathic urinary bladder stones of childhood. Aust NZ J Surg 50:18, 1980
27. Watanabe H, Watanabe K, Shiino K, et al: Micro-explosion cystolithotripsy. J Urol 129:23, 1983
28. Woodside JR, Crawford ED: Dissolution of vesical calculi with Renacidin in a paraplegic man. Paraplegia 18:69, 1980

H. Norman Noe
F. Bruder Stapleton

27

Pediatric Stone Disease

Although stone disease in children has been known through recorded history, it has not received as much attention as deserved because of the relatively low incidence compared to that of adults. The early reports were centered on documenting the occurrence of endemic calculi and cataloguing the etiologies of stone disease in children. Later observations pointed up geographic variations as to the incidence and stone type seen in the pediatric stone disease state. More recently, efforts have been made to thoroughly investigate pediatric stone patients metabolically to determine an exact etiology that could also be helpful in their long-term treatment and management. It is our purpose in this chapter to review the subject of pediatric stone disease and provide a framework in which this problem can be better understood and more effectively managed.

EPIDEMIOLOGY

In the past century, pediatric stone disease was largely limited to endemic bladder stones in children. Such bladder calculi are composed primarily of acid urates and present predominantly in males under the age of 5 years. These stones form primarily in children in whom there is neither obstruction nor infection of the lower urinary system, and once they are removed, the rate of recurrence seems to be low. These stones have gradually disappeared from industrialized and increasingly affluent populations. They still are prevalent in the developing countries of North Africa, Thailand, Indonesia, and the Middle and Far East. The disease seems to be particularly prevalent in children of low socioeconomic class. It is felt that nutrition plays a major role in the predisposition to endemic calculi. It has been suggested that human breast milk and foods such as polished rice and cereals are low in phosphates and result in high peaks of urinary ammonia excretion and low phosphate excretion, which predispose to formation of this type of calculus.

As endemic stones disappeared from Europe and, to a degree, from North America, new patterns of stone composition and geographic variations began to emerge. Infection-

STONE DISEASE: DIAGNOSIS AND MANAGEMENT ISBN 0-8089-1873-7

related stones now appear to be the most common type encountered in Europe, whereas in North America metabolic causes most commonly are given as the etiology for stone disease in a child. In populations where infection stones are common, younger children are most affected and there is a predominance of male patients over female patients. Recent reports from North America tend to show a more even distribution of stone disease from birth through adolescence, and there does not appear to be as large a male preponderance. Racial factors appear to be of some influence in that blacks and Latins have a much lower rate of stone disease. A genetic predisposition to stone disease has been noted, and it has been suggested that the inheritance is that of a polygenic pattern with variable penetrance.[68] It has also been noted that certain areas of the world and North America have predisposition to stones leading to a "stone belt" type of designation that appears to affect both adults and children. It would thus appear that such intrinsic factors as heredity, age, and sex are modified by, as yet, poorly defined extrinsic or environmental factors such as diet, water intake, and climate.

The incidence of occurrence of stone disease has been reported from various institutions as 1 of 1000 pediatric admissions up to 1 of 7600 pediatric admissions. When examined, these figures primarily reflect the population, geography, and referral nature of the reporting institution. The recurrence rate of stone disease can also be varied geographically in children. Areas such as the southeastern United States and Newfoundland report recurrence rates in the vicinity of 40–50 percent, whereas other areas report recurrence rates as low as 5–6 percent.

Factors such as hereditary renal tubular disorders and enzyme disorders can be suspected by careful history and confirmed by metabolic investigation. Other factors such as hyperparathyroidism and hyperadrenocorticism may also be identified. It must also be kept in mind that environmental factors such as dairy product intake, vitamin consumption, and steroid administration can also predispose to stone disease.

Many factors, intrinsic as well as environmental, thus come into play when attempting to define the cause of pediatric stone disease. More than one factor can play a role when determining the cause of stone disease and, more importantly, whether an individual is predisposed to a high rate of recurrence that could potentially affect morbidity or even loss of renal function.

CLINICAL ASPECTS

Presentation

Severe colicky flank pain typical of adults with stones is not as often encountered in children. In many cases, a high index of suspicion is necessary to consider the diagnosis of a stone in the pediatric patient. The common presenting signs and symptoms of children with stones are primarily those of hematuria and abdominal or flank pain. In the younger child, the abdominal pain may be vague and nonspecific, although in the older child or adolescent a more typical adult presentation can be encountered. Signs and symptoms of urinary tract infection can also accompany the presence of a urinary calculus. Gross hematuria can be the first sign of a stone in the urinary tract. The usual case, however, is for microscopic, painless hematuria to be present in the overwhelming majority of children with stones. In fact, urolithiasis should always be a consideration in the pediatric patient with painless hematuria. Pyuria may be the initial sign of stone disease in a child and may simply accompany irritative signs or symptoms of urinary tract infection. The stone may be discovered in the course of the workup for that condition. In a few instances, apparently painless passage of the calculus has been the first sign that a stone was present. This has been primarily noted in children with upper urinary stones. Calculi involving the lower urinary system, however, will typically present with a greater number of symptoms. Severe dysuria with obstructive and other irritative voiding symptoms usually are noted with lower urinary calculi. Some children report increased irritability while in the upright position but relief of pain when lying down, which removes the calculus from being impacted in the bladder neck. In a few instances, actual obstruction by impaction of a urethral calculus has been the first sign that stones were present.

Once a suspicion of stone disease is aroused, the diagnosis is primarily radiographic. Radiopaque calculi of the upper urinary system is usually defined by the plain radiograph of the abdomen or, more exactly, by the excretory urogram (Figs. 27-1*A* and 27-1*B*). In some instances, renal ultrasound has clearly shown the calculus to be present within the urinary system, especially in some cases associated with hydronephrosis (Figs. 27-2*A* and 27-2*B*). Ultrasound has proved to be a useful technique for following stones in children once the diagnosis has been made. Although stones in the urinary system in children are largely radiopaque, a small percentage of children will have lucent calculi. This usually occurs in less than 5 percent of the total number of patients. In some instances when radiolucent uric acid stones are suspected, CT scanning of the areas regional to the urinary system will show the stone when plain radiographs will not. It should be remembered, however, that the standard for diagnosis still remains the excretory urogram with oblique and delayed films used as required for documentation and localization of the stone.

Review of the Literature

Experiences with pediatric stone disease have been increasingly analytical over the past three decades. Early reports, such as those of Campbell, tend to confirm the high rate of urate stones in children.[18] In 1957 Myers made the observation that stones were no longer endemic and seemed to be changing in site, frequency, and composition in children.[50] Reports then followed that seemed to emphasize that with this change there appeared to be a high association of congenital anomalies and urinary stasis that could be responsible for the formation of stones.[5,6,22,88,91] In the 1970s, additional reports appeared regarding pediatric stone disease, and greater consideration was given to the etiology of the stone and such factors as possible metabolic considerations and stone recurrence.[8] A few series stressed the importance of infection in pediatric stone patients in the United States,[57] but this population was primarily in a myelodysplasia clinic and did not represent a general cross section of pediatric stone patients. A report concerning primarily adolescents was published by Rambar and MacKenzie, noting a high incidence of preexisting conditions such as neurogenic bladder, exstrophy, and other well-known causes of stone disease that appear to be a continuation from early childhood.[66]

In studying the recent reports on pediatric urolithiasis, it is obvious that there are geographic variations in both stone incidence and etiology. It is important to note whether the reporting institution was a referral center. Both Paulson et al.[63] and Malek and Kelalis[44] reported a large series of pediatric stone patients with varied causes, many metabolic; the most common was the so-called idiopathic stone former. In these series, attempts were made to define any metabolic abnormalities, and specific mention was

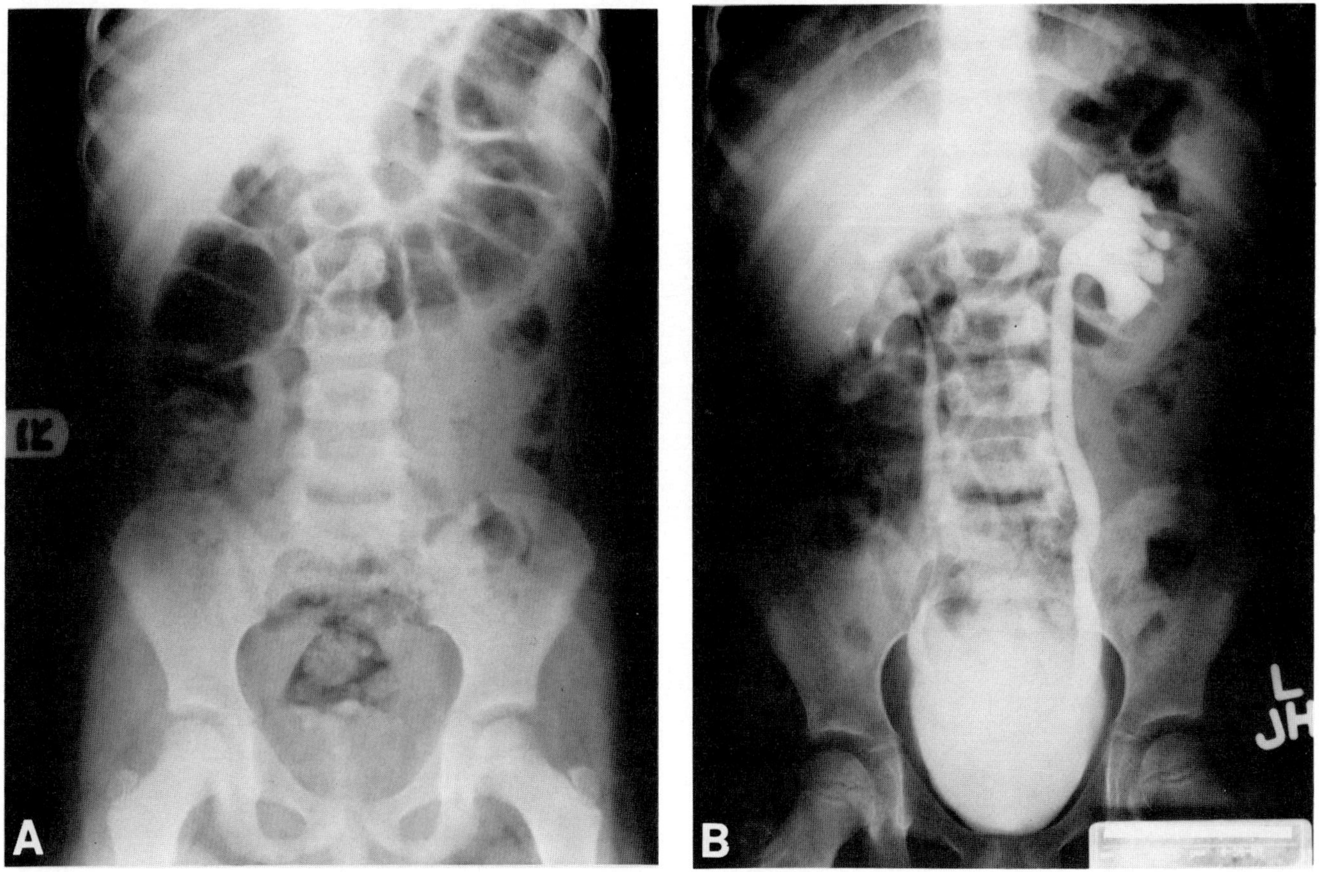

Fig. 27-1. (*A*) Plain film in a female child with hematuria and multiple calcific densities regional to the urinary tract. (*B*) Excretory urogram confirming bilateral ureteral calculi in same child proved to have hyperoxaluria.

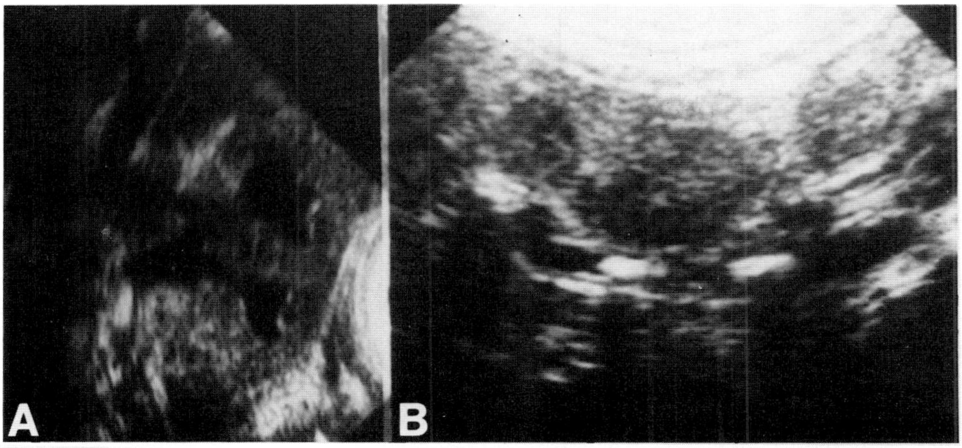

Fig. 27-2. (*A*) Coronal renal ultrasound showing ureteral calculus impacted at the ureteropelvic junction in an infant with stones (left image). (*B*) Longitudinal image of the ureter showing calculi within (right image).

made to evaluate for hypercalciuria. Sinno et al. reported a large series of patients from the Southeastern United States where there is a recognized increased incidence of stone disease in the general population.[74] They documented six children with hypercalciuria and noted also a positive family history in 56 percent of their patients and a high recurrence rate of 44 percent. Both Reiner et al.[67] and Walther et al.[90] subsequently reviewed their series from different areas of the United States. Although they attempted to define stone disease as to etiology, they did not succeed in defining the role of metabolic screening and actually felt that there was no merit in the latter.[65,90] In neither of these series, however, was there a significant attempt to define calcium excretion abnormalities. Their conclusions could reflect the different populations encountered at these centers. In contrast, in Newfoundland, Churchill, et al. studied a number of children with urolithiasis and did, indeed, find a number with hypercalciuria who had been previously classified as having idiopathic urolithiasis.[20] They also found a high percentage of children with a positive family history for stone disease, which reflects a similar finding in the adults in their area.[20] Additional reviews on the subject of childhood urolithiasis have been carried out by a number of authors.[11,55,58,86] From these reports as well as those mentioned previously, it is now obvious that the pediatric stone patient needs to be evaluated thoroughly from a metabolic standpoint as it might reflect a tendency toward recurrence and the need for long term followup and therapy.

Several recent reviews from Europe have continued to emphasize the role of infection in childhood urolithiasis at the various reporting centers. Ghazali et al. reported a high percentage of children with infection-related stones but did emphasize that other causes such as urinary stasis as well as hypercalciuria could exist as causative agents and should be sought.[28] Other reports simply confirm the role of infection in stone patients in their areas of Europe.[9,32,45,64,70]

It is thus obvious from reviewing the literature that there is a difference between the pediatric stone patient in Europe and that in North America. Additionally, there appears to be quite a variation, even within areas of North America, which has prompted many investigators to adopt different attitudes toward metabolic evaluation of the pediatric stone patient. In the southeastern United States, the series by Paulson, Sinno, and Noe tend to confirm the need for metabolic evaluation of the pediatric stone patient as it might relate to calcium excretion abnormalities. The majority of reports from North America would tend to support that contention, taking into account certain population differences or specialized centers with unusual referral patterns. It is, therefore, useful to have a classification for pediatric stone disease that might reflect both the need for diagnostic evaluation and also therapy.

Classification

When attempting to classify stone disease, a practical approach can be very helpful. Many have suggested the designation of primary (i.e., stone formed in the kidney) and secondary such as might be encountered with calcification of a foreign body within the urinary system, either iatrogenic or self-induced. In addition, stones can be classified as to their anatomic position (upper or lower urinary tract, ureteral, etc.). The most helpful classification, however, would seem to be in terms of etiology of stone disease, which would go beyond immediate treatment and could have implications for the longer term. Classification by stone composition would simply be a variation of the latter but would also be helpful in defining exact metabolic abnormalities or the role infection might play in stone disease. We prefer the classification scheme shown in Table 27-1. The scheme given is meant only as a guide, realizing that there are some areas where overlap can occur.

Structural abnormalities leading to urinary stasis may or may not be associated with infection and would obviously require, as one of the immediate therapeutic aims, that any obstruction or urodynamic abnormality be corrected. Infection-related stones unassociated with obstruction or urodynamic abnormalities do occur but seem to be infrequent in this country. This has been especially true in our patient population. When this does occur, however, it tends to affect younger children and be associated with *Proteus* urinary infections. Rendering the patient both infection-free and stone-free would be the primary goal of therapy in this group.

Metabolic causes such as tubular disorders, enzyme disorders, hypercalcemic states,

Table 27-1
General Scheme for Classifying Stone Disease
(Selected Examples Only)

Structural or urodynamic abnormalities
With infection
Without infection
Metabolic causes
Tubular disorders (RTA, cystinuria)
Enzymatic (e.g., oxaluria, xanthinuria)
Hypercalcemic states (e.g., Cushing's, hyperparathyroidism)
Calcium excretion abnormalities (e.g., renal leak, hyperabsorption)
Infection stones
Immobilization
Uric acid lithiasis
Miscellaneous (e.g., steroid medication, inflammatory bowel disease)

and endocrinopathies would require specific approaches to diagnosis and therapy depending on the cause. Of particular importance is the recent emphasis on the identification and classification of the various hypercalciuric states. This is dealt with in detail later in this chapter.

Immobilization is known to lead to stones due to calcium reabsorption and resultant hypercalcemia and hypercalciuria. Uric acid stones can occur as primary excretion abnormalities or secondary to such conditions as myeloproliferative disorders. A number of miscellaneous causes, such as inflammatory bowel disease, the milk alkali syndrome, and steroid administration, can lead to stones, although this usually accounts for only a minority of patients.

We tend to reserve the term "idiopathic" for those children in whom no cause can be found, despite a thorough historical, anatomic, and metabolic evaluation. Unfortunately, there are still some patients remaining in this category, which will, likewise, be discussed later in the text.

LeBonheur Experience

During a 7-year period, 112 children with 164 episodes of urolithiasis have been evaluated at LeBonheur Children's Medical Center. These patients were referred from six states within a 200-mile radius of Memphis, Tennessee. The age of the children ranged from 4 months to 18 years (Fig. 27-3). Three boys, one with idiopathic and two with secondary hypercalciuria, developed urolithiasis in the first year of life. Boys constituted 59 percent of the total pediatric stone population, with the ratio of boys to girls generally being similar in all age groups (Fig. 27-3). Ninety-four percent of children with urolithiasis were white, five percent of the children were black, and one was an Asian immigrant (Fig. 27-4). All the black children had calculi associated with urinary tract infection and either a neurogenic bladder or urologic abnormalities. The Asian immigrant presented with a uric acid ureteral stone shortly after arriving in the United States. The paucity of black children with urolithiasis is particularly striking since approximately 45 percent of the Memphis metropolitan area is black. Initial stone episodes occurred throughout the

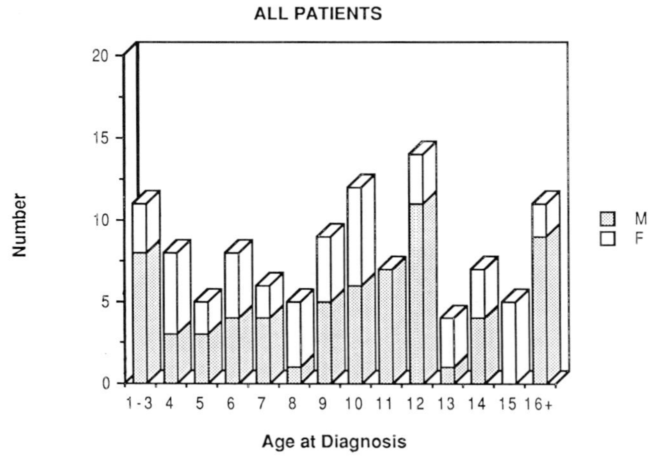

Fig. 27-3. Age at diagnosis of children with stones at LeBonheur Children's Medical Center.

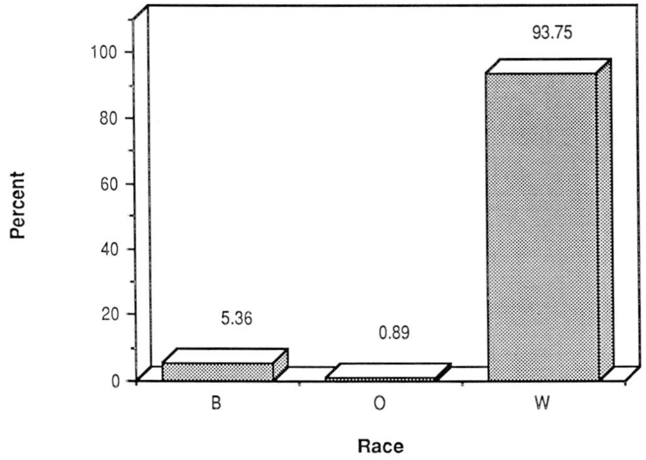

Fig. 27-4. Race distribution of stone patients at LeBonheur Children's Medical Center.

year; however, relatively few children suffered the first stone episode during the months of July and August (Fig. 27-5).

The presenting clinical manifestation of urolithiasis was pain in 60 percent of the patients. All except one child had either microscopic or macroscopic hematuria associated with episodes of urolithiasis. The single exception was an asymptomatic child with a renal calculus secondary to enteric oxaluria. In 66 stone episodes, calculi were located in the upper urinary tract; in 51 children, stones were located in the ureters (18 in the left ureter and 33 in the right ureter); 7 were found in the bladder; and 40 stones passed spontaneously without specific localization.

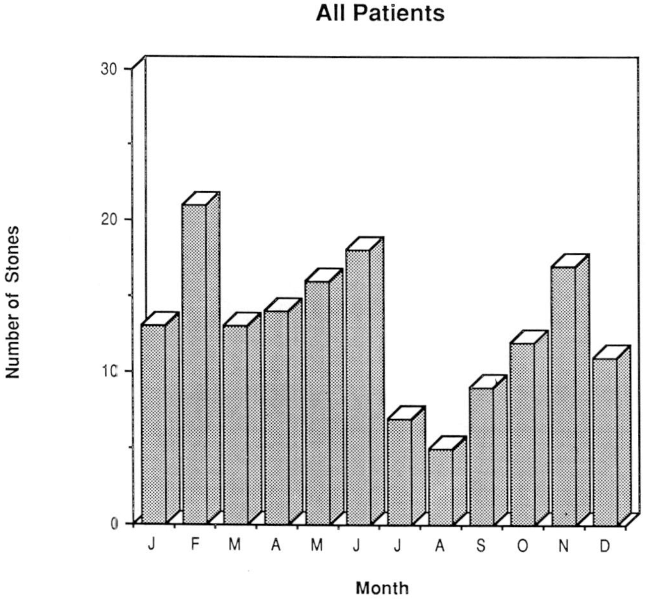

Fig. 27-5. Month of stone occurrence.

CALCULUS FORMATION

Pathogenesis

The complex physiochemical process that leads to the formation of a urinary calculus generally is the result of an imbalance between urinary stone-promoting and stone-inhibiting factors. Etiologies of calculi in our patients are shown in Fig. 27-6. Excessive excretion of lithogenic substances accounts for many of the calculi in our region. Hypercalciuria was diagnosed in 47 children (41 percent), cystinuria was noted in 5 children (4.5 percent), uric acid-related calculi were found in 4 children (3.5 percent), and hyperoxaluria was reported in 3 children (3 percent). Calculi related to urinary tract infections accounted for 13.5 percent of our patients. Despite complete evaluation, no explanation (idiopathic) of calculus formation was uncovered in 21 children (18.8 percent). Fourteen children (12.5 percent) either refused complete evaluation or failed to return to the clinic for diagnostic studies.

As noted above, the excretion of adequate amounts of crystallizable substances in the urine is a prerequisite for stone formation. Once the solution becomes supersaturated and nucleation occurs, it is felt that crystal growth and crystal aggregation can proceed. It is felt, however, that the urine must have an absence of a number of inhibitors of crystallization before stone formation can actually occur. The role of certain naturally occurring urinary inhibitory factors in the pathogenesis of childhood urolithiasis has received relatively little attention. These inhibitors are citrate, magnesium, pyrophosphate, and other organic compounds. These factors will become of primary importance in those with so-called idiopathic stone formation and are discussed under that heading, toward the end of this chapter.

The composition of urinary calculi in children is similar to that observed in adult stone patients. In our 6-year experience with pediatric urolithiasis, 101 calculi have been

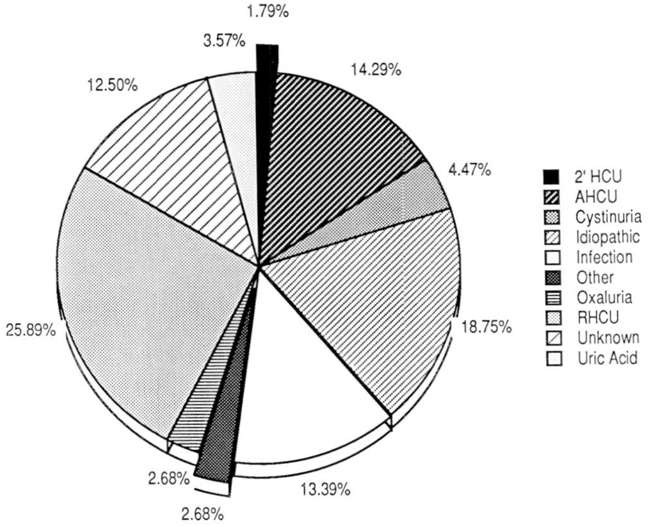

Fig. 27-6. Etiologies of calculi in LeBonheur pediatric stone patients (AHCU = absorptive hypercalciuria; RHCU = renal hypercalciuria).

subjected to chemical analysis. Of these stones, 75 (74 percent) were composed of calcium oxalate, 5 were composed of cystine, 6 were urate stones, 12 calculi contained calcium phosphate, and 3 were struvite stones.

Infection Stones

Infection stones may be of the primary or secondary type. Secondary stones are those that form in association with underlying obstruction and stasis, neurogenic bladder dysfunction, instrumentation of the urinary system, or in the presence of a foreign body. It is also possible for a noninfection type of stone to become *secondarily* infected, that is, the calcium oxalate stone that grows to produce obstruction and stasis. There apparently is more to the etiology of stone formation, however, than simple obstruction and stasis, or one would see more stones in children with congenital obstructive lesions. It has been noted by a large number of investigators that urinary obstruction or infection is most likely a promoting rather than an initiating factor in renal calculus formation.[12,91] It has been observed that approximately 1 percent of children with urinary tract infection will have a calculus present at the time of initial investigation. Likewise, the incidence of stone disease among children with the more common obstructive abnormalities is also low, in the range of 1–4 percent. It has been suggested that a possible underlying metabolic or calcium excretion abnormality might coexist before a child with an obstructed or anomalous urinary system would be prone to develop stones.[55] In general, in the child with an obstructive lesion associated with a stone, therapeutic results are favorable when the stone is removed and the obstruction corrected. A low recurrence rate usually is expected in these instances.

In the anatomically normal child in whom infection seems to be the primary factor in stone formation, the exact mechanism is unknown. One thing is clear, however, and that is the association of this type of stone with urea-splitting bacteria.[76] In the majority of cases, a *Proteus* species is present, but other bacteria such as *Klebsiella, Staphylococcus, Pseudomonas, Enterococcus, Ureaplasma urealyticum,* and some species of *Escherichia coli* can also be urease-producing. The enzyme urease produced by these bacteria splits urea in the presence of water to ammonia and carbon dioxide, leading to an alkaline urine that allows for supersaturation of the urine with magnesium ammonium phosphate, calcium phosphate, and carbonate apatite crystals. This, in essence, produces a favorable situation for stone formation. Although it has been suggested that underlying metabolic abnormalities might be present in those children with primary infection stones, no one has consistently been able to demonstrate that as yet. Once the stone is formed, bacteria can thrive in the center and are protected from eradication by antimicrobial therapy.[26] Removal of the stone is required to ensure urinary tract sterility. In many cases, bacteria other than a *Proteus* species are present once the stone is formed, but in a number of cases it has been noted that the initial urinary infection in a child with stones has been attributed to a *Proteus* organism.

These stones are composed of a large matrix element with magnesium ammonium phosphate (struvite) and calcium phosphate (apatite) as the crystalline components. In some cases, a soft, almost gelatinous type of matrix stone can be seen filling all or a portion of the collecting system of a kidney.

In children with infection stones, particularly those of the primary type, the occurrence is predominantly in males and in younger children. As stated, the majority are associated with *Proteus* infections and are not always associated with underlying abnormalities. When evaluating all children with infection stones, it has been noted that approximately one-third of the children will have some form of obstructive or urodynamic alteration of the urinary system and another third will be associated with vesicoureteral reflux. Regarding the presence of staghorn calculi, reflux appears to be more important in children than in adults.[42]

In most cases diagnosis will be based on radiographic evaluation following the initial urinary infection (Fig. 27-7). History of infections may be long-standing, and only on thorough investigation will the stone be identified as a source of persistent infection. In children with foreign-body-associated stones, such as suture material, catheter remnant, or objects placed through genital manipulation, the history may be helpful. Children with neurogenic bladder and frequent instrumentation are particularly susceptible to urinary stone disease at the bladder level. The majority of children with infection stones, however, still have them arise in the upper urinary system. Plain-film nephrotomograms may be necessary to evaluate both kidneys and to demonstrate precisely the location and extent of the calculus disease. When a stone is recovered, it should be analyzed to

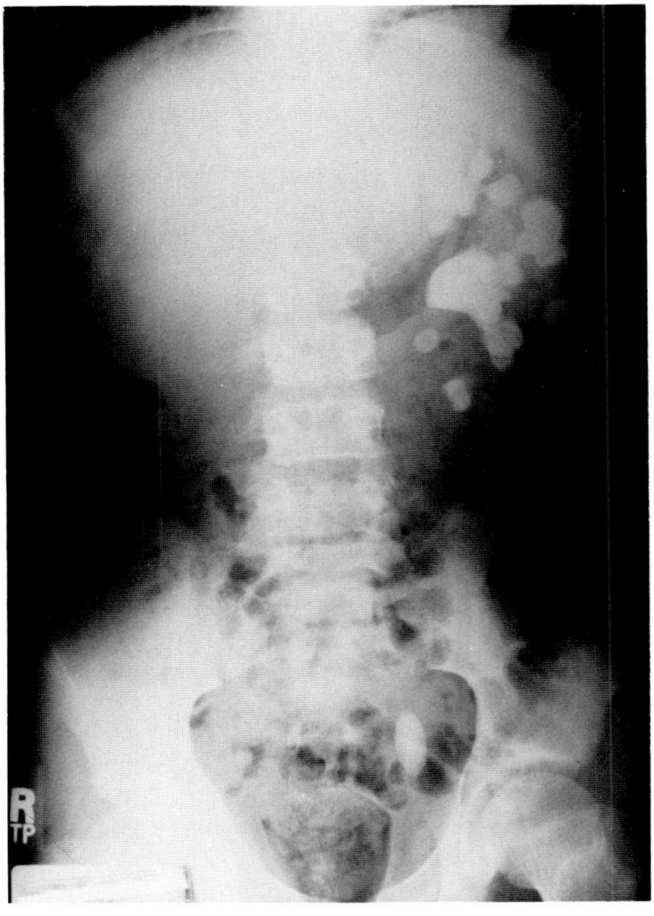

Fig. 27-7. Male child with primary infection stones in both kidney and left lower ureter.

identify its chemical composition, which can, in some cases, give a clue to the etiology of the stone.

A special form of chronic pyelonephritis known as *xanthogranulomatous pyelonephritis* has been reported in children. Usually it presents as a mass lesion, is associated with urinary tract infection, and can be associated with renal calculi.[14,36,43] It occurs more commonly on the left side with a roughly equal distribution between male and female patients. Although the condition can be segmental, in most cases it involves the entire kidney, and nephrectomy is required to affect a cure.

The treatment of infection stones must deal with removing any obstruction, rendering the urinary system stone-free, and eliminating urinary infection. In a child with an acute obstruction and infection, emergent treatment will be required. In those instances in which a studied approach to the problem is allowed, it is best to treat the child with antibiotics prior to any surgical treatment. The goal of surgery is to remove all stone material from the urinary system and correct any associated abnormalities such as ureteropelvic junction (UPJ) obstruction or megaloureter. The surgical treatment of infection stones in children is by the standard techniques, and when the child can be rendered stone and infection-free, the results have been reported to be favorable.[1,4] Even when the initial treatment is successful, it is still important to keep these children on prophylaxis to insure an infection-free urinary system for a period of at least 6 and preferably 12, months. Maintenance of an acid urine pH and a high fluid intake are also recommended to help minimize the chance of stone recurrence. Followup should be for at least 2 years in these children and preferably up to 5 years to evaluate for recurrences.

It has been noted that surgical treatment does not always render the urinary system free of stone, and residual calculi can be seen in 5–30 percent of the patients. Recurrent stones can also occur and have been found equally in those with or without urinary abnormalities. These recurrent stones are closely associated with *Proteus* infection. As reported by Androulakakis et al., recurrent stones seem to be associated more with significant symptoms and uncontrollable infection than are residual stones, particularly if the latter are small and in a caliceal position.[1] Large residual calculi of the renal pelvis, however, can pose significant problems, much the same as recurrent stones. Although in the past reoperation has been required for those with recurrent stones and symptoms and uncontrollable infections, new techniques may allow easier treatment of such patients. The development of extracorporeal shockwave lithotripsy (ESWL) and percutaneous stone extraction may provide less invasive methods for successful treatment of these patients.

Chemolysis can also be used in an attempt to dissolve any residual stone fragments following surgical therapy. The two most common agents used are Suby's Solution G and hemiacidrin. The latter is known as Renacidin (Guardian Chemical Corp., Hauppauge, Long Island, NY, 11787), and although it has been proven effective, its use has not been widely reported in children. Early reports of complications and death associated with hemiacidrin irrigations were felt to be largely associated with infected urine during the irrigation itself.[53] The guidelines and precautions have been outlined for the safe use of hemiacidrin, yet the FDA still feels that this drug is contraindicated for use in the upper urinary system. If chemolysis is to be used, this contraindication must be kept in mind, and for those reluctant to use hemiacidrin, Suby's Solution G may be an attractive alternative.

The use of acetohydroxamic acid (AHA) has been found to be helpful in treating infection stone disease in patients with persistent urinary infections.[30] This agent inhibits urease activity and, thereby, inhibits urinary alkalinization despite persistent growth of urease-producing bacteria. Acetohydroxamic acid may have a place in selected instances in treating children with infection stones, but, as yet, there has again been no widespread experience with this drug in children.

In summary, we feel that infection stones in children are quite threatening and must be treated aggressively. The goal of treatment is to eliminate any source of obstruction and stasis as well as to render the urinary tract stone and infection-free. A number of choices of therapy, both medical and surgical, can be used to achieve successful results in these patients. Careful long-term followup and maintenance of a sterile urine are essential to reduce the likelihood of recurrences.

HYPERCALCIURIA

Increased urinary excretion of calcium is the most commonly identified etiology of urolithiasis in our referral center located in the southern United States. Regional differences may explain the rather dramatically disparate reports of the role of hypercalciuria in childhood urolithiasis. Walther and associates, for instance, failed to identify hypercalciuria in any of 61 children with urinary stones in southern California.[90] Moore, on the other hand, found that 53 percent of children with urolithiasis in Chicago had hypercalciuria.[48]

The age and sex of children with hypercalciuria are shown in Figure 27-8. In general, the demographic characteristics of our children with hypercalciuria and urolithiasis mirror our total stone population. A striking racial distribution was observed, however; no black children with idiopathic hypercalciuria and urolithiasis were identified. As in the total stone population, the fewest stone episodes occurred in July through September (Fig. 27-9).

Under usual dietary conditions, the normal urinary excretion of calcium by healthy children and adults is less than 4 mg (0.1 mmol)/kg body weight daily.[27,40] Race may

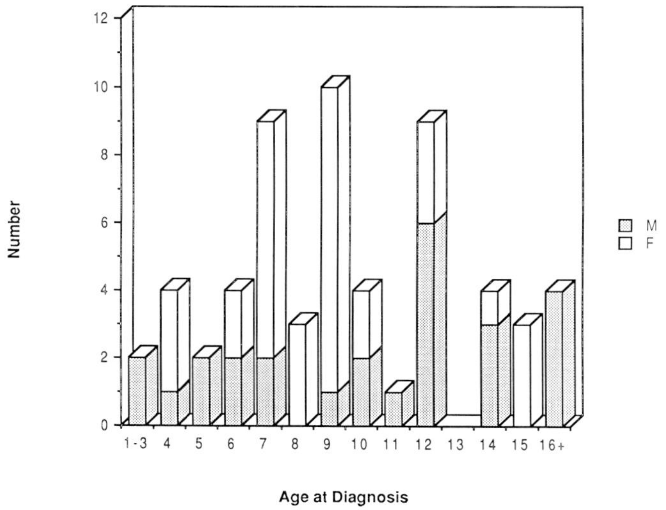

Fig. 27-8. Age at diagnosis of hypercalciuric stone patients.

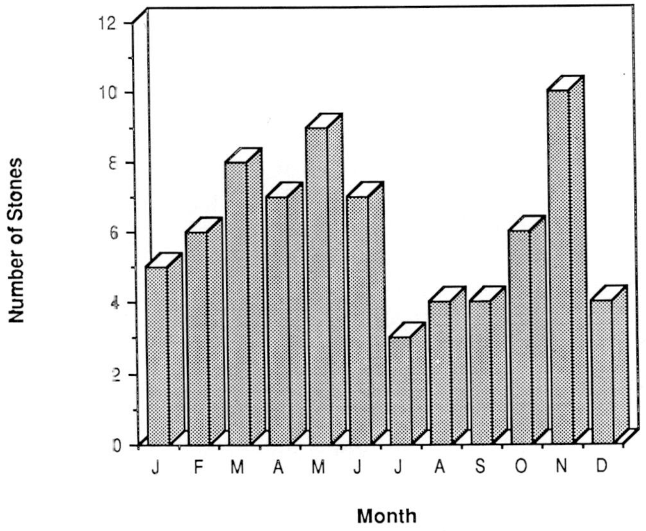

Fig. 27-9. Stone occurrence by month in hypercalciuric patients.

influence urinary calcium excretion. Urinary calcium excretion in black adults has been found to be less than in adult white individuals.[7] However, we have found 24-hour urinary calcium excretion during unrestricted dietary conditions in 41 black children (1.6 $\pm$ 0.87 mg/kg daily, mean $\pm$SE) to be similar to that in 82 white children (1.6 $\pm$ 0.86 mg/kg daily). In addition, the ratio of early morning fasting urinary calcium concentration to urinary creatinine concentration (U_{Ca}/U_{Cr}) in 14 healthy black children after 1 week of dietary calcium restriction was comparable to values in 40 white children of similar ages.[78] Thus our data do not support racial differences in urinary calcium excretion among healthy children. Further 4 mg/kg daily appears to be a valid definition of hypercalciuria in children during unrestricted dietary conditions. In 24-hour urine specimens, there is a strong relationship between urinary calcium excretion per kilogram of body weight, and the U_{Ca}/U_{Cr} ratio ($r = .83$, $P < .0001$).

Pathogenesis of Idiopathic Hypercalciuria

The pathogenesis of hypercalciuria must relate to either an increased filtered load of calcium or a decreased reabsorption of calcium in the renal tubule. Despite much investigation, the exact pathogenesis of idiopathic hypercalciuria remains unclear. It has been suggested that hypercalciuria exists as two distinct entities: renal hypercalciuria and absorptive hypercalciuria. Renal hypercalciuria is characterized by a primary renal tubular leak of calcium. A resultant mild hypocalcemia leads to leak of calcium and leads to both increased parathyroid hormone secretion and increased 1.25 $(OH)_2D_3$ formation.[60] The increased 1.25 $(OH)_2D_3$ results in an increase in calcium absorption in the gut. The condition is diagnosed by the presence of fasting hypercalciuria and theoretically requires evidence of hyperparathyroidism. Demonstration of hyperparathyroidism by measurements of radioimmunoassayable parathyroid hormone (PTH) or urinary cyclic adenosine monophosphate (AMP) have been inconsistent in children with fasting hypercalciuria.

Primary hyperabsorption of calcium from the gut or "absorptive hypercalciuria" increases the serum calcium, causing an increase in the filtered load of calcium and a decrease in parathyroid hormone secretion.[60] The lower parathyroid hormone levels result in decreased renal calcium reabsorption. Both adult and pediatric patients with absorptive hypercalciuria have increased 1.25 $(OH)_2D_3$ levels, and a primary renal phosphorus leak has been proposed in these patients as a mechanism of stimulation of 1.25 $(OH)_2D_3$ synthesis.[16,35]

A more unified theory has developed when a number of studies failed to demonstrate a clear-cut difference between patients with absorptive and renal hypercalciuria.[62] Many children with what appears to be renal hypercalciuria have normal serum PTH concentrations.[79] In addition, we recently found that serum 1.25 $(OH)_2D_3$ concentrations in children with renal hypercalciuria were not appropriately suppressed by a high calcium diet.[85]

Characterization of Hypercalciuria

Idiopathic hypercalciuria has been classified as either renal or absorptive types on the basis of oral calcium challenge tests.[34,61,79] A relatively simple outpatient calcium loading test for adult urolithiasis patients was developed by Pak and associates[63] and later modified for application in pediatric patients.[79] This oral calcium loading test requires one week of dietary calcium and sodium restriction. Patients are allowed generous hydration but no food after 6:00 P.M. the evening prior to the test. A fasting urine collection is obtained from 7.00 A.M. to 9:00 A.M. and the ratio of urinary calcium to urinary creatinine (U_{Ca}/U_{Cr}) determined. A blood sample for serum PTH concentration is drawn at 9:00 A.M. After the 9:00 A.M. urine and serum samples are obtained, a standard breakfast and 1.0-g calcium/1.73 m^2 is ingested. A postcalcium load urine sample is obtained from 9:00 A.M. to 1:00 P.M. and the U_{Ca}/U_{Cr} ratio determined. Normal *fasting* U_{Ca}/U_{Cr} ratios for children in our region are under 0.21, and normal *post*calcium challenge U_{Ca}/U_{Cr} ratios are under 0.28.

Oral calcium loading tests were performed in 45 hypercalciuric children with urolithiasis. The diagnosis of renal hypercalciuria was assigned in 29 children in whom the fasting U_{Ca}/U_{Cr} ratio exceeded 0.21 (Fig. 27-10). Most children with renal hypercalciuria also have increased gastrointestinal absorption. Absorptive hypercalciuria was diagnosed in 16 children when the fasting U_{Ca}/U_{Cr} ratio was normal and the postcalcium U_{Ca}/U_{Cr} ratio was over 0.28 (Fig. 27-11). All patients had normal parathyroid hormone values regardless of whether the child had renal or absorptive hypercalciuria. Interestingly, serum parathyroid hormone values were actually slightly greater in absorptive hypercalciuria. In three additional children, hypercalciuria and subsequent urolithiasis were secondary to medication or generalized tubular dysfunctions. Among hypercalciuric children with urolithiasis, therefore, renal hypercalciuria represented 62 percent, absorptive hypercalciuria 34 percent, and secondary hypercalciuria 4 percent of this patient population (Fig. 27-12).

The clinical manifestations of urolithiasis associated with absorptive and renal hypercalciuria were indistinguishabale. All hypercalciuric children with urinary stones have either microscopic or macroscopic hematuria. Surprisingly, flank or back pain or dysuria were prominent clinical symptoms in only 60 percent of hypercalciuric children. Bladder stones were extremely rare; 67 percent of stones were located in the ureters, and 33 percent were present in the upper urinary tract.

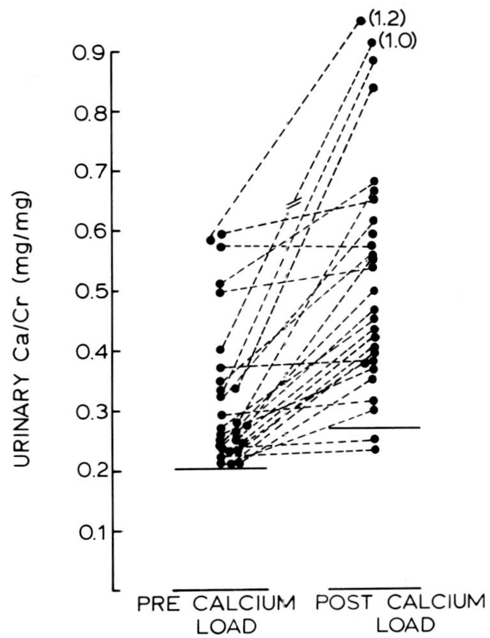

Fig. 27-10. Results of oral calcium loading tests in children with renal hypercalciuria.

Secondary Hypercalciuria

Increased urinary calcium excretion with urolithiasis has been associated with the conditions listed in Table 27-2. Most of these conditions have been associated with urolithiasis. In our series, hypercalciuria and urolithiasis were associated with generalized renal tubular dysfunction, (cystinosis),[10] furosemide therapy, and adrenocorticotropic hormone (ACTH). Of particular recent interest is the problem of urolithiasis in neonates and infants who are receiving furosemide therapy for bronchopulmonary dysplasia. Furosemide is known to be calciuric. Hufnagle and coworkers reported 10 premature infants who had renal calcifications after receiving furosemide at a dose of 2–16 mg/kg daily for 12–44 days.[33] Urinary calcium ranged from 15 to 30 mg/kg daily. We have

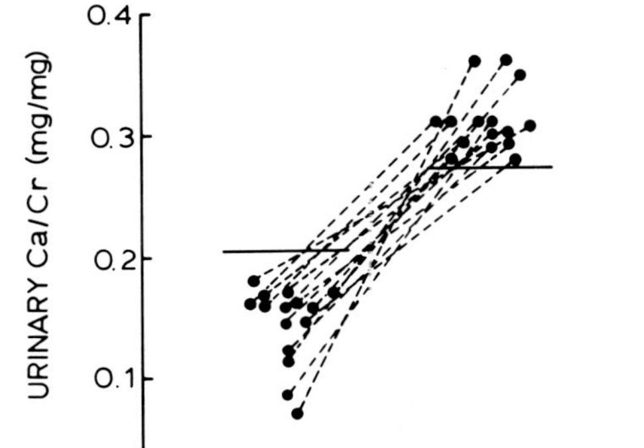

Fig. 27-11. Results or oral calcium loading tests in children with absorptive hypercalciuria.

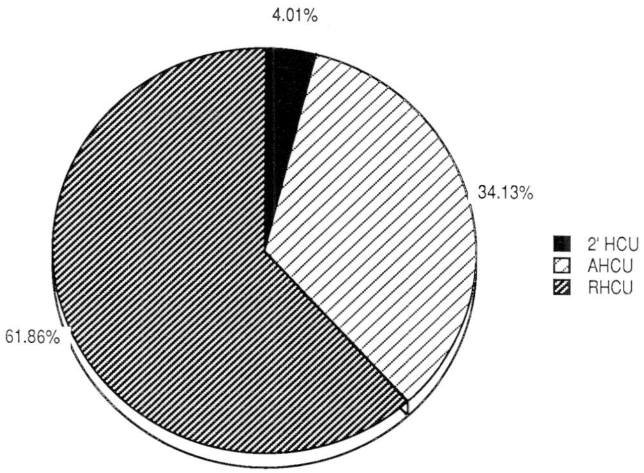

Fig. 27-12. Distribution of ypes of hypercalciuria in our observed patient population.

treated a similar patient, a 30-week-gestation male infant who was receiving furosemide for bronchopulmonary dysplasia at a daily dose of 2.5 mg/kg. After 2 months of diuretic therapy, the U_{Ca}/U_{Cr} ratio was 3.0, the child developed hematuria, and bilateral calcifications were discovered. One calculus obstructed the left ureter and multiple calcifications were observed in the right kidney.[56]

Primary hyperparathyroidism is not uncommon in adults with hypercalciuria and urolithiasis. In the past 7 years, we have not encountered a single patient with urolithiasis and primary hyperparathyroidism. In a review of 445 published examples of urolithiasis in children, only three (0.9 percent) were found to have hyperparathyroidism.[65] Nonetheless, hyperparathyroidism is a treatable condition that should be excluded in all children with hypercalcemia and/or hypercalciuria associated with urolithiasis.

Renal tubular acidosis (RTA) is another etiology of hypercalciuria and urolithiasis. Although we have not seen RTA in our stone population, it accounts for 1.3 percent of published cases of pediatric urolithiasis.[65] Chronic metabolic acidosis results in increased bone resorption and hypercalciuria. Distal RTA is much more frequently associated with

Table 27-2
Conditions Associated with Hypercalciuria

Hypercalcemia	Furosemide therapy
Hypophosphatemia	Juvenile rheumatoid arthritis
Metabolic acidosis	Endocrine
Expansion of extracellular fluid volume	Diabetes mellitus
	Hyperparathyroidism
Immobilization	Hypothyroid
Hypertension	Hyperadrenal corticism
Distal renal tubular acidosis	Vitamin D excess
Generalized renal tubular dysfunction	Sarcoidosis
	Neoplasms
Hyperalimentation	Medullary sponge kidney

nephrocalcinosis and hypercalciuria than is proximal RTA.[17] In general, urolithiasis is uncommon in appropriately managed patients with RTA. Only 2 of 27 adult patients and none of 17 patients with distal RTA had nephrolithiasis.[15]

In addition to an increased risk of urinary calculi, furosemide therapy in preterm infants has also been shown to decrease bone mineral mass and produce secondary hyperparathyroidism.[89] It has been suggested that furosemide-induced calculi might decrease in size with thiazide therapy; however, we were unable to document an improvement in our patient during hydrochlorothiazide (2 gm/kg daily) therapy. Infants who receive furosemide for chronic lung disease or congestive heart failure should be monitored with regular urinalyses, and calculi should be suspected when hematuria is discovered (Fig. 27-13).

Hematuria as a Manifestation of Hypercalciuria

In 1981 preliminary observations of five children in whom hypercalciuria was discovered after the passage of a calcium oxalate stone was reported. All five children had been evaluated months to years previously for unexplained hematuria without evidence of urinary calculi at the time of initial evaluation.[69] Similar observations were reported in Galveston, Texas.[38] To determine whether hypercalciuria without overt urolithiasis might be an etiology of unexplained hematuria in children, we prospectively examined urinary calcium excretion in 83 children referred for unexplained hematuria but without pro-

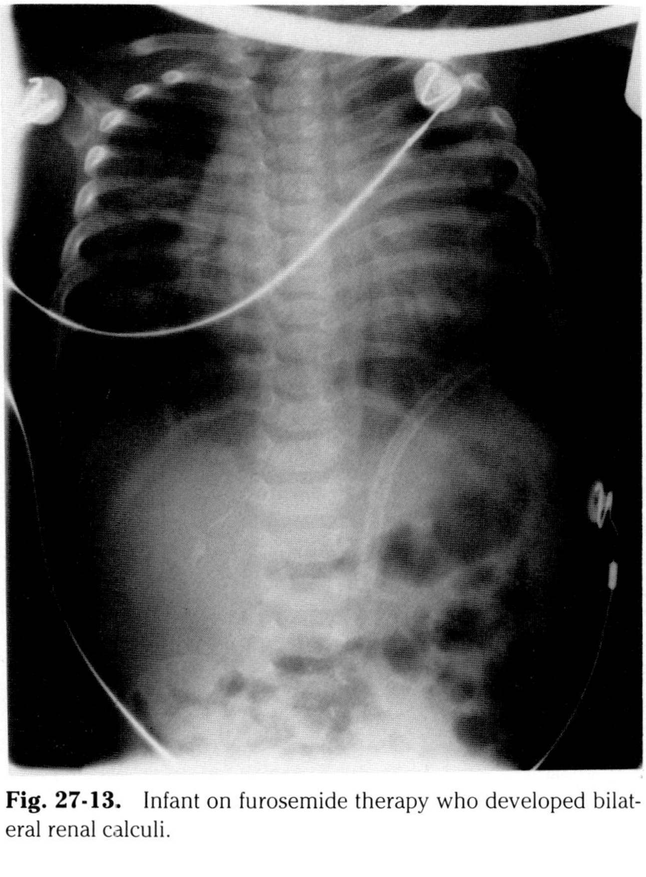

Fig. 27-13. Infant on furosemide therapy who developed bilateral renal calculi.

teinuria or previous urolithiasis. Among the 83 children (ages 3–15 years) 23 (26 percent) were found to have hypercalciuria.[81] When children with hematuria associated with hypercalciuria were compared to normocalciuric children with hematuria, several important differences emerged. Gross hematuria and a family history of urolithiasis were significantly more common in children with hypercalciuria. In fact, 87 percent of children with both hematuria and a family history of urolithiasis had hypercalciuria. These findings have been confirmed in a 12-center prospective study of 140 children with hematuria.[83] Hypercalciuria was identified in 50 of 140 (36 percent) patients. Both renal and absorptive hypercalciuria have been associated with hematuria.

The pathogenesis of the hematuria is uncertain; however, it is likely that microcrystallization develops and leads to epithelial injury. In support of this, urinary calcium oxalate crystals are found more commonly in children with hematuria and hypercalciuria than in children with unexplained hematuria. Such microcrystallization may ultimately lead to stone formation. In support of the notion of renal injury is the findings of increased urinary excretion of *n*-acetylglucosaminidase, a marker of proximal renal tubular injury in children with hypercalciuria.[82] We have now examined 20 children with urolithiasis and hypercalciuria who first presented with unexplained hematuria without evidence of calculi. This group of children represents nearly 20 percent (20 of 97) of our total hypercalciuric population.

Evaluation

When hypercalciuria is encountered, the diagnosis is confirmed with a second urine collection while the child is on an unrestricted diet. The value of distinguishing absorptive from renal hypercalciuria with an oral calcium loading test has been previously reported.[79] The initial experience found this test to be quite helpful. Recently, however, a multicenter study of children with hematuria found this test to be nondiagnostic in nearly one-third of children with hematuria and hypercalciuria.[83] For this reason, it is now recommended that a 24-hour urine calcium excretion be obtained after a week of dietary calcium and sodium restriction. If the urinary calcium excretion remains excessive during calcium restriction and the serum PTH concentrations are normal, the diagnosis is idiopathic renal hypercalciuria. If dietary calcium and sodium restriction corrects hypercalciuria, it is considered that the patient has absorptive hypercalciuria.

Therapy is tailored to each child's needs. In all children, a high fluid intake and a 2–3-g sodium diet is recommended for children with hypercalciuria because of the well-known calciuric effect of high dietary sodium intake.[49,85] For children with absorptive hypercalciuria, a reduction in dietary calcium intake to 400–600 mg/day is recommended. If urinary calcium excretion does not decline to the normal range on such dietary management, hydrochlorothiazide (2 mg/kg/daily) is added as an additional anticalciuric measure. For children with urolithiasis and renal hypercalciuria, hydrochlorothiazide (2 mg/kg/daily) is routinely administered. This therapy has resulted in a substantial reduction in the rate of stone formation in patients.[79] Because the majority of children with hypercalciuria associated with isolated hematuria do not develop urolithiasis during childhood, we do not recommend chronic hydrochlorothiazide therapy because of the attendant risks of hypokalemia and hypercalciuria. Hypokalemia occurs in 70 percent of children receiving hydrochlorothiazide. In most cases, however, serum potassium values increase to normal values with aggressive dietary management. We do recommend a high fluid intake and a low-sodium diet for children with hypercalciuria and hematuria to reduce the risk of calculus formation.

Among 45 stone patients with hypercalciuria, there have been 18 recurrent stone episodes in 10 children after the diagnosis of hypercalciuria was assigned. Seven of these patients had renal hypercalciuria, and four had absorptive hypercalciuria. In three children, the time from diagnosis to recurrence was greater than 2 years (2–4 years). In each instance, the patient had developed a false sense of security and had discontinued preventive therapeutic measures. It is well known that patients tend to be much more compliant while the memory of the acute stone episode is fresh. In most of the recurrent stone episodes, the patient was found to be noncompliant with prescribed therapy.

Oxalate Calculi

Oxalic acid is an end product of metabolism and is excreted primarily by the kidneys. Of the daily urinary oxalate excretion, 10–15 percent derives from dietary sources, and the remainder is the result of metabolism. In normal individuals, daily urinary oxalate excretion is <50 mg/1.73 m^2 body surface area.[52] Increased oxalate excretion may be caused by metabolic errors (primary hyperoxaluria), increased oxalate absorption, or excessive intake of oxalate precursors.

Primary hyperoxaluria is an uncommon metabolic disorder transmitted as an autosomal recessive trait. Two types of hyperoxaluria have been identified. Type I has excessive urinary excretion of oxalic, glyoxylic, and glycollic acids due to a deficiency of ketogluturate-glyoxylate carboxylase activity. Type II has increased excretion of oxalate and d-glycerate as a result of deficient d-glyceric dehydrogenase activity. Of the two types, type I is the most common. Both types present in early childhood, seldom after 10 years of age, with recurrent urolithiasis and early renal failure. Oxalate gradually accumulates in the kidneys and other body tissues. As renal failure becomes advanced, tissue accumulation of oxalate increases and urinary excretion decreases.

Increased urinary oxalate excretion accompanies a number of gastrointestinal disorders such as inflammatory bowel disease, pancreatitis, and surgical intestinal resection. This "enteric" hyperoxaluria is the result of increased gastrointestinal absorption of oxalate. In malabsorptive states, increased intestinal fatty acids complex with calcium, thereby leaving free oxalate available for absorption. Increased urinary oxalate excretion has been seen in children with a variety of malabsorptive disorders and after ileal resection. One of our patients was a 10-year old white female with steatorrhea from bacterial overgrowth syndrome and with hyperoxaluria and an asymptomatic renal calculus. As in previously reported cases in adults, when the steatorrhea was successfully treated, urinary oxalate excretion returned to normal.

Because of the aggressive nature of primary hyperoxaluria, intensive medical intervention is indicated. Numerous therapeutic regimens have been attempted over the years, most unsuccessfully. It is recommended that measures to decrease urinary oxalate and calcium and to increase urinary inhibition of crystallization be taken. Dietary oxalate should be further restricted. Urinary calcium excretion is further reduced by hydrochlorothiazide diuretic therapy (2 mg/kg daily) and large doses of inorganic phosphates. Pyridoxine is administered in an attempt to reduce oxalate production. Yendt and coworkers have shown that oral pyridoxine at a dose of 2–25 mg dramatically reduced urinary oxalate excretion in adults with hyperoxaluria.[94] Finally, magnesium hydroxide is given to increase the solubility of calcium oxalate. A high urine volume is maintained as with all forms of urolithiasis.

Uric Acid Calculi

The incidence of uric acid stones varies considerably in different regions of the world. In southwest Asia, for instance, uric acid stones (usually bladder) are endemic. In the United States, 7–10 percent of calculi in adults are composed of uric acid, while in pediatric patients we encountered four children (3.5 percent) with uric acid lithiasis. One child had recently immigrated from Laos, two patients had leukemia, and the other child had cystinosis with generalized renal tubular dysfunction.

Uric acid is the end product of purine metabolism in humans and is poorly soluble in biologic fluids. The kidney accounts for approximately two-thirds of the daily excretion of uric acid, with the remainder eliminated through the gastrointestinal tract. Renal urate excretion occurs through the processes of glomerular filtration, tubular reabsorption, tubular secretion, and postsecretory reabsorption. In healthy adults, the fractional excretion of uric acid is 8–12 percent, with total daily excretion at under 700 mg/day. Uric acid excretion is extremely high in neonates and remains substantially higher than adult values through early childhood.[77] Unfortunately, total urate excretion, excretion per unit body weight, and fractional excretion of uric acid all vary with age and age-related normals rather than a single normal value being used. It has been found in children older than 2 years of age that the amount of uric acid excreted per deciliter of glomerular filtrate does not vary with age in either early morning urine or in 24-hour samples.[80] A normal value of under 0.56 mg uric acid/dl glomerular filtrate may be used after 2 years of age. This value may be calculated by the following formula:

$$\frac{\text{Urine uric acid} \times \text{plasma creatinine}}{\text{Urine creatinine}}$$

Most uric acid stones result from precipitation of uric acid from supersaturated urine. Excessive urinary uric acid excretion may result from increased filtration of uric acid from excessive dietary purine intake, metabolic errors, myeloproliferative disorders, or hemolysis from tubular defects such as an isolated defect in renal tubular urate reabsorption or from generalized tubular dysfunction (Figs. 27-14*A* and 27-14*B*). An example of a metabolic error in purine metabolism that is associated with uric acid lithiasis is the Lesch-Nyhan syndrome (hypoxanthine–guanine phosphoribosyl transferase deficiency). Children appear to have a greater capacity to increase uric acid excretion than do adults. For this reason, increased production of uric acid cannot be excluded on the basis of a normal serum uric acid concentration. Uric acid excretion is increased in as many as 9 percent of adult stone patients with hypercalciuria.[21] It has been observed that a similar phenomenon exists in hypercalciuric pediatric patients.[84] In endemic areas such as Southeast Asia and the Mediterranean region, uric acid stones rarely are associated with hyperuricemia or hyperuricosuria. Often there is a familial tendency for urate stones in these regions.

Certain factors are well known to increase the risk of uric acid precipitation. These include low urine pH and low urine flow rate. Uric acid itself may play an important role in the inhibition of urinary macromolecules that normally prevent precipitation of calcium oxalate. Monosodium urate, in particular, binds glycosaminoglycans. Studies assessing the role of urate in calculus formation in children are not available and would be of interest considering their relatively high uric acid excretion per unit body weight and high fractional urate excretion.

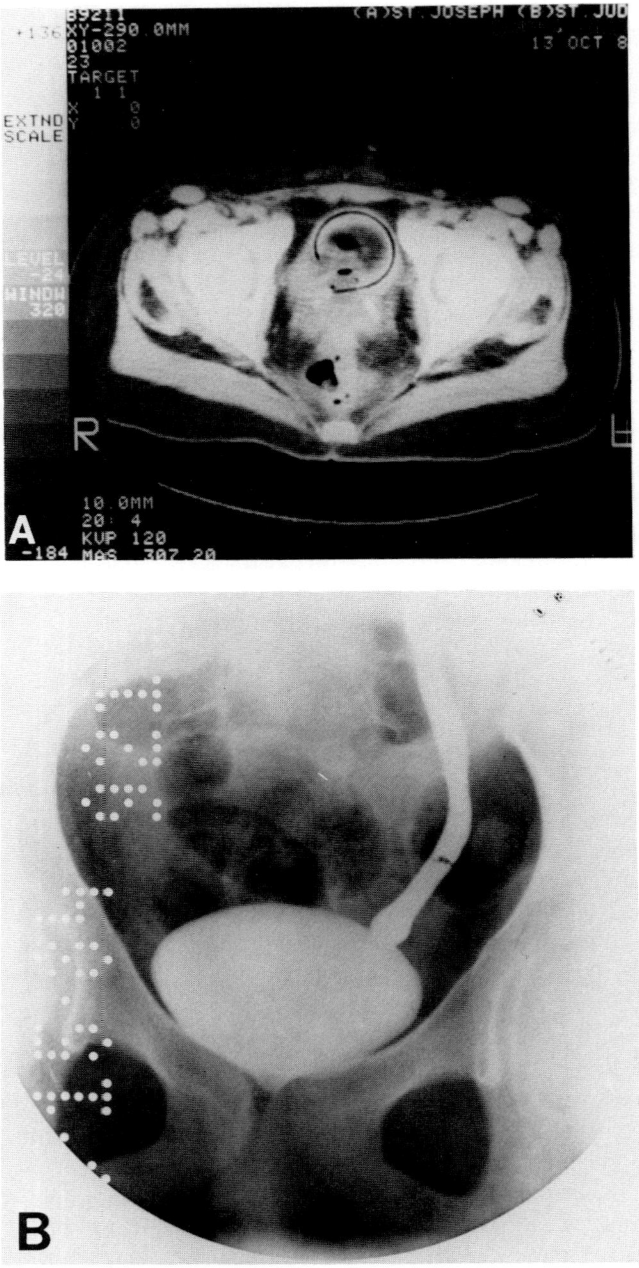

Fig. 27-14. (*A*) Child with leukemia on therapy who developed anuria and azotemia. Plain film was unrevealing, but CT scan shows uric acid sludged in both lower ureters. Note Foley balloon in catheter with bonelike density of urates in the lower ureters posteriorly. (*B*) Percutaneous nephrostogram in same patient confirming point of obstruction and providing drainage.

Therapy for uric acid calculi includes efforts to alkalinize the urine and to maintain a high urine flow rate. Diagnostic studies should determine whether a treatable etiology of hyperproduction of uric acid is present. In most instances, allopurinol therapy (5–10 mg/kg) is warranted.

Hypouricemia in the presence of decreased uric acid excretion and urinary calculi should suggest the rare condition of xanthinuria. Xanthinuria results from a deficiency in xanthine oxidase so that xanthine is not converted to uric acid. Radiolucent xanthine stones form in acidic urine. Secondary xanthinuria is an unusual complication of allopurinol therapy.

Recently a deficiency of the purine enzyme adenine phosphoribosyl transferase has been associated with urolithiasis. The metabolic defect is inherited as an autosomal recessive trait.[73] Calculi in this condition are composed of 2,8-dihydroxyadenine and are radiopaque. Special techniques such as isotachophoresis or high-performance liquid chromotography (HPLC) are required to distinguish these stones from uric acid. Moreover, alkalinization of the urine, which is indicated for urate calculi, decreases the solubility of 2,8-dihydroxyadenine. Allopurinol is effective therapy for this condition, and a low purine diet is recommended.

Cystine Calculi

Cystinuria is an autosomal recessive disorder characterized by defective renal and intestinal transport of cystine and the dibasicaminoacids (i.e., lysine, arginine, ornithine). The high urinary concentration of the relatively poorly soluble cystine results in stone formation. Patients with cystinuria have been classified into three types on the basis of intestinal amino acid transport in homozygotes and from the pattern of urinary cystine and lysine excretion in heterozygotes. In each of the three types, however, the basis of stone formation is excessive urinary excretion of cystine.

We have evaluated five children with cystinuria. All the patients were male. The age of presentation ranged from 12 to 18 years of age. These patients reported a total of nine stone episodes. Two stones were identified in the bladder, two in the ureters, and five in the upper urinary tract. Cystine crystals are usually, but not always, radiopaque as a result of the sulfur ions (Fig. 27-15). Cystinuria has been associated with hyperuricemia, uric acid urolithiasis, hemophilia, retinitis pigmentosa, muscular dystrophy, muscular hypotonia, trisomy-21, and hereditary pancreatitis.[31] A higher incidence of cystinuria has been observed in patients with mental illness or retardation. As a group, however, cystinuric patients appear to have normal intelligence. The diagnosis of cystinuria is confirmed by the recovery of a cystine stone or cystine excretion with dibasic aminoaciduria. Normal individuals excrete less than 60 mg of cystine per 1.73 m^2 body surface area per day, while cystinuria homozygotes often excrete more than 400 mg/1.73 m^2 daily.[31]Cystine crystals may be observed in the urine as flat, hexagonal, colorless crystals. Crystalluria may be absent in dilute or alkaline urine.

The basis of medical management of cystinuria is high fluid intake. Since the solubility of cystine in urine is 200–300 mg/liter, sufficient fluid should be ingested to maintain the urinary cystine concentration below 200 mg/liter. Thus, if a patient excretes 400 mg of cystine, at least 2 liters of urine will be required to assure cystine solubility. Urinary alkalinization further increases cystine solubility and is recommended for all patients. Recently a significant reduction in urinary cystine excretion was observed in four adult cystinuric patients placed on a sodium restricted diet.[37] Dietary sodium restriction thus

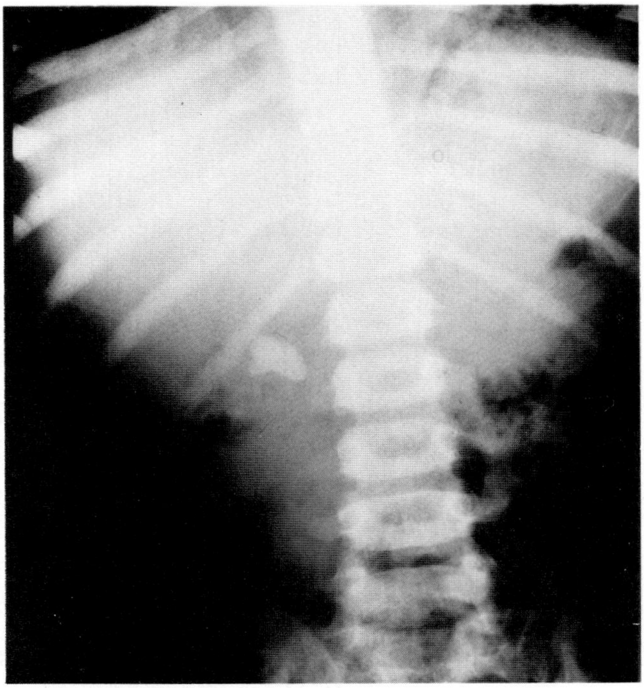

Fig. 27-15. Poorly opacified waxy-appearing pelvic cystine stone in the right kidney.

may also be very useful in preventing stones in children with cystinuria. Approximately 35 percent of patients can be successfully managed with fluid and base therapy, and the remainder will require d-penicillamine therapy. d-Penicillamine complexes with cystine and reduces both urinary cystine excretion and stone size. Unfortunately, adverse reactions may occur in as many as 50 percent of patients receiving d-penicillamine. Adverse effects include agranulocytosis, arthralgia, liver dysfunction, gastrointestinal intolerance, and proteinuria with nephrotic syndrome. Other complications include pemphigus, agnosia, and paresthesias. Potentially less toxic therapies such as α- mercaptopropionylglycine or sodium dithiosalicylate have been suggested but have not yet been subjected to critical trials.

Factitious Calculi

Surprisingly, passage of urinary calculi may be a manifestation of Munchausen's syndrome. A child has been previously reported whose mother observed a stone to pass from the penile urethra.[87] No metabolic or infectious etiology for a calculus was discovered. Analysis of the stone revealed its composition to be quartz. Careful scrutiny of this child's development revealed marked behavioral problems. This case emphasizes that when no etiology of urolithiasis is defined or when abnormal family dynamics are present, factitious disease should be considered. Analysis of the stone, if possible, may assist in this diagnosis.

Idiopathic Stones

In spite of complete metabolic and structural evaluation, some children will have stones without an explainable cause. Even though the exact mechanism of such abnormalities as hypercalciuria is not clear, it is still possible to understand that excess calcium in the urine can lead to stone formation. There are, however, a number of children in whom there is no clear explanation as to stone formation, and we prefer to designate these children as true idiopathic stone formers. The modern theories of stone formation include factors that both promote and inhibit stone formation. Although it has not always been proven, it is largely felt that idiopathic stones form because of lack of appropriate inhibitors. The majority of idiopathic stones are either calcium oxalate or calcium phosphate, and in adults usually 25 percent of these patients are normocalciuric. In the population we have studied, we noted that 18 percent of the children have not had a definable cause for stone formation even though a thorough metabolic evaluation was carried out.

Numerous inhibitors of stone formation have been noted by several investigators.[25,29,75] These have been identified primarily in adults and are citrate, pyrophosphate, magnesium, and trace elements such as zinc. Others have listed glycosaminoglycans, with some claiming that uromucoid is inhibitory and others stating that it is a promoter for stone disease. Relatively few studies have been performed to study the inhibitors of stone disease in children. Generally, citrate, glycosaminoglycans, magnesium, and pyrophosphate are thought to be the major inhibitors. Baggio et al. studied juvenile renal stone disease with particular emphasis on identifying promoting and inhibiting factors.[3] Although no specific abnormalities were identified for individual levels of promoters or inhibitors in that patient population, a significant abnormal oxalate-citrate/glycosaminoglycans ratio was noted. This was felt to be suggestive of an imbalance between promoting and inhibiting factors in children with idiopathic calcium nephrolithiasis.

Realizing urinary citrate is particularly important as a natural stone inhibitor,[50] we examined the urinary citrate excretion in a number of our children with idiopathic calcium oxalate stones.[47] We noted no statistical difference from control children in either the hypercalciuric group of patients or in patients with idiopathic stone formation. These citrate excretion data were obtained while the children were ingesting a low-calcium diet. In all groups, females had a greater urinary citrate excretion than did males, and an inverse relationship between urinary citrate excretion and age was observed. From these data in our patients, we conclude that urinary citrate excretion is rarely reduced in children with urolithiasis. It is interesting, however, to speculate that differences between urinary citrate excretion in children and adults may explain, in part, the reduced risk of calculi during childhood.

Specific treatment for children in whom there is no definable cause for urolithiasis is recommended only when metabolically or surgically active disease is felt to exist. In all patients, a high fluid intake is encouraged and dietary calcium excesses are discouraged. Treatment possibilities available include magnesium oxide with or without pyridoxine; orthophosphates either as neutral sodium, acid, or neutral potassium phosphate combinations; and potassium citrate. Selection of the appropriate agent would depend on an individual patient's circumstances. Major side effects usually are those of gastrointestinal intolerance, and treatment seldom is recommended except in those with active stone formation.

SURGICAL MANAGEMENT

The indications for surgical intervention in a child with a urinary calculus are the same as in adults. Pain, high-grade obstruction, and obstruction with infection are the usual indications. While the indications for surgical intervention have not changed, the methods for such intervention have changed greatly. In reviewing the literature regarding pediatric stone patients, it can be readily noted that a high percentage will require some form of surgical intervention with the standard forms of surgical lithotomy being listed.

Upper urinary calculi have traditionally been treated with nephrolithotomy, pyelolithotomy, or ureterolithotomy. The techniques and incisions used in these procedures are well known and are basically the same as those used in adults.[71] It should be noted, however, that usage of these techniques has been significantly reduced with the advent of percutaneous stone removal and, more importantly, ESWL. When open surgical lithotomy becomes necessary in a child, proper tissue handling techniques and respect for and preservation of blood supply to the smaller, more delicate structures of the child are mandatory. Any anatomic or functional variation in a kidney to be operated on should be taken into account as to surgical approach and the necessity of any associated procedures.

The number of pediatric stone patients to undergo surgery may vary as to the type of surgical procedure and the indications depending on the population studied. In our center, we have found that approximately 25 percent of children who present with stones will spontaneously pass the calculus. Another 25 percent will be unable to pass the calculus but are amenable to cystoscopy with basketing and extraction of a lower ureteral stone. It has been our experience that ureteral stone extraction is a safe procedure in a child when limiting the size of a calculus that one will attempt to manipulate (<5 mm) and using the smaller, more flexible ureteral stone baskets with appropriate-sized instruments. Although as yet limited in its use in pediatric patients, we have had some opportunity to utilize ureteroscopy and stone extraction in a limited number of cases. Of concern is the long-term effect of dilatation of the lower ureter and what long-term effects such as ureteral stricture might have on the child. So far, we have limited ureteroscopic treatment of stones to the older, larger child, but as instrumentation becomes smaller, the possibility of ureteroscopic stone treatment in the child could increase.

Some 10 percent of children with stones will present with an associated urologic abnormality, such as UPJ obstruction, megaureter, and caliceal diverticulum. It is in this group of children that time honored techniques of nephrolithotomy, pyelolithotomy, and ureterolithotomy may be carried out at the time the underlying obstructing abnormality is corrected. For these open procedures, control and elimination of infection with a carefully planned approach to both eliminate any underlying abnormality and completely remove the stone is required. There will continue to be a certain number of children with congenital abnormalities that will present with stone disease and will require appropriate treatment.

It is in the remaining 40 percent of pediatric stone patients that the methods of treatment are changing vary rapidly. Percutaneous techniques are, in some cases, applicable to children. The technique gained popularity in the latter part of the 1970s and the early part of the 1980s.[72,92] A few reports have been given in which children were included, and one by Woodside et al. dealt completely with application of percutaneous stone removal in children.[93] In the pediatric patient, general anesthesia usually is required, and because of the smaller nature of the kidney and the delicacy of the collecting structures, larger instruments may, in some cases, be inappropriate for use in the pediatric patient. As smaller instrumentation such as ureteroscopes is developed, the usage of percutaneous techniques in the pediatric stone patient will continue to increase. At certain times percutaneous treatment and catheter dissolution of such recalcitrant stones as cystine stones may be indicated.[24] Percutaneous procedures can also be utilized in debulking certain forms of multiple or branched staghorn calculi prior to definitive treatment with ESWL.

Extracorporeal shockwave lithotripsy has, and will continue to have, an impact on the management of pediatric stone disease, the same as in adults. With Chaussy's original report of the clinical use of ESWL, this technique has been applied in an ever-increasing number of stone patients.[19] Additional experience with ESWL has outlined the advantages as well as some potential problems with this new modality of treatment.[23,41] Experience with ESWL has even been reported in a purely pediatric population.[39,54]

One problem with ESWL in children is adjustment of the gantry to fit the smaller pediatric patient. In general, the shoulder brace must be adjusted to support the child, and shoulder rests have been recommended for replacement with plywood board covered with lead to prevent shockwave scatter and lung damage. Our experience in selected patients for ESWL has been favorable, but continued data in regard to the pediatric population for this modality will be required before more definitive information is available. Fewer shocks, between 250 and 2000, are recommended for use in children. Although the theoretical disadvantages of shock-wave therapy such as closing epiphyses or altering a growing kidney have been advanced, no such observation has been made in those children so treated. Perirenal hematomas can occur, and skin bruising at the entry and exit sites of the shock wave can be quite marked (Figs. 27-16 and 27-17).

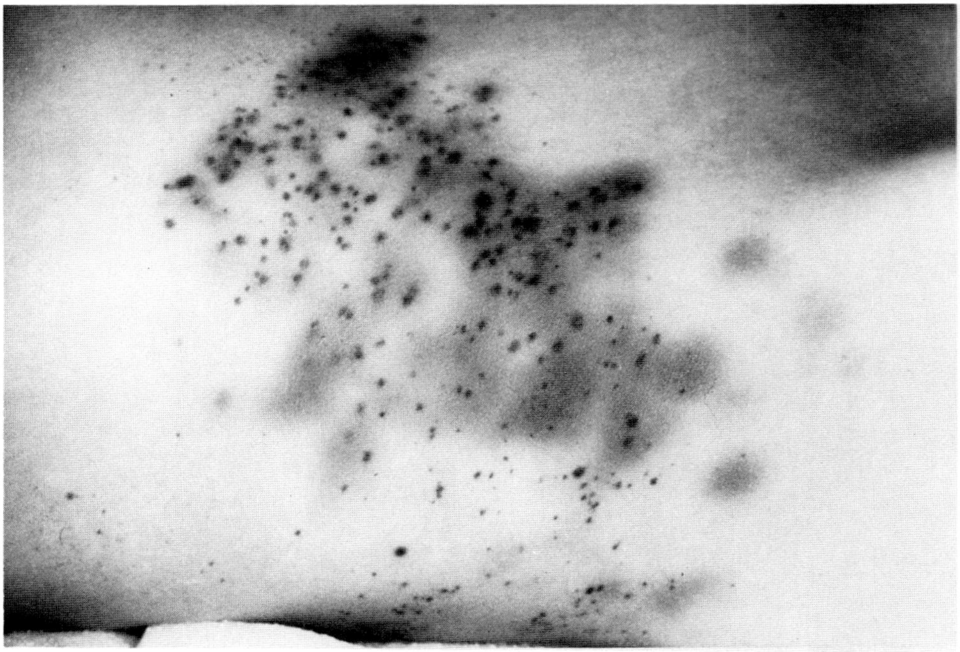

Fig. 27-16. Bruising of flank associated with ESWL used in a child. (Photograph courtesy of Dr. Larry Kroovand.)

The major potential problem of ESWL in children would be that of the smaller collecting system attempting to handle a large stone burden. As with adults with larger stones, particularly with massive staghorn calculi, it is possible that the collecting system cannot pass all the fragments, leading to obstruction and/or sepsis. Because of the need to be able to handle the problems of "Steinstrasse" ("street of stones"), it is essential that the ability to perform endoscopic treatment of an obstructed lower ureter be present. Because of the smaller size of a child and the inability to treat this phenomenon with simple basketry or passage of a catheter, extra caution seems to be appropriate in pediatric applications. Although balloon dilatation of the lower ureter with ureteroscopic management is possible in the older, larger child, in many cases percutaneous techniques would have to be used should lower ureteral obstruction develop.

Some specific contraindications for use of ESWL in children would be lower ureteral stones, bladder stones, unacceptable anesthetic risks, anatomy that precludes focusing the shock wave, and the use of this technique when distal obstruction exists. A relative contraindication would be the presence of a bleeding disorder that should be appropriately corrected before therapy is undertaken.

Some special problems associated with radiolucent calculi are encountered because of the inability to appropriately visualize them. Catheters may be placed to enhance the ability to localize a stone, but, at present, no experience or guidelines for such are

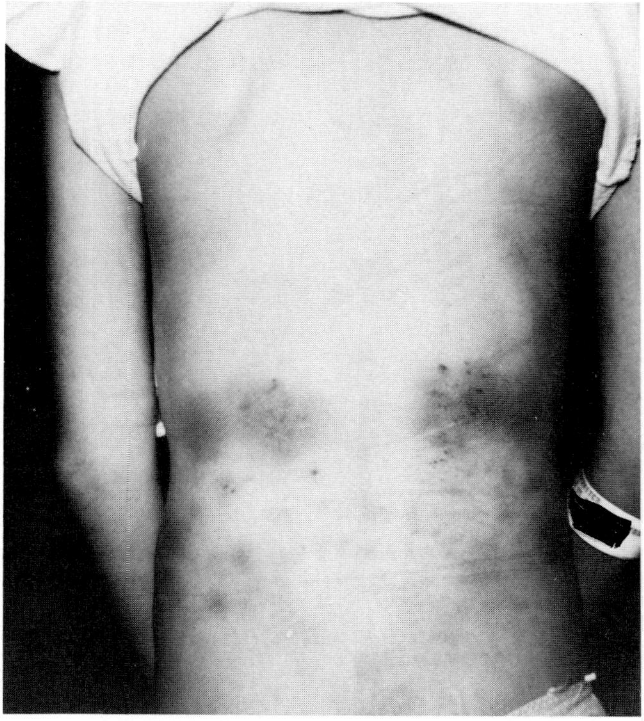

Fig. 27-17. Bruising of flank following bilateral ESWL in a child. (Photograph courtesy of Dr. David Bloom.)

available for the use in children. It has also been noted that cystine stones have been very difficult to treat with ESWL. In these cases, the aforementioned use of percutaneous techniques with stone dissolution may be appropriate.

A place for nephrolithotomy may be remaining in the pediatric population. As mentioned earlier, morbidity and success of ESWL can be directly related to the size of the stone and, thus, the stone burden. The complex staghorn calculus with its branches and infection deep within the stone itself may be such an instance where open surgical procedure would still be the most efficient method of treatment. Combined use of percutaneous debulking of the stone followed by ESWL has been recommended, although little experience has been accumulated with this in children. The use of multiple anesthetics, the potential intolerance of the nephrostomy tube in a child, and the prolongation of treatment may be the least efficient mode of treatment in such cases. Anatrophic nephrolithotomy has been demonstrated to be safely applied in children and, in our hands, still is used in children with a very large stone burden.[2,13,46] The standard surgical approach through a lumbar or flank incision is utilized, isolating the posterior segmental arterial branch and delineating the avascular line for posterior entry into the renal substance. The use of intraoperative films to assure adequate stone removal and appropriate correction of any caliceal or infundibular stenosis is always undertaken. A stent and nephrostomy catheter are left for postoperative irrigation with a chemolytic agent if necessary. Vigorous and aggressive postoperative antibiotic treatment and followup are essential if this special group of patients is to be maintained infection-free, which seems to be essential if recurrences are to be held to a low level. It is now possible, of course, that stone fragments missed by either percutaneous or open surgical techniques could be treated by ESWL, and this should be kept in mind when selecting a form of therapy.

Although it has become much easier to treat the pediatric stone patient with surgical methods, we still emphasize that the removal or treatment of a stone is only one step in the overall management of that patient. The basic metabolic or anatomic defect predisposing to stone formation in a child must always be considered and appropriately evaluated and treated to minimize recurrences with their associated morbidity. This is especially true in a child who may remain at risk for urolithiasis throughout life.

RECOMMENDATIONS FOR METABOLIC EVALUATION

When urinary calculus formation commences during childhood, one anticipates a life-long risk for stone formation with its attendant morbidity. For this reason, careful evaluation of children with urinary stones is essential in order to plan appropriate preventive therapies. Whenever possible, the evaluation should begin with analysis of the composition of the stone. In some cases, such as those presenting with cystine stones or struvite stones, stone analysis will be diagnostic. Unfortunately, the majority of calculi are composed of calcium oxalate, and, therefore, further evaluation will be required.

Appropriate initial diagnostic studies for children with urolithiasis are shown in Table 27-3. As discussed earlier in this chapter, the majority of children without infection related stones will have hypercalciuria. Subsequent evaluation of children with hypercalciuria has been discussed previously.

Table 27-3
Initial Evaluation of Children with Urolithiasis

Serum	
	Bicarbonate, calcium, phosphorus, uric acid, creatinine, parathyroid hormone
Urine	
	Urinalysis, urine culture
	24-hour calcium, uric acid, oxalate, citrate
	Urine cystine screen
Stone analysis	

REFERENCES

1. Androulakakis PA, Barratt TM, Ransley PG, et al: Urinary calculi in children. Br J Urol 54:176, 1982
2. Assimos DG, Boyce WH, Harrison LH, et al: Pediatric anatrophic nephrolithotomy. J Urol 133:233, 1985
3. Baggio B, Gambaro G, Favaro S, et al: Juvenile renal stone disease: A study of urinary promoting and inhibiting factors. J Urol 130:1133, 1983
4. Bartone FF, Johnston JH: Staghorn calculi in children. J Urol 118:76, 1977
5. Bass HN, Emanuel B: Nephrolithiasis in childhood. J Urol 95:749, 1966
6. Beane HC, Magoss IV, Staubitz WJ, et al: Urolithiasis in childhood. J Urol 97:537, 1967
7. Bell NH, Green AS, Epstein S, et al: Evidence of alteration of the vitamin D endocrine system in blacks. J Clin Invest 76:470, 1985
8. Bennett AH, Colodny AH: Urinary tract calculi in children. J Urol 109:318, 1973
9. Bensman A, Rouback L, Allouch G, et al: Urolithiasis in children. Acta Pediatr Scand 72:879, 1983
10. Black J, Stapleton FB, Roy S III, et al: Varied types of urinary calculi in a patient with cystinosis without renal tubular acidosis. Pediatrics 78:295, 1986
11. Borgmann V, Nagel R: Urolithiasis in childhood—a study of 181 cases. Urol Internatl 37:198, 1982
12. Boyce WH: The renal tubule in the genesis of renal calculi in Shreiner GE (ed): Proceedings of the Third International Congress of Nephrology, Vol 2. Basel, S Karger AG, 1967, p 354
13. Boyce WH: Nephrolithotomy, in Glenn JF (ed): Urologic Surgery, 3rd ed. Philadelphia, Lippincott, 1983, pp 181–193
14. Braun G, Moussali L, Balanzar JL: Xanthogranulomatous pyelonephritis in children. J Urol 133:236, 1985
15. Brenner RJ, Spring DB, Sebastian A, et al: Incidence of radiographically evident bone disease, nephrocalcinosis and nephrolithiasis in various types of renal tubular acidosis. New Engl J Med 307:217, 1982
16. Broadus AE, Insogna KL, Lang R, et al: Evidence for disordered control of 1.25-dihydroxyvitamin d production in absorptive hypercalciuria. New Engl J Med 311:73, 1984
17. Buckalew VM Jr, Caruana RJ: The pathophysiology of distal (type I) renal tubular acidosis, in Gonick HC, Buckalew VM Jr (eds): Renal Tubular Disorders. New York, Marcel Dekker, 1985, pp 357–386
18. Campbell MF: Urology. Philadelphia, Saunders, 1963
19. Chaussy C, Schmeidt E, Jocham D, et al: First clinical experience with extracorporeally induced destruction of kidney stones by shock waves. J Urol 127:417, 1982
20. Churchill DN, Maloney CM, Nolan R, et al: Pediatric urolithiasis in the 1970s. J Urol 123:237, 1980

21. Coe FL: Hyperuricosuric calcium oxalate nephrolithiasis. Kidney Internatl 13:418, 1978
22. Daeschner CW, Singleton EB, Curtis JC: Urinary tract calculi and nephrocalcinosis in infants and children. J Pediatr 57:721, 1960
23. Drach GW, Dretler SP, Fair W, et al: Report of the United States cooperative study of extracorporeal shock wave lithotripsy. J Urol 135:1127, 1986
24. Dretler SP, Pfister RC, Newhouse JH, et al: Percutaneous catheter dissolution of cystine calculi. J Urol 131:216, 1984
25. Fleisch H: Inhibitors and promotors of stone formation. Kidney Internatl 13:361, 1978
26. Fowler JE Jr: Bacteriology of branched renal calculi and accompanying urinary tract infection. J Urol 131:213, 1984
27. Ghazali S, Barratt TM: Urinary excretion of calcium and magnesium in children. Arch Dis Child 45:97, 1947
28. Ghazali S, Barratt TM, Williams DI: Childhood urolithiasis in Britain. Arch Dis Child 48:291, 1973
29. Goldwasser B, Weinerth JL, Carson CC III: Calcium stone disease: An overview. J Urol 135:1, 1986
30. Griffith DP, Gibson JR, Clinton GW, et al: Acetohydroxamic acid: Clinical studies of a urease inhibitor in patients with staghorn renal calculi. J Urol 119:9, 1978
31. Halpern EC, Thier SO: Cystinuria, in Coe FL, Brenner BM, Stein JH (eds): Nephrolithiasis. Contemporary Issues in Nephrology, Vol 5. New York, Churchill Livingstone, 1980, pp 208–230
32. Hodgkinson A: Composition of urinary tract calculi in children of different ages. Br J Urol 49:453, 1977
33. Hufnagle KG, Khan SN, Penn D, et al: Renal calcifications: A complication of long-term furosemide therapy in pretern infants. Pediatrics 70:360, 1982
34. Hymes LC, Warshaw BL: Idiopathic hypercalciuria: Renal and absorptive subtypes in children. Am J Dis Child 38:176, 1984
35. Hymes LC, Warshaw BL: Families of children with idiopathic hypercalciuria. Am J Dis Child 139:621, 1985
36. Izzidien AY, Al-Dewachi H, Al-Hasso TK, et al: Xanthogranulomatous pyelonephritis in childhood. J Pediatr Surg 15:686, 1980
37. Jaeger P, Portmann L, Saunders A, et al: Anticystinuric effects of glutamine and of dietary sodium restriction. New Engl J Med. 315:1120, 1986
38. Kalia A, Travis LBM, Brouhard BH: The association of idiopathic hypercalciuria and asymptomatic gross hematuria in children. J Pediatr 99:716, 1981
39. Kroovand RL, Harrison LH, McCullough DL: Extracorporeal shock wave lithotripsy in childhood. Presented, Section on Urology, American Academy of Pediatrics. Washington DC, November 1986
40. Kruse K, Kracht U, Kurse U: Reference values for urinary calcium excretion and screening for hypercalciuria in children and adolescents. Eur J Pediatr 143:25, 1984
41. Lingeman JE, Newman DM, Mertz JHO, et al: Extracorporeal shock wave lithotripsy: The Methodist Hospital of Indiana experience. J Urol 135:1134, 1986
42. Lue TF, Macchia RJ, Pastore L, et al: Vesicoureteral reflux and staghorn calculi. J Urol 127:247, 1982
43. Malek RS, Elder JS: Xanthogranulomatous pyelonephritis: A critical analysis of 26 cases and of the literature. J Urol 119:589, 1978
44. Malek RS, Kelalis PP: Pediatric nephrolithiasis. J Urol 113:545, 1975
45. Marquardt H, Nagel R: Urolithiasis in childhood. Urology 9:627, 1977
46. Middleton RG, Marshall VF: Complete longitudinal nephrolithotomy for staghorn calculi in children. J Urol 106:766, 1971
47. Miller LA, Stapleton FB: Urinary citrate excretion in children with hypercalciuria. Pediatrics 107:263, 1985

48. Moore ES: Hypercalciuria in children, in Berlyne GM, Giovannetti S, Thomas G (eds): Contributions to Nephrology. New York, Karger, 1981, pp 20–32
49. Muldowney FP, Freaney R, Moloney MF: Importance of dietary sodium in the hypercalciuria syndrome. Kidney Internatl 22:292, 1982
50. Myer JL, Smith LH: Growth of calcium oxalate crystals. II. Inhibition by natural urinary crystal growth inhibitors. Invest Urol 13:36, 1975
51. Myers NA: Urolithiasis in childhood. Arch Dis Child 32:48, 1957
52. Nash MA: Urolithiasis, in Edelmann CM Jr (ed): Pediatric Kidney Disease. Boston, Little Brown, 1978, pp 1170–1176
53. Nemoy NJ, Stamey TA: Surgical, bacteriological and biochemical management of infection stones. JAMA 215:1470, 1971
54. Newman DM, Corry T, Lingeman JE, et al: Extracorporeal shock wave lithotripsy experience in children. J Urol 136:238, 1986
55. Noe HN, Stapleton FB, Jerkins GR, et al: Clinical experience with pediatric urolithiasis. J Urol 129:1166, 1983
56. Noe HN, Bryant JF, Roy S III, et al: Urolithiasis in preterm infants associated with furosemide therapy. J Urol 133:664, 1984
57. Noronha RF, Gregory JG, Duke JJ: Urolithiasis in children. J Urol 121:487, 1979
58. O'Regan S, Homsy Y, Mongeau JG: Urolithiasis in children. Can J Surg 25:566, 1982
59. Pak CYC, Kaplan RA, Bone H, et al: A simple test for the diagnosis of absorptive, resorptive and renal hypercalciurias. New Engl J Med 292:497, 1975
60. Pak CYC: Physiological basis for absorptive and renal hypercalciurias. Am J Physiol 237:F415, 1979
61. Pak CYC, Britton F, Peterson R, et al: Ambulatory evaluation of nephrolithiasis: Classification, clinical presentation and diagnostic criteria. Am J Med 69:19, 1980
62. Pak CYC: Pathogenesis of hypercalciuria, in Peck WA (ed): Bone and Mineral Research. Amsterdam, Elsevier Science Publishers, 1986, pp 303–333
63. Paulson DF, Glenn JF, Hughes J, et al: Pediatric urolithiasis. J Urol 108:811, 1972
64. Petritsch PH, Schwarz R: Urinary calculous disease in childhood. Urology 12:407, 1978
65. Piel CF, Roof BS: Renal calculi, in Rubin M, Barratt TM (eds): Pediatric Nephrology. Baltimore, Williams & Wilkins, 1975, pp 760–766
66. Rambar AC, Mackenzie RG: Urolithiasis in adolescents. Am J Dis Child 132:1117, 1978
67. Reiner RJ, Kroovand RL, Perlmutter AD: Unusual aspects of urinary calculi in children. J Urol 121:480, 1979
68. Resnick M, Pridgen DB, Goodman HO: Genetic predisposition of formation of calcium oxalate renal calculi. New Engl J Med 278:1313, 1968
69. Roy S III, Stapleton FB, Noe HN, et al: Hematuria preceding renal calculus formation in children with hypercalciuria. J Pediatr 99:712, 1981
70. Scholten HG, Bakker NJ, Cornil C: Urolithiasis in childhood. J Urol 109:744, 1973
71. Schulze H, Hertle L, Graff J, et al: Combined treatment of branched calculi by percutaneous nephrolithotomy and extracorporeal shock wave lithotripsy. J Urol 135:1138, 1986
72. Segura JW: Endourology. J Urol 132:1079, 1984
73. Simmonds HA: 2.8-Dihydroxyadenuria—or when a uric acid stone is not a uric acid stone. Clin Nephrol 12:195, 1979
74. Sinno K, Boyce WH, Resnick MI: Childhood urolithiasis. J Urol 121:662, 1979
75. Smith LH: Urolithiasis, in Earley LE, Gottschalk CW (eds): Strauss and Welts's Diseases of the Kidney, Vol 2, 3rd ed. Boston, Little Brown, 1979, p 893
76. Stamey TA: Pathogenesis and Treatment of Urinary Tract Infections. Baltimore, Williams & Wilkins, 1980
77. Stapleton FB: Developmental aspects of uric acid excretion, in Spitzer A (ed): The Kidney During Development. New York, Masson, 1982, pp 355–361

78. Stapleton FB, Noe HN, Jerkins GR, et al: Urinary excretion of calcium following an oral calcium loading test in healthy children. Pediatrics 69:594, 1982
79. Stapleton FB, Noe HN, Jerkins GR, et al: Hypercalciuria in children with urolithiasis. Am J Dis Child 136:675, 1982
80. Stapleton FB, Nash D: A screening test for hyperuricosuria. J Pediatr 102:88, 1983
81. Stapleton FB, Roy S III, Noe HN, et al: Hypercalciuria in children with hematuria. New Engl J Med 310:1345, 1984
82. Stapleton FB, Chesney RW, Behrmann AT, et al: Increased urinary excretion of renal *n*-acetyl-B-glucosaminidase in hypercalciuria. Am J Dis Child 139:950, 1985
83. Stapleton FB: Hypercalciuria in children with hematuria: Report of the southwest pediatric nephrology study group. Kidney Internatl 29:204, 1986
84. Stapleton FB, Miller LA, McMullen P: Urinary uric acid excretion in childhood urolithiasis. Pediatr Res 20:1786, 1986
85. Stapleton FB, Langman CB, Bittle J, et al: Abnormalities of vitamin D metabolism in children with fasting hypercalciuria. J Pediatr, in press
86. Steele BT, Lowe P, Rance CP, et al: Urinary tract calculi in children. J Pediatr Nephrol 4:47, 1983
87. Stein M, Stapleton FB, Edwards D, et al: Factitious disease in pediatrics. Clinicopathologic Conference, University of San Diego. West J Med 131:219, 1979
88. Troup CW, Lawnicki CC, Bourne RB, Hodgson NB: Renal calculus in children. J Urol 107:306, 1972
89. Venkataraman PS, Han BK, Tsang RC, et al: Secondary hyperparathyroidism and bone disease in infants receiving long-term furosemide therapy. Am J Dis Child 137:1157, 1983
90. Walther PC, Lamm D, Kaplan GW: Pediatric urolithiaes: A ten-year review. Pediatrics 65:1068, 1980
91. Wenzl JE, Burke EC, Stickler GB, Utz DC: Nephrolithiasis and nephrocalcinosis in children. Pediatrics 41:57, 1968
92. White EC, Smith AD: Percutaneous stone extraction from 200 patients. J Urol 132:437, 1984
93. Woodside JR, Stevens GF, Stark GL, et al: Percutaneous stone removal in children. J Urol 134:1166, 1985
94. Yendt ER, Cohanim M: Response to a physiologic dose of pyrodoxine in type I primary hyperoxaluria. New Engl J Med 312:953, 1985

PART V

Current Trends in Urolithiasis Research

G. Alan Rose

28

Current Trends in Urolithiasis Research

Dramatic advances have undoubtedly been made in the last few years in surgical procedures for removing urinary stones. These procedures became less invasive, so that only very small incisions were required, and finally became completely noninvasive. This raises the question of how much has been accomplished in the field of prevention of further stone formation. Some might say not much. Despite all the money spent in the last 15 years on research into prevention of stone formation and the many claims to have found ways of preventing recurrences, the prevalance apparently continues to rise in the developed countries.

Some have been tempted to suggest that metabolic investigations of stone formers is hardly worthwhile when extracorporeal shock-wave lithotripsy (ESWL) is available. This is misconceived because only about one-third of stone formers ever need surgical procedures, with the remainder passing small stones often with considerable pain and grief that they have no desire to repeat. Nevertheless, despite all the money and effort spent on prevention of stone recurrences, success seems to remain small compared to the dramatic changes in surgical procedures. In reviewing urolithiasis research, it therefore seems desirable to look at the situation critically and to try and consider why the efforts of many have yielded apparently only very modest results. For these reasons, in the review that follows in this chapter, stress has been laid on the deficiencies in methods and knowledge rather than on successes.

EPIDEMIOLOGY

A number of aspects of urinary stone disease suggest that an epidemiologic approach to the subject might give some clues to the etiology:

1. In the last 100 years in the developed countries, bladder stones in children have declined from a high level to a vanishing point,[1] whereas in many undeveloped countries these stones persist. During the same hundred years the upper urinary

STONE DISEASE: DIAGNOSIS AND MANAGEMENT
ISBN 0-8089-1873-7

tract stones of adults have greatly increased and are still increasing in the developed countries.[2]

2. Both bladder and upper urinary tract stones particularly affect certain geographic areas—the "stone belts."
3. The "idiopathic" upper urinary tract stones affect males almost exclusively.[3–5]
4. Upper urinary tract stones currently are more common in the affluent portion of the population.[6]

Bladder stones in children have been shown to be due to dietary lack of phosphate[7] with low urinary pH and probably raised dietary oxalate as well leading to hyperoxaluria. In the case of upper urinary tract stones, however, the cause has proved much more elusive. Why affluence causes the common calcium oxalate–phosphate stones remains far from clear. It is still not certain whether hypercalciuria is any more frequent in stone formers than in normals. Thus, while some well-renowned medical centers find hypercalciuria to occur more frequently in stone formers,[8–11] other equally renowned centers find no difference.[12–15]

The epidemiologic search for a cause of stones has, however, centered upon five main areas, which are now considered.

Dietary Calcium

Those who do find hypercalciuria among their stone formers have assumed that the former is the cause of the latter, but even this assumption may prove to be a considerable exaggeration in view of the finding described further below that increased absorption of dietary calcium leads to increased absorption of dietary oxalate. If stone formers do have hypercalciuria, is this due to increased dietary calcium or to increased absorption of dietary calcium? The former seems untenable in view of the finding that idiopathic stone formation is an almost entirely male condition while high intake of calcium rich foods is not limited to males. Furthermore, two surveys of food intake of stone formers and matched controls[16,17] recently have concluded that there was no significant difference in calcium intake between the two groups. In fact, overabsorption of dietary calcium has been demonstrated in urolithiasis[18] and idiopathic hypercalciuria,[19] but the question that then arises is whether the overabsorption is primary or secondary to a renal leak of calcium or due to some other disturbance that causes both dietary overabsorption and increased urinary loss of calcium. An enormous amount of time, effort, and money has been spent in many countries in developing methods for testing the first two possibilities in the belief that this would assist the design of logical therapy; however, it is the present author's belief that all this research has been misconceived, as discussed in the following two paragraphs.

The idea that one can use a short-term calcium deprivation test to identify "overabsorbers" and "renal leakers" has been questioned by others[19–21] and seems to be flawed, for the following three reasons. First, since plasma calcium remains constant during fasting tests and gastrointestinal absorption is zero, patients are actually being divided into those that go into large negative balance and those that go into small negative balance—that is, those who can rapidly mobilize skeletal calcium and those who cannot. This has nothing to do with renal leak. Second, patients with calcium urolithiasis do not develop skeletal depletion of calcium on low calcium diets, and as shown long ago,[22] all subjects on low calcium diet eventually return to calcium balance. Third, if patients with renal leak of calcium were given cellulose phosphate, they would develop skeletal loss of calcium. In many clinics, including the author's, cellulose phosphate has been given for many years without any bone rarefaction developing even though no attempt has been made to divide patients into overabsorbers or renal leakers of calcium.

It therefore seems that there may be some still unidentified other factor causing a general disturbance of calcium metabolism. This is supported by the finding that bone turnover rate is increased in calcium urolithiasis.[20]

For all these reasons it seems to the author that we have paid far too much attention to calcium metabolism in the last 40 years, and it is time to seek the cause of stone formation elsewhere.

Dietary Protein

A considerable body of evidence has been accumulated[23] that shows that animal protein intake is higher in stone formers than in others and that urinary calcium and oxalate are both raised by increasing animal protein intake; however, this evidence should be interpreted with caution. First, the differences in animal protein intakes between the normals and the stone formers were remarkably small, and in fact such differences were not found by others.[16,17] Second, although raising animal protein intake did raise urinary calcium and oxalate in short-term studies,[23] there is no certainty that these changes persist in the long term. Third, there is no certainty that the risk of stone formation was increased as alleged by raising animal protein intake, because there might have been other factors operating that were not taken into account. To give one example, the urinary urea would be raised by high protein intake, and this would have increased obligatory urinary volume, which, in turn, would have reduced the maximum calcium and oxalate concentrations (and activity) products obtainable. Fourth, most of the population of the Indian stone belt are vegetarians. Fifth, showing that two variables—stone formation rate and animal protein intake—are correlated does not prove cause and effect. If both are correlated with a third factor—standard of living—and if the third factor changes, the other two factors move in parallel. It is concluded that much more direct evidence would be required to substantiate the thesis that animal protein intake is a cause of calcium oxalate stones.

Dietary Carbohydrate

There is another impressive body of evidence[24] that shows that refined carbohydrate intake has increased very greatly in the developed countries[25] and that this leads to hypercalciuria[26] and urolithiasis;[27] however, similar criticisms apply, as in the case of the animal protein hypothesis (see above). The evidence is circumstantial, and some sort of direct proof is required. It should be noted here that considerable restraint should be used before giving firm dietary advice to patients. First, if one were to instruct patients to restrict intake of animal protein, refined carbohydrate, calcium, oxalate, and purines, all of which have been propounded as factors that promote urolithiasis, most would probably give up dieting altogether. Second, giving firm dietary advice based on insufficient evidence that later proves ill founded discredits those who give it and makes it more difficult later to persuade patients to accept other advice although it may be better founded.

Dietary Fiber

At the same time as the consumption of animal protein and refined carbohydrates has increased in the developed countries, the intake of fiber has decreased, and this is yet another factor that is thought to account for rising urolithiasis.[24] Certainly a high bran intake lowers urinary calcium,[28,29] but there are no reports yet of the effect of bran on urinary oxalate or actual stone formation rate.

Water Consumption

There is much circumstantial evidence to support the view that low urinary volume favors urolithiasis and high urinary volume protects against it. Hot climate has long been associated with oxalate crystalluria[30] and urinary stone disease.[31–34] The incidence of urolithiasis was raised in bomber air crews compared to nonflying personnel on a U.S. air base in Florida.[35]

It is not self-evident that diluting urine will reduce urolithiasis, however, since there is always the theoretical possibility that the effect of diluting the inhibitors of crystal nucleation, growth, and aggregation might be more disadvantageous than the advantage due to reducing urinary ionic concentrations. Of great interest, therefore, is a prospective trial of water prophylaxis against urolithiasis that was carried out in Israel.[36] Immigrants in two desert areas at the same latitude were studied. Before settling in the areas, one group was instructed in the importance of water drinking and the other was not. The results are summarized in Table 28-1, which is a summary of the only prospective controlled trial known to the author that clearly shows that water drinking and increased urinary volume reduces the stone incidence rate. Although they can be criticized for using stone incidence rate rather than true prevalence rate, the message seems quite clear that increased urinary volume does reduce stone incidence rate. No similar study has ever been reported, but these results are consistent with the findings that urinary volume is the most important risk factor for urolithiasis (see below).

Surprisingly, many authors do not list chronic dehydration as a cause of urolithiasis. However, chronic dehydration stone disease was found in 13 percent of patients attending the author's metabolic stone clinic.[37] All except two were males, and eight have a history of chronic dehydration due to occupation alone. In this same group, 28 had lived in a hot climate, but 17 of these had subsequently been employed in occupations with

Table 28-1
Prospective Trial of Water Drinking to Prevent Urolithiasis

Only 1 trial ever reported—Arch Environ Health 13:625–630, 1966
In immigrants to 2 desert areas in Israel
Group A; instructed in water drinking
Group B; not instructed

	A	B
Mean 24-hour urine volume (ml)	1071	804
Adult stone incidence rate (%)	0.12	1.52

But
Limited to 3-year period
Not true prevalence rate

hot surroundings. The mean length of exposure to chronic dehydration was 11.2 years (3 months to 52 years).

URINARY RISK FACTORS FOR STONES

In 1978 Robertson et al.[38] devised a simple mathematical method for converting the frequency distribution curves of any given parameter in urine in normal subjects and stone formers into risk factors for stone formation. Initially, they found that calcium, oxalate, urate, and pH were significantly higher in the stone formers and thus were risk factors, while magnesium, sodium, potassium, ammonium, phosphate, citrate, and sulfate were similar in the two groups and hence were not risk factors. Acid mucopolysaccharides (AMPS) were lower in the stone formers and considered protective. Their results clearly show oxalate as the most important risk factor with AMPS second, pH and urate about equal in third place, and calcium in last place. Rather curiously, 24-hour urinary volume was omitted from the study, but this omission was corrected in a later paper[39] when it became apparent that urinary volume was the most important risk factor of all. Although this work has been very widely quoted by many authors, it has not been confirmed elsewhere. The only group to have reported an attempt to confirm it[40] were not able to do so because they were the Australian group who found urinary composition in stone formers to be the same as for their normal population and hence the risk factors could not be tested by this method. What the Australians did find, however, was that values of each of the urinary parameters were positively and significantly correlated with at least two other parameters in one or both groups. Urinary calcium and urate thus were positively correlated in both stone formers and in the normal subjects. This means that calcium and urate were not independent variables, and it may be erroneous to use both to calculate the risk of stone formation. There is a clear need for further work along these lines.

PHYSICAL CHEMISTRY

Urolithiasis is a physicochemical process that must be governed by the laws of precipitation of solids from supersaturated solutions. It is, therefore, entirely reasonable and proper to attempt to discover what these laws are and how they apply to this particular clinical situation. Unfortunately, however, urine is such a complex medium that it has been difficult to make much progress. Valiant attempts have been made, and what follows is an attempt to put into perspective what has so far been achieved. The physicochemical approach seems to be divisible into three parts: (1) calculation of degree of supersaturation, (2) the role of crystal nucleation, and (3) determinants of speed of crystal growth and aggregation.

The relationship of these aspects to one another may be illustrated by use of analogy. Consider the problems of water flowing from one tank into another at a lower level as shown in Figure 28-1. First, there must be a potential energy difference between the two tanks. This represents the thermodynamic energy difference between the states of solution and the precipitated solute suspended in the saturated solvent. Second, it is necessary to overcome a head of resistance, that is, the pressure necessary to prime the system (level B − level A). This corresponds with the level of supersaturation required to induce

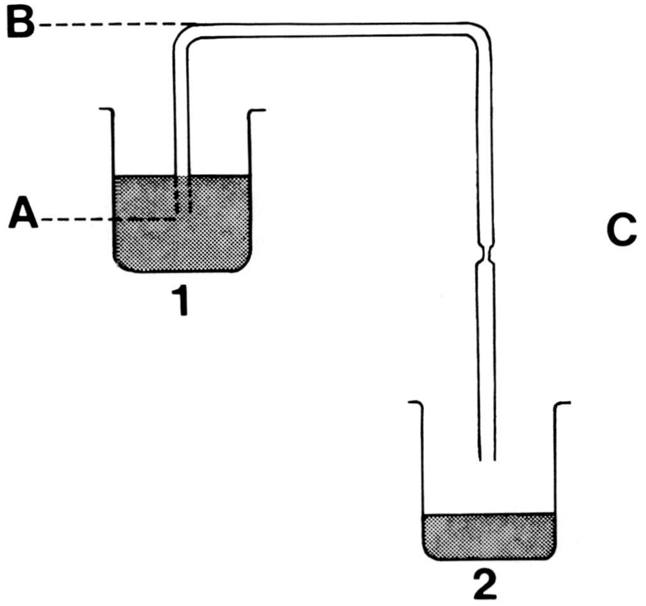

Fig. 28-1. Analogy of crystal formation. Level of water in the upper tank represents concentration of solute. Level A represents solubility (Product) in a saturated solution. Level B represents maximum supersaturation that can be achieved (so-called formation product). Level B − level A represents energy required to produce crystal nucleation. Note that although potential energy in tank 1 is greater than that in tank 2, no flow (crystal growth) will take place until water reaches level B (nucleation occurs), but then water level (solute concentration) will drop back to level A (saturation point). Once started, the rate of flow of water (crystal growth rate) may be reduced or even arrested by narrowing the constriction C (inhibition) or increased by increasing the diameter of the tube (promotion).

crystal nucleation. Third, even when the necessary head of water exists, the actual flow (rate of crystal growth) may be adjusted by changing the bore of the pipe (inhibition or promotion of crystal growth).

Degree of Supersaturation

It will be seen from the preceding sections that the physicochemical approach to urolithiasis requires first the calculation of degree of supersaturation of given urine samples. To do this, one needs to know the ionic activity concentrations of calcium, oxalate, and phosphate. To find these one needs to know:

1. Ionic strength of the sample. To calculate this, one needs to know the concentration of each of the ionic species present. Since ionic strength is proportional to the square of the charge on an ion, it is important to include all the organic acids and amino acids.
2. Dissociation constants of all the complexes of calcium, oxalate, and phosphate with each other and with any other substances. Citrate, which is sometimes measured, thus is obviously important as a complexor of calcium, but so also are certain other organic acids (e.g., isocitrate) and all the amino acids, and these seldom are measured.

If all the above data can be obtained, and total calcium and oxalate concentrations are known, it is theoretically possible to calculate the ionic activity product of calcium oxalate and hence the degree of supersaturation of calcium oxalate. Computer programs have been constructed to perform these calculations.[41–43] However, the following criticisms apply. First, it seldom is possible to know the concentrations of all the substances contributing to ionic strength in real samples of urine (see above), and this prevents calculation of the true ionic strength. Second, by making a rough estimate of ionic strength in a typical stone-forming urine sample, it can be shown (see Table 28-2) that it might easily attain a value of 0.9 *M*. Finlayson points out, however, that his equation for relating activity factor to ionic strength is valid up to an ionic strength of only 0.1 *M*.[41] Above this strength more sophisticated equations are needed,[44] of which one example is shown in Figure 28-2. Third, the extent of complexing of calcium by all the organic and amino acids in urine usually cannot be known because of lack of knowledge of their concentrations and all the dissociation constants. In some cases it is not yet certain whether complexes are formed. Urea presents a particular problem since it was considered by some[45,46] but not by others[47,48] to increase the solubility of calcium oxalate. In fact, Finlayson[47] explains this discrepancy by showing that while urea itself does reduce the calcium ion activity in a solution of low ionic strength, a compensating second effect of salt fortuitously cancels this out.

Even if it were possible to take account of all the above criticisms and obtain a true figure for the relative saturation of a given sample of urine, this would still be only a first step in predicting crystal formation. It would remain necessary to consider whether the conditions for crystal nucleation were present and also to consider how fast crystal formation and growth might occur.

Table 28-2
Calculation of Ionic Strength of a Typical Concentrated Urine Sample

Ion*	Concentration (mmol/liter)	Ionic Strength
Sodium	300	150
Potassium	80	40
Ammonium	50	25
Calcium	7	14
Magnesium	5	10
Sulfate	20	40
Citrate	5	23
Oxalate	0.5	1
Phosphate	50	225
Chloride	356	178
Amino acids	90	180†
Total		886

*For each ion, one-half of the concentration is multiplied by the square of the charge; hence, phosphate is the biggest single contributor and amino acids collectively assume considerable importance. Organic acids must also make a considerable contribution, which has been omitted except for that of citrate.

†Assumes mean charge of 2 per molecule.

LOG ACTIVITY FACTOR FOR SODIUM:-

$$\frac{-\ln 10 \,.\, A \,.\, Z^{2}_{Na} \,.\, I^{\frac{1}{2}}}{1 + \mathring{a} \,.\, B \,.\, I^{\frac{1}{2}}} + h_{Na} \,.\, M_{H_2O} \,.\, \hat{m} - \ln \left\{ 1 + M_{H_2O} \,.\, \Sigma\left[(1 - h_1) \,.\, \hat{m}_1\right] \right\}$$

Where Z = charge no. .... 1 for sodium
h = hydration no. .... 3.5 for sodium
$\hat{m}$ = osmolarity .... 288 for plasma
M_{H_2O} = molar mass of water ... 18 for water
$\mathring{a}$ = Ion-size parameter .... 0.4 n m for sodium
A = constant .... 0.5213 $(\text{mol Kg}^{-1})^{-\frac{1}{2}}$
B = constant .... 3.305 n m^{-1} $(\text{mol.ng}^{-1})^{-\frac{1}{2}}$
I = Ionic strength .... $\frac{1}{2}\Sigma I_x . Z^2$

= 0.749 for sodium in plasma.

Fig. 28-2. Equation showing how the calculation of activity factor may be considerably more complex than the simple formula $1/2\ \Sigma\ Cz^2$ that is often used. (Data from Maas AH, Siggaard-Andersen O, Weisberg HF, et al: Ion-selective electrodes for sodium and potassium: A new problem of what is measured and what should be reported. Clin Chem 31:483, 1985.)

Crystal Nucleation

Nucleation, either homogenous or heterogenous, is an essential step in crystal formation. In homogenous nucleation only the solute undergoing crystal formation is involved. How this occurs is not known with any certainty, but it is clear that energy is required. It involves the coming together of a number of ions to form an elementary crystal lattice. It is thought unlikely that this could occur by chance and must therefore proceed in a number of steps. In heterogenous nucleation the solute precipitates onto other solid particles already present in the solution, thereby lowering the energy requirement of crystal formation. Many recent crystal studies have used calcium oxalate monohydrate (COM) crystals as a seeding material in order to study calcium oxalate crystal growth rate in urine or diluted urine. Although these studies are of great interest in their own right, there are many reasons why they may not be applicable to the problem of stone growth in urine. The following two observations may be mentioned at this point. First, in idiopathic urolithiasis the calcium oxalate usually is precipitated as the di- or trihydrate,[49-56] and not as the monohydrate. Hence either the wrong crystal species (COM) is being studied or heterogenous, and not homogenous, nucleation is being studied. Second, urine contains many particles of different types—casts, cells, bacteria, and aggregated Tamm-Horsfall protein (THP)—and it is most unlikely that homogenous calcium oxalate crystal growth can ever occur. In fact, the observation that polymeric THP promotes calcium oxalate crystal formation (see below) seems to make homogenous nucleation impossible.

Crystal Growth

The rate of crystal growth has been studied by many groups of workers. The basis of the methods has usually been the seeded crystal growth technique. Crystal seeds of known composition are added to the supersaturated solution to be studied and the rate of crystal growth measured. In the earlier methods the crystal growth rate was assessed by observing the crystals themselves[57–59] or by measuring rate of depletion of the solid in the solution.[60,61] Later, calcium concentrations were monitored by suitable electrodes and the concentrations of calcium and oxalate maintained constant, and the rate of crystal growth could then be equated with rate of addition of calcium and oxalate.[62] Elegant though these methods were, they may well have been telling us very little about the problem of crystal formation in human urine in vivo for the following reasons.

First, there is no real concensus opinion on what the seeding agent should be. Should one be trying for homogenous crystal growth, in which case the secondary question raised is what crystals should be used (i.e., mono-, di-, or trihydrate of calcium oxalate)? Or should one take the view that because of all the particulate matter in urine, it is heterogenous nucleation that should be studied?

Second, as mentioned above, it is di- or even trihydrate of calcium oxalate that first precipitates in whole urine, but the seeds used usually have been monohydrate because these are stable and easier to obtain.

Third, in order to standardize the experimental conditions, it has been necessary to use either simple aqueous solutions or urine greatly diluted with simple aqueous solutions. Yet, it is clear that there are fundamental differences between crystal formation in urine and simple aqueous solutions:

1. All urinary stones contain a matrix consisting of high-molecular weight substances.[63] Also, even if calcium oxalate is precipitated from urine in vitro, a coprecipitate of mucoprotein-like substances accounts for 1–4 percent of the total precipitate.[64] Thus it may be quite misleading to consider that crystal formation in simple aqueous solution proceeds in the same fashion as in whole urine.
2. Studies of calcium oxalate crystal formation in whole urine have revealed considerable deviations from what occurs in simple aqueous systems; the transformation of calcium oxalate trihydrate to monohydrate was quite rapid in the latter but greatly retarded in the former.[65] Moreover, certain high-molecular-weight chemicals in urine induced formation of calcium phosphate onto the calcium oxalate trihydrate seeds, and whole urine has been found to contain strong inhibitors of calcium oxalate trihydrate crystal nucleation and growth, thus favoring monohydrate promotion.[66]

Fourth, even where studies of whole urine have been attempted,[61,67] compromises must be made that probably render them invalid as studies of whole urine. If a 24-hour urine is to be studied, it may be chilled or frozen to preserve it so leading to precipitation of crystals not present in the original urine. Worse, such precipitation of crystals before the study almost inevitably causes coprecipitation of the very promoters and inhibitors of crystal formation that were to have been studied.

Crystal Aggregation

Since very small calcium oxalate urinary stones have the appearance of aggregates of crystals,[68] it seems likely that crystal aggregation is an important factor in stone formation. This is made more likely by the observation that calcium oxalate stone formers pass more aggregates of calcium oxalate dihydrate crystals in the urine than do normal subjects.[69,70] Crystal aggregation is dependent on at least two factors, the zeta potential of the crystals and bridging of the gap between crystals by some other substance that glues them together. The concept of an electric double layer at a solid–liquid boundary is over 100 years old. In the case of crystals suspended in a mother liquor, the potential difference between the surface of the crystals and the bulk of the liquid is called the *zeta potential.* It arises out of the accumulation on the surface of the crystal of a net excess of either cations or anions. The zeta potential may be greatly changed by the presence of other ions in the solution including hydrogen and hydroxyl ions. When the zeta potential is high, the crystals repel one another, thus preventing crystal aggregation, but when the zeta potential is reduced, aggregation becomes possible. In a solution as complex as whole urine it is not possible with present knowledge to predict what the zeta potential might be. It is possible, however, to measure zeta potential fairly easily[71] by using the principle that if a suspension of crystals is subjected to an electrical potential difference, the rate of migration of the crystals will vary with the charge on the surface of the crystal:

$$\text{Mobility } (\mu\text{m/s}) = \frac{EZ}{4\pi TN}$$

where E is the dielectric constant of electrolyte, Z is the zeta potential, and N is the viscosity of solution.

Suitable equipment can now be purchased for this purpose (Malvern Instruments, Ltd., Framingham, MA, USA and Malvern, Worchestershire, England, WR14 1AQ). It has been shown quite recently[72] that the zeta potential on calcium oxalate crystals is increased by pyrophosphate and that this effect greatly increases as pH is shifted from 6 to 5. The same authors also showed that the zeta potential on calcium oxalate crystals in artificial urine was reduced by increasing the ionic strength and by increasing the proportion of whole urine added to the system. Tamm-Horsfall mucoprotein was shown to have a dramatic effect on lowering the zeta potential of calcium oxalate crystals in artificial urine. The message from this work is clear, namely, that although studies of the zeta potential in simple solutions is of great interest, they cannot at this stage of our science enable us to predict what might happen in whole urine. To find the solution to this, we have to study whole urine.

When the zeta potential is low, crystals may approach one another sufficiently closely to become adherent by one of the two mechanisms. First, there may be a simple bridging process involving no other materials. This is a part of the general proposition that large crystals grow at the expense of small crystals so as to reduce total surface area of the interface and hence the energy required to sustain the interface. Second, there may be bridging of two crystals by the intervention of a different molecular species. This seems to be the case when crystals of calcium oxalate in urine become stuck together by high-molecular-weight compounds.[73] Although the material coating the crystals has the appearance of mucoid, its chemical composition is still unknown and a lot more work on the physical and chemical properties of this substance is needed before we can understand the way in which crystals aggregate in whole urine.

STUDIES ON WHOLE URINE

In previous sections much criticism has been directed at the concept of extrapolating ideas to whole urine that were derived from the study of simple solutions or urine highly diluted with simple aqueous solutions. The difference between crystal formation in simple aqueous solutions, dilute urine, and concentrated urine is vividly illustrated by the following. The bipyramidal "envelope" crystals of calcium oxalate dihydrate (COD) can be produced either by evaporating dilute urine until it reaches high physiologic concentration of 1250 mOsmol/liter[74] or by adding oxalate to concentrated urine.[75] If one adds calcium and oxalate to dilute urine, dendritic or hexagonal crystals usually are obtained, but rarely envelopes,[76] although this can happen occasionally. If one evaporates a simple solution of calcium oxalate in water, it is not possible to obtain envelope crystals, and yet other forms develop. These considerations have led to a greater interest of crystals in urine and of how they form in urine.

Crystalluria

Although the study of the occurrence of crystals in urine is very old, it was not until 1967 that the importance of conducting these studies on urine maintained at 37°C was appreciated.[77] Since then several groups have found that crystalluria is more common in urolithiasis than in normal subjects and that the aggregated envelope crystals of calcium oxalate are passed in greater numbers in the stone formers.[69,70,78] There have been those who could not confirm all of these results,[79] but this is definitely a minority point of view. Rather curiously, however, when patients with primary hyperparathyroidism were studied,[78] those both with and without urolithiasis showed the same increase in crystalluria. More understandably, crystalluria was more frequent in the summer than in the winter months.[80] Two groups[70,78] have agreed that treatment of idiopathic hypercalciuria with thiazide diuretics reduced the incidence of crystalluria while the poor response to cellulose phosphate[81] seems to have been forecast by the raised incidence of hyperoxaluria to which it led. Hence the simple observation of crystals in urine samples seems to be an aid to clinical management. It must be stressed, however, that the studies must be made on fresh urine samples studied at 37°C.

Frequently, in a stone clinic, patients comply with the instruction to raise urinary volume and pass dilute random urine samples of urine in which, of course, there are no crystals. One still would like to know what crystals would have been present had the patient drunk less water. One way to determine this is to evaporate the sample to standard osmolality, say, 1250 mOsmol/liter, incubate at 37°C for a standard time, and then observe for crystals.[75]

The Role of Tamm-Horsfall Protein

In 1856 Meckel Von Hemsbach wrote a thesis,[82] a part of which was translated[83] thus: "Two factors are essential for the formation of calculi: First, an organic compound of mucus character, in which insoluble or poorly soluble material can be deposited, and second, a fluid super-saturated with petrifying or encrusting substances." This theory remained unproven until recently. It was observed that if urine was ultrafiltered and the ultrafiltrate evaporated to 1250 or 1450 mOsmol/kg, the calcium oxalate (at pH 5.3) and calcium phosphate (at pH 6.8) crystal production was very much less than when the whole urine was evaporated.[84] Furthermore, if THP was added to the ultrafiltrates, the ability to generate crystals was restored on evaporation. A second feature was that whereas the precipitates from whole urine or from ultrafiltrates plus THP were coarsely clumped, those from ultrafiltrates alone were finely divided. Although the initial observations were qualitative, quantitative measurements[85,86] confirmed the findings. They were taken to show that THP acted as a powerful promoter of crystal formation and aggregation in whole urine, and it is difficult to see how this conclusion can be avoided. Two possible criticisms were proposed but do not seem tenable. First, it was suggested that the ultrafiltration might hold back either crystals too small to detect by light microscopy, or low molecular weight ions. It was shown,[85] however, that ultrafiltration did not change the concentrations of low-molecular-weight ions. The fact that addition of THP to ultrafiltrates restored crystal formation seems conclusive proof that this explanation is not tenable. Second, it was suggested that the THP might have contained crystals of calcium oxalate or phosphate that seeded crystal growth. However, the repeated solution, dialysis, and precipitation stages used to prepare the THP makes this criticism impossible to sustain.

Although this work completely changed ideas on the possible role of THP, it has never been repeated in an independent laboratory. One group thought that they checked on the idea of THP as a promoter of crystal formation,[87] but they made a fundamental error in technique. Instead of working at high osmotic strength, which leads to the aggregation of THP,[88] they worked at low osmotic strength, when THP is disaggregated and may be an inhibitor of crystal formation rather than a promoter.[72]

It is worth mentioning here that it has recently been shown[89] that when calcium oxalate stones grow on to plastic foreign bodies in rat bladders, an essential first step is the coating of the plastic with an amorphous organic material.

Inhibitor Studies in Whole Urine by Evaporation Technique

The evaporation technique provides a method of abstracting water from dilute urine so as to make concentrated urine in a way that simulates what happens in the renal tubules. Because the process is so rapid, the rate of concentration is similar to what occurs in the renal tubules, and the only real difference is that the evaporation technique is not a continuously flowing system. Nevertheless, it does seem to offer a method of studying the ability of specific chemicals to change the propensity of urine to crystal formation. The principle of the method is illustrated in Fig. 28-3. The urine to be tested is adjusted to pH 5.3 for studying calcium oxalate or 6.8 for studying calcium phosphate crystal formation. The oxalate concentration may be slightly raised if this is thought desirable, but this is optional. In ideal studies the fresh urine is divided into three aliquots. In one aliquot the test chemical is added, in another it is removed, and the third is the control. A useful way to remove a chemical is by circulating the urine through nylon coils bearing immobilized enzyme. This worked well for urate and pyrophosphate

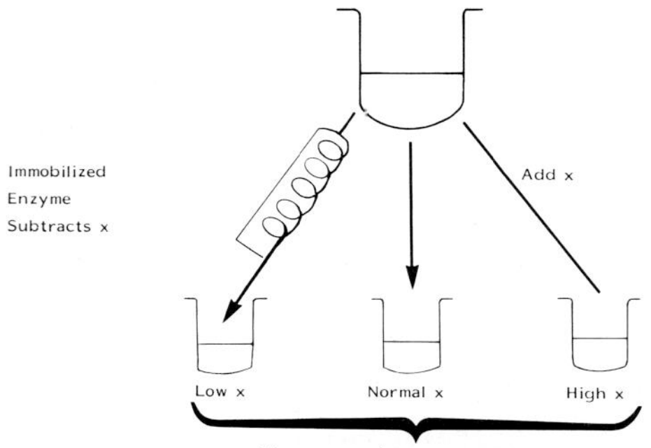

Fig. 28-3. The principle of a method used to study the effect of a given substance X on crystal formation in whole urine. A single urine sample is split into three aliquots. The substance X is added to one and removed from another preferably by immobilized enzyme. The three aliquots are evaporated to the same osmolarity (about 1250 mOsmol/liter) and crystal formations compared.

studies. All three aliquots are evaporated to the same final osmolality, and crystal formation may then be observed in several ways. Microscopy can be rendered semiquantitative[85] and will identify changes in crystal size, habit, and aggregation. Oxalate in crystals can be compared quantitatively by counting radioactive carbon-labeled oxalate,[85] or measured directly by the sensitive method now available for measurement of plasma oxalate.[90] Calcium phosphate can be measured directly in the precipitate.[86] Alternatively, crystals could be counted and sized by a Coulter counter.

With the use of these techniques it has been shown that in whole urine, citrate reduced calcium oxalate and phosphate crystal formation[91] and magnesium reduced calcium oxalate crystal formation,[91] but that pyrophosphate had no effect on calcium oxalate crystal formation.[93] It also was shown that urate, if it had any effect, reduced rather than increased calcium oxalate crystal formation.[94] More recently, it was shown that tartrate could reduce calcium oxalate crystal formation.[95] Some of these findings differ very substantially from what was found in simple aqueous solutions. Thus magnesium had been found to have little effect on calcium oxalate precipitation,[96,97] whereas there is no agreement whatsoever[98] on whether pyrophosphate is really an important inhibitor of calcium oxalate crystal formation in urine. In recent years urate has been considered to increase the risk of calcium oxalate urolithiasis,[99] and this was explained as due to reduction in the inhibitory effect of glycosaminoglycans (GAGs) in simple aqueous solution.[100] The results in whole urine described above, as well as more recent work in whole urine by others,[101] casts serious doubts on this explanation.

These differences serve to stress the case for studying whole urine rather than simple aqueous solutions. Although total crystal mass has been mainly studied to date, as mentioned above, this can be coupled with microscope techniques to identify changes in crystal size and aggregation and there is no reason why these studies should not be rendered quantitative by using Coulter counters. Others are now beginning to find ways of studying whole urine[76,101–104] and such methods should be developed further.

Other Problems in Studying Whole Urine

Timing

It has been calculated that the transit time of urine through the kidneys is about 3 minutes.[105] Transit time in the renal pelvis obviously varies greatly depending on urinary flow rate but may be of the order of minutes. Urine may remain in the bladder for several hours. It is, therefore, possible that crystals observed in random urine samples may not have been present in urine flowing through the collecting tubules and calyces of the kidneys. First, it is conceivable that of two successive lots of urine to enter the bladder, one lot was rich in calcium but poor in oxalate while the reverse was true in the second lot. Calcium oxalate crystallization might then begin only on mixing in the bladder. Second, experience with the evaporation techniques confirms that crystals take an appreciable period of time to grow in whole urine. Figure 28-4 shows how they increased in weight following evaporation to standard osmolarity of a number of urine samples. In conducting evaporation studies, it is, therefore, desirable to standardize the subsequent incubation time before the crystals are separated from mother liquor and select the time that seems appropriate for one's studies.

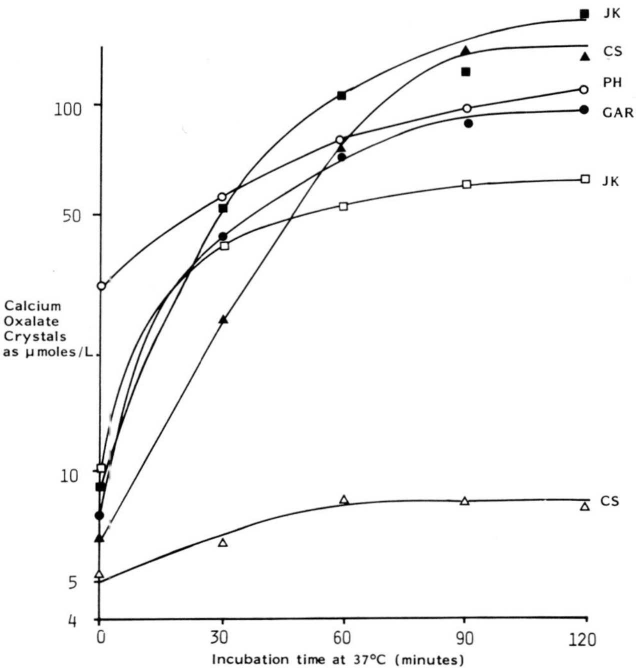

Fig. 28-4. Post-evaporation urine crystal growth at pH 5.3. Six normal samples of urine were evaporated to 1250 mOsmol/liter and calcium oxalate crystal formation measured after various times of incubation at 37°C. It is clearly important to standardize this time in any given series of observations.

Significance of Crystalluria

It is important to consider the significance of the finding of crystals in bladder urine. It certainly indicates supersaturation of urine in the recent past but not necessarily in the sample under observation, since we have sometimes observed crystals apparently dissolving in dilute urine. The finding of crystalluria cannot be equated with stone formation since ipso facto crystals that are passed no longer have the opportunity to form stones. It is the crystals that form but fail to pass and hence are not observed in bladder urine that might contribute to stone formation. Crystalluria is simply proof that one of the conditions required for stone formation—supersaturation of urine—has been a recent event. The finding of aggregated crystals is an indication that the factors required for urolithiasis have been present: supersaturation crystal nucleation, and ability to aggregate.

Fixed or Free Particles

Finlayson and Reid[105] considered the ways in which crystals of calcium oxalate might become attached to the ducts of Bellini in the kidneys. They performed calculations to show that the crystals could not, in the transit time available, grow sufficiently large to become mechanically stuck in the ducts. This calculation assumed a renal transit time of about 3 minutes. The measurement of such transit times can be made only in well-hydrated patients, however, and transit times under conditions of dehydration required for stone formation must be much larger. Nevertheless, they proposed that such "free particle" attachment was not a possible basis for stone formation within the kidneys and that the alternative "fixed particle" mechanism must operate. In support of the latter, they have found,[105] and it has been confirmed,[106] that calcium oxalate crystals may be attached to renal tubular epithelium by strands of organic material that appear to be proteinacious. They did not, however, consider the third possibility suggested by Rose[76] and Hallson and Rose[107] that calcium oxalate and THP might be precipitated together and that the sticky mass so produced might become stuck in the renal tubules.

The Role of Urinary Citrate

Urinary citrate has long been considered to protect against calcigerous urolithiasis. Thus citrate forms a negatively charged complex with calcium ions,[108] so making them unavailable for precipitation as calcium oxalate or phosphate. Since the normal urinary citrate may be up to 6 mmol per 24-hour period compared with about 9 mmol of calcium per 24-hour period, this could be an important factor in reducing calcium and oxalate (and phosphate) products. Furthermore, there is the additional possibility that citrate might be an inhibitor of calcium oxalate or phosphate crystal growth[109,110] or aggregation. It is important, therefore, to know whether urinary citrate is normal or low in urolithiasis. A number of papers have been published on this subject, and yet this simple piece of information is still not unequivocably available. Older papers inevitably used rather nonspecific methods based on formation of pentobromacetone.[111] In recent years specific enzyme methods have been developed[112] and used in a number of papers, and yet the answer is still not clear. Possible reasons for this will now be considered.

Normal Urinary Citrate

Urinary citrate is dependent on a number of factors. First, it is important to appreciate that certain bacteria that may be found in urine can metabolize citrate with the result that if urine is allowed to stand at room temperature for some hours before it is measured, the results may be too low.[113,114] Figure 28-5 shows how urinary citrate values may fall in this way. It is important, therefore, to avoid studying patients with urinary infection and to chill urine soon after collection. It may be better to measure citrate/creatinine ratios in fresh random samples of urine than 24-hour urinary citrate levels. Second, urinary citrate is correlated with urinary pH in healthy individuals when subjected to loading with acid or alkali[115] as shown in Figure 28-6. The same correlation exists for spontaneous fluctuations in urinary pH (see Fig. 28-7), although this was not found by others.[116] Third, urinary citrate falls with decreasing GFR[117,118] as shown in Figures 28-8 and 28-9. Fourth, there may be a sex differential in urinary excretion of citrate. In several studies, 24-hour urinary citrate was found to be higher in women than men by some[117,119–122] but not by others.[123–124] A possible explanation for this discrepancy is offered by a recent paper[125] reaffirming an earlier finding[126] that urinary citrate is higher in young females than males. A rising urinary citrate with age was found in normal subjects of both sexes,[124] however, so the matter must still be regarded as unresolved.

This failure to form a consensus of the effect of sex on urinary citrates could well be due to the failure of some papers to analyze the data for variables such as urinary pH and GFR, but there might be other causes as well. If estrogen production is a factor, it might be

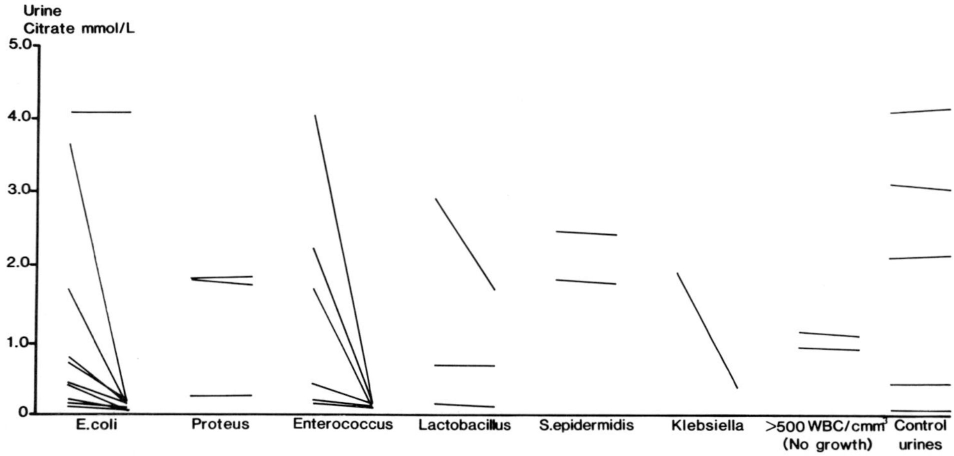

Fig. 28-5. A series of urine samples, each of which showed more than 10^6 organisms/ml, was incubated at 37°C overnight. In some cases the citrate level was raised before the incubation. Citrate concentration was measured before and after the incubation. It is seen that certain bacteria frequently led to a marked fall in urinary citrate, but this was not observed in the control urines or sterile pyuria.

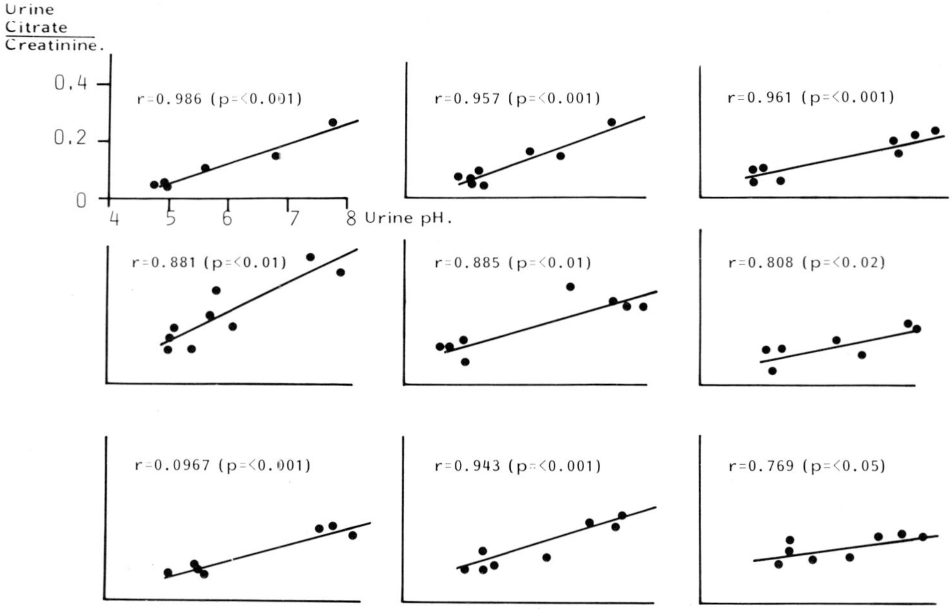

Fig. 28-6. Urinary citrate and creatinine concentrations and pH were measured on normal subjects before and after loading with ammonium chloride and sodium bicarbonate. In each subject the citrate/creatinine ratio was correlated with pH, although the slopes varied considerably.

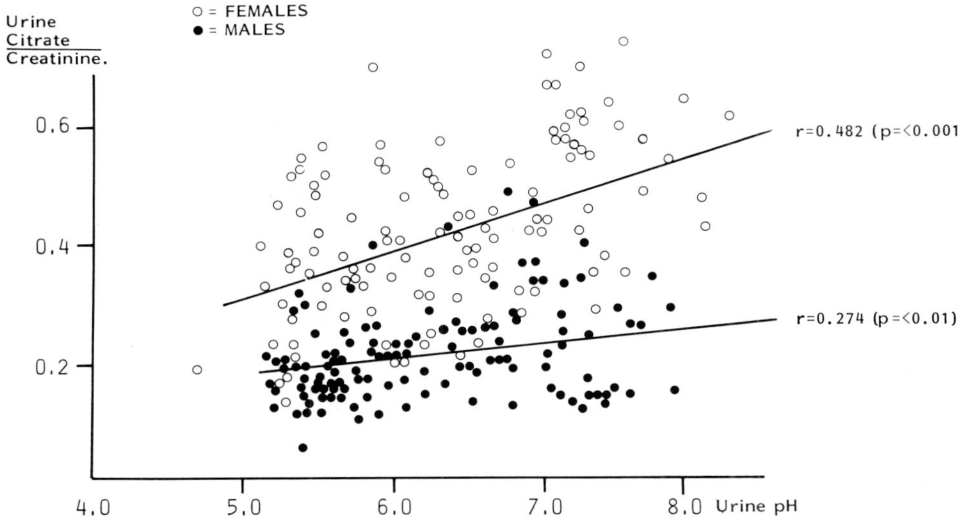

Fig. 28-7. Repeated measurements of urinary citrate and creatinine concentrations and pH were made on a group of normal subjects without any medication. The levels, correlation and slope are all greater for females than for males.

important to consider whether there are variations in urinary citrate during the female menstrual cycle. If these are present, allowance would have to be made for this factor as well. Our own experience is that there is a clear difference between the sexes as shown in Figures 28-7 and 28-9 when results are expressed per mmol of creatinine. The difference is reduced when expressed per 24-hour urine, but it does not disappear.

Urinary Citrate in Calcium Stone Formers

There is no doubt that hypocitraturia does occur in a number of conditions that are associated with calcium urolithiasis. These conditions include steatorrhea,[127-129] presum-

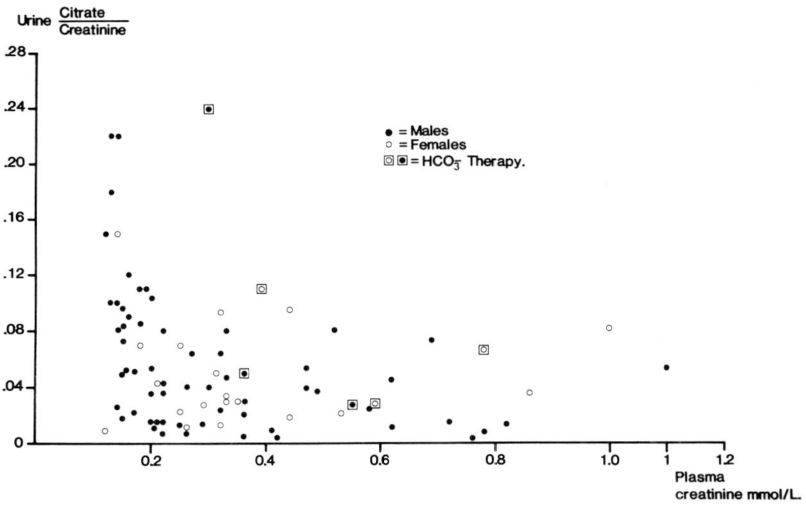

Fig. 28-8. Negative correlation between urinary citrate/creatinine ratio and plasma creatinine.

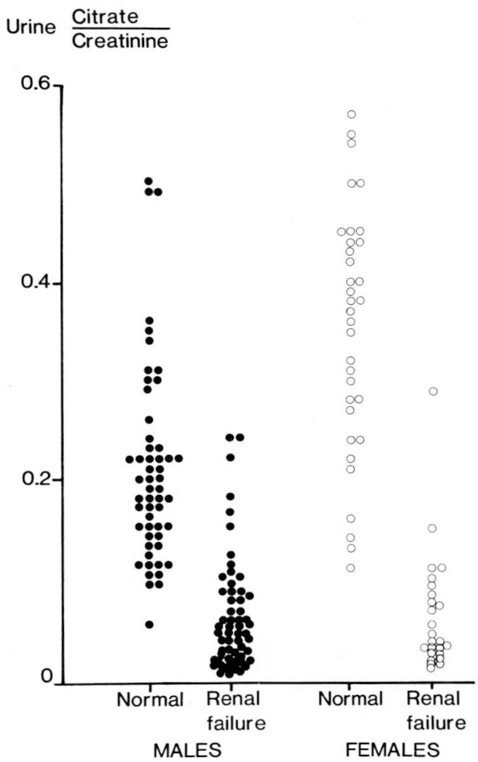

Fig. 28-9. Urinary citrate/creatinine ratio is lower in normal males than in normal females and lower in chronic renal failure.

ably as a result of magnesium depletion,[127] and the classical distal tubular variety of renal tubular acidosis (RTA).[115,130,131] The metabolic abnormalities in these conditions are complex, however, and it does not necessarily follow that the cause of the urolithiasis is the low urinary citrate. It is of great interest, therefore, to know whether it is possible to identify low urinary citrate as the sole metabolic abnormality in calcium urolithiasis and whether urinary citrate is low in idiopathic calcium stone formation. Again it must be stated that there is no general agreement about these points at the present time. Thus, although urinary citrate was found to be low by some[119,123,125,132,133,143] in most of the papers making this claim, there has not been rigorous exclusions of factors such as infection and low GFR, which might have caused low urinary citrate in a nonspecific way, and properly matched controls. These problems were largely excluded in a recent paper[124] in which, although some of the stone formers had hypocitraturia, the effect was really rather small. Even this paper, however, failed to take account of urinary pH values, and moreover some of the patients could have had incomplete RTA. Yet other papers have found little or no hypocitraturia in stone formers.[122,135]

Is Urinary Citrate Important?

Again opinions vary concerning whether citrate plays an important part in affecting calcium oxalate and phosphate crystal formation. Three points should be made, however. First, evaporation studies showed clearly that raising urinary citrate reduced both calcium oxalate and calcium phosphate crystal formation,[91] although these studies do not reveal the mechanism whereby this occurred. Second, urinary stone risk is increased in RTA and acetazolamide (Diamox; Lederle) therapy,[136] both of which are characterized by low urinary citrate. Third, certain citrate metal complexes seem to act as powerful inhibitors of calcium oxalate and phosphate crystal formation,[137,138] although the importance of this in urine still has to be assessed. The author's view is that citrate is very important in reducing crystal formation in urine, but further work is required on many of the points mentioned above.

INCREASING INTEREST IN URINARY OXALATE

In recent years there has been increasing recognition that the urinary calcium is much less significant than urinary oxalate in the problem of calcium oxalate (phosphate) urolithiasis.[139] The evidence has come from a number of different fields, which are summarized here.

Theoretical Physical Chemistry

It was shown by Robertson[140] that a given percentage rise in total urinary oxalate was much more effective in increasing calcium oxalate ion activity product than the same percentage rise in total urinary calcium. In brief, this is because whereas most of the additional oxalate remains as free ions, most of the additional calcium is complexed and does not remain as free ions. This means that hyperoxaluria should be a more potent risk factor than hypercalciuria for urolithiasis.

Observed Risk Factors

As described above, it has been shown,[38,39] although not yet confirmed elsewhere, that urinary oxalate is in fact a more important risk factor for urolithiasis than urinary calcium.

Incidence of Hyperoxaluria

There are now many reports in the literature showing that idiopathic calcium formation or idiopathic hypercalciuria is accompanied by raised urinary oxalate.[141–145] Others have not made this observation, but it must be said here that methods of measuring urinary oxalate are prone to errors in many laboratories for a number of reasons, not least of which is interference by ascorbate.[146,147] Nevertheless, some centers have made particular efforts to overcome these problems, and it is the author's opinion, supported by his own unpublished data, that hyperoxaluria does indeed commonly occur in idiopathic calcium oxalate urolithiasis. To find it, however, one requires a precise and reliable method that can handle large numbers of samples with ease. In the author's laboratory, urinary oxalate is assayed by automated enzyme method[148] more frequently than urinary calcium, as a result of which a new syndrome has been uncovered in which there is mild metabolic hyperoxaluria with raised urinary glycollate, which is (usually) responsive to vitamin B_6, although the dose required is variable.[149,150] This interesting condition is discussed further in Chapter 16 and is not considered further here.

It now appears that although the finding of hypercalciuria is of interest in urolithiasis, it is not the cause, but merely an indicator that hyperoxaluria may be present as a result of low intestinal calcium, with the hyperoxaluria as the main cause of the stone formation.

THERAPEUTIC METHODS

Although therapy is covered in Chapters 7–17, certain aspects should be considered in a chapter devoted to current trends in urolithiasis research, and these are mentioned below.

Stone Clinic Effects

One interesting finding of the small number of controlled trials of therapy for urolithiasis has been the beneficial effects of placebo.[151–153] It may well be that at least a part of this effect is due to increase in water intake and restriction of calcium and oxalate intake.[154] There is no doubt that increasing urinary volume reduces risk of urolithiasis (see above), and it is very difficult for patients with urolithiasis to avoid being advised to take these measures. First, it would seem to be ethically wrong to withhold advice to increase water intake. Second, even if the physician withheld such advice, it would be offered by others gratuitously. As a consequence, it may be very difficult to assess the effects of specific drug therapy unless a double-blind study is performed. Charts showing reduction in stone formation rate when patients begin attending a particular clinic may not necessarily indicate that the specific drug given is responsible. Perhaps partly as a consequence of this problem, some of the claims to have found a cure for idiopathic calcium urolithiasis have not withstood the test of time. There are other problems, however; it may be very difficult to assess stone formation rate, and many workers have instead used stone passage rate. Some trials have been too short, and very few have been double-blind.

Strategy

This section concentrates mainly on the problem of calcium oxalate (phosphate) stones, although the principles of water therapy apply to all stone formers. With regard to calcium oxalate stones, one needs to decide whether to give first priority to reducing urinary calcium or oxalate. Until some years ago, most would have tried to reduce urinary calcium, but this strategy now requires a bit more thought. First, the method chosen for lowering urinary calcium should not lead to a rise in urinary oxalate, or else the end state may be worse than the first state, with patients developing calcium oxalate crystalluria[79] and stone recurrences.[81] Hence methods that reduce gastrointestinal free calcium should be avoided unless a low oxalate diet is also advocated. Second, it seems that overabsorption of calcium from the gastrointestinal tract leads to secondary overabsorption of oxalate;[155] thus the finding of "idiopathic hypercalciuria" should be regarded as a warning to look for hyperoxaluria. Of the two conditions, the hyperoxaluria is a greater risk of urolithiasis than the hypercalciuria. Hence it is more important to treat the former than the latter. Nevertheless, hypercalciuria remains a risk factor, albeit not a very strong one (see above). The clinician, therefore, must consider both the urinary calcium and oxalate values before deciding which to treat most aggressively. Perhaps the most important lesson is never to reduce gastrointestinal free calcium without also restricting dietary oxalate.

Water

This is a panacea for all urinary stone problems. For the doubters, it should be pointed out that dilution of urine reduces all urinary ionic concentrations so that the effect for calcium oxalate relates to the square of urinary volume, while for magnesium ammonium phosphate, it is related to the cube of the urinary volume. Even if the water supply is rich in calcium, the effect will still be to reduce urinary oxalate just as well as will soft water, and even urinary calcium concentration will be reduced[156] unless all the water is lost in sweat. The problem with high water intake is mainly to persuade patients to take it day and night and to take more when exposed to heat. To this end they should be given written instructions on "good water drinking"—setting out aims and how to achieve them, the hazards, and ways of checking on urinary volume (color of urine, frequency of micturition, measuring urinary volume).

Diet

The aim of a diet (for calcium oxalate urolithiasis) should be to lower urinary oxalate and calcium in that order. This is best achieved by low oxalate and calcium diets (see below). Bran may have a part to play in lowering urinary calcium,[28,29,157] but one might expect this to raise urinary oxalate, as does cellulose phosphate (see below). A recent report, however, revealed that one type of bran actually lowered urinary oxalate,[158] and this would be helpful if confirmed. A case can also be made for restriction of dietary carbohydrate, protein (see above), purines, and ascorbic acid (see below), but to insist on restricting all these items is clearly impractical and it is probably more effective to ignore these aspects and concentrate on restriction of calcium and oxalate intake alone.

Lowering of Urinary Calcium

There are now highly effective ways of lowering urinary calcium. The diet should be low in milk, cheese, and products thereof. Moderate restriction of salt may be helpful, as may addition of bran (see above). Thiazide diuretics lower urinary calcium[81,159–161] by acting on the renal tubules[162] and cellulose phosphate reduces calcium absorption from the intestinal tract. Lowering urinary calcium does not necessarily mean reduced risk of urolithiasis, however, and it is necessary to consider whether this occurs in each case. Thiazides have been said to reduce stone recurrence rate by some,[163,164] but others have disagreed.[159,165] Unfortunately, all these studies are open to criticism either because of lack of proper controls or because of the short duration of the trial. A recent study[154] had a mean followup time of over 11 years and showed that patients on bendrofluazide had a definite stone recurrence rate of 58 percent and a possible, but not certain, recurrence rate of a further 27 percent. While these results appear to be very poor, they were not as bad as they seemed because even the smallest detectable stone growth in a period of 20 years was accepted as a recurrence. More, better-controlled, and longer studies are clearly required, but at the present time it seems that thiazides probably do reduce stone recurrence rate, although not sufficiently.

Cellulose phosphate therapy seems clearly discredited as a means of reducing stone recurrence rate. Although success was reported with this treatment when used in conjunction with magnesium supplements for 1.5–4.8 years,[166] others who did not use magnesium supplements reported no success.[154,167] Cellulose phosphate certainly reduces urinary calcium[154] but can lead to increased calcium oxalate crystalluria,[79] presumably as a result of reduction in urinary magnesium[168,169] and rise in urinary oxalate, unless dietary oxalate is severely restricted.[169] The author now considers that cellulose phosphate is best avoided. Although it might be used together with dietary oxalate restriction and magnesium supplements, there are two further side effects: (1) up to a quarter of the patients may develop diarrhea or offensive stools;[4] and (2) after many years of therapy, patients may develop metabolic hyperoxaluria.[150]

In 1981 it was reported independently from two centers[170,171] that the prostaglandin synthesis inhibitor indomethacin lowered urinary calcium, although the reports differed in certain important details. The effect seemed to be mediated through depression of prostaglandin synthesis[171] and was also shown by flurbiprofen (Froben, Boots, Shreveport, LA).[173] Others have been unable to confirm the effect,[174,175] however, and there must be some doubt as to (1) whether urinary calcium can be lowered in the long term by indomethacin and (2) whether this would reduce stone recurrence rate. Again, more work is required.

Ways of Lowering Urinary Oxalate

Diet

Although there is a common belief that most normal urinary oxalate is endogenous, this is probably incorrect (see above), and the best way to reduce urinary oxalate is to restrict dietary intake. There are, however, other factors that should be mentioned.

Oxalate restriction. It has been shown that intake of certain oxalate-rich foods does lead to increased urinary oxalate.[176,177] These foods are, in order of importance, rhubarb, nuts, chocolate, beetroot, strawberries, spinach, tea (especially iced), instant coffee, and celery. Notable ommissions are tomatoes and Coca Cola (in England).

Ascorbate restriction. Because ascorbate converts to oxalate nonenzymatically in vitro,[146,178,179] many assays for urinary oxalate are invalid in the presence of ascorbate. Consequently, much of the work purporting to show in vivo conversion of ascorbate to oxalate could be invalid. Nevertheless, some such nonenzymatic conversion must take place in the bloodstream,[90] and recently it has been shown[180] that stone formers have delayed gastrointestinal absorption of ascorbate with consequential increased conversion to oxalate. It is probable, therefore, that there is merit in restricting high ascorbate intake to reduce urinary oxalate.

Purine restriction. It has been known for a long time (but largely forgotten) that there is a metabolic pathway from purines to oxalate.[181,182] High purine intake can lead to a significant increase in urinary oxalate;[183] therefore, high dietary purine should be avoided in calcium oxalate urolithiasis.

Allopurinol

There is a certain amount of evidence that allopurinol lowers urinary oxalate.[183–185] The effect is rather small, and in order to see it, the subject should be on a low-oxalate, high-purine diet. If these observations are correct, it offers a rational explanation for the alleged effect of allopurinol in reducing calcium oxalate stone recurrences as claimed by some[186–188] but denied by others.[189,190] The alternative idea that allopurinol could have such an effect through reduction of urinary urate seems untenable in the light of the observations that urate does not increase calcium oxalate crystal formation in whole urine.[94,101] The effect of allopurinol in reducing urinary urate is much smaller than can be obtained by restriction of dietary oxalate, however, and it is suggested that the former should only be used in conjunction with the latter, and not as an alternative.

Pyridoxine

It has been known for a long time that pyridoxine deficiency causes hyperoxaluria in animals and humans; thus, use of pyridoxine was advised for calcium oxalate urolithiasis as a means of lowering urinary oxalate.[187] This was thought to be accomplished,[191] but it seems doubtful that the methods then in use for measuring urinary oxalate could have detected the small reduction claimed. This work should be repeated with modern proven methods of high precision. In the author's laboratory it was shown[149] that giving pyridoxine to normal subjects had no effect on urinary oxalate, but there is always the possibility, albeit a remote one, that idiopathic stone formers might behave differently.

In cases of metabolic hyperoxaluria (see Chapter 16), the situation is quite different; in such cases, pyridoxine therapy is clearly indicated.

Magnesium

Magnesium hydroxide (or oxide) by mouth has been advocated for some 20 years as a preventive measure for urolithiasis. The claims in earlier papers were not convincing[187,192] because there were no proper controls. It was also claimed that magnesia was helpful in primary hyperoxaluria,[193,194] and more recent papers with controlled trials do seem to show that magnesia is effective.[195–197] These observations seem to be in keeping with the finding (see above) that raising urinary magnesium reduces calcium oxalate and phosphate crystal formation when dilute urine is concentrated by evaporation.[92] It does seem at the present time that magnesium therapy should be used more often than in the past.

Phosphate

The use of inorganic phosphate to prevent urolithiasis has been reviewed recently,[198] and it does not seem necessary to repeat this here. Certain points need to be made, however. First, only neutral phosphate should be used since the acid phosphate seems to be ineffective.[199] Second, neutral phosphate does seem to reduce calcium oxalate stone formation in primary hyperoxaluria[193,198] and idiopathic stone disease.[198,200,201] Third, neutral phosphate affects urine composition in many ways, and which of these are beneficial and which are simply coincidental is still not quite clear. Initially, authors stressed the rise in pyrophosphate, but it is unlikely that this actually reduces calcium oxalate crystal formation in whole urine.[93] Urinary calcium falls, and presumably this must be a factor. Perhaps more important is the rise in urinary citrate consequent to rise in urinary pH caused by giving a neutral salt of considerable buffering power. Fourth, the treatment is not without side effects. Diarrhea forces a reduction in dose in a considerable proportion of cases. The considerable sodium load can cause or aggravate hypertension. Nevertheless, the treatment remains useful and of great interest.

Alkalis

The idea of treating calcium oxalate urolithiasis by alkalinization of the urine is rather novel. It seems to have originated from a report in 1981[202] with the purpose of raising urinary citrate.

Alkalinization can be achieved equally well with sodium or potassium bicarbonate or citrates or mixtures thereof and with similar effects on urinary pH and citrate. However, the effects on other substances in the urine does depend on the form of the alkali given. Thus, while a mixture of sodium and potassium citrates and citric acid raised urinary pH and citrate,[203] oral citrate also seems to reduce urinary calcium in both rats[204] and human stone formers.[205] The use of potassium citrate has been advocated[205] to avoid the hypertensive and hypercalciuric effects of sodium. There are claims that such alkali therapy reduces calcium oxalate urolithiasis,[206] but so far the trials have been uncontrolled and more studies are needed.

Thiosulfate

A recent paper from Greece[207] reports that when 20 mmol/day of thiosulfate was given orally, about 25 percent of the load appeared in the urine and there was a marked fall in ionized calcium. During a 4-year period of treatment 34 patients with idiopathic calcium urolithiasis showed a fall to a ninth in stone recurrence rate compared to the 3 previous years of observation. This seems to merit further observation.

PREDICTING THE OUTCOME OF THERAPY

One major problem in treating stone formers is to how to know, without waiting for 5 or 10 years, whether the treatment used is effective. There are at least three ways in which this might be done: (1) measurement of ion activity products in urine, (2) observation of crystals in urine, and (3) observation of the "discriminant index."

The first of these is not considered further. It is difficult to perform and of doubtful significance for reasons that have been considered in the section on physical chemistry. The other two methods are considered below.

Observations of Crystals in Urine

Several groups of investigators have shown that patients with calcium oxalate (phosphate) urolithiasis excrete more calcium oxalate crystals in the urine and that the crystals are larger and more aggregated than is the case with normal subjects.[69,70,78] Furthermore, treatment of stone formers with bendrofluazide lowers calcium oxalate crystal excretion.[70,78] Cellulose phosphate therapy without dietary oxalate restriction causes hyperoxaluria with increase in calcium oxalate crystalluria,[70] but when dietary oxalate was restricted, both the hyperoxaluria and calcium oxalate crystalluria were reduced.[208] All this strongly suggests that observations of crystalluria might be a good predictor of stone recurrence and be a means of judging efficiency of treatment without having to wait and see whether stone recurrence actually occurred; however, it will obviously take a long time to prove that this is so. Not the least of the problems of such research is to know what sort of urine sample should be studied. Samples should be examined fresh and at 37°C, and 24-hour collections are not suitable (see above). Samples at different times of day may give different results.[70]

Use of the Discriminant Index

The so-called discriminant index (DI) was devised in Israel.[209] Striking claims have been made for the use of this technique (see below), and it is important to have a clear understanding of what the technique does. Fresh early-morning urine is filtered to remove cell fragments or other solid matter. Then 20 ml of urine is mixed with 75 ml of distilled water and the calcium (ion) concentration then raised to 4 m*M*. An equal volume of 6 m*M* oxalate solution is added and rapidly mixed. The calcium ion concentration is measured continually with a calcium electrode with a 20-second response time. Precipitation of calcium oxalate begins immediately and the calcium ion concentration recorded at 30 seconds and 10 minutes. The log of the ratio of the two calcium ion concentrations is the DI, and the normal range is -0.4 to 2.8. The lower the DI, the greater the inhibitory potential of the urine.

In a recent paper[210] it was claimed that the DI can be used to monitor the efficiency of treatment in preventing stone recurrences. This is a remarkable claim, and it is important that it be evaluated by an independent group. The present author, however, sees two problems. First, it is difficult to understand how one can properly record a rapidly changing calcium ion concentration 30 seconds after the mixing when the electrode used has a response time of 20 seconds. Second, the DI appears to be measuring inhibitors of crystal formation, and not calcium ion activities. Hence, if the DI signals a decreased risk of stone formation in response to thiazides, allopurinol, or inorganic phosphate therapy, the implications must be that these drugs act by changing the inhibitors of crystal formation, and this is rather surprising.

REFERENCES

1. Anderson DA: Environmental factors in the aetiology of urolithiasis, in Delatte LC, Rapado A, Hodgkinson A (eds): Urinary Calculi. Karger, Basel, 1973, pp 130–144,
2. Andersen DA: A survey of the incidence of urolithiasis in Norway from 1853 to 1960. J Oslo City Hosp 16:101–147, 1966
3. Henneman PH, Benedict PH, Forbes AP, et al: Idiopathic hypercalciuria. New Engl J Med 259:802–807, 1958
4. Rose GA, Harrison AR: The incidence, investigation and treatment of idiopathic hypercalciuria. Br J Urol 46:261–274, 1974
5. Pak CYC, Ohato M, Lawrence E, et al: The hypercalciurias. Causes, parathyroid functions and diagnostic criteria. J Clin Invest 54:387–400, 1974
6. Robertson WG, Peacock M, Heyburn PJ, et al: The risk of calcium stone formation in relation

to affluence and dietary animal protein, in Brockis JG, Finlayson B (eds): Urinary Calculus. Littleton, MA, PSG Publishing Co, 1981, pp 3–12

7. Valyasevi A, Dhanamitta S: Studies of bladder stone disease in Thailand. Urinary studies in newborn and infants of hypo and hyperendemic areas. Am J Clin Nutr 20:1369–1377, 1967
8. Flocks RH: Calcium and phosphate excretion in the urine of patients with renal or ureteric calculi. JAMA 113:1466–1471, 1939
9. Hodgkinson A, Pyrah LN: The urinary excretion of calcium and inorganic phosphate in 344 patients with calcium stone of renal origin. Br J Surg 46:10–18, 1958
10. Bulusu L, Hodgkinson A, Nordin BEC, Peacock M: Urinary secretion of calcium and creatinine in relation to age and body weight in normal subjects and patients with renal calculus. Clin Sci 38:601–612, 1970
11. Robertson WG, Morgan DB: The distribution of urinary calcium in normal persons and stone formers. Clin Chim Acta 37:503–508, 1972
12. King JS, O'Connor FJ, Smith MJU, et al: The urinary calcium/magnesium ratio in calcinogenous stone formers. Invest Urol 6:60–65, 1968
13. Welshman SG, McGeown MG: The relationship of the urinary cations, calcium, magnesium, sodium and potassium in patients with renal calculi. Br J Urol 47:237–242, 1978
14. Tiselius HG, Alvigard LE, Larsson GL, et al: A biochemical basis for grouping of patients with urolithiasis. Eur Urol 4:241–249, 1978
15. Ryall RL, Marshall VR: The value of the 24 hour urine analysis in the assessment of stone formers attending a general hospital out-patient clinic. Br J Urol 55:1–5, 1983
16. Griffith HM, O'Shea B, Kevany JP, et al: A control study of dietary factors in renal stone formation. Br J Urol 53:416–420, 1981
17. Power C, Barker DJP, Nelson M, et al: Diet and renal stones: a case-control study. Br J Urol 56:456–459, 1984
18. Blacklock NJ, Macleod MA: Calcium-47 absorption in urolithiasis. Br J Urol 46:377–383, 1979
19. Dunscombe VM, Watts RWE, Peters TJ: Studies on intestinal calcium absorption in patients with idiopathic hypercalciuria. Quart J Med 53:69–79, 1984
20. Liverman UA, Sperling O, Atsmon A, et al: Metabolic and calcium kinetic studies in idiopathic hypercalciuria. J Clin Invest 47:2580–2590, 1968
21. Aladjem M, Modan M, Lusky A, et al: Idiopathic hypercalciuria: A familial generalised renal hyperexcretory state. Kidney Internatl 24:549–554, 1983
22. Nicolaysen R: The calcium requirement of man as related to diseases of the skeleton. Clin Orthop 17:226–234, 1960
23. Robertson WG, Peacock M, Heyburn PJ, et al: Should recurrent calcium oxalate stone formers become vegetarians? Br J Urol 51:427–431, 1979
24. Blacklock NJ: Epidemiology, in Chisholm GD, Williams DI (eds): Scientific Foundations of Urology. London, Heinemann, 1982, Chapter 32
25. Cleave TL: The Saccharine Disease. Bristol, Wright, 1974
26. Lemann J, Piering WF, Lennon EJ: Possible role of carbohydrate induced calciuria in calcium oxalate kidney stone formation. New Engl J Med 280:232–237, 1969
27. Yoshido O: Epidemiology of urolithiasis in Japan. Jap J Urol 70:975–983, 1979
28. Shah PJR, Williams G, Green NA: Idiopathic hypercalciuria: Its control with unprocessed bran. Br J Urol 52:426–429, 1980
29. Okawa T, Ebisuno S, Kitagawa M, et al: Rice bran for hypercalciuria patients with urinary calculous disease. J Urol 129:1009–1011, 1983
30. Black JM: Oxaluria in British troups in India. Br Med J 1:590–592, 1945
31. Pierce LW, Bloom B: Observations in urolithiasis among American troops in a desert area. J Urol 54:466–470, 1945
32. Frank M, deVries A, Lazebnik I, et al: Epidemiological investigations of urolithiasis in Israel. J Urol 81:497–504, 1959

33. von Boshamer K: The calculus areas of the world, in von Boshamer K, Handbuch der urologie, Vol 10. Berlin, Stringer, 1961, p 34
34. Blacklock NJ: The pattern of urolithiasis in the Royal Navy. in Hodgkinson A, Nordin BEC (eds): Proceedings of the Renal Stone Research Symposium. London, Churchill Livingstone, 1969, pp 33–47
35. Kohler FP: Asymptomatic upper urinary tract lithiasis in flying personnel. J Urol 86:370–372, 1961
36. Frank M, deVries A: Prevention of urolithiasis. Arch Environ Health 13:625–630, 1966
37. Rose GA: Hot climate or chronic-dehydration stone disease, in Rose GA: Urinary Stones: Clinical and Laboratory Aspects. Lancaster, England, MTP Press, 1982, pp 234–238
38. Robertson WG, Peacock M, Heyburn PJ, et al: Risk factors in calcium stone disease of the urinary tract. Br J Urol 50:449–454, 1978
39. Robertson WG, Peacock M, Heyburn PJ, et al: Risk factors in calcium stone disease, in Brockis JG, Finlayson B (eds): Urinary Calculus. Littleton, MA, PSG Publishing Co, 1981, pp 265–273
40. Ryall RL, Darroch JN, Marshall VR: The evaluation of risk factors in male stone-formers attending a general hospital out-patient clinic. Br J Urol 56:116–121, 1984
41. Robertson WG, Peacock M, Nordin BEC: Activity products in stone-forming and non-stone forming urine. Clin Sci 34:579–594, 1968
42. Finlayson B: Calcium stones: Some physical and clinical aspects, in David DS (ed): Calcium Metabolism in Renal Failure and Nephrolithiasis. New York, Wiley, 1977, pp 337–382
43. Werness PG, Brown CB, Smith LH, et al: Equil 2: A basic computer programme for the calculation of urinary saturation. J Urol 134:1242–1244, 1985
44. Horvath AL: Handbook of aqueous electrolyte solution. Chichester, England, Ellis Horwood, 1985
45. Miller GH, Vermeulen CW, Moore JD: Calcium oxalate solubility in urine: experimental urolithiasis XIV. J Urol 79:607–612, 1958
46. Elliott JS, Eusebio E: Calcium oxalate solubility: The effect of inorganic salts, urea, creatinine, and organic acids. Invest Urol 3:72–76, 1965
47. Finlayson B, Rotha A, Dubois LG: Perturbation of calcium ion activity by urea. Invest Urol 10:138–140, 1972
48. Hodgkinson A: Solubility of calcium oxalate in human urine, simulated urine and water. Invest Urol 18:123–126, 1980
49. Robertson WG, Peacock M, Nordin BEC: Calcium crystalluria in recurrent renal stone formers. Lancet 2:21–24, 1969
50. Werness PG, Bergert JH, Smith LH: Crystalluria. J Crystal Growth 53:166–181, 1981
51. Hesse A, Berg W, Schneider HJ, et al: A contribution to the formation mechanism of calcium oxalate urinary calculi. I. Stabilizing urinary constituents in the formation of Weddelite urinary calculi. Urol Res 4:125–128, 1976
52. Hesse A, Berg W, Schneider HJ, et al: A contribution to the formation mechanism of calcium oxalate urinary calculi. II. In vitro experiments concerning the theory of the formation of Whewellite urinary calculi. Urol Res 4:157–160, 1976
53. Hesse A, Berg W, Schneider HJ, et al: A contribution to the formation mechanism of calcium oxalate urinary calculi. III. On the role of magnesium in the formation of oxalate calculi. Urol Res 4:161–167, 1976
54. Bellanato J, Delatte LC, Hidalgo A, et al: Application of infra red spectroscopy to the study of renal stones, in Delatte LC, Rapado A, Hodgkinson (eds): Urinary Calculi. Basel, Karger, 1973, pp 237–246
55. Rose GA, Woodfine C: The thermogravimetric analysis of renal stones (in clinical practice). Br J Urol 48:403–412, 1976
56. Heijnen W, Jellinghaus W, Klee WE: Calcium oxalate trihydrate in urinary calculi. Urol Res 13:281–283, 1985

57. Lyon ES, Vermeulen CW: Crystallization concepts and calculogenesis: Observations on an artificial oxalate concentration. Invest Urol 3:309–320, 1965
58. Robertson WG, Peacock M, Nordin BEC: Inhibitors of the growth and aggregation of calcium oxalate crystals in vivo. Clin Chim Acta 43:31–37, 1973
59. Coe FL, Lawton RL, Goldstein RB, et al: Sodium urate accelerates precipitation of calcium oxalate in vitro. Proc Soc Exp Biol Med 149:926–929, 1975
60. Meyer JL: Nucleation kinetics in the calcium oxalate-sodium urate monohydrate system. Invest Urol 19:197–201, 1981
61. Baumann JM, Wacker M: The direct measurement of inhibitory capacity to crystal growth of calcium oxalate in undiluted urine and in other inhibitor containing solutions. Urol Res 8:171–175, 1980
62. Sheeham ME, Nancollas GH: Calcium oxalate crystal growth: A new constant composition method for modelling urinary stone formation. Invest Urol 17:446–450, 1980
63. Boyce WH, Garvey FK: The amount and nature of organic matrix in urinary calculi: a review. J Urol 76:213–227, 1956
64. Finlayson B, Vermeulen CW, Stewart EJ: Stone matrix and mucoprotein from urine. J Urol 86:355–363, 1961
65. Tomazic BB, Nancollas GH: A study of the phase transformation of calcium oxalate trihydrate-monohydrate. Invest Urol 16:329–335, 1979
66. Gardner GL, Doremus RH: Crystal growth inhibitors in human urine. Effect of calcium oxalate kinetics. Invest Urol 15:478–485, 1978
67. Tiselius HG: Inhibition of calcium oxalate crystal growth in urine during treatment with allopurinol. Br J Urol 52:189–192, 1980
68. Sengbusch RV, Timmermann A: Die Bildung von Calcium-oxalat Mikrosteinen im menschlichen Harn und Ihre Veranderung Durch Diatetsche und Medikomentose Massnahmen. Urol Internatl 5:218–231, 1957
69. Robertson WG, Peacock M, Nordin BEC: Calcium oxalate crystalluria and urine saturation in recurrent renal stone formers. Clin Sci 40:365–374, 1971
70. Hallson PC, Rose GA: Crystalluria in normal subjects and in stone formers with and without thiazide and cellulose phosphate treatment. Br J Urol 48:515–524, 1976
71. Nash RA, Haeger BE: Zeta potential in the development of pharmaceutical suspensions. J Pharm Sci 55:829–837, 1966
72. Robertson WG, Scurr DS, Sergeant VJ: Ionic and macromolecular modifiers of crystallisation of calcium salts in urine, in Gasser G, Vahlensieck W (eds): Pathogenese und Klinik der Harnsteine, Vol 11. Darmstadt, Steinkopff Verlag, 1985, pp 1–11
73. Rushton HG, Spector M, Rodgers AL, et al: Developmental aspects of calcium oxalate tubular deposits and calculi induced by rat kidneys. Invest Urol 19:52–57, 1981
74. Hallson PC, Rose GA: A new urinary test for "stone activity." Br J Urol 50:442–448, 1978
75. Ryall RL, Hibberd CM Marshall VR: A method of studying inhibitory activity in whole urine. Urol Res 13:285–289, 1985
76. Rose GA: Urinary Stones: Clinical and Laboratory Aspects. Lancaster, MTP Press, 1982, pp 10–11
77. Dyer R, Nordin BEC: Urinary crystals and their relation to stone formation. Nature 215:751–752, 1967
78. Werness PG, Bergert JH, Smith LH: Crystalluria J Cryst Growth 53:166–181, 1981
79. Elliott JS, Rabinowitcz IN: Calcium oxalate crystalluria: Crystal size in urine. J Urol 123:324–327, 1980
80. Hallson PC, Rose GA: Seasonal variations in urinary crystals. Br J Urol 49:227–284, 1977
81. Marickar YMF, Rose GA: Relationship of stone growth and urinary biochemistry in long-term follow-up of stone patients with idiopathic hypercalciuria. Br J Urol 57:613–617, 1985
82. Von Hemsbach M: Mikrogealogie. Berlin, 1856
83. Lichwitz L: In Alexander J (ed): Colloid Chemistry, Vol. 5. New York City, Chemical Catalogue Co. 1944, p 1063

84. Hallson PC, Rose GA: Uromucoids and urinary stone formation. Lancet 1:1000–1002, 1979
85. Rose GA, Sulaiman S: Tamm-Horsfall mucoproteins promote calcium oxalate crystal formation in urine: Quantitative studies. J Urol 127:177–179, 1982
86. Rose GA, Sulaiman S: Tamm-Horsfall mucoproteins promote calcium phosphate crystal formation in whole urine: quantitative studies. Urol Res 12:217–221, 1984
87. Kitamura T, Pak CYC: Tamm and Horsfall glycoprotein does not promote spontaneous precipitation and crystal growth of calcium oxalate in vitro. J Urol 127:1024–1026, 1982
88. Kasidas GP, Rose GA: Measurement of plasma oxalate in healthy subjects and in patients with chronic renal failure using immobilised oxalate oxidase. Clin Chim Acta 154:49–58, 1986
89. Khan SR, Hackett RL: Developmental morphology of calcium oxalate foreign body stones in rats. Calc Tissue Internatl 37:165–173, 1985
90. Hallson PC, Rose GA, Samuell CT: The role of uromucoids in urinary stone formation, in Brockis JG, Finlayson B (eds): Urinary Calculus, Littleton, MA, PSG Publishing Co, 1981, pp 285–295
91. Hallson PC, Rose GA, Sulaiman S: Raising urinary citrate lowers calcium and oxalate and calcium phosphate crystal formation in whole urine. Urol Internatl 38:179–181, 1983
92. Hallson PC, Rose GA, Sulaiman S: Magnesium reduces calcium oxalate crystal formation in human whole urine. Clin Sci 62:17–19, 1982
93. Hallson PC, Rose GA, Sulaiman S: Pyrophosphate does not influence calcium oxalate or calcium phosphate crystal formation in concentrated whole human urine. Urol Res 11:151–154, 1983
94. Hallson PC, Rose GA, Sulaiman S: Urate does not influence the formation of calcium oxalate crystals in whole human urine at pH 5.3. Clin Sci 62:421–425, 1982
95. Hallson PC, Rose GA: The additive effects of magnesium and tartrate upon inhibition of calcium oxalate crystal formation in whole urine, in Schwille PO, Smith LH, Robertson WG, et al (eds): Urolithiasis and Related Clinical Research. New York, Plenum Press, 1984, pp 847–850
96. Welshman SG, McGeown MG: A quantitative investigation of the effects on the growth of calcium oxalate crystals on potential inhibitors. Br J Urol 44:677–680, 1972
97. Meyer JL, Smith LH: Growth of calcium oxalate crystals. II. Inhibition by natural urinary crystal growth inhibitors. Invest Urol 13:36–39, 1975
98. Drach GW, Robertson WG, Scurr DS, et al: Pyrophosphate inhibition of calcium oxalate dihydrate crystallisation in simulated urine: Continuous flow studies. World. J Urol 1:146–149, 1983
99. Coe FL: Hyperuricosuric calcium oxalate nephrolithiasis. Kidney Internatl 13:418–426, 1978
100. Pak CYC, Holt K, Zerwekh J: Attenuation by monosodium urate of the inhibitory effect of mucopolysaccharide on calcium oxalate nucleation. Invest Urol 17:138–140, 1979
101. Ryall RL, Hibberd CM, Marshall VR: The effect of crystalline monosodium urate on the crystallisation of calcium oxalate in whole human urine. Urol Res 14:63–65, 1986
102. Tiselius HG, Berg C, Larsson L: Evaluation of crystallisation risk in calcium stone formers. Urol Res 14:91, 1986
103. Ackerman D, Baumann JM, Wacker M: The relation between chemical composition and crystallisation conditions in whole urine of calcium stone formers. Urol Res 14:91, 1986
104. Joost J, Kleboth K: Measurements of inhibitory activity in the urine of calcium oxalate stone formers. Urol Res 14:91, 1986
105. Finlayson B, Reid F: The expectation of free and fixed particles in urinary stone disease. Invest Urol 15:442–448, 1978
106. Rushton HG, Spector M, Rodgerson AL, et al: Developmental aspects of calcium oxalate tubular deposits and calculi induced in rat kidneys. Invest Urol 19:52–57, 1981
107. Hallson PC, Rose GA, Samuell CT: The role of uromucoids in urinary stone formation, in Brockis JG, Finlayson B (eds): Urinary Calculus, Littleton, MA, PSG Publishing Co, 1981, pp 285–295

108. Hastings AB, McLean FC, Eichelberger L, et al: The ionisation of calcium, magnesium and strontium citrates. J Biol Chem 107:351–370, 1934
109. Ryall RL, Hibberd CM, Marshall VR: A method for studying inhibitory activity in whole urine. Urol Res 13:285–289, 1985
110. Kok CJ, Papapoulos SE, Bijvoet OLM: A physicochemical exploration for the role of citrate in recurrent stone disease. Urol Res 14:94, 1986
111. Natelson S, Pincus JB, Lugovoy JK: Microestimation of citric acid: A new colourimetric method for pentabromacetome. J Biol Chem 175:745–750, 1948
112. Moellering H, Gruber W: Determination of citrate by citrate lyase. Anal Biochem 17:369–376, 1966
113. Burr RG, Nuseibeh I, Abiaka CD: Biochemical studies in paraplegic renal stone patients. 2. Urinary excretion of citrate, inorganic pyrophosphate, silica and urate. Br J Urol 57:275–278, 1985
114. Graef V, Schmidtman H, Jarrar K: On the preservation of urines for the determination of citrate, in Schwille PO, Smith LH, Robertson WG, et al (eds): Urolithiasis and Related Clinical Research. New York, Plenum Press, 1985, pp 689–692
115. Dedmon RE, Wrong O: The excretion of organic anion in renal tubular acidosis with particular reference to citrate. Clin Sci 22:19–32, 1962
116. Nordin BEC, Smith DA: Citric acid excretion in patients with renal calculi. J Urol 129:1158–1160, 1983
117. Hodgkinson A: Citric acid excretion in normal adults and in patients with renal calculus. Clin Sci 23:203–212, 1962
118. Fraser AK, Gregory MC, Rose GA, et al: A study of factors affecting urinary citrate levels, in Schwille PO, Smith LH, Robertson WG (eds): Urolithiasis and Related Clinical Research. New York, Plenum Press, 1985, pp 249–252
119. Welshman SG, McGeown MG: Urinary citrate excretion in stone formers and normal controls. Br J Urol 48:7–11, 1976
120. Tiselius HG: Urinary excretion of citrate in normal subjects and in patients with urolithiasis, in Smith LH, Robertson WG, Finlayson B (eds): Urolithiasis: Clinical and Basic Research. New York, Plenum Press, 1985, pp 39–44
121. Lux B, Braun J, May P, et al: Ausscheidung von citrat, calcium und magnesium bei Harnsteinbildern. Fortschr Urol Nephrol 20:92–95, 1982
122. May P, Braun J, Lux B, et al: Citratkonzentration im serum und urine bei Gesunden und Harnsteinbildern. Fortschr Urol Nephrol 20:198–201, 1982
123. Menon M, Mahle CJ: Urinary citrate excretion in patients with renal calculi. J Urol 129:1158–1160, 1983
124. Hosking PH, Wilson JWL, Kiedtke RR, et al: Urinary citrate excretion in normal persons and patients with idiopathic calcium urolithiasis. J Lab Clin Med 106:682–689, 1985
125. Schwille PO, Scholz D, Schwille K, et al: Citrate in urine and serum and dissociated variables in sub-groups of urolithiasis. Nephron 31:194–202, 1982
126. Shorr E, Berscheim AR, Taussky H: The relation between urinary citric acid excretion to the menstrual cycle and the steroidal reproductive hormones. Science 95:606–607, 1942
127. Rudman D, Dedonis JL, Fountain MT, et al: Hypocitraturia in patients with gastrointestinal malabsorption. New Engl J Med 303:657–661, 1980
128. Hagmaier V, Werness P, Schmidt K, et al: Enteric hyperoxaluria risk factors for urolithiasis in addition to hyperoxaluria, in Ryall R, Brokis JG, Marshall V, et al (eds): Urinary Stone. London, Churchill Livingstone, 1984, pp 241–247
129. Backman L, Backman U, Danielson GB, et al: Renal tubular function in patients following intestinal by-pass operations, in Schwille PO, Smith LH, Robertson WG, et al (eds): Urolithiasis and Related Clinical Research. New York, Plenum Press, 1985, pp 143–146
130. Royer P, Lestradet H, Nordmann R, et al: Etudes sur quatre cas d'acidose tubulaire clinique idiopathique avec hypocitraturia. Sem Hop 38:808–829, 1962

131. Morrissey JF, Ochoa M, Lotspeich WD, et al: Citrate excretion in renal tubular acidosis. Ann Intern Med 58:159–166, 1963
132. Elliott JS, Ribeiro ME: The urinary excretion of citric, hippuric and lactic acid in normal adults and in patients with calcium oxalate urinary calculus disease. Invest Urol 10:102–106, 1972
133. Rudman D, Kutner MH, Redd SC II, et al: Hypocitraturia in calcium nephrolithiasis. J Clin Endocrinol Metab 55:1052–1057, 1982
134. Nicar MJ, Skurla C, Sakhaee K, et al: Low urinary citrate excretion in nephrolithiasis. Urology 21:8–14, 1983
135. Huber RD: Matouschek, Citratausscheidung und Konzentration im 24 h Harn bei Kalziumoxatsteintragein und stein—frein patienten, in Pathogenese und Klinik der Harnsteine X. Darmstadt, Steinkopff, 1984, pp 116–118
136. Kass MA, Kolker AE, Gordon M, et al: Acetazolamide and urolithiasis. Ophthalmology 88:261–265, 1981
137. Meyer JL, Thomas WC Jr: Trace metal citric acid complexes as inhibitors of calcification and crystal growth. II. Effects of Fe(III), Cr(III) and Al (III) complexes on calcium phosphate crystal growth. J Urol 128:1372–1375, 1982
138. Meyer JL, Thomas WC Jr: Trace metal citric acid complexes as inhibitors of calcification and crystal growth. III. Effects of Fe(III), Cr(III) and Al (III) complexes on calcium oxalate crystal growth. J Urol 128:1376–1378, 1982
139. Roberson WG, Peacock M: The cause of idiopathic calcium stone disease, hypercalciuria or hyperoxaluria? Nephron 26:105–110, 1980
140. Robertson WG, Nordin BEC: Activity products in urine, in Hodgkinson A, Nordin BEC (eds): Renal Stone Research Symposium. London, Churchill Livingstone, 1969, pp 221–232
141. Wallace MR, Mason K, Gray J: Urine oxalate and calcium in idiopathic renal stone formers. NZ Med J 2:87–89, 1981
142. Marangella M, Fruttero B, Bruno M, et al: Hyperoxaluria in idiopathic calcium stone disease: Further evidence of intestinal hyperabsorption of oxalate. Clin Sci 63:381–385, 1982
143. Pinto B, Ruisz-Marcellan FJ, Bernshtam J: Effect of a 5-year treatment program in patients with hyperoxaluric stones. J Urol 130:943–944, 1983
144. Baggio B, Gambaro G, Favaro S, et al: Prevalence of hyperoxaluria in idiopathic calcium oxalate kidney stone disease. Nephron 35:11–14, 1983
145. Etoide T, Bowyer RC, Brockis JG: Comparison of urinary oxalate excretion in urolithiasis patients with and without hypercalciuria. Br J Urol 57:505–509, 1985
146. Rose GA: Advances in analysis of urinary oxalate: The ascorbate problem solved, in Schwille PO, Smith LH, Robertson WG, et al (eds): Urolithiasis and Related Clinical Research. New York, Plenum Press, 1985, pp 634–644
147. Kasidas GP, Rose GA: Spontaneous in vitro generation of oxalate from l-ascorbate in some assays for urinary oxalate and its prevention, in Schwille PO, Smith LH, Robertson WG, et al (eds): Urolithiasis and Related Clinical Research. New York, Plenum Press, 1985, pp 653–656
148. Kasidas GP, Rose GA: Continuous flow assay for urinary oxalate using immobilised oxalate oxidase. Ann Clin Biochem 22:412–419, 1985
149. Kasidas GP, Rose GA: Metabolic hyperoxaluria and its response to pyridoxine, in Ryall R, Brockis JG, Marshall V, et al (eds): Urinary Stone. London, Churchill Livingstone, 1983, pp 138–147
150. Kasidas GP, Rose GA, Samuell CT: Mild but clinically significant metabolic hyperoxaluria and its response to pyridoxine, in Gasser G, Vahlensieck W (eds): Pathogenese und Klinik der Harnsteine XI. Darmstadt, Steinkopff, 1985, pp 394–399
151. Ettinger B: Recurrent nephrolithiasis: natural history and effect of phopshate therapy. A double-blind controlled study. Am J Med 61:200–206, 1976
152. Smith MJV: Placebo versus allopurinol for renal calculi. J Urol 117:690–692, 1977

153. Brocks P, Dahl C, Wolf H, et al: Do thiazides prevent recurrent idiopthic renal calcium stones. Lancet 2:124–125, 1981
154. Hosking DH, Erickson SB, Van Den Berg CJ, et al: The stone clinic effect in patients with idiopathic calcium urolithiasis. J Urol 130:1115–1118, 1983
155. Erickson SB, Cooper K, Broadus AE, et al: Oxalate absorption and postprandial urine supersaturation in an experimental human model of absorptive hypercalciuria. Clin Sci 67:131–138, 1984
156. Rose GA: The medical treatment of renal lithiasis, in Wickham EJW (ed): Urinary Calculus Disease. Edinburgh, Churchill Livingstone, 1979
157. Macleod MA, Blacklock NJ: The influence of glucose and crude fibre (wheat bran) on the rate of intestinal 47 Ca absorption. J Roy Navy Med Serv 65:143–146, 1979
158. Stromaier WL, Bichler KH: Calcium metabolism under therapy with Farnolith in patients with hypercalciuria and normal persons. Urol Res 14:94, 1986
159. Yendt ER, Guay GF, Garcia PA: The use of thiazides in the prevention of renal calculi. Can Med Assoc J 28:614–620, 1970
160. Rose GA, Harrison AR: The incidence, investigation, and threatment of idiopathic hypercalciuria. Br J Urol 54:578–583, 1974
161. Gill HS, Rose GA: Idiopathic hypercalciuria. Urate and other ions in urine before and on various long-term treatments. Urol Res 13:291–275, 1985
162. Jorgensen FS: Effect of thiazide diuretics upon calcium metabolism. Dan Med Bull 23:223–230, 1976
163. Backman U, Danielson BG, Johansson G, et al: Effect of therapy with bendrofluazide in patients with recurrent renal calcium stones. Br J Urol 51:175–180, 1979
164. Laerum E, Larson S: Thiazide prophylaxis of urolithiasis. Acta Med Scand 215:383–389, 1984
165. Scholz D, Schwille PO, Sigel A: Double-blind study with thiazides in recurrent urolithiasis. J Urol 128:903–907, 1982
166. Pak CYC, Delea CS, Bartter FC: Successful treatment of recurrent nephrolithiasis (calcium stones) with cellulose phosphate. New Engl J Med 290:175–180, 1974
167. Backman U, Danielson BG, Johansson G, et al: Treatment of recurrent calcium stone formation with cellulose phosphate. J Urol 123:9–13, 1980
168. Dent CE, Harper CM, Parfitt AM: The effect of cellulose phosphate on calcium metabolism in patients with idiopathic hypercalciuria. Clin Sci 27:417–425, 1964
169. Hallson PC, Kasidas GP, Rose GA: The treatment of idiopathic hypercalciuria and stone formation, in Brockis JG, Finlayson B (eds): Urinary Calculus. Littleton, MA, PSG Publishing Co, 1981, pp 435–445
170. Carter WC, Halushka PV, Jones D, et al: Indomethacin lowers urinary calcium excretion in normal volunteers and normocalciuric stone formers, in Smith LH, Robertson WG, Finlayson B (eds): Urolithiasis: Clinical and Basic Research. New York, Plenum Press, 1981, pp 723–725
171. Buck AC, Sampson WF, Lote CJ, et al: The influence of renal prostoglandins on glomerular filtration rate (GFR) and calcium excretion in urolithiasis. Br J Urol 53:485–491, 1981
172. Buck AC: Renal prostoglandins and calcium excretion in urolithiasis. J Intern Med Res 11(Suppl 21):18–23, 1983
173. Rao PN, Blacklock NJ: An interim report of Flurbiprofen for the control of idiopathic hypercalciuria. J Intern Med Res 11(Suppl 2):24–27, 1983
174. Rocco VK, Sakhaee K, Pak CYC, et al: Lack of effect of prostaglandin inhibition on calcium excretion in normal volunteers. J Urol 133:1093–1094, 1985
175. Shah PJR, Rose GA: Prostaglandin synthesase inhibitors and their effect on urinary calcium excretion and other parameters in idiopathic hypercalciuria. Br J Urol 56:1–8, 1984
176. Finch AM, Kasidas GP, Rose GA: Urine composition in normal subjects after oral ingestion of oxalate-rich foods. Clin Sci 60:411–418, 1981
177. Hesse A, Strenge A, Vahlensieck W: Oxalic acid excretion of calcium oxalate stone formers

and of healthy persons, in Ryall R, Brockis JG, Marshall V, et al (eds): Urinary Stone. Edinburgh, Churchill Livingstone, 1984, pp 57–62
178. Mazzachi BC, Teubner JK, Ryall RL: The effect of ascorbic acid on urine oxalate measurement, in Schwille PO, Smith LH, Robertson WG, et al (eds): Urolithiasis and Related Clinical Research. New York, Plenum Press, 1985, pp 649–652
179. Scurr DS, Januzovich N, Smith A, et al: A comparison of three methods for measuring urinary oxalate, in Schwille PO, Smith LH, Robertson WG, et al (eds): Urolithiasis and Related Clinical Research. New York, Plenum Press, 1985, pp 645–648
180. Chalmers AH, Cowley DM, Brown JM: A possible etiological role for ascorbate in calculi formation. Clin Chem 32:333–336, 1986
181. Aponte GE, Fetter TR: Familial idiopathic oxalate nephrocalcinosis. Am J Clin Pathol 24:1363–1373, 1954
182. Zarembski PA, Hodgkinson A: Some factors influencing the urinary excretion of oxalic acid in man. Clin Chim Acta 25:1–101, 1969
183. Simmonds HA, VanAcker KJ, Potter CF, et al: Influence of purine content of diet and allopurinol on uric acid and oxalate excretion levels, in Smith LH, Robertson WG, Finlayson B (eds): Urolithiasis: Clinical and Basic Research. New York, Plenum Press, 1981, pp 363–367
184. Scott R, Paterson PJ, Mathieson A, et al: The effect of allopurinol on urinary oxalate excretion in stone formers. Br J Urol 50:455–458, 1978
185. Tomlinson B, Cohen SL, Al-Khader A, Kasidas GP, Rose GA: Further reduction of oxalate excretion by allopurinol in stone formers on low purine diet, in Schwille PO, Smith LH, Robertson WG, et al (eds): Urolithiasis and Related Clinical Research. New York, Plenum Press, 1985, pp 561–564
186. Smith MJV: Placebo versus allopurinol for renal calculi. J Urol 117:690–692, 1977
187. Gershoff SN, Prien EL: Effect of daily magnesium and vitamin B_6 administration to patients with recurring calcium oxalate kidney stones. Am J Clin Nutr 20:393–399, 1967
188. Fellström B, Backman U, Danielson BG, et al: Allopurinol treatment of renal calcium stone disease. Br J Urol 57:375–379, 1985
189. Marangella M, Tricerri A, Ronzani M, et al: The relationship between clinical outcome and urine biochemistry during various forms of therapy for idiopathic calcium stone disease, in Schwille PO, Smith LH, Robertson WG, et al (eds): Urolithiasis and Related Clinical Research. New York, Plenum Press, 1985, pp 561–564
190. Robertson WG, Peacock M, Selby PL, et al: A multicentre trial to evaluate three treatments for recurrent idiopathic calcium stone disease—a preliminary report, in Schwille PO, Smith LH, Robertson WG, et al (eds): Urolithiasis and Related Clinical Research. New York, Plenum Press, 1985, pp 545–548
191. Gershoff SN, Mayer AL, Kulczycki LL: Effect of pyridoxine administration on the urinary excretion of oxalic acid, pyridoxine, and related compounds in mongoloids and non-mongoloids. Am J Clin Nutr 7:76–79, 1959
192. Moore CA, Bunce GE: Reduction in frequency of renal calculus formation by oral magnesium administration. A preliminary report. Invest Urol 2:7–13, 1964
193. Dent CE, Stamp TCB: Treatment of primary hyperoxaluria. Arch Dis Child 45:735–745, 1970
194. Silver L, Brendler H: Use of magnesium oxide in management of hyperoxaluria. J Urol 106:274–279, 1971
195. Melnick I, Landes RR, Hoffman AA, et al: Magnesium therapy for recurring calcium oxalate urinary calculi. J Urol 105:119–122, 1971
196. Johansson G, Backman U, Danielson BG, et al: Biochemical and clinical effects of the prophylactic treatment of renal calcium stones with magnesium hydroxide. J Urol 124:770–774, 1980
197. Danielson BG: Drugs against kidney stones. Effects of magnesium and alkali, in Schwille PO, Smith LH, Robertson WG, et al (eds): Urolithiasis and Related Clinical Research. New York, Plenum Press, 1985, pp 525–532

198. Smith LH: The effects of orthophosphate and ion binders, in Schwille PO, Smith LH, Robertson WG, et al (eds): Urolithiasis and Related Clinical Research. New York, Plenum Press, 1985, pp 483–489
199. Ettinger B, Kolb FO: Inorganic phosphate treatment of nephrolithiasis. Am J Med 55:32–37, 1973
200. Bernstein DS, Newton R: The effect of oral sodium phosphate on the formation of renal calculi and on idiopathic hypercalciuria. Lancet 2:1105–1107, 1966
201. Oliver I, Weinberger A, Bar-Meir S, et al: Orthophosphate treatment of calcium lithiasis associated with idiopathic hypercalicuria. Urol Internatl 29:414–420, 1974
202. Butz M, Dulce HJ: Enhancement of urinary citrate in oxalate stone formers by the intake of alkaline salts, in Smith LH, Robertson WG, Finlayson B (eds): Urolithiasis: Clinical and Basic Research. New York, Plenum Press 1981, pp 881–884
203. Tiselius HG: Urine composition in calcium oxalate stone formers during treatment with alkalis, in Schwille PO, Smith LH, Robertson WG, et al (eds): Urolithiasis and Related Clinical Research. New York, Plenum Press, 1985, pp 533–536
204. Rumenapf G, Kalkum M, Schwille PO: Citrate and intestinal calcium absorption (CaA). In situ perfusion studies in the rat. Urol Res 14:94, 1986
205. Pak CYC, Fuller C, Sakhaee K, et al: Long term treatment of calcium nephrolithiasis with potassium citrate. J Urol 134:11–19, 1985
206. Pak CYC, Fuller C: Idiopathic hypocitraturia calcium oxalate nephrolithiasis successfully treated with potassium citrate. Ann Intern Med 104:33–37, 1986
207. Yatzidis H: Successful sodium thiosulphate treatment for recurrent calcium urolithiasis. Clin Nephrol 23:63–67, 1985
208. Hallson PC, Kasidas GP, Rose GA: The treatment of idiopathic hypercalciuria and stone formation, in Brockis JG, Finlayson B (eds): Urinary Calculus. Littleton, MA, PSG Publishing Co, 1981, pp 435–446
209. Sarig S, Garti N, Azoury R, et al: A method for discrimination between calcium oxalate stone formers and normals. J Urol 128:645–649, 1982
210. Perlberg S, Azoury R, Garti N, et al: Use of the discriminant index in dynamic treatment to reduce recurrence of calcium oxalate kidney stones. Br J Urol 57:500–504, 1985

Index